AMERICAN MEDICAL ASSOCIATION

Netter's ATLAS of SURGICAL ANATOMY for CPT® CODING

Sheri Poe Bernard

ILLUSTRATIONS BY
Frank H. Netter, MD

CONTRIBUTING ILLUSTRATORS
John A. Craig, MD
Carlos A.G. Machado, MD

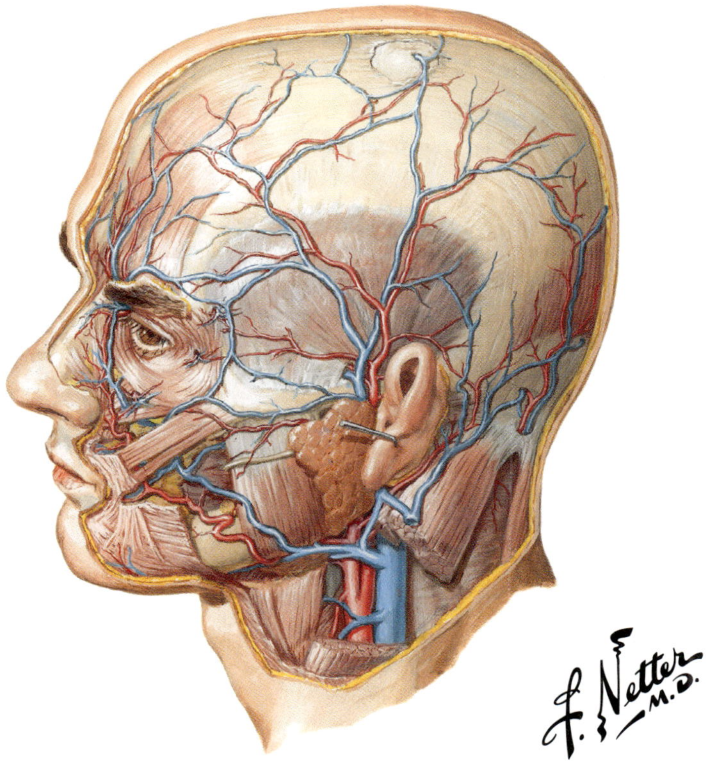

Executive Vice President, Chief Executive Officer: James L. Madara, MD
Chief Operating Officer: Bernard L. Hengesbaugh
Vice President, Business Operations: Vanessa Hayden
Vice President, Coding and Reimbursement Products Portfolio: Jay Ahlman
Vice President, Sales and Marketing: Lisa Manoogian
Vice President, Product Development: Mason Meadows
Director, Print and Digital Products: Richard W. Newman
Senior Acquisition Editor: Elise Schumacher
Manager, Book and Product Development and Production: Nancy Baker
Senior Developmental Editor: Lisa Chin-Johnson
Production Specialist: Mary Ann Albanese
Director, Sales: Susan Wilson
Director, Key Account Management: Joann Skiba
Director, Product Marketing: Karen Christensen-Araujo
Director, Channel Sales: Erin Kalitowski
Marketing Manager: Rachel Dunn
Internal Reviewer: Marie Mindeman, Director, CPT Coding and Regulatory Services

Printed in the United States of America. 15 16 17 18 19 20 / TB-WI / 9 8 7 6 5 4 3 2 1

Additional copies of this book may be ordered by calling 800-621-8335 or AMA|Store at *amastore.com*. Refer to product number OP495015.

AMA publication and product updates, errata, and addendum can be found at ama-assn.org/go/ProductUpdates.

ISBN: 978-1-62202-030-0
AC33:03/15

Contents

About Sheri Poe Bernard, CCS-P, CPC, COC

Sheri Poe Bernard, CCS-P, CPC, COC, is one of the nation's leading developers of medical coding curricula and referential material. With more than 20 years of experience in coding and reimbursement publishing, training, and test development, she is an expert communicator of coding concepts.

Bernard is currently a risk adjustment consultant in coding, training, and clinical documentation improvement, as well as a freelance writer. She is a sought-after public speaker on topics including coding, reimbursement, risk adjustment, and anatomy. She pioneered training labs in which medical coders learn anatomy using physiologically similar organs from farm animals. She served for 15 years as a coding content developer at the company now known as Optum360 and was instrumental in the development of the *Coders' Desk Reference*, Encoder Pro, and additive features of the Optum360 International Classification of Diseases and Healthcare Common Procedure Coding System Level II coding books. She was vice president of training and certification at the AAPC, where she implemented processes for content quality control and oversaw the rewrite and review of certification tests and curricula for three years. Before her employment at AAPC, Bernard served as a member of the AAPC National Advisory Board for eight years, six years as an officer. She worked for two years as a senior technical advisor for the Step-By-Step coding curriculum developed by Carol J. Buck, published by Elsevier, Inc.

Early in her career, Bernard spent 10 years as a daily news journalist and editor, including a stint as a medical reporter. Those years served to hone her research, writing, and editing skills in preparation for a career in training, education, and curriculum development for medical coding professionals.

About Frank H. Netter, MD

Frank H. Netter, MD, was an American surgeon and renowned medical illustrator. He was born in 1906 in New York City. He studied art at the Art Student's League and National Academy of Design before entering medical school at New York University, where he received his MD degree in 1931. During his student years, Netter's notebook sketches attracted the attention of the medical faculty and other physicians, allowing him to augment his income by illustrating articles and textbooks. He continued illustrating as a sideline after he established his medical practice in 1933. Ultimately, he gave up his practice in favor of a full-time commitment to art. During World War II, Netter served in the United States (US) Army and played a major role in illustrating training manuals used by the Armed Forces. After his services in the US Army during World War II, Netter began his long collaboration with the CIBA Pharmaceutical Company (now Novartis Pharmaceuticals). This 45-year partnership resulted in the production of the extraordinary collection of medical art so familiar to physicians and other medical professionals worldwide.

In 2005, Elsevier, Inc., purchased the Netter Collection and all publications from Icon Learning Systems. More than 50 publications that feature Netter's art are now available through Elsevier, Inc. Netter's works are among the finest examples of the use of illustration in the teaching of medical concepts. The 13-book *Netter Collection of Medical Illustrations*, which includes the greater part of the more than 20,000 paintings created by Netter, became and remains one of the most famous medical works ever published. The *Netter Atlas of Human Anatomy*, first published in 1989 and now in its Sixth Edition, presents a selection of anatomical paintings from the Netter Collection. Now translated into 11 languages, it is the anatomy atlas of choice among thousands of medical and health professions students the world over.

The Netter illustrations are appreciated not only for their aesthetic qualities but, more importantly, for their intellectual content. As Netter wrote in 1949, ". . . clarification of a subject is the aim and goal of illustration. No matter how beautifully painted, how delicately and subtly rendered a subject may be, it is of little value as a medical illustration if it does not serve to make clear some medical point." Netter's planning, conception, point of view, and approach are what inform his paintings and what makes them so intellectually valuable.

Frank H. Netter, physician and artist, died in 1991. Learn more about the *Netter Collection of Medical Illustrations* at www.netterimages.com.

Reviewers

The American Medical Association and the author would like to thank the following reviewers, who have graciously taken the time to review the illustrations and/or manuscript.

Bernard R. Blais, MD

Brian P. Foley, MD

Mark H. Hyman, MD, FACP, FAADEP

Randolph E. Soo-Hoo, MD, MPH, FACOEM

Karin VanMeter, PhD

Illustrations List

FIGURE A. Body Planes—3/4 View

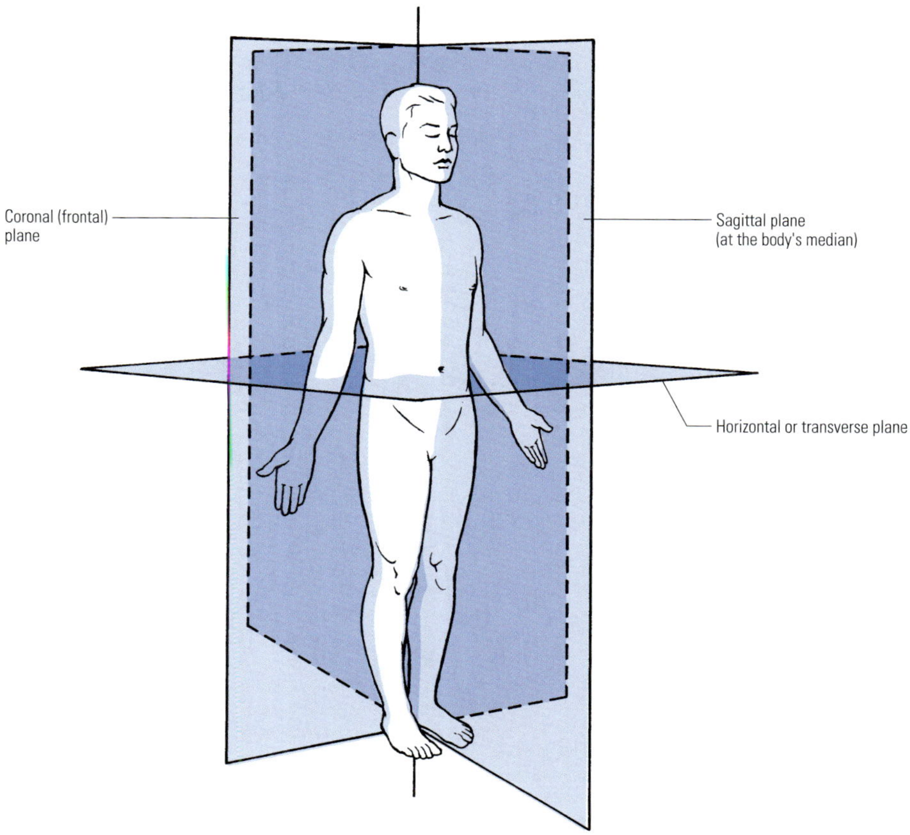

FIGURE B. Body Aspects—Side View

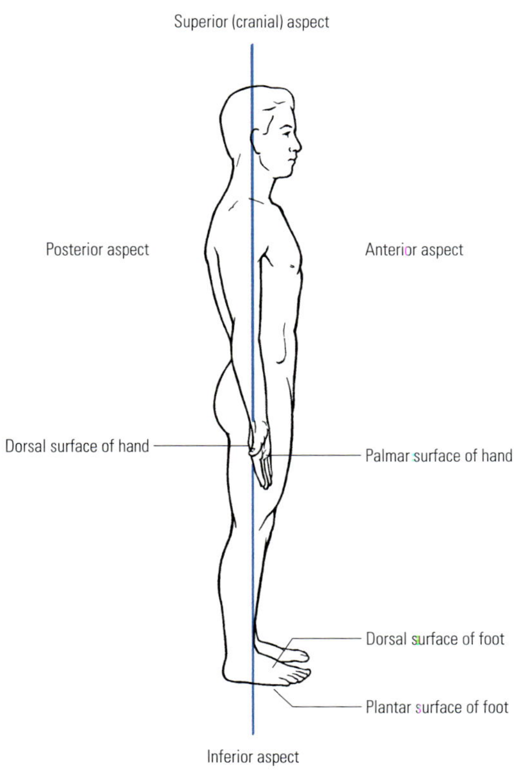

FIGURE C. Body Planes—Front View

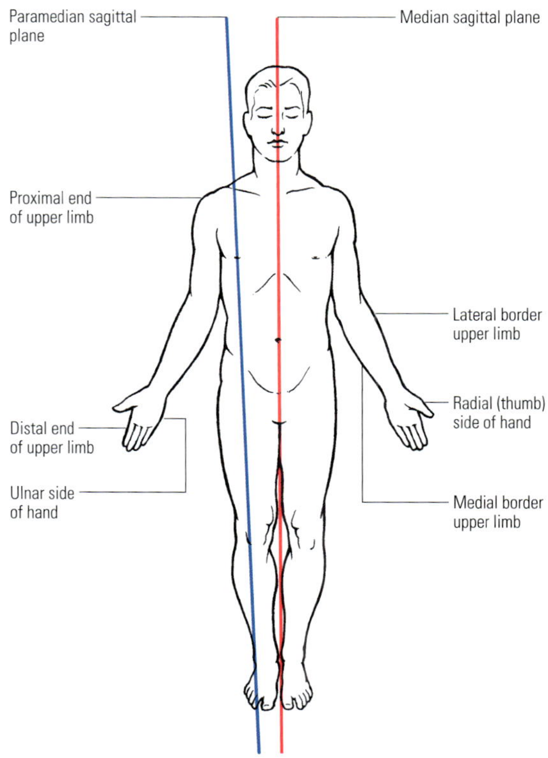

Introduction

Netter's Atlas of Surgical Anatomy for CPT Coding (Netter's Surgical Coding Atlas) unites annotated CPT® codes and code descriptors from the CPT® Surgery section with clinically and significant renderings by renowned medical illustrator, Frank H. Netter, MD. This book is designed to simplify the navigation through complex operative reports for CPT code abstraction. For this book, the CPT Surgery codes are paired with corresponding Netter illustrations in a user-friendly format that includes anatomical annotations and an extensive glossary of medical terms. While the Netter's Surgical Coding Atlas does not replace the CPT codebook, it is an ideal tool for readers who wish to boost their anatomical knowledge within the context of CPT codes as they abstract codes from operative reports.

The book is simply organized to match the CPT codebook: official codes and descriptions from the Surgery section of the CPT codebook are organized in numeric order, from code 10021 through code 69990. Note that unlisted codes are the only codes that are not included in the Netter's Surgical Coding Atlas. Subsections (eg, Integumentary System, Musculoskeletal System, and Respiratory System) in the CPT Surgery section are separated as individual chapters in the Netter's Surgical Coding Atlas for easy access and reference. Smaller Surgery sections from the CPT code set (including General, Hemic and Lymphatic Systems, Mediastinum and Diaphragm, Intersex Surgery, and Endocrine System) are combined into adjacent chapters.

The Netter's Surgical Coding Atlas is an invaluable resource for CPT surgical coding with integrated anatomical instruction and illustrations. It is an incomparable book that brings anatomical and coding concepts together to serve as a reference and educational resource for both new and seasoned coders, as well as coding students. The Netter's Surgical Coding Atlas can be used by a new coder who is trying to understand the relationship of anatomy and coding and who is learning to apply and translate their understanding of anatomy in the context of CPT codes, or by a seasoned coder who is trying to glean and extract important information from an operative report to physician notes—all in context of anatomy and CPT codes simultaneously.

Features of the Netter's Surgical Coding Atlas

The Netter's Surgical Coding Atlas should not be used as a primary CPT coding reference as it contains none of the guidelines, parenthetical instructions, modifiers, and appendices found in the most current edition of the official CPT codebook. Instead, it contains, with the exception of unlisted codes, all of the official CPT codes and code descriptors from the CPT Surgery section, together with their corresponding headings, subheadings, and subsections. The code groupings are paired with corresponding Netter illustrations, captions about the illustrations, and coding annotations. The Netter's Surgical Coding Atlas is an ideal supplement and companion to the CPT codebook.

Each chapter in this book begins with an introduction and overview of the anatomical system(s) within the chapter to provide a basic understanding of pathophysiology that may affect code selection. Seven hundred Netter's illustrations are paired with specific CPT codes in the Netter's Surgical Coding Atlas. Throughout the book, a unique feature, "Coding Atlas," provides additional information and details of anatomy related to procedures within specific CPT code ranges.

Throughout the Netter's Surgical Coding Atlas, selected procedural and medical terms are set in **purple** type to indicate that definitions of these words are available in the Glossary. This comprehensive, alphabetized glossary of procedural and anatomical terms simplifies complex terminology to promote further understanding.

Coding Atlas

Coding Atlas is a unique feature of the Netter's Surgical Coding Atlas, which combines related information about CPT codes, anatomy, and pathophysiology for the group of codes that will be covered in that section of the chapter. See the following example.

Endovascular Repair of Descending Thoracic Aorta

Coding Atlas

In endovascular repair of the descending thoracic aorta, an endoprosthesis is carried through a scope to the site of an aneurysm, ulcer, or other abnormality and secured over the defect endoscopically. The thoracic aorta is the origin of several paired arteries: bronchial, mediastinal, esophageal, and pericardial. The superior phrenic artery also branches from the thoracic aorta, as do the posterior intercostal arteries. In some cases, an aneurysm bridges an area with an arterial branch, and prosthetic extension(s) are placed in the artery forking from the aorta to complete the repair.

Illustrations and Captions

Both medical procedures and human anatomy drawings from Netter are used in this book to help illustrate both the procedures and the anatomical parts relative to the specific CPT codes. The detailed labels and annotations from Netter are reproduced in the Netter's Surgical Coding Atlas as well. Note that some of the procedural illustrations from Netter may be out-of-date in terms of the depicted tools used for a procedure and for this reason, you will find that a footnote has been included for all procedural illustrations: **Note: Tools, implants, and/or equipment depicted in the illustration may be outdated but the procedural approach is valid.** An illustration of body planes is reproduced from the *CPT Professional* codebook as well. There are over 700 illustrations in this book and to help readers find these easily, an illustrations list is provided in the Front Matter of this book.

Captions serve to tie the illustrations to the codes on surrounding pages, augmenting the readers' understanding of the application of CPT codes.

Appendices

The Netter's Surgical Coding Atlas has three appendices: Glossary, Surgical Acronyms, and Procedural Eponyms. The Glossary is an alphabetized compilation of terms that are colorized throughout the book. In the glossary, these terms are defined using terms that apply across all specialties. The second appendix is entitled, Surgical Acronyms, which is a compilation of common surgical acronyms and their meanings. Finally, the third appendix is a compilation of surgical procedure eponyms and a brief description of the procedure. In addition, a subject index, which is organized alphabetically to help readers locate procedural and anatomical information, is provided as well.

CPT Code Set Nomenclature

A basic understanding of CPT code set nomenclature is required to use this book. This nomenclature is briefly outlined here, but more information is available in the CPT codebook. The Netter's Surgical Coding Atlas was developed using the 2015 CPT code set.

Parent and Child Codes Relationship

Understanding the relationship between the parent and child codes is critical to reading CPT code descriptions. In an effort to save space on the printed page, the parent and child code's shared or common description is not listed or repeated in the child code's descriptor. The shared content appears before the semicolon in the parent code. In addition, the child code's descriptor is physically indented beneath the parent code's descriptor to show this relationship. A parent code may be followed by several child codes. See the following examples.

35901 Excision of infected graft; neck

35903   extremity

35905   thorax

35907   abdomen

Based on the example above, code 35901 is a parent code, while the other 3 codes are child codes. The common or shared part of code 35901 (the part before the semicolon) should also be considered as part of codes 35903, 35905, and 35907. Therefore, the complete descriptions for the child codes are:

35903 Excision of infected graft; extremity

35905 Excision of infected graft; thorax

35907 Excision of infected graft; abdomen

CPT Code Symbols

Many of the symbols from the CPT codebook are used in the Netter's Surgical Coding Atlas and similar to the CPT codebook, a legend is provided to explain the symbols. The following is a list of the CPT code symbols, which are presented together with the examples used in the Netter's Surgical Coding Atlas. For more information about these symbols, refer to the CPT codebook.

⊙ **Moderate sedation code.** Conscious sedation is inherent in many surgical procedures. The moderate sedation symbol is applied to those CPT codes for which moderate sedation services are included. Codes with this symbol should not be reported in conjunction with moderate sedation codes. For example:

⊙ **50200** Renal biopsy; percutaneous, by trocar or needle

+ Add-on code. Some surgical procedures are performed in conjunction with a primary procedure, never alone. The add-on symbol indicates that the procedure represented by the code is an additive procedure and never a primary procedure. These add-on codes often include language such as "each additional" or "List separately in addition to primary procedure" in their descriptions. Here is an example of an add-on code:

+ 66990 Use of ophthalmic endoscope (List separately in addition to code for primary procedure)

Resequenced code. Some codes in the CPT code set appear out of numerical order. Resequencing allows placement of new codes within a family of related codes, regardless of the availability of numbers for sequential code placement. Numerically placed references (ie, Code is out of numerical sequence. See . . . .) are used as navigational alerts to direct the user to the location of an out-of-sequence code.

26111 Code is out of numerical sequence. See 26100-26262

26113 Code is out of numerical sequence. See 26100-26262

26115 Excision, tumor or vascular malformation, soft tissue of hand or finger, subcutaneous; less than 1.5 cm

26111 1.5 cm or greater

26116 Excision, tumor, soft tissue, or vascular malformation, of hand or finger, subfascial (eg, intramuscular); less than 1.5 cm

26113 1.5 cm or greater

⦸ **Modifier 51 exempt code.** When multiple procedures are performed during the same surgical session and by the same physician, modifier 51 is appended to any secondary procedures.

⦸ **31500** Intubation, endotracheal, emergency procedure

Unlisted Codes

Unlisted codes are not used in the Netter's Surgical Coding Atlas becasue they are nonspecific and cannot be annotated or illustrated. Refer to the CPT codebook for unlisted codes.

Using This Book

A good foundation in anatomy and pathophysiology is essential for any coding professional. However, there are times when documentation in an operative report challenges the limits of even the most seasoned coder. At those times, an anatomy reference is invaluable. Most anatomy references focus on clinical elements required by physicians, nurses, and other clinicians. These detailed clinical elements may not provide a coder with quick and easy answers. The Netter's Surgical Coding Atlas is designed to pair appropriate anatomical illustrations, annotations, and captions with CPT surgical code ranges for a convenient look-up anatomy reference that will save time and enhance coding accuracy.

The following operative report and Netter's Surgical Coding Atlas excerpts serve to illustrate how the book will assist coders with understanding the nomenclature of medical documentation and CPT codes to make the correct coding choices. On the facing page, two illustrations and their captions have been reproduced. These illustrations appear in the book near the codes in column 2 of the facing page. A Coding Atlas that further informs the coding decision for the operative report is included with the codes. Each element (illustrations, caption, Coding Atlas notation, codes, descriptions, and glossary terms) contributes to coder decision making. Final code selection should be verified using the CPT codebook, as key guidelines, coding notes, rules, and modifiers are available only in the official codebook.

Regular use of the Netter's Surgical Coding Atlas will enable the reader to further understand the relationship between human anatomy and surgical procedures and all in context of their appropriate CPT codes. It is also a useful tool for students who are studying anatomy and pathophysiology.

Shoulder Hemiarthroplasty

Preoperative Diagnosis
Comminuted fracture, dislocation right proximal humerus

Postoperative Diagnosis
Same

Procedure
Hemiarthroplasty of right shoulder using #8 mm cemented humeral stem and 48 × 21 mm modular head replacement.

Technique
The anesthesiologist administered general anesthesia. The patient was positioned in modified beach chair position. The right shoulder was prepped and draped in the usual manner. A longitudinal incision was made extending from lateral to the coracoid down toward the deltoid tuberosity of the humerus. This incision was taken down through the skin and subcutaneous tissues were split. Hemostasis was achieved with electrocautery. The deltoid fascia was identified. The deltopectoral interval was identified and the deltoid split just lateral to the cephalic vein. The deltoid was then retracted. There was marked hematoma and swelling within the subdeltoid bursa. This was removed. The biceps brachii tendon was identified as the landmark for the rotator interval. Mayo scissors were used to split the remaining portion of the rotator interval. The greater tuberosity portion with the rotator cuff was identified. Excess bone was removed from the greater tuberosity side to allow for closure later. The lesser tuberosity portion with the subscapularis was still attached to the humeral head, therefore, osteotome was utilized to separate the lesser tuberosity from the humeral head fragment.

Excess bone was removed from the lesser tuberosity as well. The humeral head was delivered out of the wound. It was localized to the area of the anteroinferior glenoid region. The glenoid was then inspected and noted to be intact. The fracture was at the level of the surgical neck on the proximal humerus. The canal was repaired with the broaches. The 48 x 21 mm head was the most appropriate size, matching the patient's as well as the soft tissue tension on the shoulder. The cement gun was filled and the canal was filled with the cement. The #8 stem was then impacted into place and held in position in appropriate retroversion until the cement had cured. Excess cement was removed by sharp dissection. Prior to cementation of the stem, a hole was drilled in the shaft of proximal humerus and #2 fiber wires were placed through this hole for closure later. Once the cement was cured, the modular head was impacted on to the Morse taper. The lesser tuberosity was then reapproximated back to the original site utilizing the #2 fiber wire suture that was placed in the humeral shaft as well as the holes in the humeral implant. The greater tuberosity portion with rotator cuff was also attached to the implant as well as the shaft of the humerus utilizing #2 fiber wires as well. The rotator interval was closed with #2 fiber wire in an interrupted fashion. The biceps brachii tendon was inspected within this closure. The deltoid fascia was then approximated with interrupted #2-0 Vicryl suture. Subcutaneous layer was approximated with interrupted #2-0 Vicryl and skin approximated with staples. Subcutaneous tissues were infiltrated with 0.25% Marcaine solution.

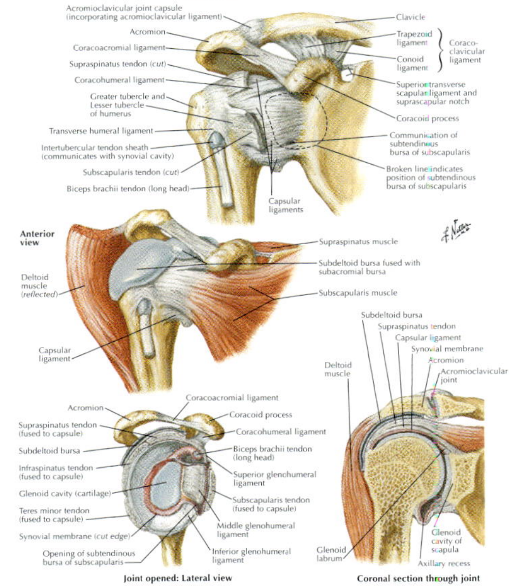
Musculoskeletal System — Netter's Atlas of Surgical Anatomy for CPT Coding

FIGURE 2-21. Shoulder Girdle

The shoulder girdle contains multiple joints. The major joint is the glenohumeral joint (GHJ), articulating the head of the humerus in the glenoid fossa of the scapula. The sternoclavicular (SC) joint stabilizes the clavicle by joining it to the superior sternum. The scapulothoracic (ST) joint is a small attachment between the scapula and rib. The acromioclavicular (AC) joint connects the clavicle to the acromion, an extension of the scapula. Together, the joints of the shoulder provide the body's widest range of motion.

58 ⊙=Moderate sedation ✚=Add-on code ⊘=Modifier 51 exempt #=Resequenced code

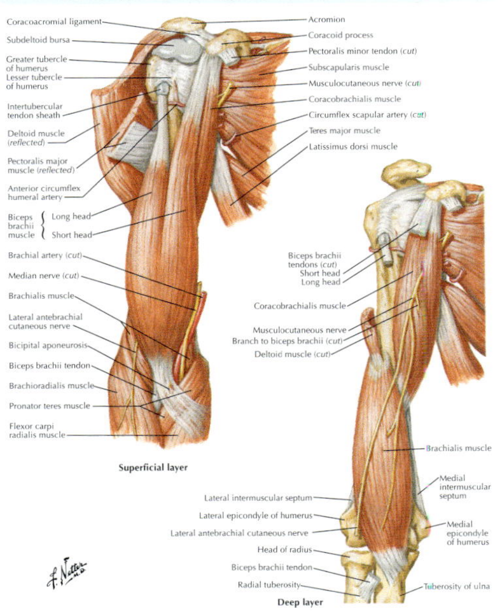
Musculoskeletal System — Netter's Atlas of Surgical Anatomy for CPT Coding

FIGURE 2-25. Muscles of the Upper Arm

The biceps and triceps muscles of the upper arm work as antagonistic muscles to bend and straighten the elbow. Antagonistic muscles are muscles that work in opposition to each other, ie, when the triceps contract, the biceps are stretched and the elbow straightens. Conversely, when the biceps contract, the triceps are stretched and the elbow bends. It is because of this push-and-pull action that these and similarly paired muscles are called **antagonist muscles**.

64 ⊙=Moderate sedation ✚=Add-on code ⊘=Modifier 51 exempt #=Resequenced code

Repair, Revision, and/or Reconstruction

Coding Atlas

In **hemiarthroplasty** of the shoulder, the head of the humerus bone is replaced. In total arthroplasty, both the head of the humerus (ball) and the glenoid (socket) are replaced. In the revision of a total arthroplasty, removal of existing hardware is inherent in the procedure and not reported separately.

23440	Resection or transplantation of long tendon of biceps
23450	Capsulorrhaphy, anterior; Putti-Platt procedure or Magnuson type operation
23455	with labral repair (eg, Bankart procedure)
23460	Capsulorrhaphy, anterior, any type; with bone block
23462	with coracoid process transfer
23465	Capsulorrhaphy, glenohumeral joint, posterior, with or without bone block
23466	Capsulorrhaphy, glenohumeral joint, any type multi-directional instability
23470	Arthroplasty, glenohumeral joint; hemiarthroplasty
23472	total shoulder (glenoid and proximal humeral replacement (eg, total shoulder))
23473	Revision of total shoulder arthroplasty, including allograft when performed; humeral **or** glenoid component
23474	humeral **and** glenoid component

Glossary

allograft. Tissue for grafting from a donor of the same species.

arthroplasty. Reconstructive surgery of a joint or joints to restore motion because of ankyloses or trauma or to prevent excessive motion; this repair and reconstruction may use silicone, metallic, or other implants.

capsulorrhaphy. Suture repair of a capsule, especially a joint capsule.

hemiarthroplasty. Joint reconstruction in which only one of the two surfaces of the joint is replaced with a prosthesis.

resection. Surgical removal of a section or segment of an organ or structure; in the case of muscle or tendon, this will result in the muscle being more lax than it was before surgery.

transplantation. Surgical transfer and grafting of tissue from one location to another or from one entity to another.

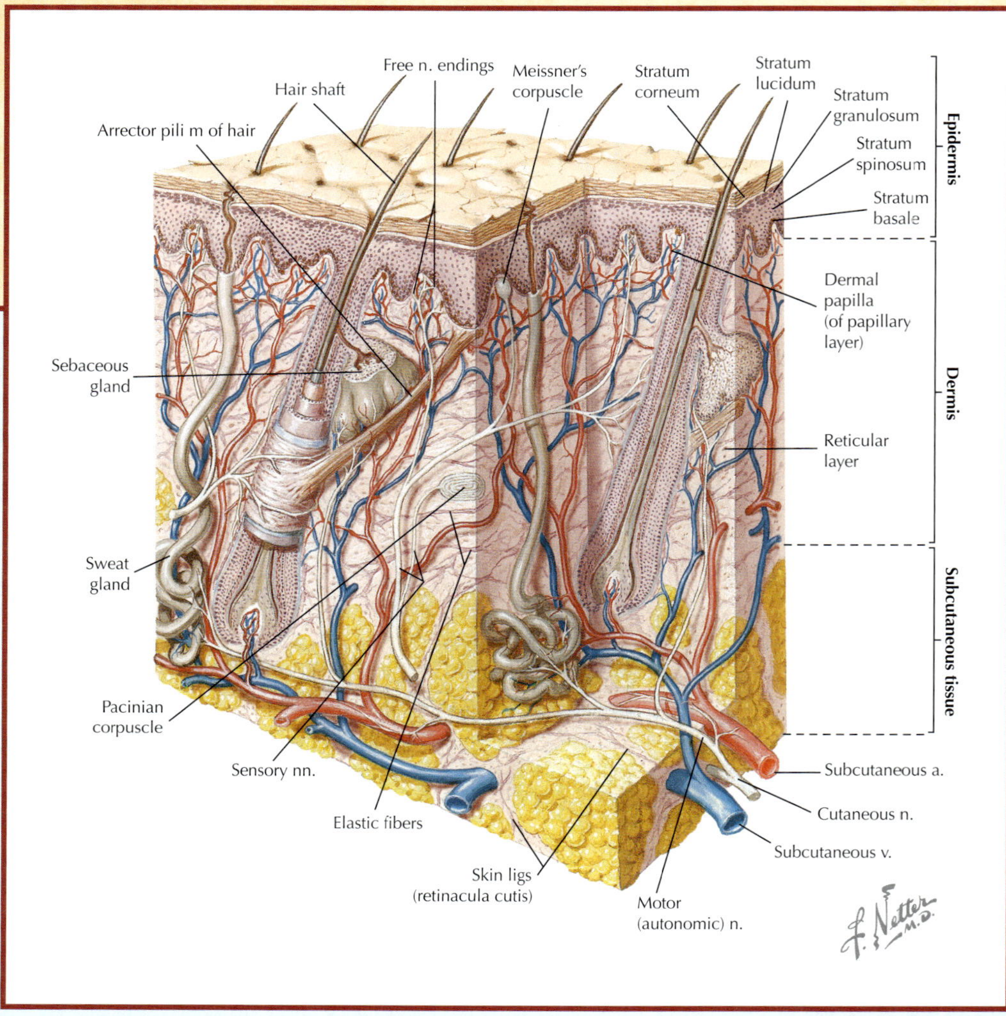
Free n. endings
Meissner's corpuscle
Stratum corneum
Stratum lucidum
Hair shaft
Stratum granulosum
Arrector pili m of hair
Stratum spinosum
Stratum basale
Epidermis
Dermal papilla (of papillary layer)
Sebaceous gland
Dermis
Reticular layer
Sweat gland
Subcutaneous tissue
Pacinian corpuscle
Subcutaneous a.
Sensory nn.
Cutaneous n.
Elastic fibers
Subcutaneous v.
Skin ligs (retinacula cutis)
Motor (autonomic) n.
F. Netter M.D.

CHAPTER 1

Integumentary System

The integumentary system includes skin, nails, hair, sebaceous and sudoriferous glands, and breast. The skin is a covering that protects other parts of the body. Skin also serves as the sensory organ of touch and is important in the regulation of body temperature. Vitamin D, which is essential to bone health, is absorbed through the skin.

The skin has three layers: epidermis, dermis, and **hypodermis**. The epidermis is the outermost protective layer of skin. It contains melanin, which gives the skin its color. The top layer of epidermis, the stratum corneum, is composed of dead cells that are shed approximately every two weeks. The epidermis is **avascular**. Underlying the epidermis is the dermis, rich with nerves, blood vessels, hair follicles, and glands. Sebaceous glands produce lubricating oil, and apocrine glands, which are associated with hair follicles, produce scent. The **eccrine glands** produce sweat that helps us regulate our body temperature. Underlying the dermis is the fatty hypodermis, also referred to as **subcutaneous** tissue. As the thickest layer of skin, the hypodermis provides insulation and absorbs shocks.

Because the skin is the body's first line of defense, it is often the site of injury. Many CPT codes in the Integumentary System are used to report treatments for injuries including wounds, burns, ulcers, and abnormal skin growths. Sometimes skin repairs require more complex procedures, such as adjacent tissue transfers, grafts, or the use of skin replacement therapies.

Skin changes as we age. The dermis contains **collagen** and elastic tissues that contribute to a youthful appearance. With age, the epidermal cells become thinner and less able to retain moisture. The dermal layer also becomes thinner. Less collagen is produced, and the elastin fibers that prevent sagging of skin lose their elasticity. Sebaceous and sweat glands slow their production of oils and sweat. A significant number of CPT codes are used to report procedures that are performed on the integumentary system for **cosmesis**, eg, to lift or tighten skin or breast tissue or to remove subcutaneous fat, rather than for therapeutic reasons.

Toenails and fingernails are integumentary structures with six components: nail root, bed, nail plate, eponychium (cuticle), **perionychium**, and **hyponychium**. The nail root (germinal **matrix**) lies under the skin at the **proximal** nail. This is where new nail is produced. The nail plate is the exposed nail, from cuticle to fingertip, while the nail bed is the vascular tissue directly beneath the nail plate. The eponychium provides a seal between the skin and the nail plate at its base, while the perionychium is the skin boundary at the sides of the nail bed. The hyponychium is the junction between the **distal** edge nail plate and the fingertip.

The female breast is considered part of the integumentary system. It is composed primarily of **adipose** tissue with a network of **ducts** that run from the lobules, where milk is produced during lactation, to the nipple, where the milk is expressed. The breast overlies the pectoralis major muscle between the second and sixth ribs and is anchored in place by the Cooper suspensory ligaments. These ligaments stretch over time, leading to **ptosis**. The nipple is centered on the areola, which contains sebaceous glands for lubrication. A tail of adipose breast tissue, the tail of Spence, extends into the armpit. Procedures on the breast may involve more complex structures such as chest wall, ribs, or pectoral muscles. CPT codes used to report biopsy and excision associated with breast tumors do not differentiate between the sexes.

General

Coding Atlas

In fine needle aspiration (FNA), matter is suctioned (aspirated) through a syringe's long, slender needle (gauge 18-23) to obtain a sample of a suspicious mass. The sample then undergoes separately reported pathological examination. No tissue is cut in FNA. In some cases, imaging guidance is necessary to ensure the correct site is sampled.

10021 Fine needle aspiration; without imaging guidance

10022 with imaging guidance

Integumentary System

Skin, Subcutaneous, and Accessory Structures

Introduction and Removal

Coding Atlas

Catheter drainage allows for outflow of fluid from the body into a collection device. Typically, gravity facilitates the drainage. In some cases, image guidance may be required to access the site to be drained. Code 10030 is reported once for each separate catheter placed, using image guidance, in soft tissue, excluding peritoneal, retroperitoneal, transvaginal, transrectal, and visceral collections.

⊙ **10030** Image-guided fluid collection drainage by catheter (eg, abscess, hematoma, seroma, lymphocele, cyst), soft tissue (eg, extremity, abdominal wall, neck), percutaneous

Incision and Drainage

Coding Atlas

Integumentary incision and drainage (I&D) is performed to release purulent or pressurized fluids under or within the skin. The intent of I&D procedures is incision, not excision. These codes represent procedures in which the physician actively drains the area incised using techniques such as cavity exploration, swabbing, lavage, and irrigation. I&D is also used to extract foreign bodies from the skin or subcutaneous tissue. Integumentary codes for I&D are chosen based on the type of defect (eg, foreign body, pilonidal cyst, abscess, hematoma) and whether the physician has documented that the procedure was complicated.

10040 Acne surgery (eg, marsupialization, opening or removal of multiple milia, comedones, cysts, pustules)

10060 Incision and drainage of abscess (eg, carbuncle, suppurative hidradenitis, cutaneous or subcutaneous abscess, cyst, furuncle, or paronychia); simple or single

10061 complicated or multiple

10080 Incision and drainage of pilonidal cyst; simple

10081 complicated

10120 Incision and removal of foreign body, subcutaneous tissues; simple

10121 complicated

10140 Incision and drainage of hematoma, seroma or fluid collection

10160 Puncture aspiration of abscess, hematoma, bulla, or cyst

10180 Incision and drainage, complex, postoperative wound infection

Debridement

Coding Atlas

Debridement is the removal of contaminated or damaged tissue. CPT codes 11000-11047 are used to report debridement of wounds to depths that involve subcutaneous tissue, muscle or fascia, and bone. Debridement to the level of the epidermis and dermis is reported with CPT codes 97597 and 97598. The depth reported for debridement is the deepest depth of tissue removed. When determining body surface, measure only the area that undergoes debridement. Debridement of burns is reported with codes 16020-16030. The difference between debridement and excision is that an excision requires closure. The debridement site is not closed unless the debridement is related to a repair that is the primary goal of the encounter.

11000 Debridement of extensive eczematous or infected skin; up to 10% of body surface

✚ **11001** each additional 10% of the body surface, or part thereof (List separately in addition to code for primary procedure)

11004 Debridement of skin, subcutaneous tissue, muscle and fascia for necrotizing soft tissue infection; external genitalia and perineum

11005 abdominal wall, with or without fascial closure

11006 external genitalia, perineum and abdominal wall, with or without fascial closure

+ 11008 Removal of prosthetic material or mesh, abdominal wall for infection (eg, for chronic or recurrent mesh infection or necrotizing soft tissue infection) (List separately in addition to code for primary procedure)

11010 Debridement including removal of foreign material at the site of an open fracture and/or an open dislocation (eg, excisional debridement); skin and subcutaneous tissues

11011 skin, subcutaneous tissue, muscle fascia, and muscle

11012 skin, subcutaneous tissue, muscle fascia, muscle, and bone

11042 Debridement, subcutaneous tissue (includes epidermis and dermis, if performed); first 20 sq cm or less

#+ 11045 each additional 20 sq cm, or part thereof (List separately in addition to code for primary procedure)

11043 Debridement, muscle and/or fascia (includes epidermis, dermis, and subcutaneous tissue, if performed); first 20 sq cm or less

#+ 11046 each additional 20 sq cm, or part thereof (List separately in addition to code for primary procedure)

11044 Debridement, bone (includes epidermis, dermis, subcutaneous tissue, muscle and/or fascia, if performed); first 20 sq cm or less

11045 Code is out of numerical sequence. See 11000-11047

11046 Code is out of numerical sequence. See 11000-11047

+ 11047 each additional 20 sq cm, or part thereof (List separately in addition to code for primary procedure)

Paring or Cutting

Coding Atlas

The integumentary system is composed of three layers: epidermis, dermis, and subcutaneous tissue or **hypodermis**. Epidermis is generated at its innermost layer and becomes increasingly flatter and drier as it matures and reaches the skin surface. The top layer of epidermis is composed of dead cells that shed and are replaced every two weeks. The dermis is a complex layer that contains nerves, vessels, hair follicles, and glands. **Hyperkeratotic** lesions are thickened skin that result from overgrowth of epidermis to protect against local irritation (**corns** and calluses), inflammation (chronic **eczema**), and other immune system reactions. Codes in the range 11055-11057 are used to report procedures that seldom require local anesthesia or chemical cauterization. Report only one code according to the number of lesions treated during the encounter.

11055 Paring or cutting of benign hyperkeratotic lesion (eg, corn or callus); single lesion

11056 2 to 4 lesions

11057 more than 4 lesions

Biopsy

Coding Atlas

The intent of a skin biopsy code is to report a diagnostic procedure in which the tissue removed undergoes separately reported pathological examination. When the skin is sampled for biopsy as part of a larger surgical procedure, the biopsy service is considered part of the larger surgical procedure. The codes in this range are used to report biopsy and simple closure of dermis and epidermis or mucous membrane.

11100 Biopsy of skin, subcutaneous tissue and/or mucous membrane (including simple closure), unless otherwise listed; single lesion

+ 11101 each separate/additional lesion (List separately in addition to code for primary procedure)

Removal of Skin Tags

Coding Atlas

An **acrochordon**, or **skin tag**, is a fleshy dermal stalk that forms on the skin, especially in areas where the skin creases, such as the neck, axilla, groin, and eyelid. These tags may be chronically irritated by clothing or shaving. Skin tag removal by any method is reported using CPT codes 11200 and 11201. Excision of anal tags that are the **sequelae** of **hemorrhoids** is reported using codes 46220 and 46230.

11200 Removal of skin tags, multiple fibrocutaneous tags, any area; up to and including 15 lesions

+ 11201 each additional 10 lesions, or part thereof (List separately in addition to code for primary procedure)

Shaving of Epidermal or Dermal Lesions

Coding Atlas

Shaving may be selected as the method for removing benign lesions that exist completely within the dermis and epidermis. When shaving, the scalpel is held parallel to the skin to undercut the lesion. For traditional excisions, the scalpel is held perpendicular to the skin, and the edges of the skin are cut before the tissue to be removed is undermined. After shaving a lesion, the remaining wound does not require closure.

11300 Shaving of epidermal or dermal lesion, single lesion, trunk, arms or legs; lesion diameter 0.5 cm or less

11301 lesion diameter 0.6 to 1.0 cm

11302 lesion diameter 1.1 to 2.0 cm

11303 lesion diameter over 2.0 cm

11305 Shaving of epidermal or dermal lesion, single lesion, scalp, neck, hands, feet, genitalia; lesion diameter 0.5 cm or less

11306 lesion diameter 0.6 to 1.0 cm

11307 lesion diameter 1.1 to 2.0 cm

11308 lesion diameter over 2.0 cm

11310 Shaving of epidermal or dermal lesion, single lesion, face, ears, eyelids, nose, lips, mucous membrane; lesion diameter 0.5 cm or less

11311 lesion diameter 0.6 to 1.0 cm

11312 lesion diameter 1.1 to 2.0 cm

11313 lesion diameter over 2.0 cm

Excision—Benign Lesions

Coding Atlas

Benign lesions are contained, ie, they lack the ability to invade neighboring tissues, or metastasize. Skin lesions that are considered benign include lipomas, cysts, fibromas, nevi, and some moles. The codes in this series are used to report the excision of benign lesions that originate in the integumentary system. The actual lesion and excision may extend beyond the integumentary system. A margin of healthy full-thickness skin is usually excised with the benign lesion. The diameter of the entire excision (including margin) is used to calculate the measurement necessary for CPT code selection. Any repair of the surgical site that requires layered closure, extensive undermining, or retention sutures may be reported separately. When the morphology of a lesion is ambiguous, the coder should choose the excision code category (malignant vs benign) based on the physician's approach to the lesion rather than the final pathology report. In this way, the coding will reflect the physician's knowledge, skill, time, and effort, regardless of the pathology report. For example, a lesion suspected of being benign would be excised with relatively smaller margins than a lesion suspected of being malignant.

11400 Excision, benign lesion including margins, except skin tag (unless listed elsewhere), trunk, arms or legs; excised diameter 0.5 cm or less

11401 excised diameter 0.6 to 1.0 cm

11402 excised diameter 1.1 to 2.0 cm

11403 excised diameter 2.1 to 3.0 cm

11404 excised diameter 3.1 to 4.0 cm

11406 excised diameter over 4.0 cm

11420 Excision, benign lesion including margins, except skin tag (unless listed elsewhere), scalp, neck, hands, feet, genitalia; excised diameter 0.5 cm or less

11421 excised diameter 0.6 to 1.0 cm

11422 excised diameter 1.1 to 2.0 cm

11423 excised diameter 2.1 to 3.0 cm

11424 excised diameter 3.1 to 4.0 cm

11426 excised diameter over 4.0 cm

11440 Excision, other benign lesion including margins, except skin tag (unless listed elsewhere), face, ears, eyelids, nose, lips, mucous membrane; excised diameter 0.5 cm or less

11441 excised diameter 0.6 to 1.0 cm

11442 excised diameter 1.1 to 2.0 cm

11443 excised diameter 2.1 to 3.0 cm

11444 excised diameter 3.1 to 4.0 cm

11446 excised diameter over 4.0 cm

11450 Excision of skin and subcutaneous tissue for hidradenitis, axillary; with simple or intermediate repair

11451 with complex repair

11462 Excision of skin and subcutaneous tissue for hidradenitis, inguinal; with simple or intermediate repair

11463 with complex repair

11470 Excision of skin and subcutaneous tissue for hidradenitis, perianal, perineal, or umbilical; with simple or intermediate repair

11471 with complex repair

Excision—Malignant Lesions

Coding Atlas

Malignant lesions have the ability to invade neighboring tissues, or metastasize. Skin neoplasms that are considered malignant include melanoma; basal cell, squamous cell, and Merkel cell carcinoma; and Kaposi sarcoma. The CPT codes in this series are used to report the excision of malignant lesions of cutaneous origin in the integumentary system. The actual malignancy and excision may extend beyond the integumentary system. A wide margin of healthy full-thickness skin or other surrounding tissue also is excised with the malignant lesion. Any repair of the surgical site that requires layered closure, extensive undermining, retention sutures, or flaps and grafts may be reported separately.

FIGURE 1-1. Excision of Lesion

During the excision of a skin lesion, the physician determines how much margin of healthy skin should be removed based on the lesion's appearance. The resultant defect may be closed simply or may require intermediate or complex closure, which can be reported in addition to the CPT code for the excision. Note: Tools, implants, and/or equipment depicted in the illustration may be outdated but the procedural approach is valid.

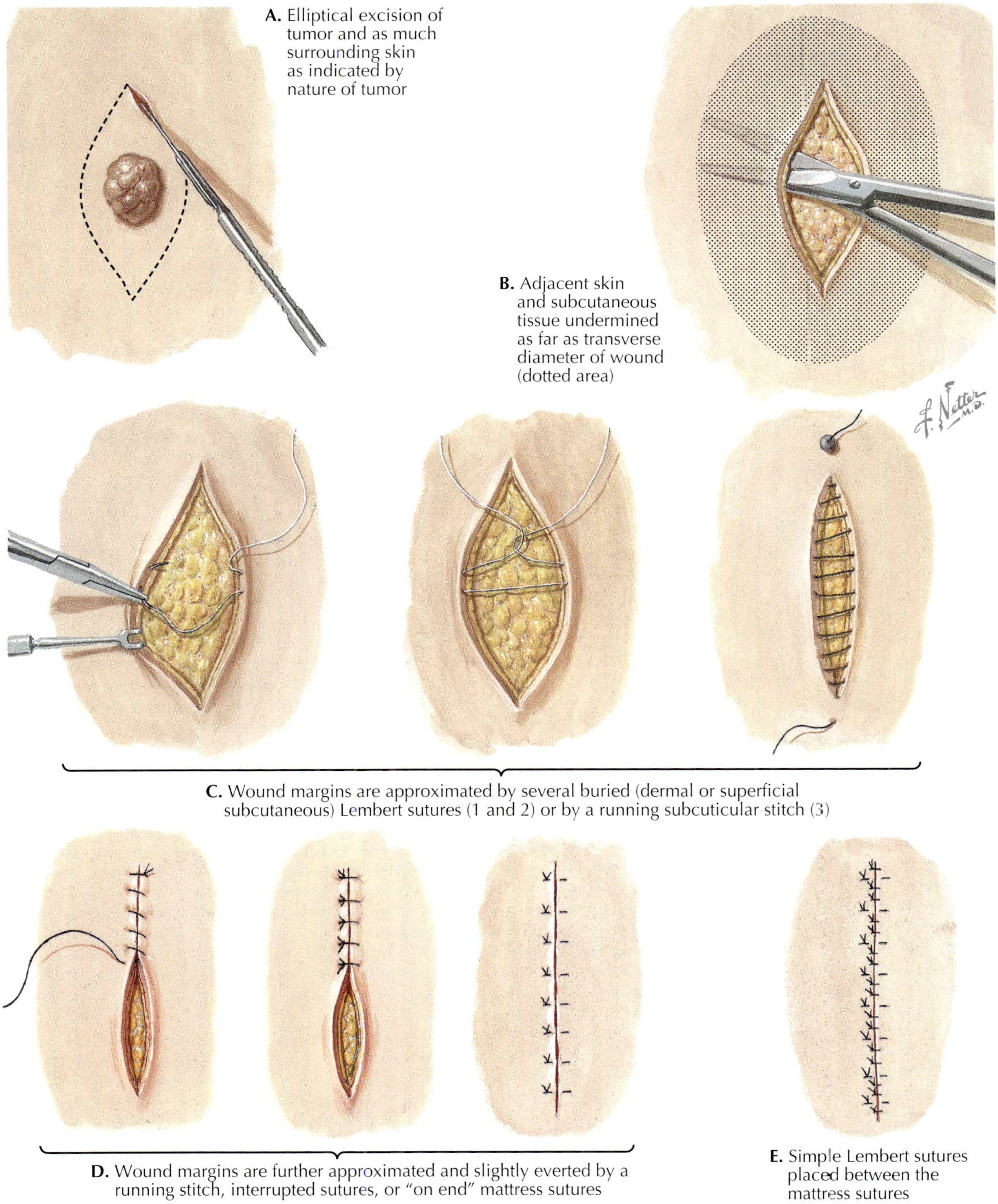

FIGURE 1-2. Ingrown Toenail

Nail growth occurs under the skin within the matrix at the nail's **proximal** end. To cure a chronic or recurrent **onychocryptosis** (ingrown toenail), the physician may remove a portion of nail along the affected **perionychium**, extending to include that portion of nail matrix. For an **acute** ingrown nail, the physician may remove only the affected skin and nail, without removing the **matrix**.

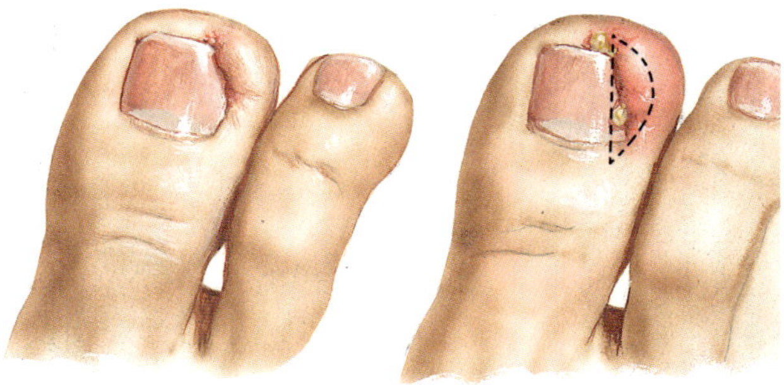

11600 Excision, malignant lesion including margins, trunk, arms, or legs; excised diameter 0.5 cm or less

11601 excised diameter 0.6 to 1.0 cm

11602 excised diameter 1.1 to 2.0 cm

11603 excised diameter 2.1 to 3.0 cm

11604 excised diameter 3.1 to 4.0 cm

11606 excised diameter over 4.0 cm

11620 Excision, malignant lesion including margins, scalp, neck, hands, feet, genitalia; excised diameter 0.5 cm or less

11621 excised diameter 0.6 to 1.0 cm

11622 excised diameter 1.1 to 2.0 cm

11623 excised diameter 2.1 to 3.0 cm

11624 excised diameter 3.1 to 4.0 cm

11626 excised diameter over 4.0 cm

11640 Excision, malignant lesion including margins, face, ears, eyelids, nose, lips; excised diameter 0.5 cm or less

11641 excised diameter 0.6 to 1.0 cm

11642 excised diameter 1.1 to 2.0 cm

11643 excised diameter 2.1 to 3.0 cm

11644 excised diameter 3.1 to 4.0 cm

11646 excised diameter over 4.0 cm

Nails

Coding Atlas

Nails that are **hypertrophic**, **mycotic**, or **dystrophic** may be treated with **debridement**. In debridement, the physician uses instruments (eg, nail splitters, elevators, or electrical burrs) to remove extraneous tissue from the nail. Chronic **onychocryptosis**, or ingrown toenail, results when the nail grows into the **perionychium**, or skin at the side of the nail bed. This can cause chronic pain and infection and may be treated by surgical, **laser**, **electrocautery**, or chemical techniques that destroy or excise all or part of the nail and nail matrix. Removal or destruction of the **matrix** ensures that its corresponding nail cannot grow back.

11719 Trimming of nondystrophic nails, any number

11720 Debridement of nail(s) by any method(s); 1 to 5

11721 6 or more

11730 Avulsion of nail plate, partial or complete, simple; single

✚ **11732** each additional nail plate (List separately in addition to code for primary procedure)

11740 Evacuation of subungual hematoma

11750 Excision of nail and nail matrix, partial or complete (eg, ingrown or deformed nail), for permanent removal;

11752 with amputation of tuft of distal phalanx

11755 Biopsy of nail unit (eg, plate, bed, matrix, hyponychium, proximal and lateral nail folds) (separate procedure)

11760 Repair of nail bed

11762 Reconstruction of nail bed with graft

11765 Wedge excision of skin of nail fold (eg, for ingrown toenail)

Pilonidal Cyst

Coding Atlas

A pilonidal cyst or sinus forms when hair becomes embedded in the skin near the tailbone at the top of the buttock cleft. Pilonidal cysts are prone to infection and recurrence. Codes 11770-11772 are used to report the excision of the cyst (pilonidal cystectomy). CPT code choice is dependent on how extensive the excision is and whether the excision is complicated by infection or other conditions, eg, multiple fistulas. If an infected pilonidal cyst is treated only with incision and drainage (I&D), report code 10080 or code 10081.

11770 Excision of pilonidal cyst or sinus; simple

11771 extensive

11772 complicated

Introduction

Coding Atlas

Codes 11900 and 11901 are used to report treatment of integumentary lesions including keloids, psoriasis, and acne by direct injection of a therapeutic agent into the defect. Code selection is based on the number of lesions treated, not on the number of injections, as a single lesion may be treated with multiple injections. Codes 11900 and 11901 should not be reported together. Chemotherapeutic lesion injection is reported with code 96405 or code 96406.

11900 Injection, intralesional; up to and including 7 lesions

11901 more than 7 lesions

11920 Tattooing, intradermal introduction of insoluble opaque pigments to correct color defects of skin, including micropigmentation; 6.0 sq cm or less

11921 6.1 to 20.0 sq cm

✚ **11922** each additional 20.0 sq cm, or part thereof (List separately in addition to code for primary procedure)

11950 Subcutaneous injection of filling material (eg, collagen); 1 cc or less

11951 1.1 to 5.0 cc

11952 5.1 to 10.0 cc

11954 over 10.0 cc

11960 Insertion of tissue expander(s) for other than breast, including subsequent expansion

11970 Replacement of tissue expander with permanent prosthesis

11971 Removal of tissue expander(s) without insertion of prosthesis

11976 Removal, implantable contraceptive capsules

11980 Subcutaneous hormone pellet implantation (implantation of estradiol and/or testosterone pellets beneath the skin)

11981 Insertion, non-biodegradable drug delivery implant

11982 Removal, non-biodegradable drug delivery implant

11983 Removal with reinsertion, non-biodegradable drug delivery implant

Repair (Closure)

Repair—Simple

Coding Atlas

Integumentary repair codes are used to report procedures in which the skin is closed using sutures, staples, or tissue adhesives in any combination or alone. A repair performed using only adhesive strips should be reported using the appropriate Evaluation and Management (E/M) service code. A simple repair is reported for wound closure that is single layer and without significant wound contamination. Local anesthesia and cauterization are included in simple repair.

12001 Simple repair of superficial wounds of scalp, neck, axillae, external genitalia, trunk and/or extremities (including hands and feet); 2.5 cm or less

12002 2.6 cm to 7.5 cm

12004 7.6 cm to 12.5 cm

12005 12.6 cm to 20.0 cm

12006 20.1 cm to 30.0 cm

12007 over 30.0 cm

12011 Simple repair of superficial wounds of face, ears, eyelids, nose, lips and/or mucous membranes; 2.5 cm or less

12013 2.6 cm to 5.0 cm

12014 5.1 cm to 7.5 cm

12015 7.6 cm to 12.5 cm

12016 12.6 cm to 20.0 cm

12017 20.1 cm to 30.0 cm

12018 over 30.0 cm

12020 Treatment of superficial wound dehiscence; simple closure

12021 with packing

Repair—Intermediate

Coding Atlas

An intermediate repair is reported for wound closure that is documented as having more than one layer or that has a single layer but requires extensive cleaning. Any wounds of similar classification (simple, intermediate, complex) that are classified to the same anatomical grouping (eg, for code 12036, intermediate wounds of the scalp, axillae, trunk, and extremities, excluding hands and feet) may be combined into a single code by adding the wound lengths documented.

12031 Repair, intermediate, wounds of scalp, axillae, trunk and/or extremities (excluding hands and feet); 2.5 cm or less

12032 2.6 cm to 7.5 cm

12034 7.6 cm to 12.5 cm

12035 12.6 cm to 20.0 cm

12036 20.1 cm to 30.0 cm

12037 over 30.0 cm

12041 Repair, intermediate, wounds of neck, hands, feet and/or external genitalia; 2.5 cm or less

12042 2.6 cm to 7.5 cm

12044 7.6 cm to 12.5 cm

12045 12.6 cm to 20.0 cm

12046 20.1 cm to 30.0 cm

12047 over 30.0 cm

12051 Repair, intermediate, wounds of face, ears, eyelids, nose, lips and/or mucous membranes; 2.5 cm or less

12052 2.6 cm to 5.0 cm

12053 5.1 cm to 7.5 cm

12054 7.6 cm to 12.5 cm

12055 12.6 cm to 20.0 cm

12056 20.1 cm to 30.0 cm

12057 over 30.0 cm

Repair—Complex

Coding Atlas

Complex repairs include layered closure of deeper tissues such as subcutaneous tissue and superficial fascia, **debridement**, extensive **undermining**, **stents**, and **retention sutures**. Repair of any nerves, vessels, or **tendons** is reported separately. Simple exploration of the wound is included in any wound repair. Debridement is separately reported only when prolonged cleaning is required or when significant amounts of tissue are removed during a complex repair.

13100 Repair, complex, trunk; 1.1 cm to 2.5 cm

13101 2.6 cm to 7.5 cm

✚ **13102** each additional 5 cm or less (List separately in addition to code for primary procedure)

13120 Repair, complex, scalp, arms, and/or legs; 1.1 cm to 2.5 cm

13121 2.6 cm to 7.5 cm

✚ **13122** each additional 5 cm or less (List separately in addition to code for primary procedure)

13131 Repair, complex, forehead, cheeks, chin, mouth, neck, axillae, genitalia, hands and/or feet; 1.1 cm to 2.5 cm

13132 2.6 cm to 7.5 cm

✚ **13133** each additional 5 cm or less (List separately in addition to code for primary procedure)

13151 Repair, complex, eyelids, nose, ears and/or lips; 1.1 cm to 2.5 cm

13152 2.6 cm to 7.5 cm

✚ **13153** each additional 5 cm or less (List separately in addition to code for primary procedure)

13160 Secondary closure of surgical wound or dehiscence, extensive or complicated

Adjacent Tissue Transfer or Rearrangement

Coding Atlas

When skin **undermining** is combined with additional skin incisions to cover a defect, codes for adjacent tissue transfer or rearrangement are reported. The skin in an adjacent tissue transfer or rearrangement always remains connected to one or more of its borders. Codes are chosen based on the site of the defect and its size. When a lesion excision repair requires adjacent tissue transfer, the lesion excision is included in the adjacent tissue transfer and is not reported separately. Flaps differ from adjacent tissue transfer because flaps are transferred to a nonadjacent recipient site.

FIGURE 1-3. Adjacent Tissue Transfer

The repair of a wound after the excision of a defect can usually be performed simply or with layered sutures. An adjacent tissue transfer involves an additional incision or incisions and the undermining and advancement of adjacent skin so that the defect may be covered adequately. Common procedures include rotation, advancement, double pedicle flap, and Z-, W-, and V-Y plasties. Note: Tools, implants, and/or equipment depicted in the illustration may be outdated but the procedural approach is valid.

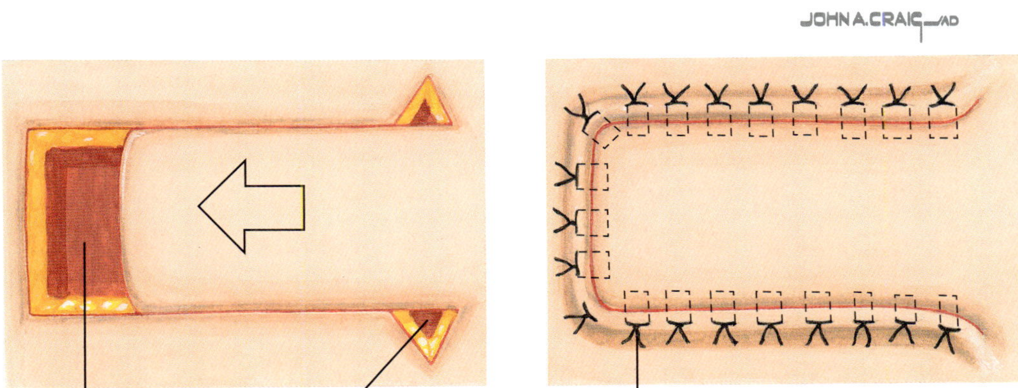

Design of flap for transfer into primary defect. Triangles of tissue excised to prevent bunching (Burow's triangles)

Flap is advanced into primary defect. No secondary defect is created

14000 Adjacent tissue transfer or rearrangement, trunk; defect 10 sq cm or less

14001 defect 10.1 sq cm to 30.0 sq cm

14020 Adjacent tissue transfer or rearrangement, scalp, arms and/or legs; defect 10 sq cm or less

14021 defect 10.1 sq cm to 30.0 sq cm

14040 Adjacent tissue transfer or rearrangement, forehead, cheeks, chin, mouth, neck, axillae, genitalia, hands and/or feet; defect 10 sq cm or less

14041 defect 10.1 sq cm to 30.0 sq cm

14060 Adjacent tissue transfer or rearrangement, eyelids, nose, ears and/or lips; defect 10 sq cm or less

14061 defect 10.1 sq cm to 30.0 sq cm

14301 Adjacent tissue transfer or rearrangement, any area; defect 30.1 sq cm to 60.0 sq cm

+ 14302 each additional 30.0 sq cm, or part thereof (List separately in addition to code for primary procedure)

14350 Filleted finger or toe flap, including preparation of recipient site

Skin Replacement Surgery

Coding Atlas

Skin replacement may provide a permanent solution to skin loss or damage or it may provide a temporary covering for a burn or nonhealing wound. The following two coding components are required for skin replacement: surgical site preparation and application of the graft material. Skin grafts are essentially **autotransplantations**; skin from one part of the body is excised and placed at another site on the same body. A full-thickness skin graft (FTSG) is comprised of all of the epidermis and dermis. A split-thickness skin graft (STSG) is comprised of all of the epidermis and part of the dermis. Grafts may also be created from skin substitutes or skin cultures.

Surgical Preparation

15002 Surgical preparation or creation of recipient site by excision of open wounds, burn **eschar**, or scar (including subcutaneous tissues), or incisional release of scar contracture, trunk, arms, legs; first 100 sq cm or 1% of body area of infants and children

+ 15003 each additional 100 sq cm, or part thereof, or each additional 1% of body area of infants and children (List separately in addition to code for primary procedure)

15004 Surgical preparation or creation of recipient site by excision of open wounds, burn eschar, or scar (including subcutaneous tissues), or incisional release of scar contracture, face, scalp, eyelids, mouth, neck, ears, orbits, genitalia, hands, feet and/or multiple digits; first 100 sq cm or 1% of body area of infants and children

+ 15005 each additional 100 sq cm, or part thereof, or each additional 1% of body area of infants and children (List separately in addition to code for primary procedure)

Autografts/Tissue Cultured Autograft

15040 **Harvest** of skin for tissue cultured skin autograft, 100 sq cm or less

15050 Pinch graft, single or multiple, to cover small ulcer, tip of digit, or other minimal open area (except on face), up to defect size 2 cm diameter

15100 Split-thickness **autograft**, trunk, arms, legs; first 100 sq cm or less, or 1% of body area of infants and children (except 15050)

+ 15101 each additional 100 sq cm, or each additional 1% of body area of infants and children, or part thereof (List separately in addition to code for primary procedure)

15110 Epidermal autograft, trunk, arms, legs; first 100 sq cm or less, or 1% of body area of infants and children

+ 15111 each additional 100 sq cm, or each additional 1% of body area of infants and children, or part thereof (List separately in addition to code for primary procedure)

15115 Epidermal autograft, face, scalp, eyelids, mouth, neck, ears, orbits, genitalia, hands, feet, and/or multiple digits; first 100 sq cm or less, or 1% of body area of infants and children

+ 15116 each additional 100 sq cm, or each additional 1% of body area of infants and children, or part thereof (List separately in addition to code for primary procedure)

15120 Split-thickness autograft, face, scalp, eyelids, mouth, neck, ears, orbits, genitalia, hands, feet, and/or multiple digits; first 100 sq cm or less, or 1% of body area of infants and children (except 15050)

+ 15121 each additional 100 sq cm, or each additional 1% of body area of infants and children, or part thereof (List separately in addition to code for primary procedure)

15130 Dermal autograft, trunk, arms, legs; first 100 sq cm or less, or 1% of body area of infants and children

+ 15131 each additional 100 sq cm, or each additional 1% of body area of infants and children, or part thereof (List separately in addition to code for primary procedure)

15135 Dermal autograft, face, scalp, eyelids, mouth, neck, ears, orbits, genitalia, hands, feet, and/or multiple digits; first 100 sq cm or less, or 1% of body area of infants and children

+ 15136 each additional 100 sq cm, or each additional 1% of body area of infants and children, or part thereof (List separately in addition to code for primary procedure)

15150 Tissue cultured skin autograft, trunk, arms, legs; first 25 sq cm or less

+ 15151 additional 1 sq cm to 75 sq cm (List separately in addition to code for primary procedure)

+ 15152 each additional 100 sq cm, or each additional 1% of body area of infants and children, or part thereof (List separately in addition to code for primary procedure)

15155 Tissue cultured skin autograft, face, scalp, eyelids, mouth, neck, ears, orbits, genitalia, hands, feet, and/or multiple digits; first 25 sq cm or less

+ 15156 additional 1 sq cm to 75 sq cm (List separately in addition to code for primary procedure)

+ 15157 each additional 100 sq cm, or each additional 1% of body area of infants and children, or part thereof (List separately in addition to code for primary procedure)

15200 Full thickness graft, free, including direct closure of donor site, trunk; 20 sq cm or less

+ 15201 each additional 20 sq cm, or part thereof (List separately in addition to code for primary procedure)

15220 Full thickness graft, free, including direct closure of donor site, scalp, arms, and/or legs; 20 sq cm or less

+ 15221 each additional 20 sq cm, or part thereof (List separately in addition to code for primary procedure)

15240 Full thickness graft, free, including direct closure of donor site, forehead, cheeks, chin, mouth, neck, axillae, genitalia, hands, and/or feet; 20 sq cm or less

+ 15241 each additional 20 sq cm, or part thereof (List separately in addition to code for primary procedure)

15260 Full thickness graft, free, including direct closure of donor site, nose, ears, eyelids, and/or lips; 20 sq cm or less

+ 15261 each additional 20 sq cm, or part thereof (List separately in addition to code for primary procedure)

Skin Substitute Grafts

15271 Application of skin substitute graft to trunk, arms, legs, total wound surface area up to 100 sq cm; first 25 sq cm or less wound surface area

+ 15272 each additional 25 sq cm wound surface area, or part thereof (List separately in addition to code for primary procedure)

15273 Application of skin substitute graft to trunk, arms, legs, total wound surface area greater than or equal to 100 sq cm; first 100 sq cm wound surface area, or 1% of body area of infants and children

+ 15274 each additional 100 sq cm wound surface area, or part thereof, or each additional 1% of body area of infants and children, or part thereof (List separately in addition to code for primary procedure)

15275 Application of skin substitute graft to face, scalp, eyelids, mouth, neck, ears, orbits, genitalia, hands, feet, and/or multiple digits, total wound surface area up to 100 sq cm; first 25 sq cm or less wound surface area

+ 15276 each additional 25 sq cm wound surface area, or part thereof (List separately in addition to code for primary procedure)

15277 Application of skin substitute graft to face, scalp, eyelids, mouth, neck, ears, orbits, genitalia, hands, feet, and/or multiple digits, total wound surface area greater than or equal to 100 sq cm; first 100 sq cm wound surface area, or 1% of body area of infants and children

+ 15278 each additional 100 sq cm wound surface area, or part thereof, or each additional 1% of body area of infants and children, or part thereof (List separately in addition to code for primary procedure)

Flaps (Skin and/or Deep Tissues)

Coding Atlas

The objective of a **pedicle flap** is to move tissue to a new site without compromising blood supply to the relocated tissue. At the new site, the pedicle flap covers a defect. In some cases, the physician creates a tubed bridge of tissue between the donor site and the recipient site. Over time, a blood supply is established at the recipient site, and the donor end of the pedicle can be severed from its vascular supply. A pedicle flap may also be called an **interpolation flap.**

15570 Formation of direct or tubed pedicle, with or without transfer; trunk

15572 scalp, arms, or legs

15574 forehead, cheeks, chin, mouth, neck, axillae, genitalia, hands or feet

15576 eyelids, nose, ears, lips, or intraoral

15600 Delay of flap or sectioning of flap (division and inset); at trunk

15610 at scalp, arms, or legs

15620 at forehead, cheeks, chin, neck, axillae, genitalia, hands, or feet

15630 at eyelids, nose, ears, or lips

15650 Transfer, intermediate, of any pedicle flap (eg, abdomen to wrist, Walking tube), any location

15731 Forehead flap with preservation of vascular pedicle (eg, axial pattern flap, paramedian forehead flap)

15732 Muscle, myocutaneous, or fasciocutaneous flap; head and neck (eg, temporalis, masseter muscle, sternocleidomastoid, levator scapulae)

15734 trunk

15736 upper extremity

15738 lower extremity

Other Flaps and Grafts

Coding Atlas

Microvascular anastomosis is the joining of vessels less than 2 mm in diameter and performed with the aid of an operating microscope. A composite graft includes more than one type of tissue, eg, the cartilaginous skin mix found in the nostrils and ear. This mix of tissues may be used to fill a skin defect and provide skin with structural support. Derma-fascia-fat grafts are similarly used to fill defect pockets and restore the flesh to normal positioning.

15740 Flap; island pedicle requiring identification and dissection of an anatomically named axial vessel

15750 neurovascular pedicle

15756 Free muscle or myocutaneous flap with microvascular anastomosis

15757 Free skin flap with microvascular anastomosis

15758 Free fascial flap with microvascular anastomosis

15760 Graft; composite (eg, full thickness of external ear or nasal ala), including primary closure, donor area

15770 derma-fat-fascia

15775 Punch graft for hair transplant; 1 to 15 punch grafts

15776 more than 15 punch grafts

+ 15777 Implantation of biologic implant (eg, acellular dermal matrix) for soft tissue reinforcement (ie, breast, trunk) (List separately in addition to code for primary procedure)

Other Procedures

Coding Atlas

Chemical peel describes a procedure in which exfoliation is accomplished by applying therapeutically caustic agents to the skin. This causes a chemical reaction that results in a reduction of lines and a more uniform coloring of the skin known as improving **cosmesis**. **Dermabrasion** provides similar results manually.

15780 Dermabrasion; total face (eg, for acne scarring, fine wrinkling, rhytids, general keratosis)

15781 segmental, face

15782 regional, other than face

15783 superficial, any site (eg, tattoo removal)

15786 Abrasion; single lesion (eg, keratosis, scar)

+ 15787 each additional 4 lesions or less (List separately in addition to code for primary procedure)

15788 Chemical peel, facial; epidermal

15789 dermal

15792 Chemical peel, nonfacial; epidermal

15793 dermal

15819 Cervicoplasty

15820 Blepharoplasty, lower eyelid;

15821 with extensive herniated fat pad

15822 Blepharoplasty, upper eyelid;

15823 with excessive skin weighting down lid

15824 Rhytidectomy; forehead

15825 neck with platysmal tightening (platysmal flap, P-flap)

15826 glabellar frown lines

15828 cheek, chin, and neck

15829 superficial musculoaponeurotic system (SMAS) flap

15830 Excision, excessive skin and subcutaneous tissue (includes lipectomy); abdomen, infraumbilical panniculectomy

15832 thigh

15833 leg

15834 hip

15835 buttock

15836 arm

15837 forearm or hand

15838 submental fat pad

15839 other area

15840 Graft for facial nerve paralysis; free fascia graft (including obtaining fascia)

15841 free muscle graft (including obtaining graft)

15842 free muscle flap by microsurgical technique

15845 regional muscle transfer

+ 15847 Excision, excessive skin and subcutaneous tissue (includes lipectomy), abdomen (eg, abdominoplasty) (includes umbilical transposition and fascial plication) (List separately in addition to code for primary procedure)

15850 Removal of sutures under anesthesia (other than local), same surgeon

15851 Removal of sutures under anesthesia (other than local), other surgeon

15852 Dressing change (for other than burns) under anesthesia (other than local)

15860 Intravenous injection of agent (eg, fluorescein) to test vascular flow in flap or graft

15876 Suction assisted lipectomy; head and neck

15877 trunk

15878 upper extremity

15879 lower extremity

Pressure Ulcers (Decubitus Ulcers)

Coding Atlas

Decubitus ulcers are localized injuries that result from pressure on the skin over time. The typical decubitus ulcer is seen in a patient who is bedridden, wheelchair-bound, or otherwise immobile. When blood supply is compromised by constant pressure, the skin begins to break down, and an ulcer may result. Typically, the ulcer develops over a bony prominence. If an ulcer does not respond to more conservative treatment, it may be excised. Surgical excision of the ulcer may be performed in conjunction with the creation of a skin flap to facilitate wound closure. In some cases, bone is removed.

15920 Excision, coccygeal pressure ulcer, with coccygectomy; with primary suture

15922 with flap closure

15931 Excision, sacral pressure ulcer, with primary suture;

15933 with ostectomy

15934 Excision, sacral pressure ulcer, with skin flap closure;

15935 with ostectomy

15936 Excision, sacral pressure ulcer, in preparation for muscle or myocutaneous flap or skin graft closure;

15937 with ostectomy

FIGURE 1-4. Blepharoplasty

Excess skin on the upper eyelid (**dermatochalasia**) may impede the **visual field**, reducing the **superior** visual field substantially. In upper eyelid **blepharoplasty**, this excessive skin is excised to improve vision. Upper and lower blepharoplasties also are performed for cosmetic reasons, with the excision of excess skin and fat deposits improving the patient's aesthetic appearance. Note: Tools, implants, and/or equipment depicted in the illustration may be outdated but the procedural approach is valid.

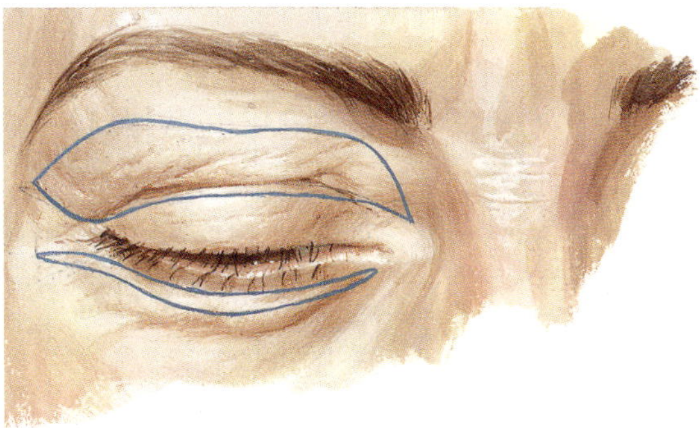

A. Areas of proposed skin excision marked out by methylene blue

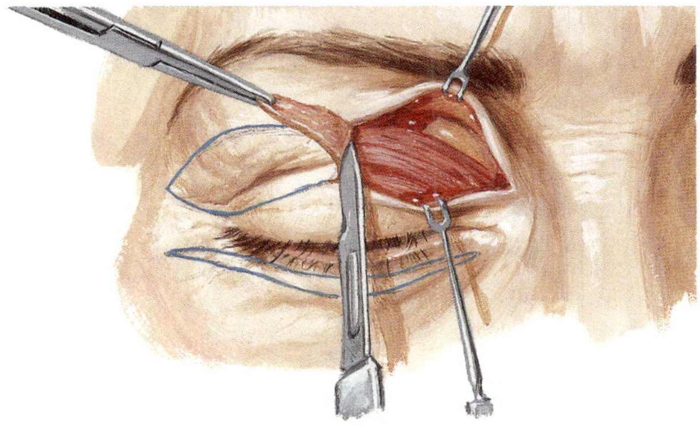

B. Strip of skin excised from upper lid; fat pad shining through orbital fascia and orbicularis oculi muscle

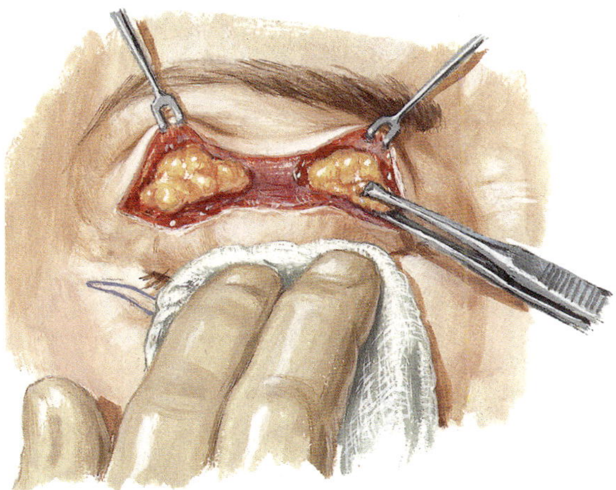

C. Orbital fascia opened in two places (medially and laterally). Pressure on eyeball causes fat pads to bulge. They are teased out meticulously

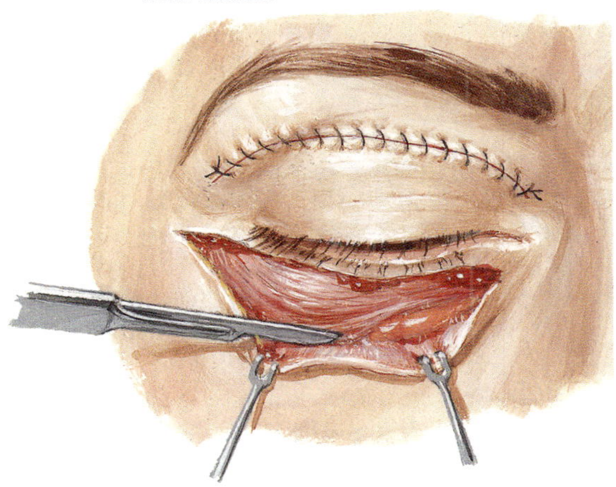

D. Upper lid incision sutured with 6-zero silk continuous stitches. Orbicularis oculi fibers are being separated from skin

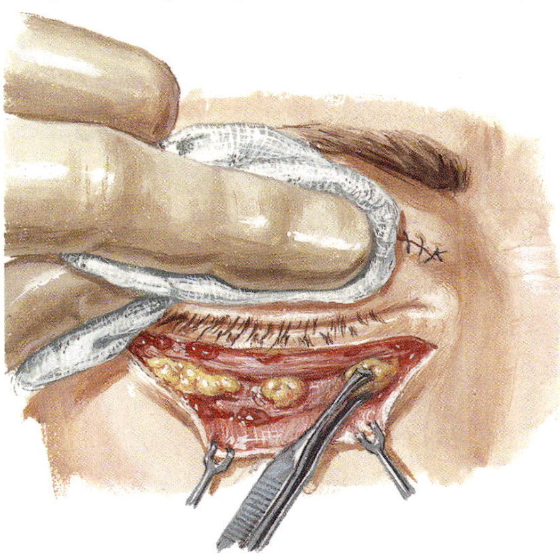

E. Orbital fascia opened; fat pads bulge due to digital pressure and are teased out meticulously

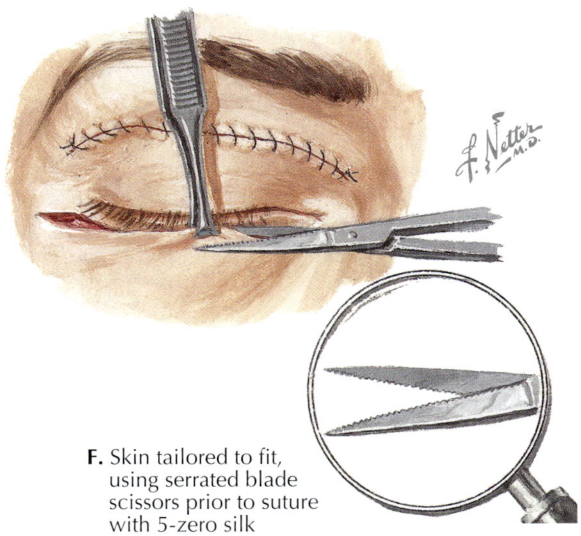

F. Skin tailored to fit, using serrated blade scissors prior to suture with 5-zero silk

15940 Excision, ischial pressure ulcer, with primary suture;

15941 with ostectomy (ischiectomy)

15944 Excision, ischial pressure ulcer, with skin flap closure;

15945 with ostectomy

15946 Excision, ischial pressure ulcer, with ostectomy, in preparation for muscle or myocutaneous flap or skin graft closure

15950 Excision, trochanteric pressure ulcer, with primary suture;

15951 with ostectomy

15952 Excision, trochanteric pressure ulcer, with skin flap closure;

15953 with ostectomy

15956 Excision, trochanteric pressure ulcer, in preparation for muscle or myocutaneous flap or skin graft closure;

15958 with ostectomy

Burns, Local Treatment

Coding Atlas

Burns occur when a heat source injures the skin. Among common burn-causing heat sources are electrical current, chemicals, fire, hot liquid, and radiation. The burn may affect only the outermost skin, subcutaneous tissue, or it may penetrate to the bronchial tubes and lungs or other organs. The codes in this series are used to report only the local treatment of the burned surface.

16000 Initial treatment, first degree burn, when no more than local treatment is required

16020 Dressings and/or debridement of partial-thickness burns, initial or subsequent; small (less than 5% total body surface area)

16025 medium (eg, whole face or whole extremity, or 5% to 10% total body surface area)

16030 large (eg, more than 1 extremity, or greater than 10% total body surface area)

16035 Escharotomy; initial incision

✚ 16036 each additional incision (List separately in addition to code for primary procedure)

Destruction

Destruction, Benign or Premalignant Lesions

Coding Atlas

Some skin lesions can be successfully destroyed by electrodesiccation, electrofulguration, liquid nitrogen freeze, laser, or chemical treatment. The codes in this section are used to report the destruction of benign or premalignant lesions including condylomata, papillomata, molluscum contagiosum, herpetic lesions, plantar and flat warts, milia, and actinic keratoses. These destructions may be performed in conjunction with curetting. The mouth, genitalia, anus, eyelid, and conjunctiva have been assigned site-specific skin destruction codes in other chapters within the CPT code set. Those codes would be reported instead of 17000-17250, as appropriate. There are also specific codes for corns and callouses (11055-11057).

17000 Destruction (eg, laser surgery, electrosurgery, cryosurgery, chemosurgery, surgical curettement), premalignant lesions (eg, actinic keratoses); first lesion

✚ 17003 second through 14 lesions, each (List separately in addition to code for first lesion)

⦸ 17004 Destruction (eg, laser surgery, electrosurgery, cryosurgery, chemosurgery, surgical curettement), premalignant lesions (eg, actinic keratoses), 15 or more lesions

17106 Destruction of cutaneous vascular proliferative lesions (eg, laser technique); less than 10 sq cm

17107 10.0 to 50.0 sq cm

17108 over 50.0 sq cm

17110 Destruction (eg, laser surgery, electrosurgery, cryosurgery, chemosurgery, surgical curettement), of benign lesions other than skin tags or cutaneous vascular proliferative lesions; up to 14 lesions

17111 15 or more lesions

17250 Chemical cauterization of granulation tissue (proud flesh, sinus or fistula)

FIGURE 1-5. Lund-Browder Diagram and Classification Method Table for Burn Estimations

The Lund-Browder Classification Method is used for estimating the extent, depth, and percentage of burns, allowing for the varying proportion of body surface in persons of different ages.

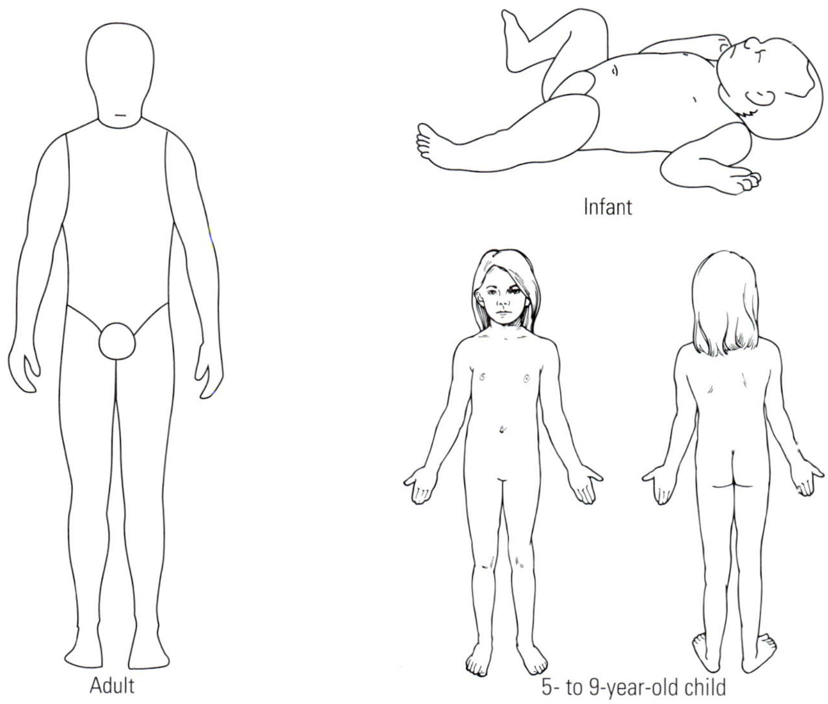

Area	Birth 1 year	1-4 years	5-9 years	10-14 years	15 years	Adult	2 degrees	3 degrees	Total	Donor areas
Head	19	17	13	11	9	7				
Neck	2	2	2	2	2	2				
Ant. trunk	13	13	13	13	13	13				
Post. trunk	13	13	13	13	13	13				
R. buttock	2 1/2	2 1/2	2 1/2	2 1/2	2 1/2	2 1/2				
L. buttock	2 1/2	2 1/2	2 1/2	2 1/2	2 1/2	2 1/2				
Genitalia	1	1	1	1	1	1				
R. U. arm	4	4	4	4	4	4				
L. U. arm	4	4	4	4	4	4				
R. L. arm	3	3	3	3	3	3				
L. L. arm	3	3	3	3	3	3				
R. hand	2 1/2	2 1/2	2 1/2	2 1/2	2 1/2	2 1/2				
L. hand	2 1/2	2 1/2	2 1/2	2 1/2	2 1/2	2 1/2				
R. thigh	5 1/2	6 1/2	8	8 1/2	9	9 1/2				
L. thigh	5 1/2	6 1/2	8	8 1/2	9	9 1/2				
R. leg	5	5	5 1/2	6	6 1/2	7				
L. leg	5	5	5 1/2	6	6 1/2	7				
R. foot	3 1/2	3 1/2	3 1/2	3 1/2	3 1/2	3 1/2				
L. foot	3 1/2	3 1/2	3 1/2	3 1/2	3 1/2	3 1/2				
Total										

FIGURE 1-6. Escharotomy

An **escharotomy** is a surgical incision through necrotic skin that resulted from a burn injury. Escharotomy relieves tension caused by **edema** in subcutaneous tissues in the acute phase of a burn. High **interstitial pressure** can cause **compartment syndrome** and **ischemia**, worsening tissue loss around the burn site. An escharotomy incision typically follows the length of the burn. Note: Tools, implants, and/or equipment depicted in the illustration may be outdated but the procedural approach is valid.

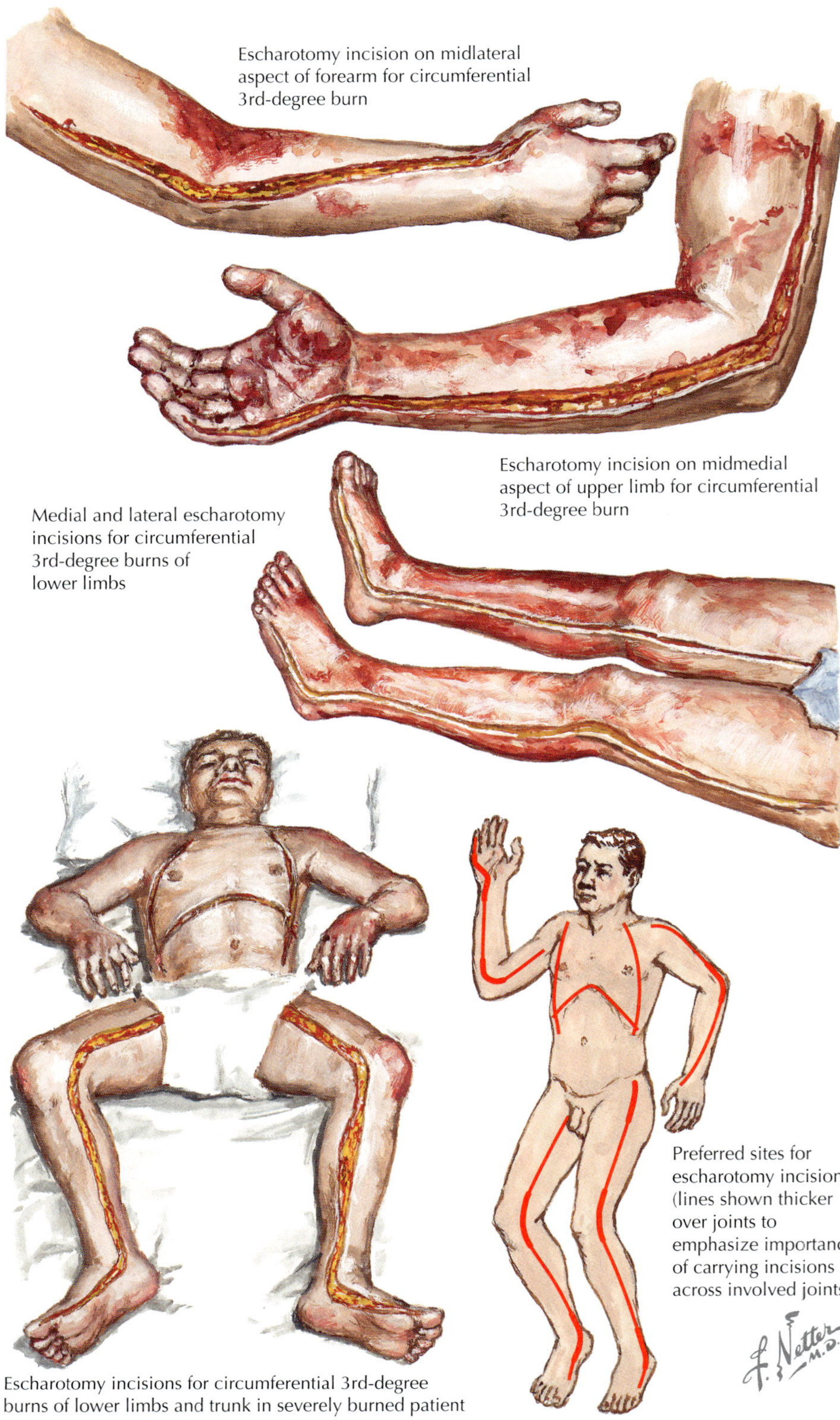

Destruction, Malignant Lesions, Any Method

Coding Atlas

Any combination of electrosurgery, cryosurgery, laser, or chemical treatment can be used with curettage to accomplish surgical destruction of a malignant lesion. Code choice is based on the anatomical location and the size of the malignant lesion, eg, basal or squamous cell carcinoma. Application of topical fluorouracil is not reported as destruction but may be included in services provided with an evaluation and management service.

17260 Destruction, malignant lesion (eg, laser surgery, electrosurgery, cryosurgery, chemosurgery, surgical curettement), trunk, arms or legs; lesion diameter 0.5 cm or less

17261 lesion diameter 0.6 to 1.0 cm

17262 lesion diameter 1.1 to 2.0 cm

17263 lesion diameter 2.1 to 3.0 cm

17264 lesion diameter 3.1 to 4.0 cm

17266 lesion diameter over 4.0 cm

17270 Destruction, malignant lesion (eg, laser surgery, electrosurgery, cryosurgery, chemosurgery, surgical curettement), scalp, neck, hands, feet, genitalia; lesion diameter 0.5 cm or less

17271 lesion diameter 0.6 to 1.0 cm

17272 lesion diameter 1.1 to 2.0 cm

17273 lesion diameter 2.1 to 3.0 cm

17274 lesion diameter 3.1 to 4.0 cm

17276 lesion diameter over 4.0 cm

17280 Destruction, malignant lesion (eg, laser surgery, electrosurgery, cryosurgery, chemosurgery, surgical curettement), face, ears, eyelids, nose, lips, mucous membrane; lesion diameter 0.5 cm or less

17281 lesion diameter 0.6 to 1.0 cm

17282 lesion diameter 1.1 to 2.0 cm

17283 lesion diameter 2.1 to 3.0 cm

17284 lesion diameter 3.1 to 4.0 cm

17286 lesion diameter over 4.0 cm

Mohs Micrographic Surgery

Coding Atlas

Mohs micrographic surgery (MMS) is a surgical technique in which repeated excisions and microscopic examinations ensure that an entire lesion is removed with the best cosmetic and therapeutic effect. The surgeon acts as the pathologist during the surgical encounter and examines each layer that is removed. Layers are removed until the entire lesion and a margin of healthy tissue has been excised. An MMS "block" is a slice of tissue prepared and embedded in a mounting medium and examined microscopically.

17311 Mohs micrographic technique, including removal of all gross tumor, surgical excision of tissue specimens, mapping, color coding of specimens, microscopic examination of specimens by the surgeon, and histopathologic preparation including routine stain(s) (eg, hematoxylin and eosin, toluidine blue), head, neck, hands, feet, genitalia, or any location with surgery directly involving muscle, cartilage, bone, tendon, major nerves, or vessels; first stage, up to 5 tissue blocks

✚ **17312** each additional stage after the first stage, up to 5 tissue blocks (List separately in addition to code for primary procedure)

17313 Mohs micrographic technique, including removal of all gross tumor, surgical excision of tissue specimens, mapping, color coding of specimens, microscopic examination of specimens by the surgeon, and histopathologic preparation including routine stain(s) (eg, hematoxylin and eosin, toluidine blue), of the trunk, arms, or legs; first stage, up to 5 tissue blocks

✚ **17314** each additional stage after the first stage, up to 5 tissue blocks (List separately in addition to code for primary procedure)

✚ **17315** Mohs micrographic technique, including removal of all gross tumor, surgical excision of tissue specimens, mapping, color coding of specimens, microscopic examination of specimens by the surgeon, and histopathologic preparation including routine stain(s) (eg, hematoxylin and eosin, toluidine blue), each additional block after the first 5 tissue blocks, any stage (List separately in addition to code for primary procedure)

Other Procedures

17340 Cryotherapy (CO2 slush, liquid N2) for acne

17360 Chemical exfoliation for acne (eg, acne paste, acid)

17380 Electrolysis epilation, each 30 minutes

Breast

Incision

Coding Atlas

Puncture **aspiration** of a breast **cyst** is a **diagnostic** procedure that may also have **therapeutic** benefits for the patient, since the process decompresses what may be a painful cyst.

19000 Puncture aspiration of cyst of breast;

+ 19001 each additional cyst (List separately in addition to code for primary procedure)

19020 Mastotomy with exploration or drainage of abscess, deep

19030 Injection procedure only for mammary ductogram or galactogram

Excision

Coding Atlas

In a breast **biopsy**, all or a portion of a lesion is removed without consideration of the adequacy of **surgical margins**. In breast excision, there is documentation of attention to surgical margins. Chest wall tumor codes 19260-19272 are reported with codes from the Breast section even when there is no breast involvement.

19081 Biopsy, breast, with placement of breast localization device(s) (eg, clip, metallic pellet), when performed, and imaging of the biopsy specimen, when performed, percutaneous; first lesion, including stereotactic guidance

+ 19082 each additional lesion, including stereotactic guidance (List separately in addition to code for primary procedure)

19083 Biopsy, breast, with placement of breast localization device(s) (eg, clip, metallic pellet), when performed, and imaging of the biopsy specimen, when performed, percutaneous; first lesion, including ultrasound guidance

+ 19084 each additional lesion, including ultrasound guidance (List separately in addition to code for primary procedure)

19085 Biopsy, breast, with placement of breast localization device(s) (eg, clip, metallic pellet), when performed, and imaging of the biopsy specimen, when performed, percutaneous; first lesion, including magnetic resonance guidance

+ 19086 each additional lesion, including magnetic resonance guidance (List separately in addition to code for primary procedure)

19100 Biopsy of breast; percutaneous, needle core, not using imaging guidance (separate procedure)

19101 open, incisional

19105 Ablation, cryosurgical, of fibroadenoma, including ultrasound guidance, each fibroadenoma

19110 Nipple exploration, with or without excision of a solitary lactiferous duct or a papilloma lactiferous duct

19112 Excision of lactiferous duct fistula

19120 Excision of cyst, fibroadenoma, or other benign or malignant tumor, aberrant breast tissue, duct lesion, nipple or areolar lesion (except 19300), open, male or female, 1 or more lesions

19125 Excision of breast lesion identified by preoperative placement of radiological marker, open; single lesion

+ 19126 each additional lesion separately identified by a preoperative radiological marker (List separately in addition to code for primary procedure)

19260 Excision of chest wall tumor including ribs

19271 Excision of chest wall tumor involving ribs, with plastic reconstruction; without mediastinal lymphadenectomy

19272 with mediastinal lymphadenectomy

Introduction

Coding Atlas

Prior to a breast **biopsy**, a wire, clip, or pellet may be inserted into the lesion so that lesion is easier to identify during the excision procedure. This placement may require radiological guidance. Code choice is determined by type of guidance and number of lesions localized.

19281 Placement of breast localization device(s) (eg, clip, metallic pellet, wire/needle, radioactive seeds), percutaneous; first lesion, including mammographic guidance

+ 19282 each additional lesion, including mammographic guidance (List separately in addition to code for primary procedure)

19283 Placement of breast localization device(s) (eg, clip, metallic pellet, wire/needle, radioactive seeds), percutaneous; first lesion, including stereotactic guidance

+ 19284 each additional lesion, including stereotactic guidance (List separately in addition to code for primary procedure)

FIGURE 1-7. Breast

The breast contains an extensive network of lymphatic channels that collect excess fluids and return them to the bloodstream. These channels also provide a means of transportation for **metastatic** cancers. Lymph nodes along the lymph channels filter out harmful substances and may be the first site of metastasis in breast cancer.

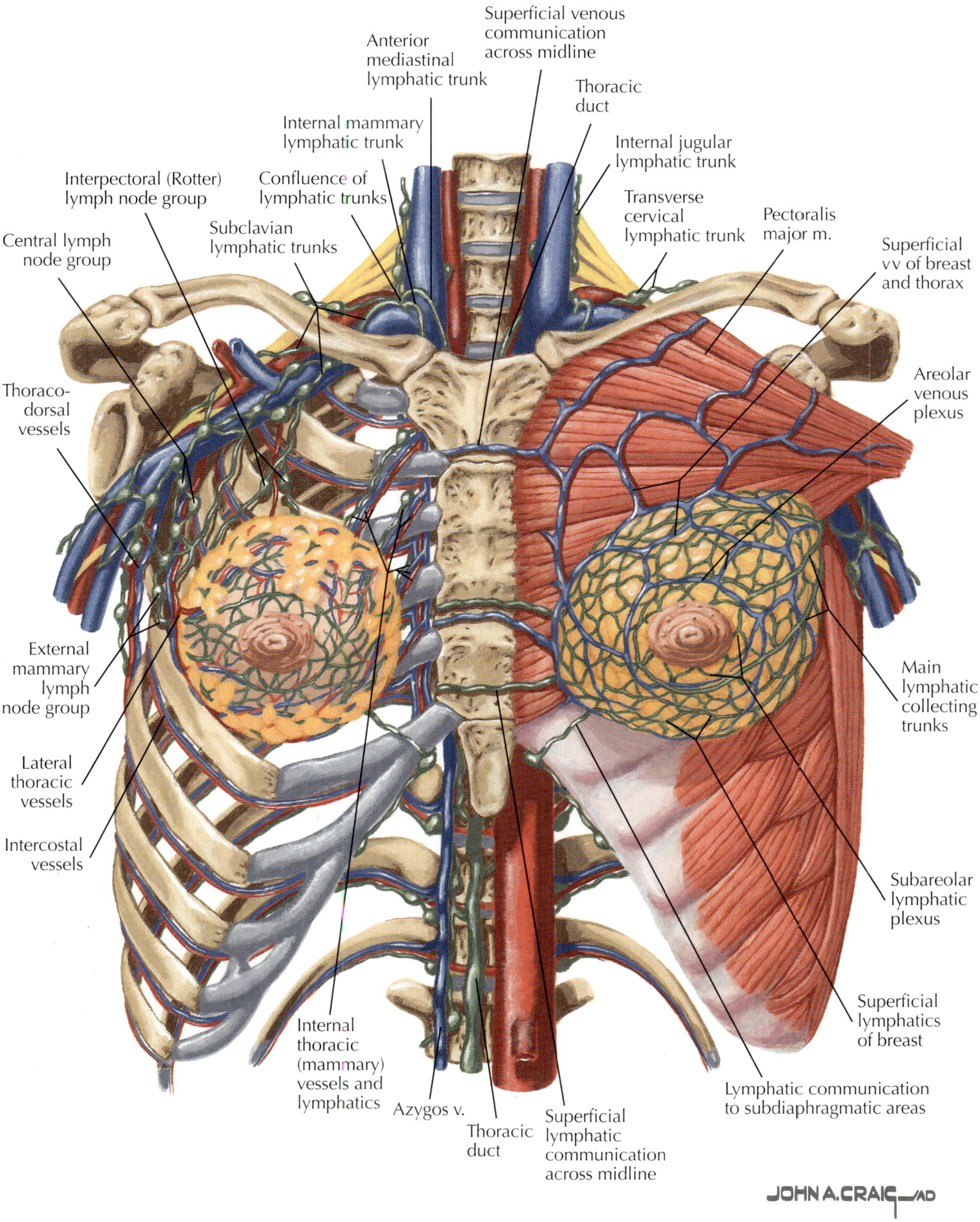

FIGURE 1-8. Puncture Aspiration

Puncture **aspiration** differs from **fine-needle aspiration** (FNA) in that fine needles (gauge 18–23) are used to draw cells from the targeted mass, while puncture aspiration is used to draw fluid from a cyst with a larger needle. Breast cysts usually form due to a **benign** duct obstruction and are common in women of reproductive age. Note: Tools, implants, and/or equipment depicted in the illustration may be outdated but the procedural approach is valid.

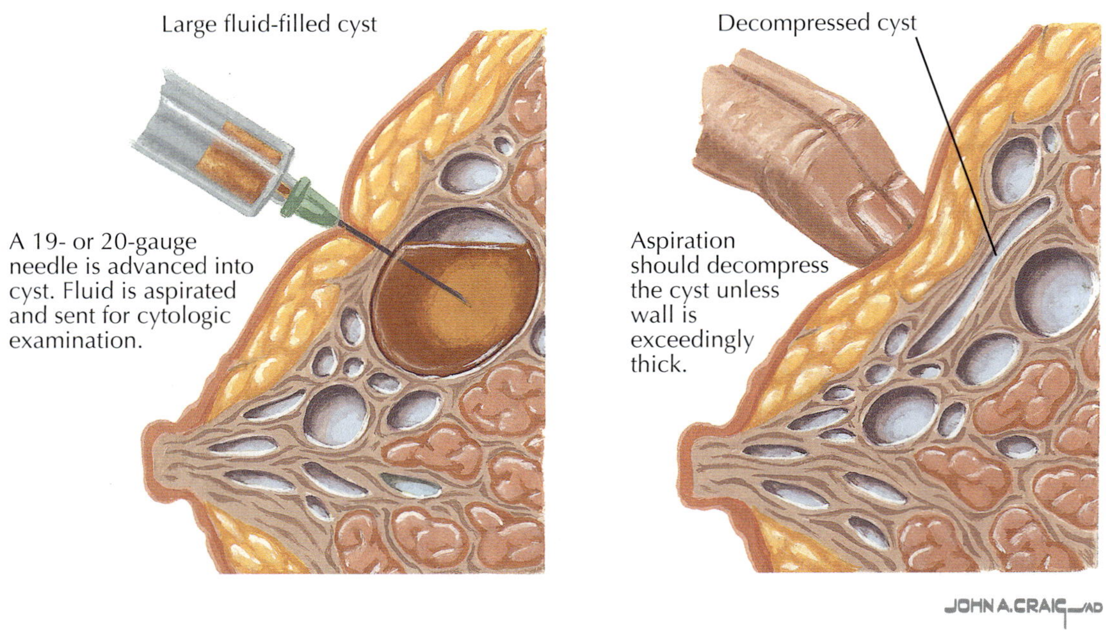

19285 Placement of breast localization device(s) (eg, clip, metallic pellet, wire/needle, radioactive seeds), percutaneous; first lesion, including ultrasound guidance

+ 19286 each additional lesion, including ultrasound guidance (List separately in addition to code for primary procedure)

19287 Placement of breast localization device(s) (eg clip, metallic pellet, wire/needle, radioactive seeds), percutaneous; first lesion, including magnetic resonance guidance

+ 19288 each additional lesion, including magnetic resonance guidance (List separately in addition to code for primary procedure)

19296 Placement of radiotherapy **afterloading** expandable **catheter** (single or multichannel) into the breast for **interstitial** radioelement application following partial **mastectomy**, includes imaging guidance; on date separate from partial mastectomy

+ 19297 concurrent with partial mastectomy (List separately in addition to code for primary procedure)

⊙ 19298 Placement of radiotherapy afterloading **brachytherapy** catheters (multiple tube and button type) into the breast for interstitial radioelement application following (at the time of or subsequent to) partial mastectomy, includes imaging guidance

Mastectomy Procedures

Coding Atlas

In a partial **mastectomy**, a large amount of breast tissue and some skin are removed. In a simple, complete mastectomy, the entire breast is removed, but lymph nodes and surrounding muscles are spared. **Subcutaneous** mastectomy describes surgery in which the **tumor** and breast tissue are removed, but the nipple and skin of the breast are spared. Radical mastectomy codes are selected based on which lymph nodes and muscles are excised with the breast. A total mastectomy should be reported using a code from the code range 19303-19307 based on the excision described in the operative report.

FIGURE 1-9. Needle Core Biopsy

When a needle core **biopsy** of the breast is performed, a plug of tissue is drawn into a hollow needle that is inserted into a **lesion**. Multiple plugs may be taken from a single **lesion**. Needle core biopsies are reported once for each lesion sampled, regardless of the number of plugs sampled from each lesion. Note: Tools, implants, and/or equipment depicted in the illustration may be outdated but the procedural approach is valid.

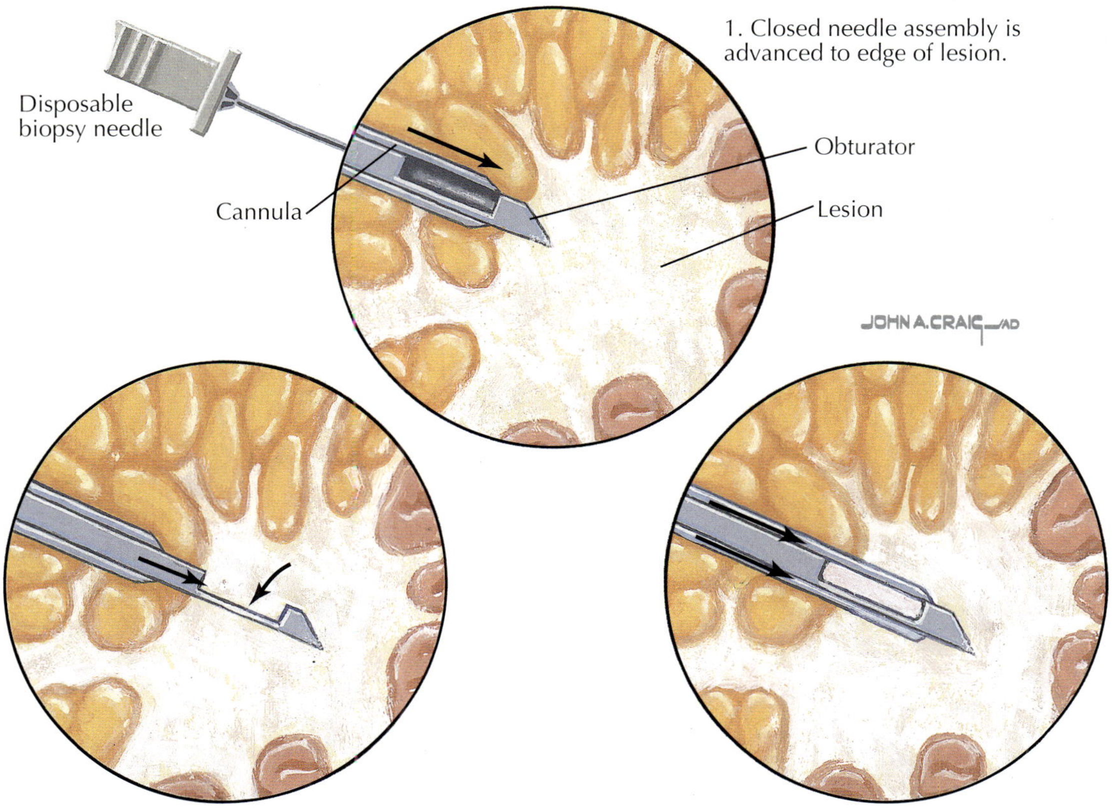

19300 Mastectomy for gynecomastia

19301 Mastectomy, partial (eg, lumpectomy, tylectomy, quadrantectomy, segmentectomy);

19302 with axillary lymphadenectomy

19303 Mastectomy, simple, complete

19304 Mastectomy, subcutaneous

19305 Mastectomy, radical, including pectoral muscles, axillary lymph nodes

19306 Mastectomy, radical, including pectoral muscles, axillary and internal mammary lymph nodes (Urban type operation)

19307 Mastectomy, modified radical, including axillary lymph nodes, with or without pectoralis minor muscle, but excluding pectoralis major muscle

Repair and/or Reconstruction

Coding Atlas

Breast shapes may be surgically changed for cosmetic or therapeutic reasons. In **mastopexy**, a breast with **ptosis** is surgically lifted, with the nipple relocated to a higher position on the breast. In **mammaplasty**, fat, tissue, and skin may be removed to reduce the size of breasts or may be rearranged to enhance the appearance of the breast. In some mammaplasties, implants are inserted to increase breast size.

FIGURE 1-10. Nipple Reconstruction

Code 19350 is reported for many types of nipple reconstruction. Any **cartilage** harvest, **flaps, grafts,** or tattooing performed in the reconstruction of the nipple are considered inherent in code 19350. Nipple reconstruction is often performed as part of the reconstruction postmastectomy.

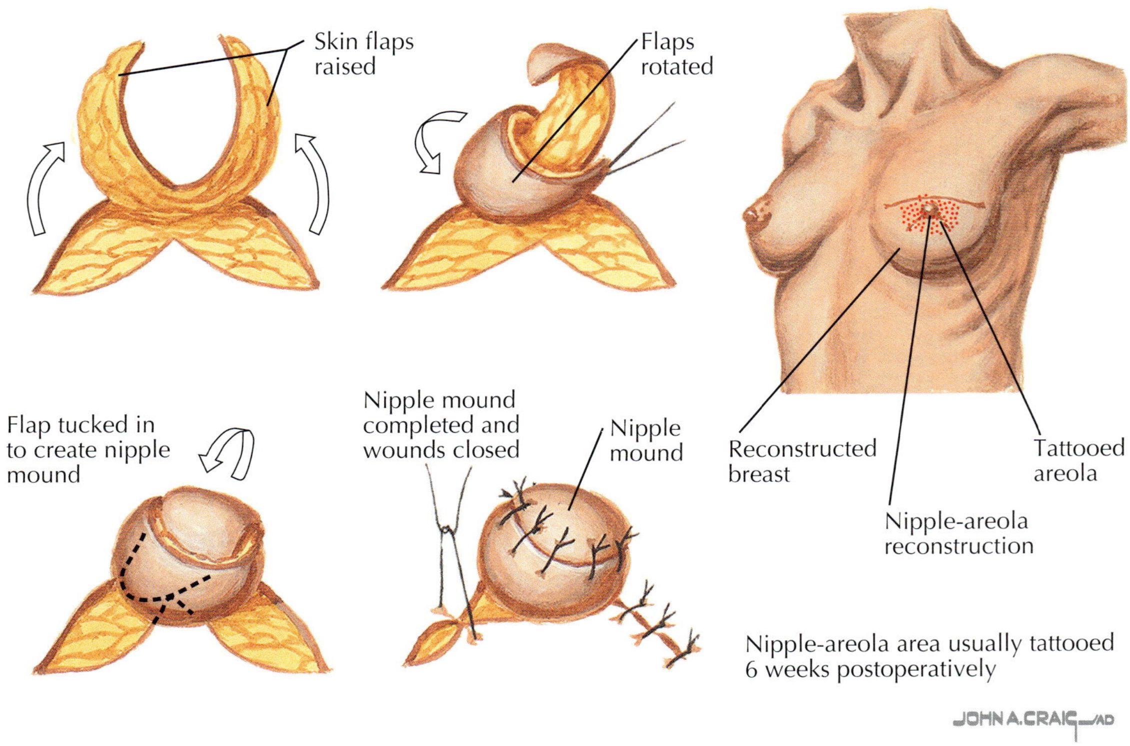

19316 Mastopexy

19318 Reduction mammaplasty

19324 Mammaplasty, augmentation; without prosthetic implant

19325 with prosthetic implant

19328 Removal of intact mammary implant

19330 Removal of mammary implant material

19340 Immediate insertion of breast prosthesis following mastopexy, mastectomy or in reconstruction

19342 Delayed insertion of breast prosthesis following mastopexy, mastectomy or in reconstruction

19350 Nipple/areola reconstruction

19355 Correction of inverted nipples

19357 Breast reconstruction, immediate or delayed, with tissue expander, including subsequent expansion

19361 Breast reconstruction with latissimus dorsi flap, without prosthetic implant

19364 Breast reconstruction with free flap

19366 Breast reconstruction with other technique

19367 Breast reconstruction with transverse rectus abdominis myocutaneous flap (TRAM), single pedicle, including closure of donor site;

19368 with microvascular anastomosis (supercharging)

19369 Breast reconstruction with transverse rectus abdominis myocutaneous flap (TRAM), double pedicle, including closure of donor site

19370 Open periprosthetic capsulotomy, breast

19371 Periprosthetic capsulectomy, breast

19380 Revision of reconstructed breast

19396 Preparation of moulage for custom breast implant

FIGURE 1-11. Tissue Expander

At the time of a mastectomy or during a later reconstruction, a tissue expander may be inserted under the skin and chest muscle. The expander is a balloon-like device that is expanded over time. The expander is attached to a portal through which fluid can be injected to increase the balloon's size, allowing for gradual stretching of the overlying tissue. Note: Tools, implants, and/or equipment depicted in the illustration may be outdated but the procedural approach is valid.

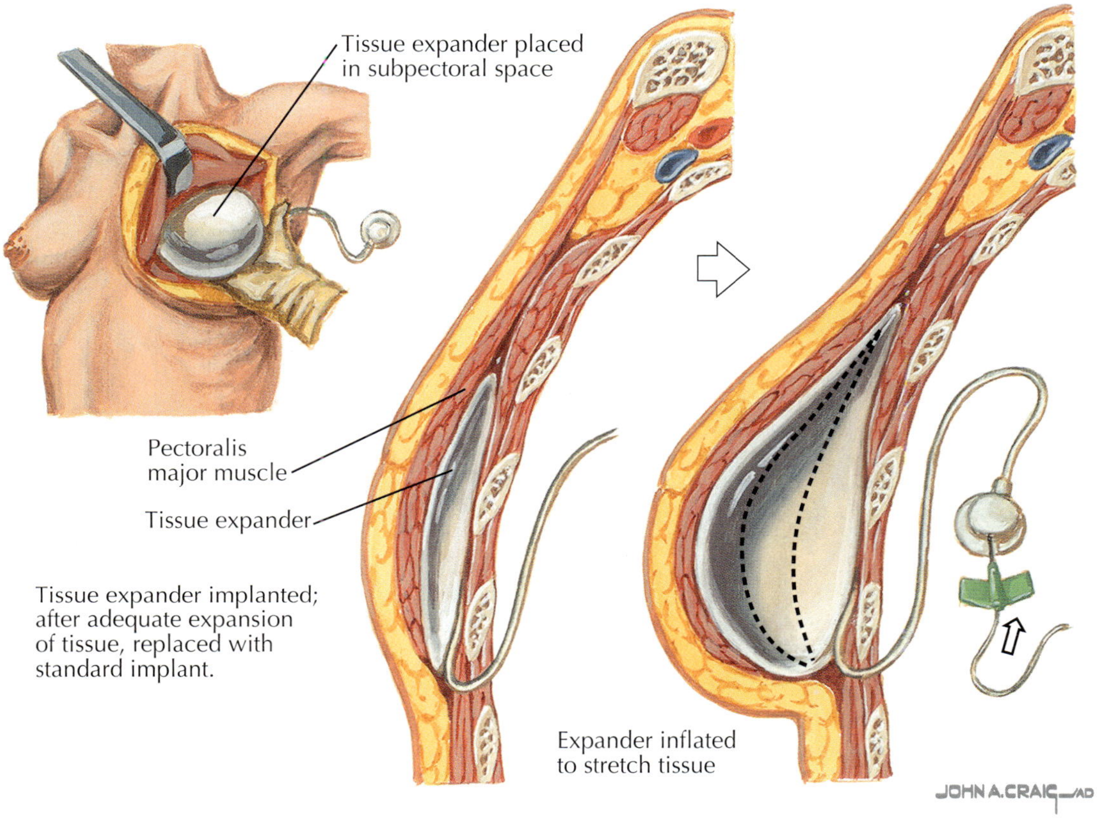

FIGURE 1-12. Flaps in Breast Reconstruction

The transfer of tissue from other parts of the body to the breast area can help a patient achieve an acceptable cosmetic outcome following mastectomy. Sometimes, the flap remains attached at the donor site to maintain blood flow, ie, a **transverse rectus abdominis myocutaneous flap** (TRAM flap). Other times, a **free flap** of skin and subcutaneous tissue may be transplanted, with its blood vessels attached to vessels at the mastectomy site through **microanastomosis**.

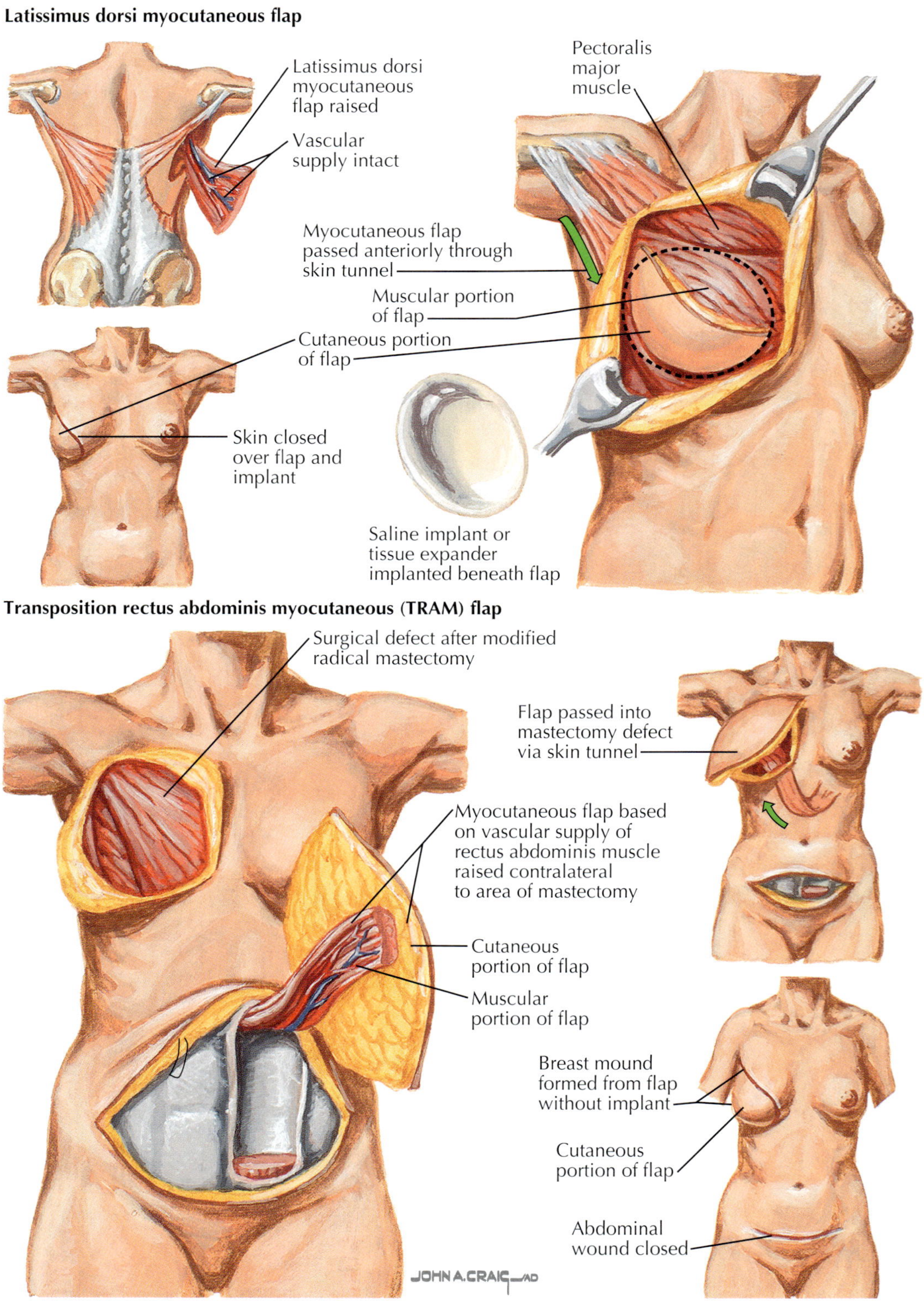

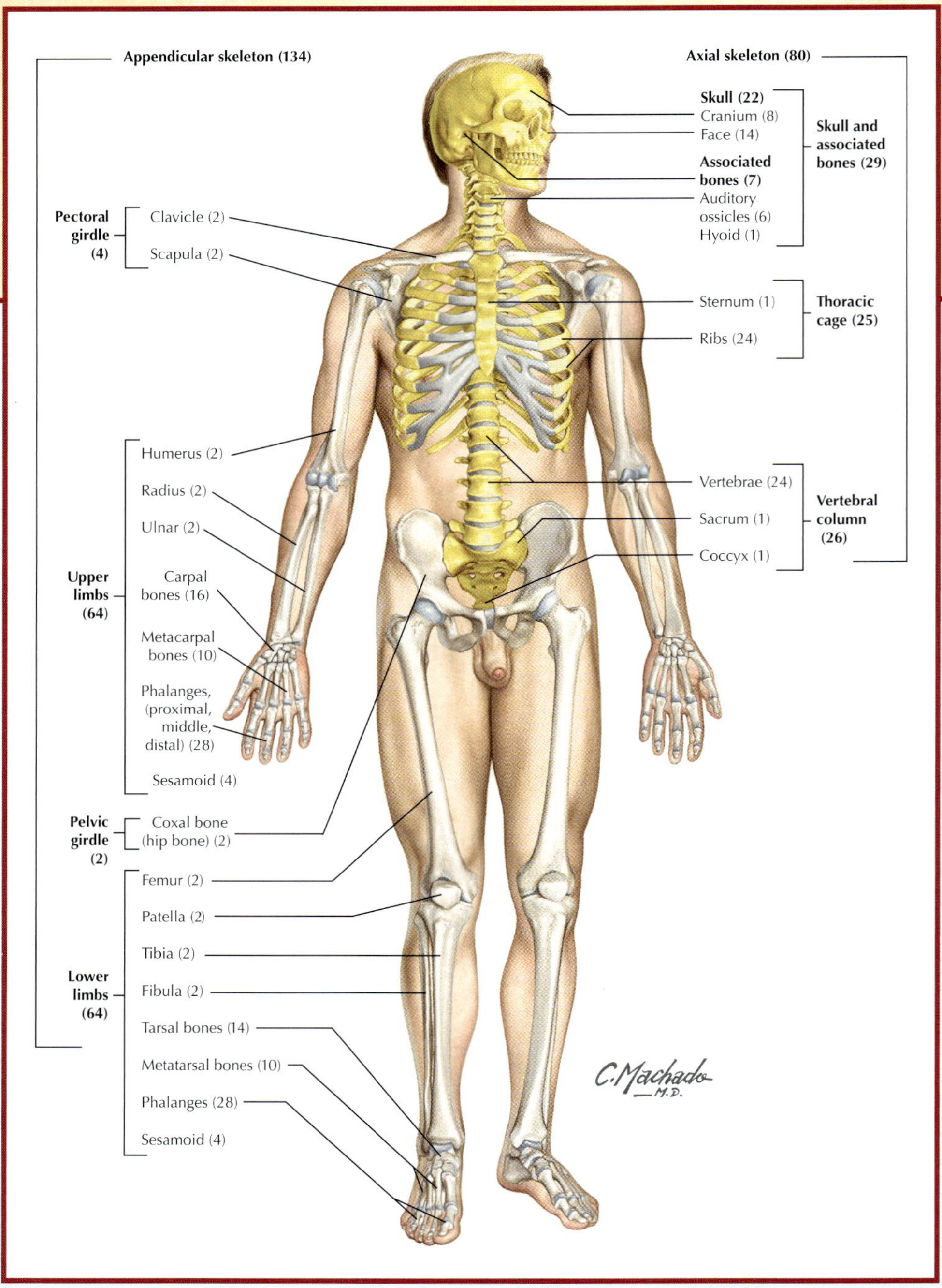
Appendicular skeleton (134)
Axial skeleton (80)
Skull (22)
Cranium (8)
Face (14)
Associated bones (7)
Auditory ossicles (6)
Hyoid (1)
Skull and associated bones (29)
Pectoral girdle (4)
Clavicle (2)
Scapula (2)
Sternum (1)
Ribs (24)
Thoracic cage (25)
Humerus (2)
Radius (2)
Ulnar (2)
Carpal bones (16)
Metacarpal bones (10)
Phalanges, (proximal, middle, distal) (28)
Sesamoid (4)
Upper limbs (64)
Vertebrae (24)
Sacrum (1)
Coccyx (1)
Vertebral column (26)
Pelvic girdle (2)
Coxal bone (hip bone) (2)
Femur (2)
Patella (2)
Tibia (2)
Fibula (2)
Tarsal bones (14)
Metatarsal bones (10)
Phalanges (28)
Sesamoid (4)
Lower limbs (64)
C. Machado M.D.

CHAPTER 2

Musculoskeletal System

The musculoskeletal system is composed of muscle, bone, and other connective tissue. An adult body contains more than 200 bones that, when articulated, give it structure and mobility. Bones also function to protect organs, eg, the skull protects the brain and the sternum protects the heart. Bones provide a reservoir for calcium and phosphorus, essential minerals for cellular activities throughout the body. Bones are remodeled in response to physical stress or damage (such as exercise or simply from the weight of our bodies) and to hormones and other chemicals circulating in the blood throughout life. Bone remodeling adjusts bone architecture to meet changing mechanical needs and helps to repair microdamages in bone matrix to prevent the accumulation of old bone. It also plays an important role in maintaining plasma calcium homeostasis.

Sites on bone are identified by their purpose or shape. A process is a bony projection or prominence. There are several types of processes that help form joints. A condyle is a large and rounded prominence at a joint; a facet is a flat and smooth bone surface; a head is the enlarged end of a bone at a joint; and the ramus is a branch of bone. Other processes provide an environment for attachment of muscle or ligament. A crest is a narrow ridge; a epicondyle is a secondary prominence above a condyle; a linea is a narrow ridge; a spinous process is a pointy or sharp prominence; a trochanter is an irregular process found only on the femur; a tubercle is a small knobby process; and a tuberosity is a large knobby process.

Bones accommodate blood vessels and nerves along depressions or openings. These anatomic sites are also named according to their function. For example, a fissure is a narrow passageway; a fontanel is a space between skull bones; a foramen is a round opening; a fossa is a shallow depression; a fovea is a small, deep depression; a sinus is a bony tube; and a sulcus is a long and narrow groove.

Tendons flow from muscle and secure to bone. **Cartilage** extends from the surface of a bone at a joint to reduce friction during movement.

Joints flex to varying degrees. Fibrous joints are immobile; cartilaginous joints have limited movement; and synovial joints have a high degree of movement. The fibrous joints in the skull, eg, provide flexibility during birth but are immobile in adulthood. Costal cartilages connect ribs numbered 8 through 10 to the sternum. The joint between the rib and sternum has limited movement, allowing for expansion of the rib cage during respiration. Vertebrae are also connected by cartilaginous joints. Synovial joints are the most common joints in the body. These joints are sealed in a synovial membrane that creates lubricating fluid and are wrapped in tough **ligaments** to give the joint strength and support. A bursa is a fluid-filled sac that functions to reduce friction between two structures in a synovial joint

Each muscle or muscle grouping is encased in **fascia**, allowing it to move independently from surrounding tissue. Skeletal muscle contracts in response to electrical stimuli from motor neurons of the spinal cord. When a muscle contracts, its tendons pull on the bone to which it is attached, causing bone movement. A muscle may be named based on its attachments, eg, sternocleidomastoid muscle connects the sternum and clavicle to the mastoid process. Others are named based on their location, eg, the orbicularis oculi muscle is located at the orbit.

All procedures using arthroscopic approach are segregated in the Musculoskeletal System code set, appearing toward the end of the section. Excluded from the Musculoskeletal System code set are codes used to report procedures performed on bone marrow. These procedures are reported using codes from the Hemic and Lymphatic Systems code set.

FIGURE 2-1. Percutaneous Needle Biopsy

A tissue sample is obtained by inserting a large-bore needle into a targeted muscle defect or, for some diagnoses, simply into the muscle to obtain a sample of muscle tissue. A muscle **biopsy** may be performed to diagnose the **etiology** of a lesion, a neuromuscular disorder, or some infectious processes such as toxoplasmosis. Note: Tools, implants, and/or equipment depicted in the illustration may be outdated but the procedural approach is valid.

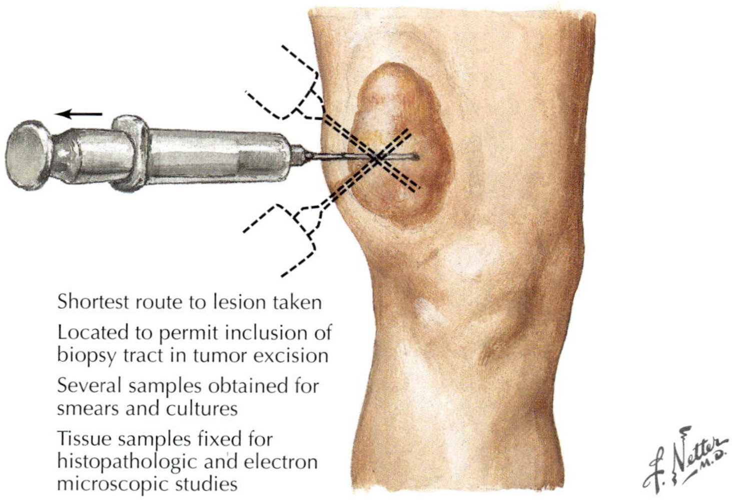

General

Incision

Coding Atlas

A subfascial **abscess** is a pocket of pus that has formed along the deep muscle tissues such as muscle sheaths or deep blood vessels. These abscesses may be incised, explored, and cleansed. The wounds are sometimes packed and usually are not closed or they are closed around a drain.

20005 Incision and drainage of soft tissue **abscess**, subfascial (ie, involves the soft tissue below the deep **fascia**)

Wound Exploration—Trauma (eg, Penetrating Gunshot, Stab Wound)

Coding Atlas

The codes in this section are used to describe procedures in which a traumatic wound is explored, but no major repairs are required. For example, if a knife or bullet penetrates the patient's abdomen but misses all major structures, a **thoracotomy/laparotomy** is not required. However, small repairs, cleansing, and **debridement** may be performed.

20100 Exploration of penetrating wound (separate procedure); neck

20101 chest

20102 abdomen/flank/back

20103 extremity

Excision

Coding Atlas

In a bone **biopsy**, representative cancellous bone and samples of one or two cortical plates are removed to establish the pathology of a bone lesion or metabolic derangement. Cancellous bone is a latticework of spongy, vascular tissue found in vertebrae and toward the ends of long bones. Cortical bone is the compact osseous tissue that forms the outer shell of most bones. Any removal of bone marrow during bone biopsy is incidental.

20150 Excision of epiphyseal bar, with or without **autogenous** soft tissue graft obtained through same fascial incision

20200 Biopsy, muscle; superficial

20205 deep

20206 **Biopsy**, muscle, **percutaneous** needle

FIGURE 2-2. Carpal Tunnel Injection

To treat symptoms of carpal tunnel syndrome, a combination of anesthetic and corticosteroid may be injected at the wrist to reduce inflammation of **tendons** in this area. Carpal tunnel syndrome occurs when pressure on the medial nerve causes symptoms such as weakness and numbness in the hand. The medial nerve shares space in the carpal tunnel with tendons and other soft tissue. Inflammation can cause these soft tissues to swell, compressing the nerve. Note: Tools, implants, and/or equipment depicted in the illustration may be outdated but the procedural approach is valid.

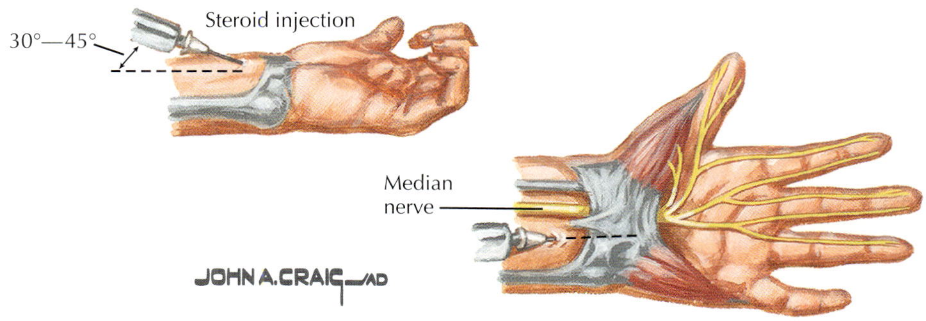

20220 Biopsy, bone, trocar, or needle; superficial (eg, ilium, sternum, spinous process, ribs)

20225 deep (eg, vertebral body, femur)

20240 Biopsy, bone, open; superficial (eg, ilium, sternum, spinous process, ribs, trochanter of femur)

20245 deep (eg, humerus, ischium, femur)

20250 Biopsy, vertebral body, open; thoracic

20251 lumbar or cervical

Introduction or Removal

Coding Atlas

The injection of contrast into an abnormal muscle tract for X-ray study allows the physician to map and treat the abnormality. In other instances, a **sinus tract** may be injected with a **therapeutic** agent, eg, an antibiotic.

20500 Injection of sinus tract; therapeutic (separate procedure)

20501 diagnostic (sinogram)

20520 Removal of foreign body in muscle or tendon sheath; simple

20525 deep or complicated

20526 Injection, therapeutic (eg, local anesthetic, corticosteroid), carpal tunnel

20527 Injection, enzyme (eg, collagenase), palmar fascial cord (ie, Dupuytren's contracture)

20550 Injection(s); single tendon sheath, or ligament, aponeurosis (eg, plantar "fascia")

20551 single tendon origin/insertion

20552 Injection(s); single or multiple trigger point(s), 1 or 2 muscle(s)

20553 single or multiple trigger point(s), 3 or more muscle(s)

20555 Placement of needles or catheters into muscle and/or soft tissue for subsequent interstitial radioelement application (at the time of or subsequent to the procedure)

20600 Arthrocentesis, aspiration and/or injection, small joint or bursa (eg, fingers, toes); without ultrasound guidance

20604 with ultrasound guidance, with permanent recording and reporting

20605 Arthrocentesis, aspiration and/or injection, intermediate joint or bursa (eg, temporomandibular, acromioclavicular, wrist, elbow or ankle, olecranon bursa); without ultrasound guidance

20606 with ultrasound guidance, with permanent recording and reporting

20610 Arthrocentesis, aspiration and/or injection, major joint or bursa (eg, shoulder, hip, knee, subacromial bursa); without ultrasound guidance

20611 with ultrasound guidance, with permanent recording and reporting

20612 Aspiration and/or injection of ganglion cyst(s) any location

20615 Aspiration and injection for treatment of bone cyst

20650 Insertion of wire or pin with application of skeletal traction, including removal (separate procedure)

20660 Application of cranial tongs, caliper, or stereotactic frame, including removal (separate procedure)

FIGURE 2-3. Joint Arthrocentesis, Aspiration, or Injection

Joint aspiration (**arthrocentesis**) may be performed on **synovial joints** for **diagnostic** or **therapeutic** reasons. The needle penetrates the joint capsule or **bursa**, and fluid within is withdrawn. Codes for arthrocentesis are based on the size of the targeted joint or bursa. Note: Tools, implants, and/or equipment depicted in the illustration may be outdated but the procedural approach is valid.

Techniques for Aspiration of Joint Fluid

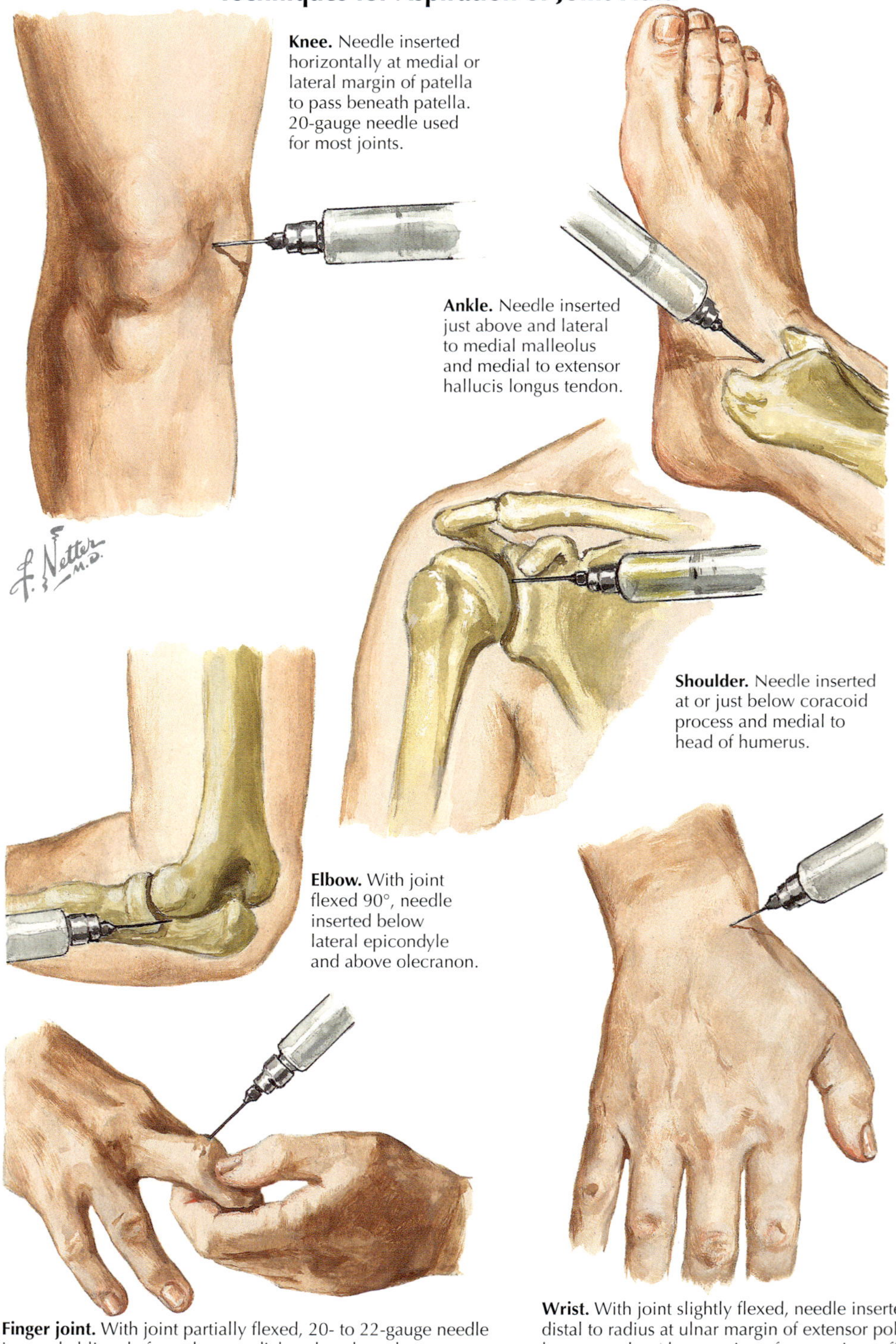

Knee. Needle inserted horizontally at medial or lateral margin of patella to pass beneath patella. 20-gauge needle used for most joints.

Ankle. Needle inserted just above and lateral to medial malleolus and medial to extensor hallucis longus tendon.

Shoulder. Needle inserted at or just below coracoid process and medial to head of humerus.

Elbow. With joint flexed 90°, needle inserted below lateral epicondyle and above olecranon.

Finger joint. With joint partially flexed, 20- to 22-gauge needle inserted obliquely from dorsomedial or dorsolateral aspect.

Wrist. With joint slightly flexed, needle inserted just distal to radius at ulnar margin of extensor pollicis longus tendon (demarcation of anatomic snuffbox).

FIGURE 2-4. Application of Halo or Tongs

Application of cranial tongs (code 20660) is often part of a larger procedure. Cranial tongs may be placed to stabilize a fracture pending definitive fracture care and would be reportable. Codes 20661 and 20664 are used to report the connection of cranial rings, also called halos, to a body brace or cast; work associated with alignment and connection to the brace or cast is included with the code. Note: Tools, implants, and/or equipment depicted in the illustration may be outdated but the procedural approach is valid.

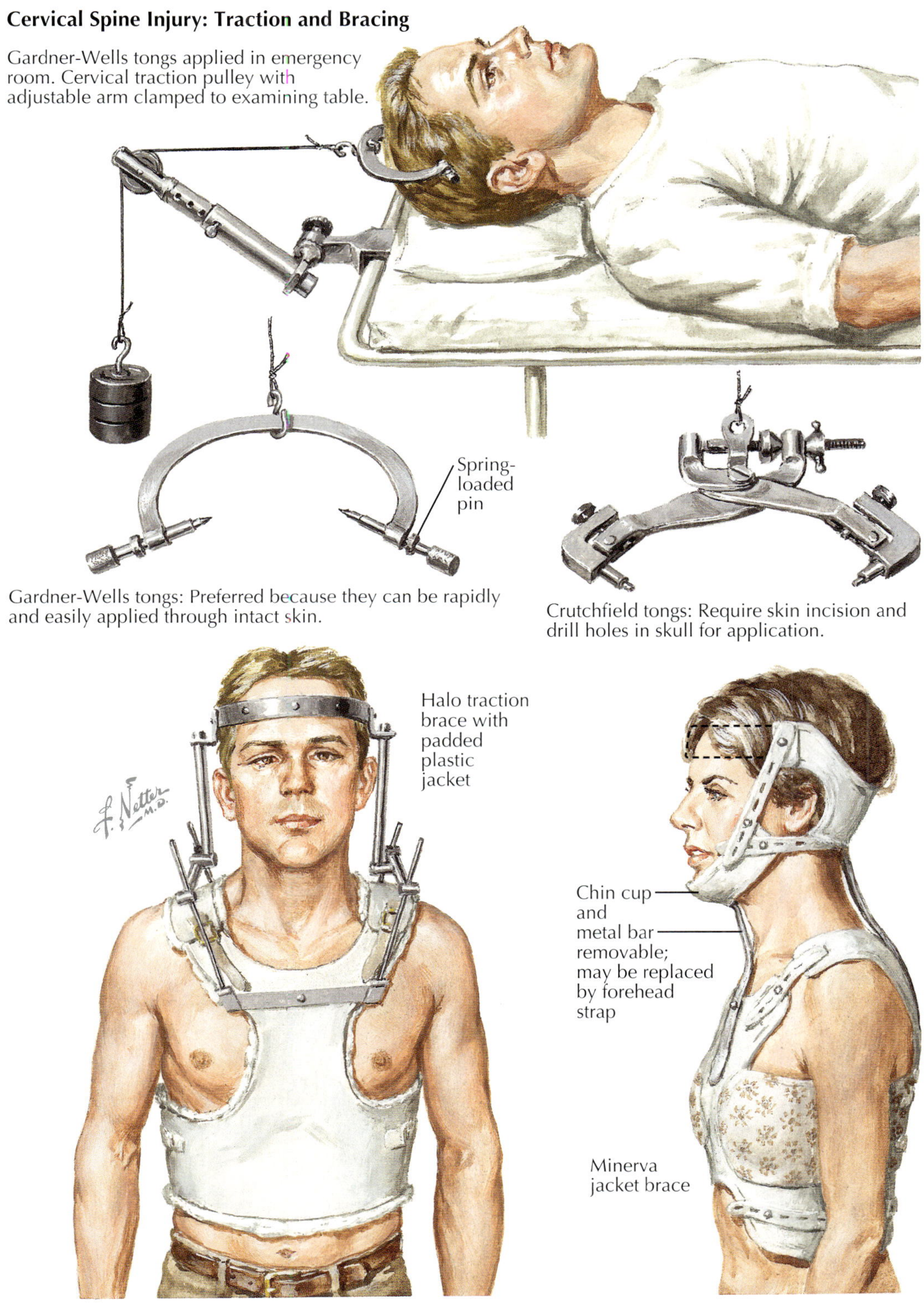

20661 Application of halo, including removal; cranial

20662 pelvic

20663 femoral

20664 Application of halo, including removal, cranial, 6 or more pins placed, for thin skull osteology (eg, pediatric patients, hydrocephalus, osteogenesis imperfecta)

20665 Removal of tongs or halo applied by another individual

20670 Removal of implant; superficial (eg, buried wire, pin or rod) (separate procedure)

20680 deep (eg, buried wire, pin, screw, metal band, nail, rod or plate)

20690 Application of a uniplane (pins or wires in 1 plane), unilateral, external fixation system

20692 Application of a multiplane (pins or wires in more than 1 plane), unilateral, external fixation system (eg, Ilizarov, Monticelli type)

20693 Adjustment or revision of external fixation system requiring anesthesia (eg, new pin[s] or wire[s] and/or new ring[s] or bar[s])

20694 Removal, under anesthesia, of external fixation system

20696 Application of multiplane (pins or wires in more than 1 plane), unilateral, external fixation with stereotactic computer-assisted adjustment (eg, spatial frame), including imaging; initial and subsequent alignment(s), assessment(s), and computation(s) of adjustment schedule(s)

⊘ **20697** exchange (ie, removal and replacement) of strut, each

Replantation

Coding Atlas

In **replantation**, an extremity that has been completely severed is reattached. The severed ends are **debrided**, and the bone is reconnected with pins or plates. Muscles, tendons, arteries, veins, and nerves are then **reanastomosed**, many on a **microsurgical** level. If the injured extremity is not completely severed, the repair of bone(s), **ligament**(s), vessel(s), and nerve(s) is reported separately, rather than by using replantation codes.

20802 Replantation, arm (includes surgical neck of humerus through elbow joint), complete amputation

20805 Replantation, forearm (includes radius and ulna to radial carpal joint), complete amputation

20808 Replantation, hand (includes hand through metacarpophalangeal joints), complete amputation

20816 Replantation, digit, excluding thumb (includes metacarpophalangeal joint to insertion of flexor sublimis tendon), complete amputation

20822 Replantation, digit, excluding thumb (includes distal tip to sublimis tendon insertion), complete amputation

20824 Replantation, thumb (includes carpometacarpal joint to MP joint), complete amputation

20827 Replantation, thumb (includes distal tip to MP joint), complete amputation

20838 Replantation, foot, complete amputation

Grafts (or Implants)

Coding Atlas

When grafting material is harvested through a separate incision, the harvest can be reported in addition to the primary procedure, unless the description for the primary procedure code states that it includes obtaining the graft material. Types of grafts may be used similarly, eg, a **tendon** graft may repair a damaged tendon. In other cases, the graft material may be used in a manner different from its origin, eg, **fascia lata** may be used to correct eyelid retraction. Codes 20930-20938 apply only to bone grafts for spinal surgery.

20900 Bone graft, any donor area; minor or small (eg, dowel or button)

20902 major or large

20910 Cartilage graft; costochondral

20912 nasal septum

20920 Fascia lata graft; by stripper

20922 by incision and area exposure, complex or sheet

20924 Tendon graft, from a distance (eg, palmaris, toe extensor, plantaris)

20926 Tissue grafts, other (eg, paratenon, fat, dermis)

✚ **20930** Allograft, morselized, or placement of osteopromotive material, for spine surgery only (List separately in addition to code for primary procedure)

✚ **20931** Allograft, structural, for spine surgery only (List separately in addition to code for primary procedure)

✚ **20936** Autograft for spine surgery only (includes harvesting the graft); local (eg, ribs, spinous process, or laminar fragments) obtained from same incision (List separately in addition to code for primary procedure)

✚ **20937** morselized (through separate skin or fascial incision) (List separately in addition to code for primary procedure)

✚ **20938** structural, bicortical or tricortical (through separate skin or fascial incision) (List separately in addition to code for primary procedure)

FIGURE 2-5. Replantation of the Forearm

Advances in **microsurgical** technique have led to an increase in **replantation** procedures. The goal of replantation is restoration of function. Replantations are classified in the CPT code set according to the level of amputation: forearm, upper arm, hand, digit excluding thumb, or thumb. Replantation codes are used to report repair following complete amputation. Note: Tools, implants, and/or equipment depicted in the illustration may be outdated but the procedural approach is valid.

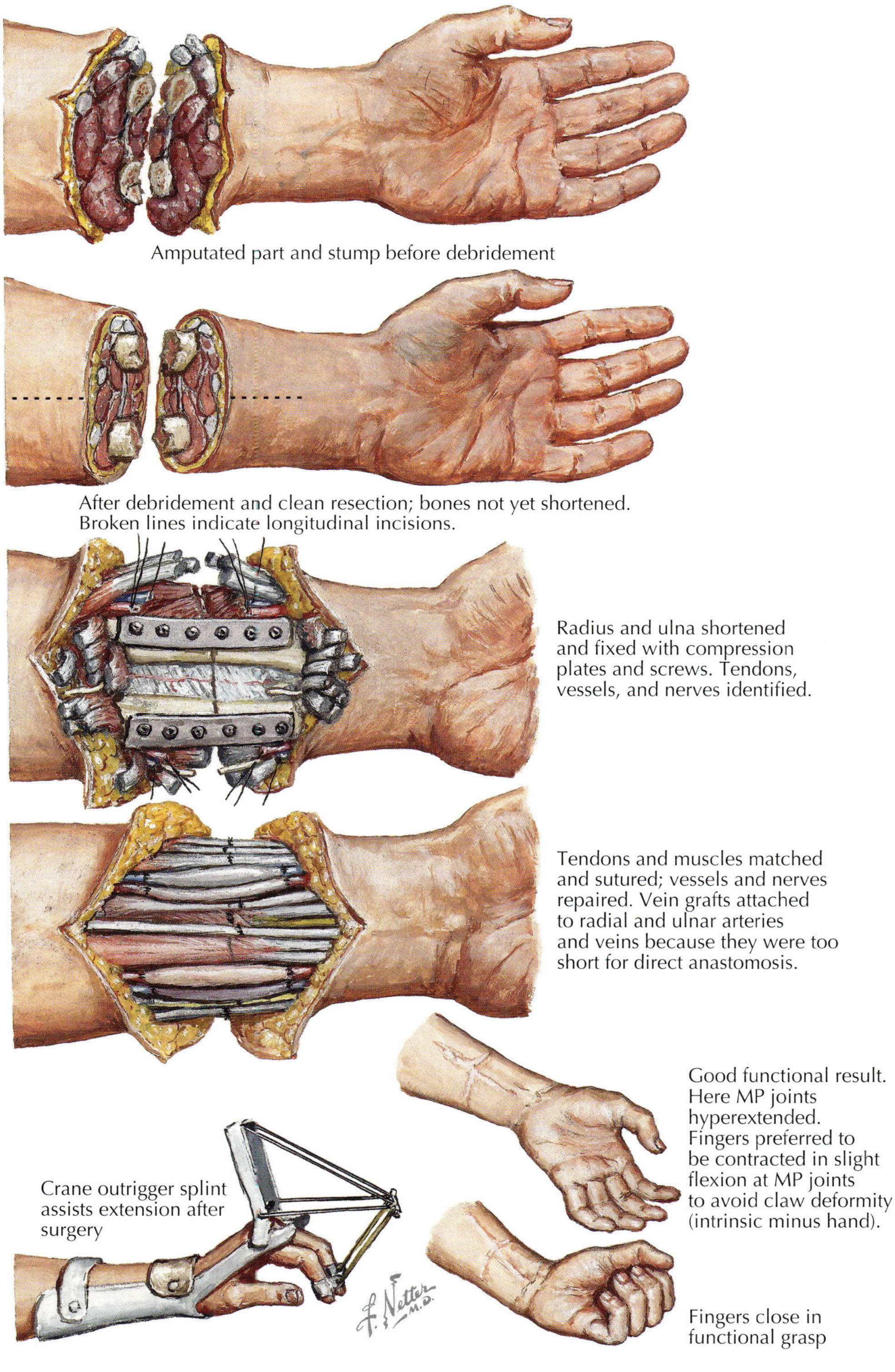

Other Procedures

Coding Atlas

Vascularized bone grafts are used to repair defects that cannot be adequately treated with nonvascularized bone. Codes 20955-20973 report the harvest of vascularized bone from the sites described. The placement of the graft is reported separately.

20950 Monitoring of interstitial fluid pressure (includes insertion of device, eg, wick catheter technique, needle manometer technique) in detection of muscle compartment syndrome

20955 Bone graft with microvascular anastomosis; fibula

20956 iliac crest

20957 metatarsal

20962 other than fibula, iliac crest, or metatarsal

20969 Free osteocutaneous flap with microvascular anastomosis; other than iliac crest, metatarsal, or great toe

20970 iliac crest

20972 metatarsal

20973 great toe with web space

⊘ **20974** Electrical stimulation to aid bone healing; noninvasive (nonoperative)

⊘ **20975** invasive (operative)

20979 Low intensity ultrasound stimulation to aid bone healing, noninvasive (nonoperative)

⊙ **20982** Ablation therapy for reduction or eradication of 1 or more bone tumors (eg, metastasis) including adjacent soft tissue when involved by tumor extension, percutaneous, including imaging guidance when performed; radiofrequency

⊙ **20983** cryoablation

✚ **20985** Computer-assisted surgical navigational procedure for musculoskeletal procedures, image-less (List separately in addition to code for primary procedure)

Head

Incision

Coding Atlas

The temporomandibular joint (TMJ) is a hinged joint that links the mandible to the rest of the skull. Cartilage within the joint absorbs stress and allows the mandible to move easily. In TMJ arthrotomy, the joint capsule is incised.

21010 Arthrotomy, temporomandibular joint

Excision

Coding Atlas

Size and tumor origin play a role in code selection for excision of soft tissue tumor. The entire resection is measured, not the diameter of the lesion itself, to determine the excision size. Excision of a tumor originating in the integument, eg, melanoma, is reported with an integumentary excision code even if it extends into muscle tissue.

21011 Excision, tumor, soft tissue of face or scalp, subcutaneous; less than 2 cm

21012 2 cm or greater

21013 Excision, tumor, soft tissue of face and scalp, subfascial (eg, subgaleal, intramuscular); less than 2 cm

21014 2 cm or greater

21015 Radical resection of tumor (eg, sarcoma), soft tissue of face or scalp; less than 2 cm

21016 2 cm or greater

21025 Excision of bone (eg, for osteomyelitis or bone abscess); mandible

21026 facial bone(s)

21029 Removal by contouring of benign tumor of facial bone (eg, fibrous dysplasia)

21030 Excision of benign tumor or cyst of maxilla or zygoma by enucleation and curettage

21031 Excision of torus mandibularis

21032 Excision of maxillary torus palatinus

21034 Excision of malignant tumor of maxilla or zygoma

21040 Excision of benign tumor or cyst of mandible, by enucleation and/or curettage

21044 Excision of malignant tumor of mandible;

21045 radical resection

21046 Excision of benign tumor or cyst of mandible; requiring intra-oral osteotomy (eg, locally aggressive or destructive lesion[s])

21047 requiring extra-oral osteotomy and partial mandibulectomy (eg, locally aggressive or destructive lesion[s])

21048 Excision of benign tumor or cyst of maxilla; requiring intra-oral osteotomy (eg, locally aggressive or destructive lesion[s])

FIGURE 2-6. Muscles of the Head

Many muscles of the face are small and thin and do not function to move bone. Instead, they move integumentary tissues for facial expression and move the cheeks and lips while eating. The larger masseter, buccinator, medial/lateral pterygoid, and temporalis muscles of the head contribute to **mastication**, the most robust muscular function of the face.

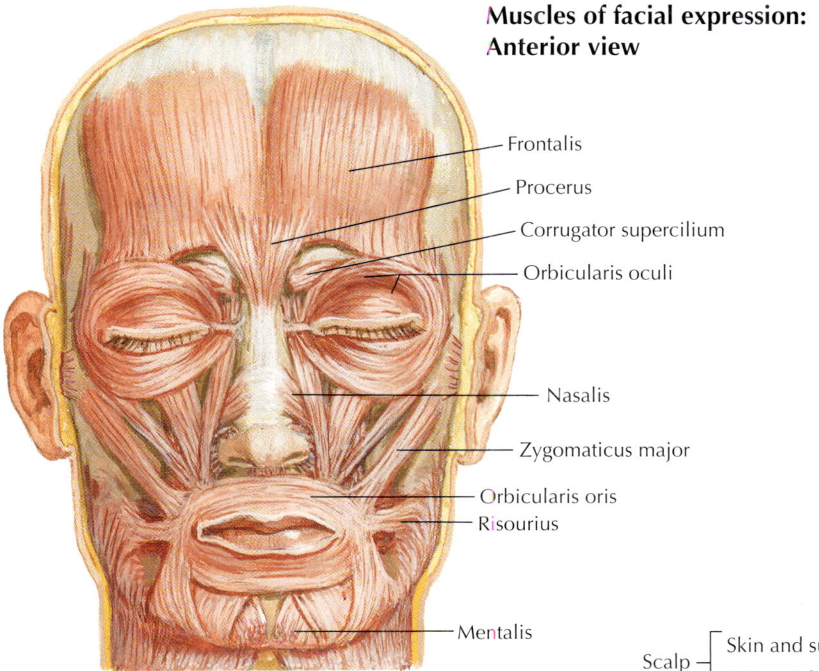

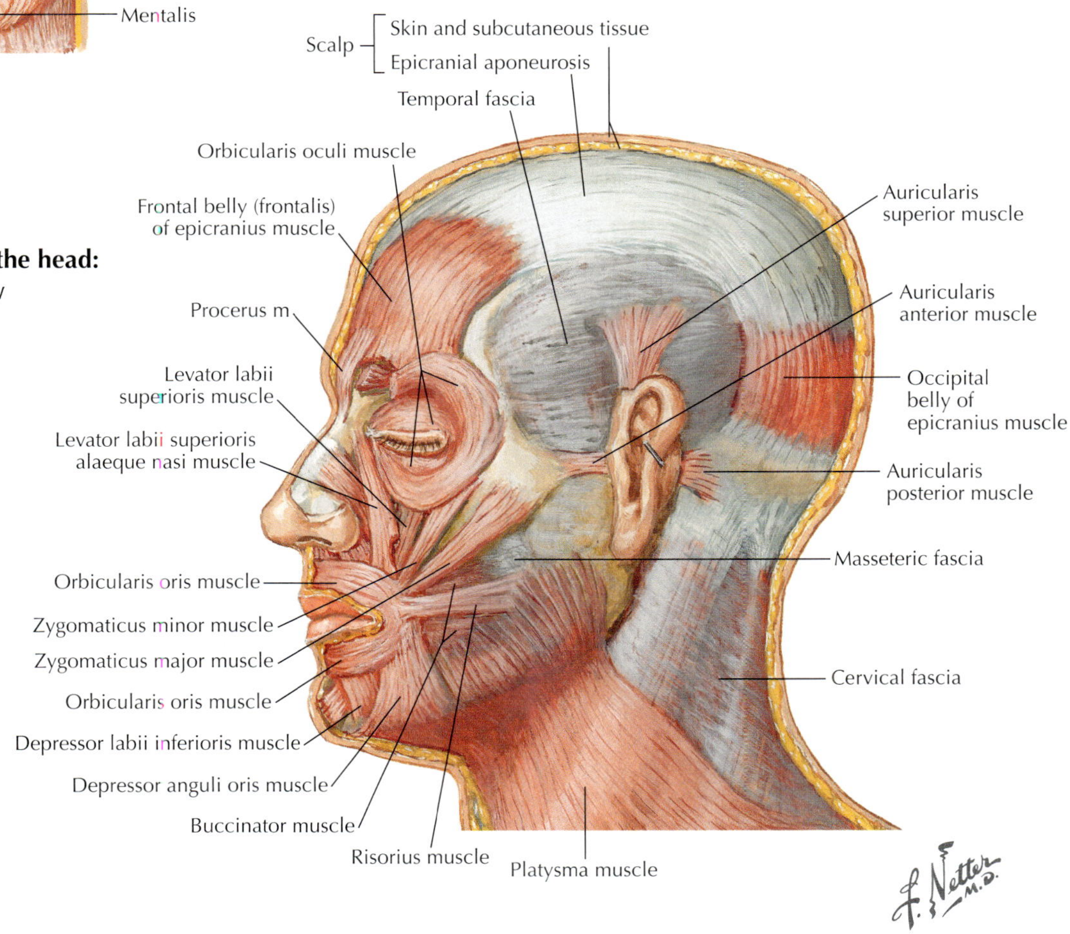

FIGURE 2-7. Temporomandibular Joint and Muscles

The temporomandibular joint is a **bilateral** synovial joint with two condylar surfaces and an **intra-articular** disc. Four muscles are primarily responsible for movement of the mandible: masseter, medial pterygoid, lateral pterygoid, and temporalis. Pain or dysfunction of the temporomandibular joint is commonly referred to as TMJ, but TMJ is actually an acronym for the joint itself.

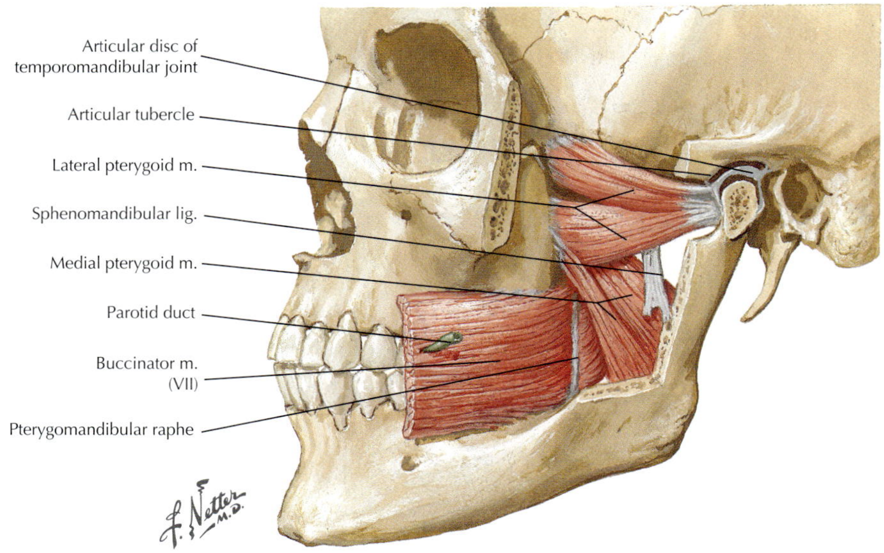

Lateral view

21049 requiring extra-oral osteotomy and partial maxillectomy (eg, locally aggressive or destructive lesion[s])

21050 Condylectomy, temporomandibular joint (separate procedure)

21060 Meniscectomy, partial or complete, temporomandibular joint (separate procedure)

21070 Coronoidectomy (separate procedure)

Manipulation

Coding Atlas

TMJ disorders may include, but are not limited to, inflammation, fibrosis, **hypermobility**, arthritis, and disc displacement. Code 21073 is used to report a therapeutic **manipulation** of the TMJ joint that requires anesthesia. Code 21073 is not appropriate for a diagnostic manipulation.

21073 Manipulation of temporomandibular joint(s) (TMJ), therapeutic, requiring an anesthesia service (ie, general or monitored anesthesia care)

Head Prosthesis

Coding Atlas

Services in this section describe preparation of **prosthetic** structures for the head to treat **congenital** or acquired deformities or to provide support to structures that are essential to functions such as speech and swallowing. They may be secured to the skin or attached to teeth or other oral structures. In most cases, they are removable. Codes 21076-21089 are used to report services only when the physician designs and fabricates the prosthesis.

21076 Impression and custom preparation; surgical obturator prosthesis

21077 orbital prosthesis

21079 interim obturator prosthesis

21080 definitive obturator prosthesis

21081 mandibular resection prosthesis

21082 palatal augmentation prosthesis

21083 palatal lift prosthesis

21084 speech aid prosthesis

21085 oral surgical splint

21086 auricular prosthesis

21087 nasal prosthesis

21088 facial prosthesis

Introduction or Removal

Coding Atlas

In the application of an **interdental** fixation device for conditions other than fracture or dislocation, the device is more permanent than wiring and has no moveable parts. An example of a device placement reported using code 21110 is an interdental fixation device that is secured to the teeth, sometimes called an arch bar, to prevent teeth migration.

21100 Application of halo type appliance for maxillofacial fixation, includes removal (separate procedure)

21110 Application of interdental fixation device for conditions other than fracture or dislocation, includes removal

21116 Injection procedure for temporomandibular joint arthrography

Repair, Revision, and/or Reconstruction

Coding Atlas

Implants in the chin or cheek may change facial proportions. Similarly, reductions in the chin, forehead, or cheek may alter the structural appearance of the face. In some cases, bones in the face are surgically broken and realigned to treat **malocclusions** or other functional defects or for **cosmesis**.

21120 Genioplasty; augmentation (autograft, allograft, prosthetic material)

21121 sliding osteotomy, single piece

21122 sliding osteotomies, 2 or more osteotomies (eg, wedge excision or bone wedge reversal for asymmetrical chin)

21123 sliding, augmentation with interpositional bone grafts (includes obtaining autografts)

21125 Augmentation, mandibular body or angle; prosthetic material

21127 with bone graft, onlay or interpositional (includes obtaining autograft)

21137 Reduction forehead; contouring only

21138 contouring and application of prosthetic material or bone graft (includes obtaining autograft)

21139 contouring and setback of anterior frontal sinus wall

21141 Reconstruction midface, LeFort I; single piece, segment movement in any direction (eg, for Long Face Syndrome), without bone graft

21142 2 pieces, segment movement in any direction, without bone graft

21143 3 or more pieces, segment movement in any direction, without bone graft

21145 single piece, segment movement in any direction, requiring bone grafts (includes obtaining autografts)

21146 2 pieces, segment movement in any direction, requiring bone grafts (includes obtaining autografts) (eg, ungrafted unilateral alveolar cleft)

21147 3 or more pieces, segment movement in any direction, requiring bone grafts (includes obtaining autografts) (eg, ungrafted bilateral alveolar cleft or multiple osteotomies)

21150 Reconstruction midface, LeFort II; anterior intrusion (eg, Treacher-Collins Syndrome)

21151 any direction, requiring bone grafts (includes obtaining autografts)

21154 Reconstruction midface, LeFort III (extracranial), any type, requiring bone grafts (includes obtaining autografts); without LeFort I

21155 with LeFort I

21159 Reconstruction midface, LeFort III (extra and intracranial) with forehead advancement (eg, mono bloc), requiring bone grafts (includes obtaining autografts); without LeFort I

21160 with LeFort I

21172 Reconstruction superior-lateral orbital rim and lower forehead, advancement or alteration, with or without grafts (includes obtaining autografts)

(For frontal or parietal craniotomy performed for craniosynostosis, use 61556)

21175 Reconstruction, bifrontal, superior-lateral orbital rims and lower forehead, advancement or alteration (eg, plagiocephaly, trigonocephaly, brachycephaly), with or without grafts (includes obtaining autografts)

21179 Reconstruction, entire or majority of forehead and/or supraorbital rims; with grafts (allograft or prosthetic material)

21180 with autograft (includes obtaining grafts)

21181 Reconstruction by contouring of benign tumor of cranial bones (eg, fibrous dysplasia), extracranial

21182 Reconstruction of orbital walls, rims, forehead, nasoethmoid complex following intra- and extracranial excision of benign tumor of cranial bone (eg, fibrous dysplasia), with multiple autografts (includes obtaining grafts); total area of bone grafting less than 40 sq cm

FIGURE 2-8. Lateral View of the Skull

Skull bones protect the brain and sense organs. The primary bones of the face are maxilla, mandible, frontal bone, nasal bones, and zygoma. The mandible is the only moveable bone in the face and it contains the lower teeth. The maxilla contains the upper teeth, forms the roof of the mouth, and also contributes to the bony structures of the orbit, maxillary sinus, and nasal cavity. Sutures are fibrous connections between adjacent bones of the skull.

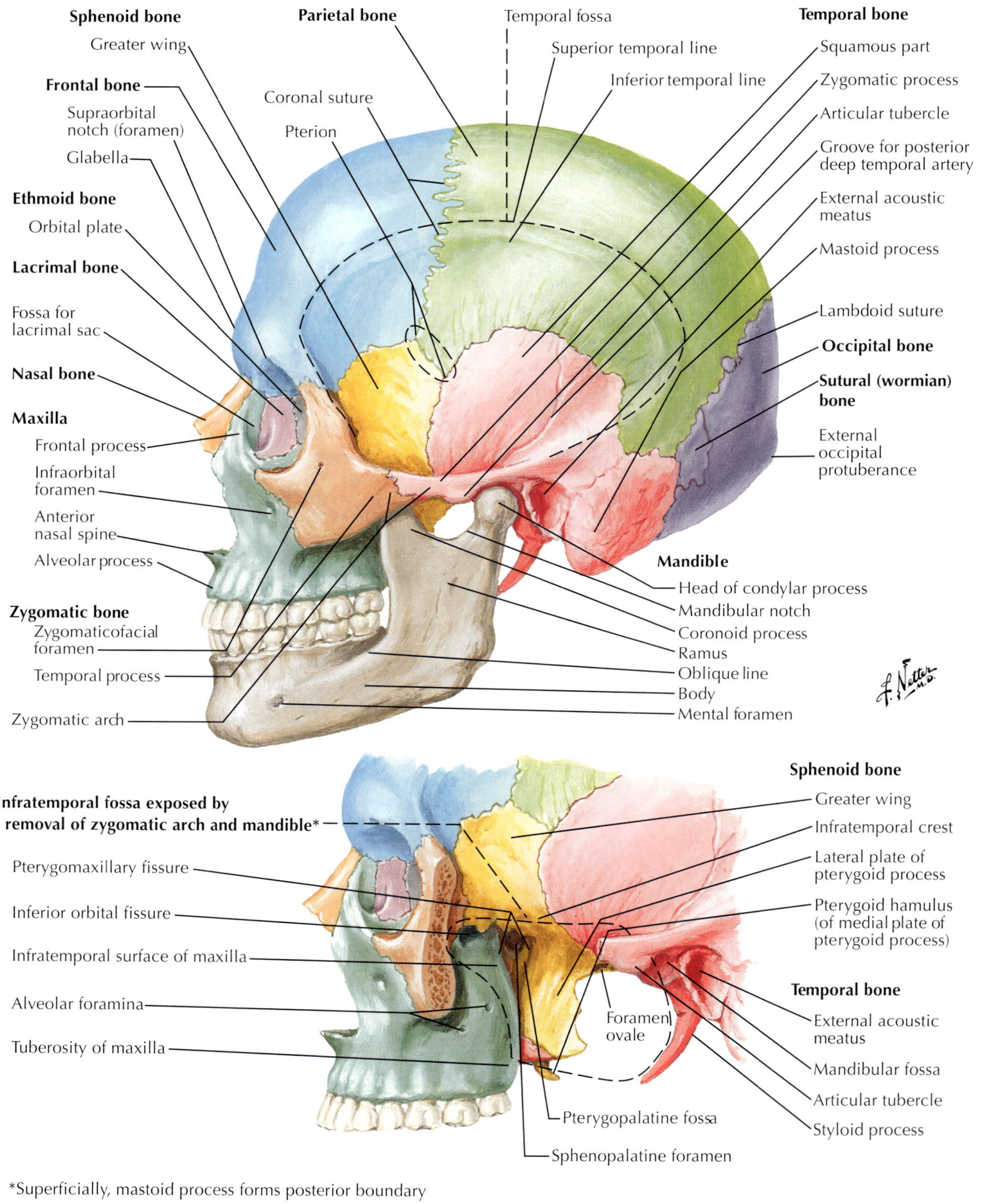

*Superficially, mastoid process forms posterior boundary

FIGURE 2-9. Anterior View of the Skull

Seven bones form the orbit: frontal, lacrimal, maxillary, palatine, zygomatic, sphenoid, and ethmoid. The eyeball and many components of the ocular **adnexa** are protected in the bony socket, which is lined in fat. Reconstruction of the orbital bone may correct a **congenital** malformation or a defect resulting from trauma or surgical excision. In documentation, "orbit" may describe the bony orbit or soft tissue orbital contents.

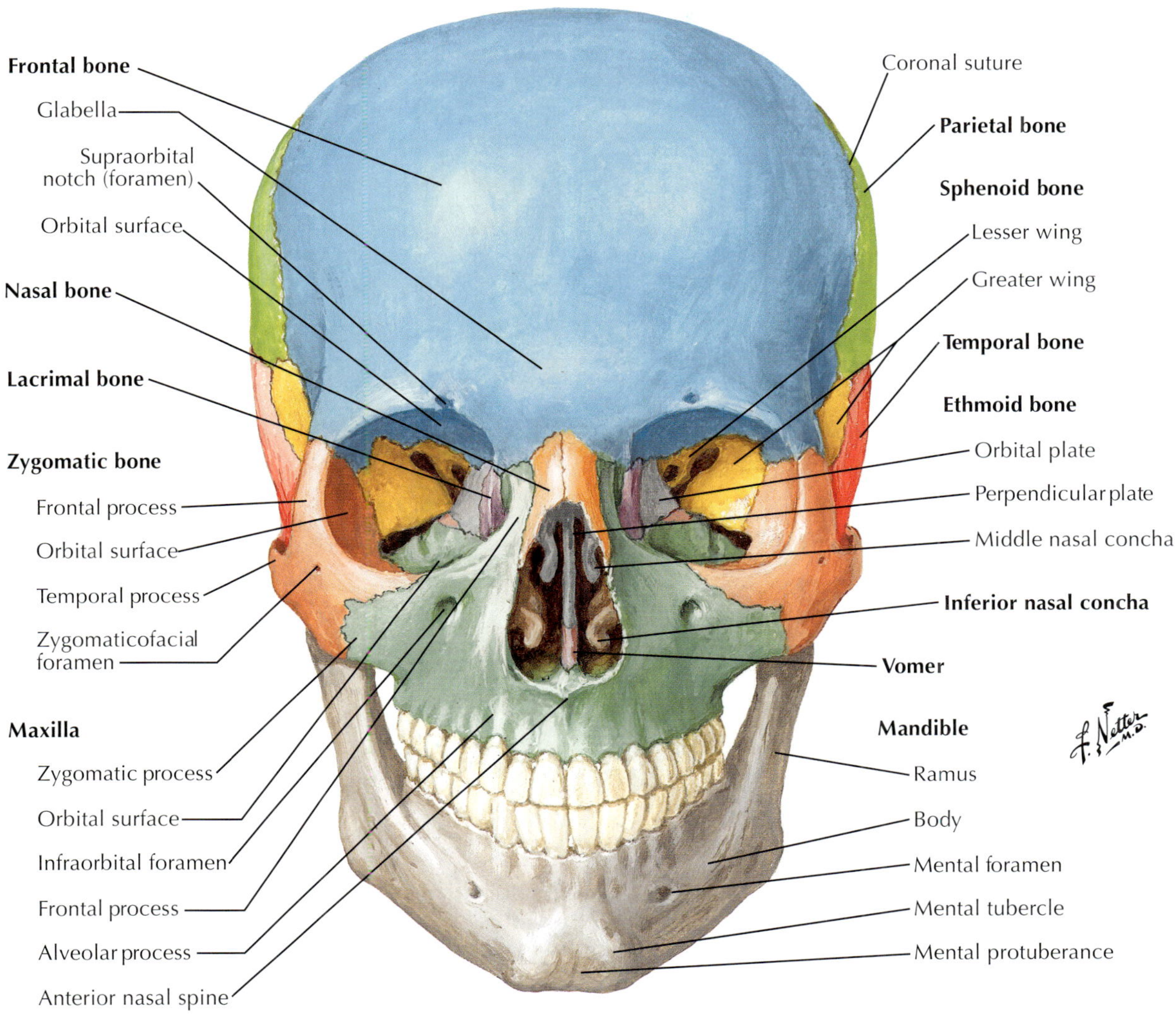

Right orbit: frontal and slightly lateral view

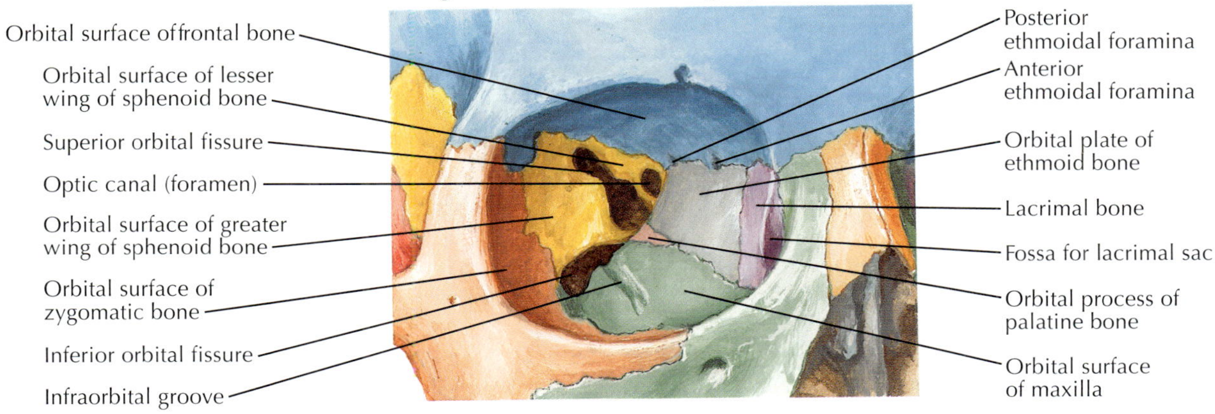

21183 total area of bone grafting greater than 40 sq cm but less than 80 sq cm

21184 total area of bone grafting greater than 80 sq cm

21188 Reconstruction midface, osteotomies (other than LeFort type) and bone grafts (includes obtaining autografts)

21193 Reconstruction of mandibular rami, horizontal, vertical, C, or L osteotomy; without bone graft

21194 with bone graft (includes obtaining graft)

21195 Reconstruction of mandibular rami and/or body, sagittal split; without internal rigid fixation

21196 with internal rigid fixation

21198 Osteotomy, mandible, segmental;

21199 with genioglossus advancement

21206 Osteotomy, maxilla, segmental (eg, Wassmund or Schuchard)

21208 Osteoplasty, facial bones; augmentation (autograft, allograft, or prosthetic implant)

21209 reduction

21210 Graft, bone; nasal, maxillary or malar areas (includes obtaining graft)

21215 mandible (includes obtaining graft)

21230 Graft; rib cartilage, autogenous, to face, chin, nose or ear (includes obtaining graft)

21235 ear cartilage, autogenous, to nose or ear (includes obtaining graft)

21240 Arthroplasty, temporomandibular joint, with or without autograft (includes obtaining graft)

21242 Arthroplasty, temporomandibular joint, with allograft

21243 Arthroplasty, temporomandibular joint, with prosthetic joint replacement

21244 Reconstruction of mandible, extraoral, with transosteal bone plate (eg, mandibular staple bone plate)

21245 Reconstruction of mandible or maxilla, subperiosteal implant; partial

21246 complete

21247 Reconstruction of mandibular condyle with bone and cartilage autografts (includes obtaining grafts) (eg, for hemifacial microsomia)

21248 Reconstruction of mandible or maxilla, endosteal implant (eg, blade, cylinder); partial

21249 complete

21255 Reconstruction of zygomatic arch and glenoid fossa with bone and cartilage (includes obtaining autografts)

21256 Reconstruction of orbit with osteotomies (extracranial) and with bone grafts (includes obtaining autografts) (eg, micro-ophthalmia)

21260 Periorbital osteotomies for orbital hypertelorism, with bone grafts; extracranial approach

21261 combined intra- and extracranial approach

21263 with forehead advancement

21267 Orbital repositioning, periorbital osteotomies, unilateral, with bone grafts; extracranial approach

21268 combined intra- and extracranial approach

21270 Malar augmentation, prosthetic material

21275 Secondary revision of orbitocraniofacial reconstruction

21280 Medial canthopexy (separate procedure)

21282 Lateral canthopexy

21295 Reduction of masseter muscle and bone (eg, for treatment of benign masseteric hypertrophy); extraoral approach

21296 intraoral approach

Fracture and/or Dislocation

Coding Atlas

Because of its projection on the face, the nose is the most common site of facial bone fracture. The nasal septum divides the cavities of the right and left nostril and is comprised of the thin, midline vomer bone and cartilage. A fracture of the vomer bone or nasal cartilage may lead to a deviated nasal septum (DNS).

21310 Closed treatment of nasal bone fracture without manipulation

21315 Closed treatment of nasal bone fracture; without stabilization

21320 with stabilization

21325 Open treatment of nasal fracture; uncomplicated

21330 complicated, with internal and/or external skeletal fixation

21335 with concomitant open treatment of fractured septum

21336 Open treatment of nasal septal fracture, with or without stabilization

21337 Closed treatment of nasal septal fracture, with or without stabilization

21338 Open treatment of nasoethmoid fracture; without external fixation

21339 with external fixation

21340 Percutaneous treatment of nasoethmoid complex fracture, with splint, wire or headcap fixation, including repair of canthal ligaments and/or the nasolacrimal apparatus

FIGURE 2-10. Le Fort I Fracture

Le Fort fractures are fractures in which the maxilla separates from the skull base. In a Le Fort I fracture, the fracture line is through the alveolar ridge, lateral nose, and inferior wall of the maxillary sinus. The upper **dentition** is essentially sheared from the upper face. Codes 21421-21423 are used to report repair of a traumatic fracture but are not used to report **therapeutic** Le Fort fractures that occur as part of a facial reconstruction. Note: Tools, implants, and/or equipment depicted in the illustration may be outdated but the procedural approach is valid.

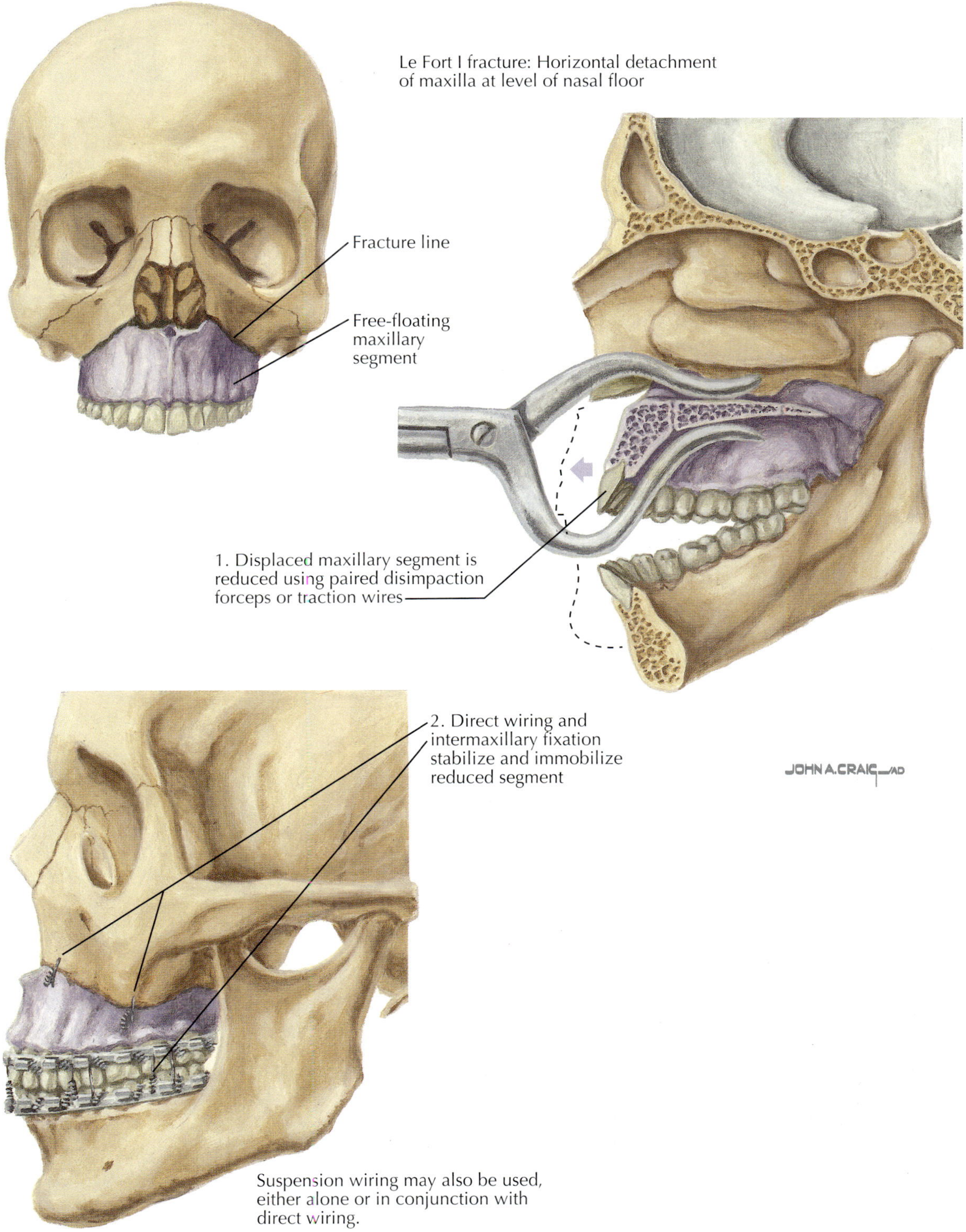

FIGURE 2-11. Le Fort III Fracture

In a Le Fort III fracture, the fracture line is through the nasofrontal **suture**, maxilla-frontal suture, orbital wall, and zygomatic arch. The facial bones are essentially sheared from the cranial bones. Codes 21432-21435 are used to report repair of a traumatic fracture; they are not used to report **therapeutic** Le Fort fractures that occur as part of a facial reconstruction. Note: Tools, implants, and/or equipment depicted in the illustration may be outdated but the procedural approach is valid.

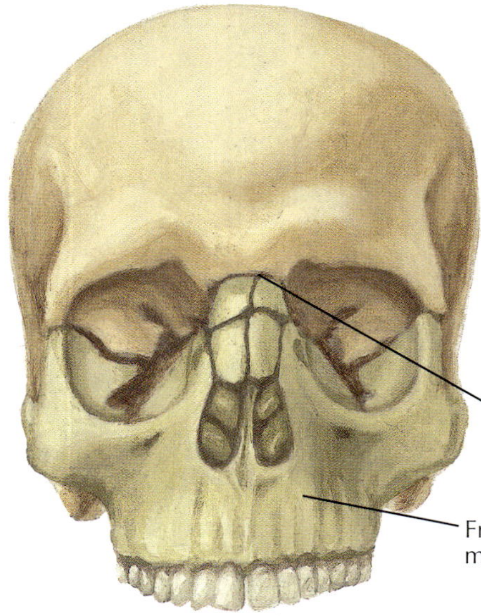

Le Fort III fracture: Fracture through zygomatic bones and orbits, separating facial bones from cranial vault.

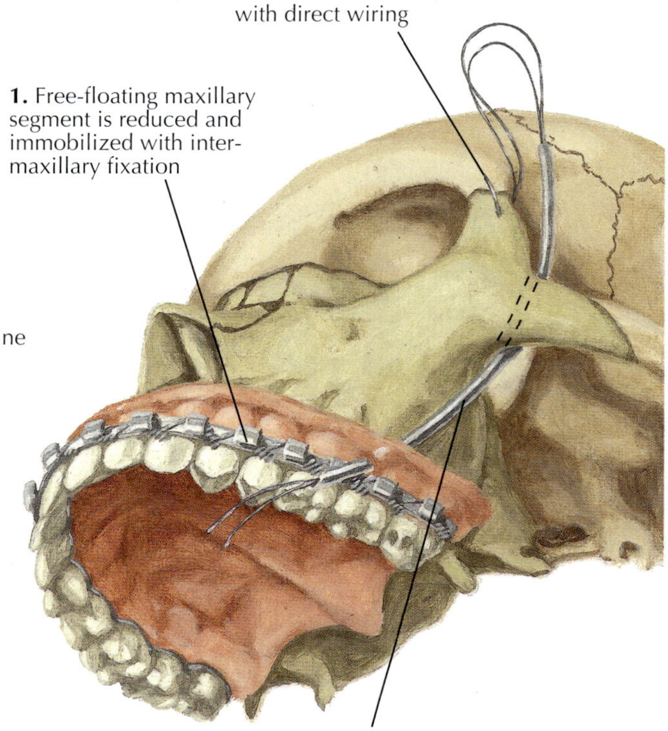

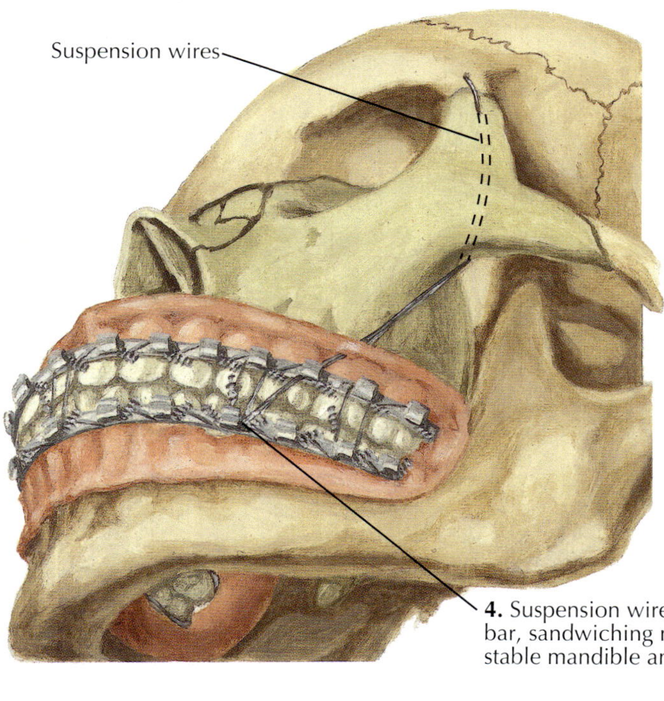

21343 Open treatment of depressed frontal sinus fracture

21344 Open treatment of complicated (eg, comminuted or involving posterior wall) frontal sinus fracture, via coronal or multiple approaches

21345 Closed treatment of nasomaxillary complex fracture (LeFort II type), with interdental wire fixation or fixation of denture or splint

21346 Open treatment of nasomaxillary complex fracture (LeFort II type); with wiring and/or local fixation

21347 requiring multiple open approaches

21348 with bone grafting (includes obtaining graft)

21355 Percutaneous treatment of fracture of malar area, including zygomatic arch and malar tripod, with manipulation

21356 Open treatment of depressed zygomatic arch fracture (eg, Gillies approach)

21360 Open treatment of depressed malar fracture, including zygomatic arch and malar tripod

21365 Open treatment of complicated (eg, comminuted or involving cranial nerve foramina) fracture(s) of malar area, including zygomatic arch and malar tripod; with internal fixation and multiple surgical approaches

21366 with bone grafting (includes obtaining graft)

21385 Open treatment of orbital floor blowout fracture; transantral approach (Caldwell-Luc type operation)

21386 periorbital approach

21387 combined approach

21390 periorbital approach, with alloplastic or other implant

21395 periorbital approach with bone graft (includes obtaining graft)

21400 Closed treatment of fracture of orbit, except blowout; without manipulation

21401 with manipulation

21406 Open treatment of fracture of orbit, except blowout; without implant

21407 with implant

21408 with bone grafting (includes obtaining graft)

21421 Closed treatment of palatal or maxillary fracture (LeFort I type), with interdental wire fixation or fixation of denture or splint

21422 Open treatment of palatal or maxillary fracture (LeFort I type);

21423 complicated (comminuted or involving cranial nerve foramina), multiple approaches

21431 Closed treatment of craniofacial separation (LeFort III type) using interdental wire fixation of denture or splint

21432 Open treatment of craniofacial separation (LeFort III type); with wiring and/or internal fixation

21433 complicated (eg, comminuted or involving cranial nerve foramina), multiple surgical approaches

21435 complicated, utilizing internal and/or external fixation techniques (eg, head cap, halo device, and/or intermaxillary fixation)

21436 complicated, multiple surgical approaches, internal fixation, with bone grafting (includes obtaining graft)

21440 Closed treatment of mandibular or maxillary alveolar ridge fracture (separate procedure)

21445 Open treatment of mandibular or maxillary alveolar ridge fracture (separate procedure)

21450 Closed treatment of mandibular fracture; without manipulation

21451 with manipulation

21452 Percutaneous treatment of mandibular fracture, with external fixation

21453 Closed treatment of mandibular fracture with interdental fixation

21454 Open treatment of mandibular fracture with external fixation

21461 Open treatment of mandibular fracture; without interdental fixation

21462 with interdental fixation

21465 Open treatment of mandibular condylar fracture

21470 Open treatment of complicated mandibular fracture by multiple surgical approaches including internal fixation, interdental fixation, and/or wiring of dentures or splints

21480 Closed treatment of temporomandibular dislocation; initial or subsequent

21485 complicated (eg, recurrent requiring intermaxillary fixation or splinting), initial or subsequent

21490 Open treatment of temporomandibular dislocation

21495 Open treatment of hyoid fracture

21497 Interdental wiring, for condition other than fracture

FIGURE 2-12. Lateral View of Muscles of the Neck

The muscles of the neck are responsible for gross motor movement of the head and neck, working in paired sets on the right and left side of the body. The sternocleidomastoid (SCM) muscle extends from the thorax to the base of the skull behind the ear. The SCM and trapezius muscles are the largest muscles in the neck.

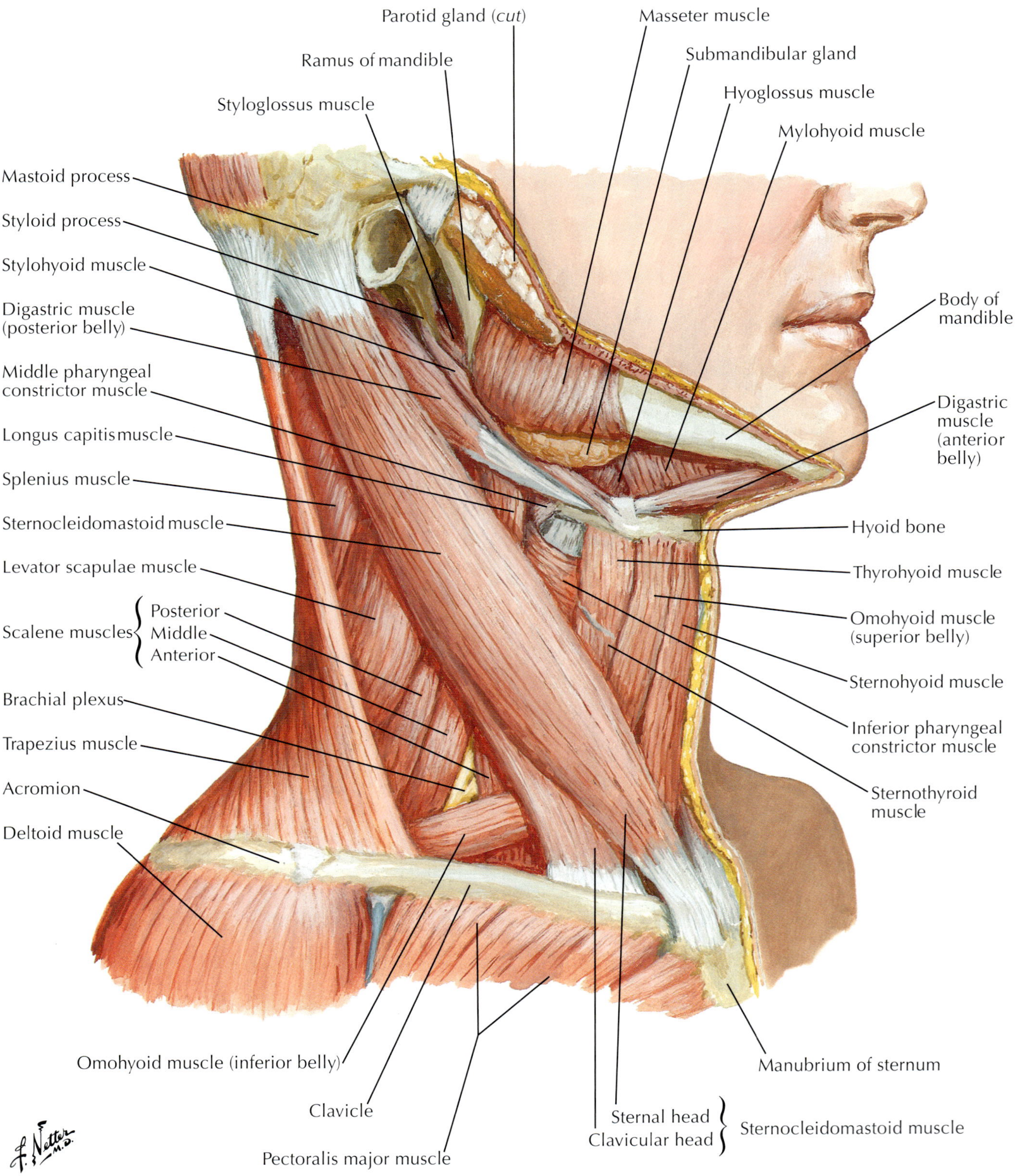

Neck (Soft Tissues) and Thorax

Incision

Coding Atlas

A deep abscess is a pocket of pus that has formed within deep soft tissues such as muscle sheaths. These abscesses may be incised, explored, and irrigated. The wounds are sometimes packed and usually are not closed, or they may be closed around a drain.

21501 Incision and drainage, deep abscess or hematoma, soft tissues of neck or thorax;

21502 with partial rib ostectomy

21510 Incision, deep, with opening of bone cortex (eg, for osteomyelitis or bone abscess), thorax

Excision

Coding Atlas

The neck is a narrow conduit upon which many bodily functions depend. Structures in the neck send oxygen to the lungs and food to the stomach; they send oxygenated blood to the brain and nerve impulses to and from the peripheral nervous system (PNS) and central nervous system (CNS). Lymph nodes from the head drain through the neck. Size and tumor origin play a role in code selection for reporting excision of soft tissue tumors of the neck. The proximity of so many critical structures makes **radical resection** for sarcoma in the neck a very complex procedure.

21550 Biopsy, soft tissue of neck or thorax

21552 Code is out of numerical sequence. See 21550-21632

21554 Code is out of numerical sequence. See 21550-21632

21555 Excision, tumor, soft tissue of neck or anterior thorax, subcutaneous; less than 3 cm

21552 3 cm or greater

21556 Excision, tumor, soft tissue of neck or anterior thorax, subfascial (eg, intramuscular); less than 5 cm

21554 5 cm or greater

21557 Radical resection of tumor (eg, sarcoma), soft tissue of neck or anterior thorax; less than 5 cm

21558 5 cm or greater

21600 Excision of rib, partial

21610 Costotransversectomy (separate procedure)

21615 Excision first and/or cervical rib;

21616 with sympathectomy

21620 Ostectomy of sternum, partial

21627 Sternal debridement

21630 Radical resection of sternum;

21632 with mediastinal lymphadenectomy

Repair, Revision, and/or Reconstruction

Coding Atlas

To help correct obstructive sleep apnea, the **retrolingual/hypopharyngeal** airway may be enlarged in a procedure referred to as hyoid **myotomy** and suspension. In this procedure, which is reported using code 21685, the hyoid bone is repositioned and fixed to improve the airway.

21685 Hyoid myotomy and suspension

21700 Division of scalenus anticus; without resection of cervical rib

21705 with resection of cervical rib

21720 Division of sternocleidomastoid for torticollis, open operation; without cast application

21725 with cast application

21740 Reconstructive repair of pectus excavatum or carinatum; open

21742 minimally invasive approach (Nuss procedure), without thoracoscopy

21743 minimally invasive approach (Nuss procedure), with thoracoscopy

21750 Closure of median sternotomy separation with or without debridement (separate procedure)

FIGURE 2-13. Ribcage Injuries

The ribcage protects underlying organs from injury and is also necessary for normal respiration. Rib fractures compromise normal respiration because pain associated with breathing leads to reduced inspiratory effort (**splinting**), which can lead to pneumonia or **atelectasis**. Multiple fractures of the ribs impact the musculature important to respiration, and fractures can also lead to penetration injuries from bone fragments.

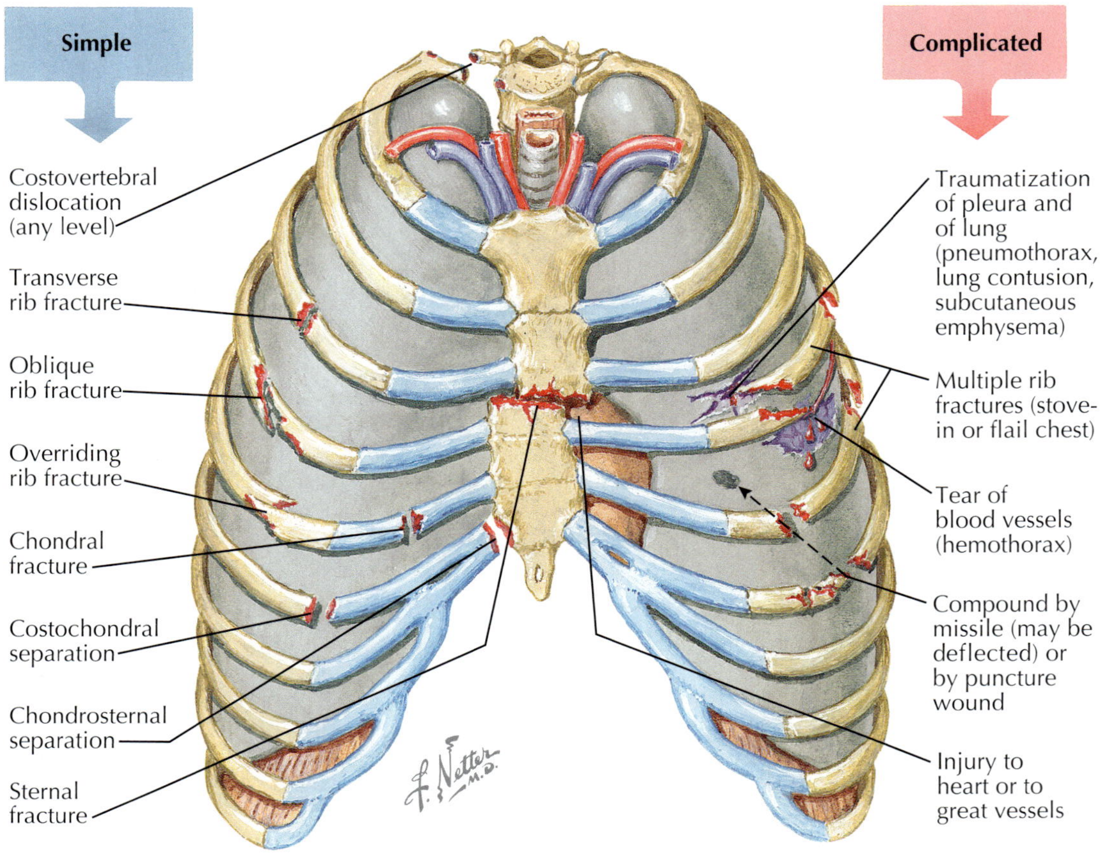

Fracture and/or Dislocation

Coding Atlas

Most fractures of the sternum are the result of motor vehicle accidents. They are most notable because when an impact is forceful enough to break the sternum, it may also be forceful enough to cause injuries to the heart, lungs, or other thoracic structures. As with rib fractures, sternal fractures can impede breathing because of the pain associated with inspiration. The appropriate level of Evaluation and Management code is used to report services when an uncomplicated rib fracture receives closed treatment.

21805 Open treatment of rib fracture without fixation, each

21811 Open treatment of rib fracture(s) with internal fixation, includes thoracoscopic visualization when performed, unilateral; 1-3 ribs

21812 4-6 ribs

21813 7 or more ribs

21820 Closed treatment of sternum fracture

21825 Open treatment of sternum fracture with or without skeletal fixation

FIGURE 2-14. Posterior Thoracic Wall

The multilayered muscles of the back provide support and movement to the head, neck, and spine. Back muscles are divided into two groups: **intrinsic** and **extrinsic**. Intrinsic muscles affect movement of the vertebral column, while extrinsic muscles form the musculature of the upper back that connect the extremities to the trunk and assist with respiration.

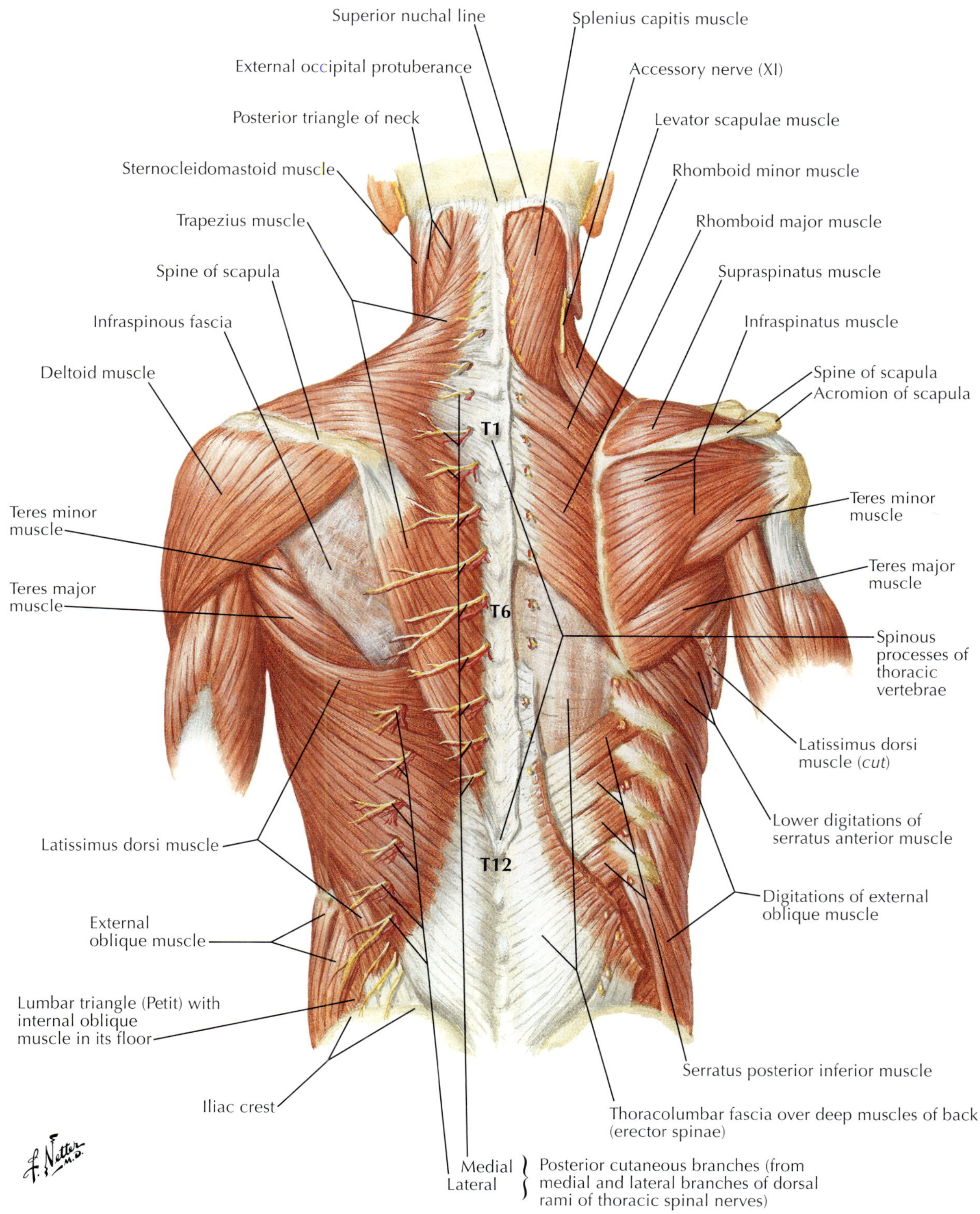

Back and Flank

Excision

Coding Atlas

Size and tumor origin play a role in code selection for excision of soft tissue tumors. The entire resection is measured, not the diameter of the lesion itself, to determine the excision size. Excision of a tumor that originates in the integument, eg, melanoma, is reported using codes for Integumentary System excision.

21920 Biopsy, soft tissue of back or flank; superficial

21925 deep

21930 Excision, tumor, soft tissue of back or flank, subcutaneous; less than 3 cm

21931 3 cm or greater

21932 Excision, tumor, soft tissue of back or flank, subfascial (eg, intramuscular); less than 5 cm

21933 5 cm or greater

21935 Radical resection of tumor (eg, sarcoma), soft tissue of back or flank; less than 5 cm

21936 5 cm or greater

Spine (Vertebral Column)

Incision

Coding Atlas

A deep soft tissue abscess of the spine lies below the fascia in muscle or other soft tissue and is accessed through an incision overlying the site on the patient's back. If the abscess is located at the thoracolumbar junction, the procedure is reported using the code that represents the area in which the majority of work was performed.

22010 Incision and drainage, open, of deep abscess (subfascial), posterior spine; cervical, thoracic, or cervicothoracic

22015 lumbar, sacral, or lumbosacral

Excision

Coding Atlas

The codes in this section are used to report therapeutic excision of a small portion of a vertebra. If the excision of the vertebral body is complete or nearly complete (corpectomy), use codes 63081-63091. If the excision is performed to correct a spinal misalignment, use osteotomy codes 22206-22226.

22100 Partial excision of posterior vertebral component (eg, spinous process, lamina or facet) for intrinsic bony lesion, single vertebral segment; cervical

22101 thoracic

22102 lumbar

+ 22103 each additional segment (List separately in addition to code for primary procedure)

22110 Partial excision of vertebral body, for intrinsic bony lesion, without decompression of spinal cord or nerve root(s), single vertebral segment; cervical

22112 thoracic

22114 lumbar

+ 22116 each additional vertebral segment (List separately in addition to code for primary procedure)

Osteotomy

Coding Atlas

An osteotomy is an excision of bone. Vertebral osteotomy is performed in order to correct a misalignment of the spine. Correction may require arthrodesis, bone graft, or placement of spinal instrumentation. Any one of these procedures is reported in addition to the osteotomy procedure.

22206 Osteotomy of spine, posterior or posterolateral approach, 3 columns, 1 vertebral segment (eg, pedicle/vertebral body subtraction); thoracic

22207 lumbar

+ 22208 each additional vertebral segment (List separately in addition to code for primary procedure)

22210 Osteotomy of spine, posterior or posterolateral approach, 1 vertebral segment; cervical

22212 thoracic

22214 lumbar

+ 22216 each additional vertebral segment (List separately in addition to primary procedure)

FIGURE 2-15. Anatomy of the Spine

The bony spine can be divided into five segments: cervical (neck), thoracic (upper back), lumbar (lower back), sacrum (base of spine), and coccyx (tailbone). Bones of the spine are called vertebrae. The space between vertebrae is filled with a cushioning intervertebral disc. The discs have a tough outer shell (annulus) and a gel-filled center (nucleus). The spinal cord runs through the vertebral column. Procedures on the spinal cord are reported using codes for the Nervous System.

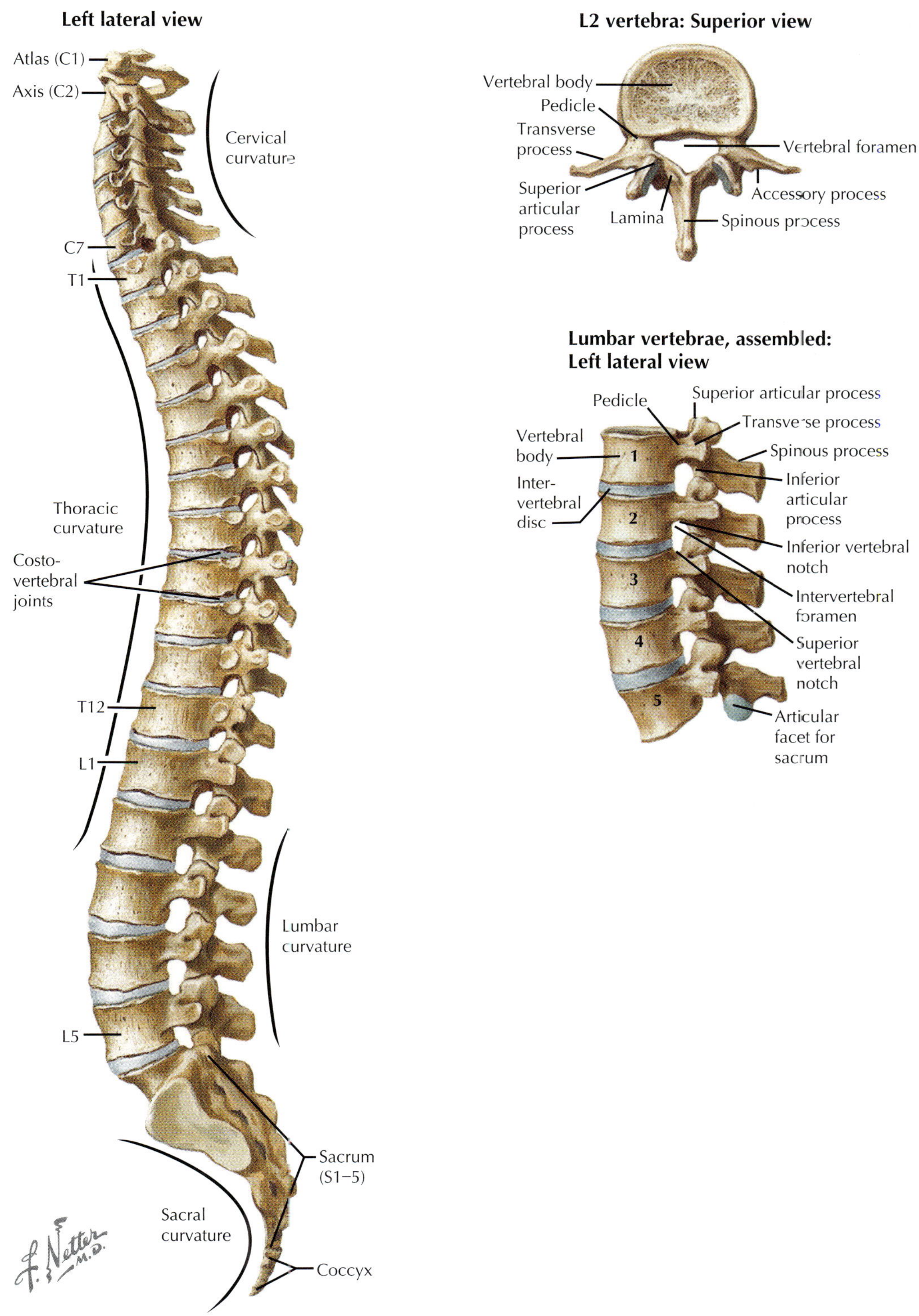

Continued on next page

FIGURE 2-15. Anatomy of the Spine *(continued)*

Muscles of the back: Intermediate layers

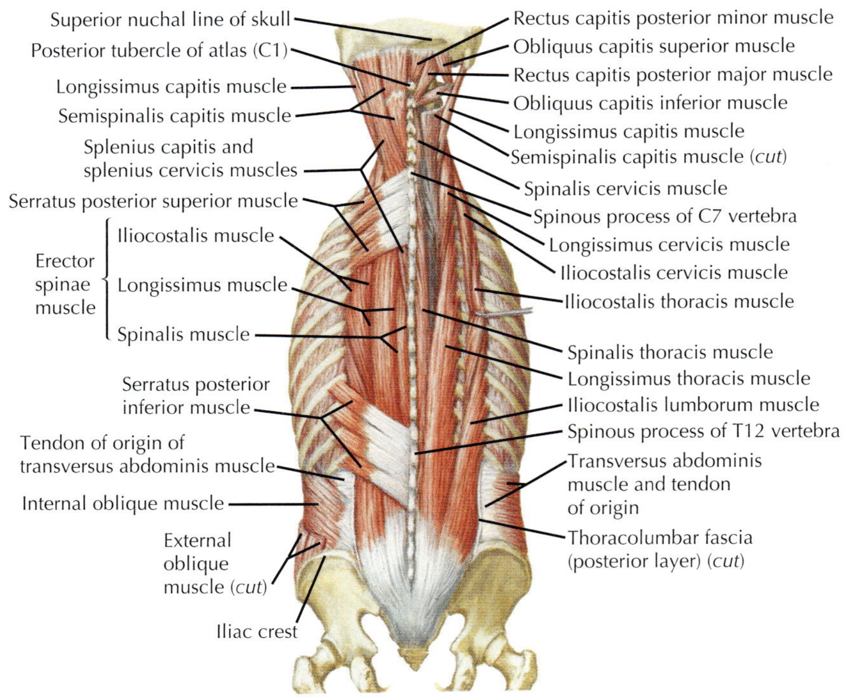

Posterior superior view

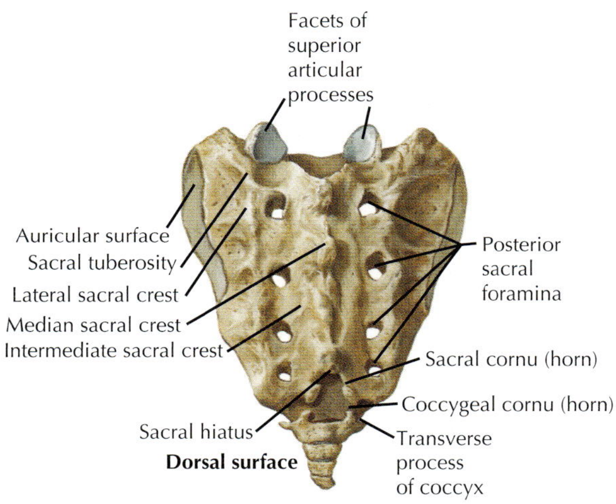

Spinal cord and ventral rami in situ

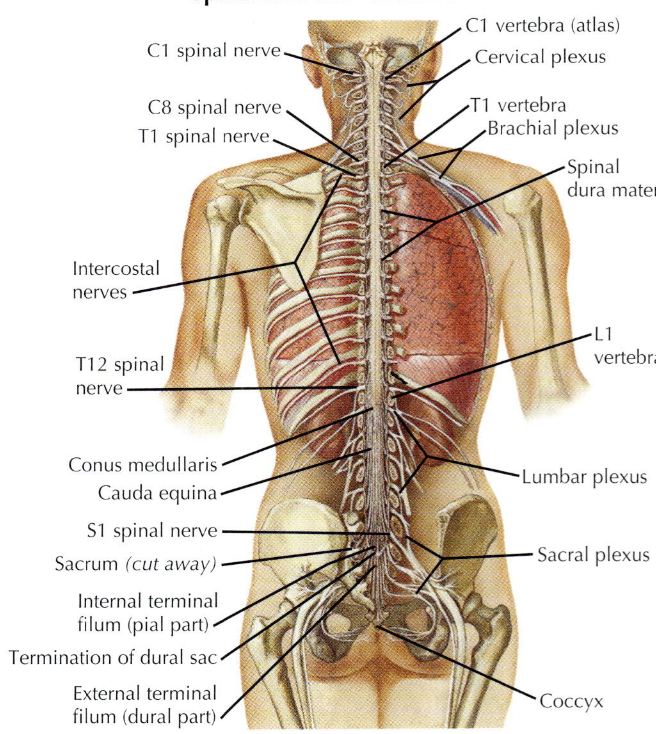

Left lateral view (partially sectioned *in median plane*)

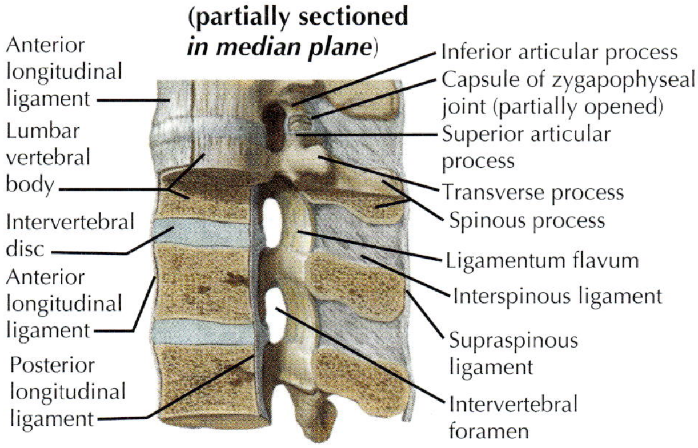

FIGURE 2-16. Posterior Approach to the Cervical Spine

One advantage to the posterior approach to the spine is the proximity of the spine to the surface of the skin. The posterior approach for spinal surgery is the most common approach, and the length of the incision is dependent on the size of the defect and the purpose of the surgery. Note: Tools, implants, and/or equipment depicted in the illustration may be outdated but the procedural approach is valid.

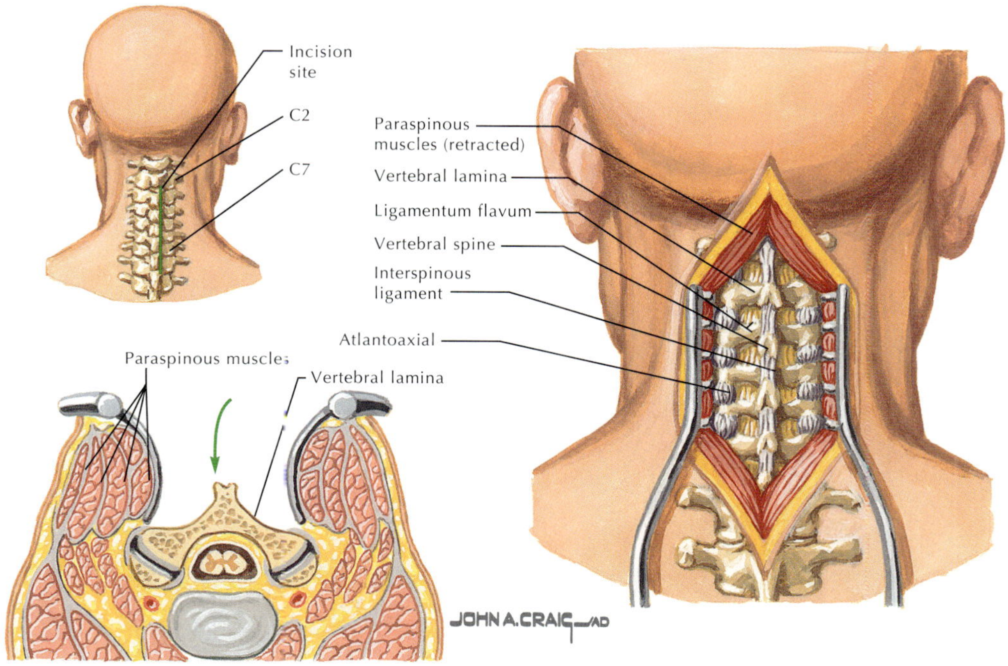

22220 Osteotomy of spine, including discectomy, anterior approach, single vertebral segment; cervical

22222 thoracic

22224 lumbar

+ 22226 each additional vertebral segment (List separately in addition to code for primary procedure)

Fracture and/or Dislocation

Coding Atlas

Vertebral fractures sometimes occur in combination with vertebral **dislocations** because when the bone is broken, ligaments holding the bone in place may be severed and the bone may dislodge when it becomes unmoored. In many cases, fracture or dislocation reduction is combined with **arthrodesis**, bone **graft**, or placement of spinal instrumentation to complete the correction. Any one of these procedures is reported in addition to the reduction.

22305 Closed treatment of vertebral process fracture(s)

22310 Closed treatment of vertebral body fracture(s), without manipulation, requiring and including casting or bracing

22315 Closed treatment of vertebral fracture(s) and/or dislocation(s) requiring casting or bracing, with and including casting and/or bracing by manipulation or traction

22318 Open treatment and/or reduction of odontoid fracture(s) and or dislocation(s) (including os odontoideum), anterior approach, including placement of internal fixation; without grafting

22319 with grafting

22325 Open treatment and/or reduction of vertebral fracture(s) and/or dislocation(s), posterior approach, 1 fractured vertebra or dislocated segment; lumbar

22326 cervical

22327 thoracic

+ 22328 each additional fractured vertebra or dislocated segment (List separately in addition to code for primary procedure)

FIGURE 2-17. Fractures of the Cervical Spine

Vertebral fractures can occur anywhere along the spine, with 10% or fewer occurring in the cervical spine. A fracture can be caused by an acute injury or by compression. Vertebral compression fractures (VCFs) are most common in patients with osteoporosis or other pathologies that weaken bones. The most common cause of acute fractures is motor vehicle accidents.

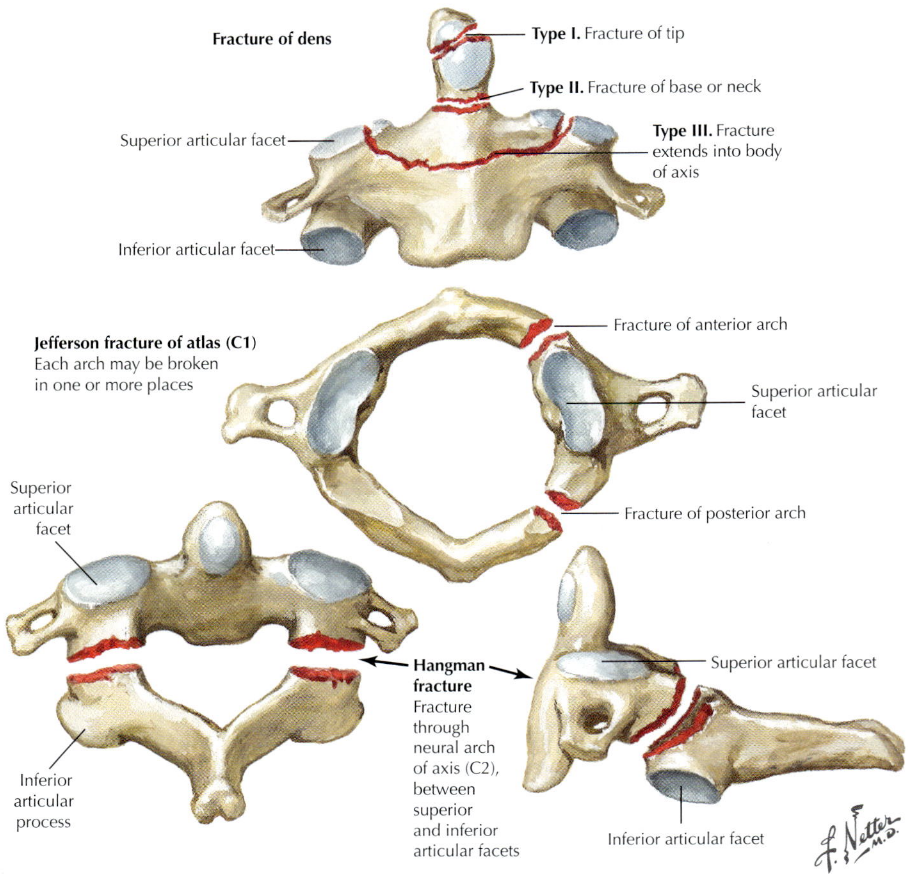

Manipulation

22505 Manipulation of spine requiring anesthesia, any region

Percutaneous Vertebroplasty and Vertebral Augmentation

Coding Atlas

In percutaneous vertebroplasty, methyl methacrylate or another similar cementing agent is injected into one or both sides of a vertebral body to reinforce the fractured or collapsed vertebra, typically in a patient with a vertebral compression fracture (VCF) from osteoporosis. The vertebral body is the round, flat portion of nearly all vertebrae. In vertebral augmentation, a cavity is first created and then injected with cement. The paired spinal processes arise from the vertebral body of all vertebrae, except the atlas.

⊙ **22510** Percutaneous vertebroplasty (bone biopsy included when performed), 1 vertebral body, unilateral or bilateral injection, inclusive of all imaging guidance; cervicothoracic

⊙ **22511** lumbosacral

⊙+ **22512** each additional cervicothoracic or lumbosacral vertebral body (List separately in addition to code for primary procedure)

FIGURE 2-18. Anterior Approach to the Cervical Spine

The anterior approach to the cervical spine may be transoral or extraoral. Extraoral is illustrated here. In the anterior approach, the surgeon may achieve better access to the targeted defect. However, the anterior approach often involves dissection through or around more anatomical structures than does the posterior approach. Note: Tools, implants, and/or equipment depicted in the illustration may be outdated but the procedural approach is valid.

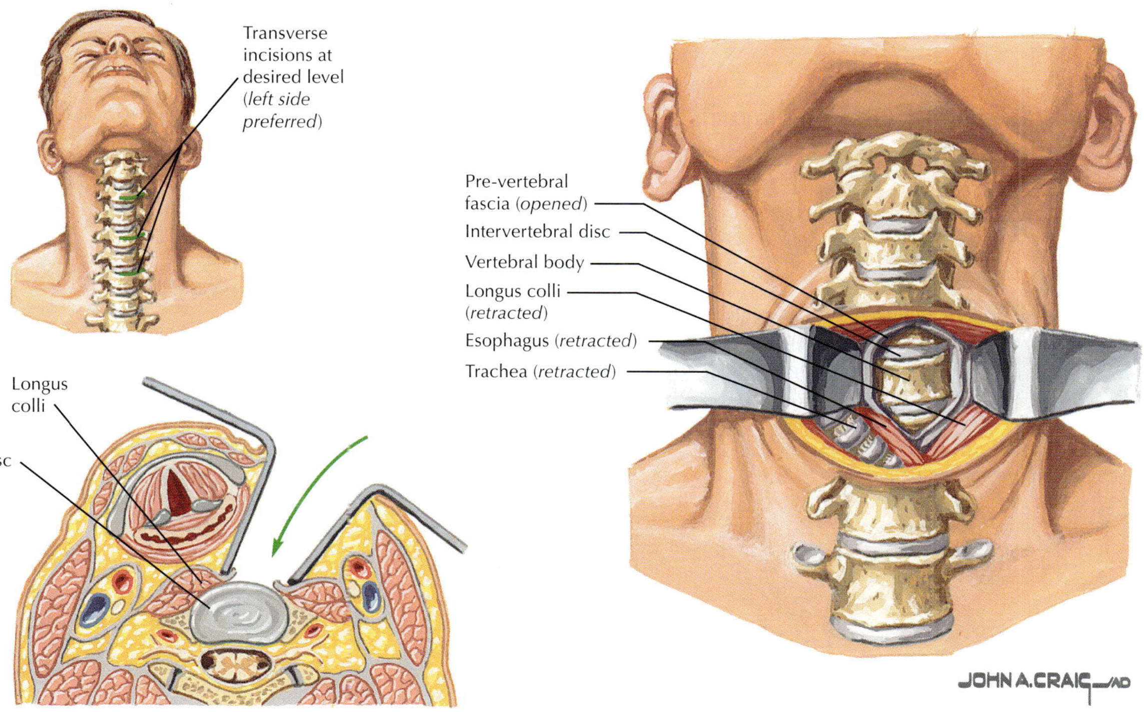

⊙ **22513** Percutaneous vertebral augmentation, including cavity creation (fracture reduction and bone biopsy included when performed) using mechanical device (eg, kyphoplasty), 1 vertebral body, unilateral or bilateral cannulation, inclusive of all imaging guidance; thoracic

⊙ **22514** lumbar

⊙+ **22515** each additional thoracic or lumbar vertebral body (List separately in addition to code for primary procedure)

⊙ **22526** Percutaneous intradiscal electrothermal annuloplasty, unilateral or bilateral including fluoroscopic guidance; single level

⊙+ **22527** 1 or more additional levels (List separately in addition to code for primary procedure)

Percutaneous Augmentation and Annuloplasty

Coding Atlas

Intradiscal electrothermal annuloplasty (IDEA), also known as intradiscal electrothermal therapy (IDET), describes a minimally invasive treatment for chronic low back pain. A flexible catheter is inserted into the disc, and a thermal device within the catheter heats the annulus to shrink and destroy tissue within.

Arthrodesis

Coding Atlas

Spinal fusion (arthrodesis) is reported according to approach, site treated, and number of interspaces or vertebral segments treated. An interspace is described as the area between two vertebrae. A vertebral segment is described as two vertebrae attached by ligaments and the intervertebral disc between them. In many cases, arthrodesis is combined with bone graft or placement of spinal instrumentation to complete the correction, and these procedures would be reported in addition to the reduction.

Lateral Extracavitary Approach Technique

22532 Arthrodesis, lateral extracavitary technique, including minimal discectomy to prepare interspace (other than for decompression); thoracic

22533 lumbar

+ 22534 thoracic or lumbar, each additional vertebral segment (List separately in addition to code for primary procedure)

Anterior or Anterolateral Approach Technique

22548 Arthrodesis, anterior transoral or extraoral technique, clivus-C1-C2 (atlas-axis), with or without excision of odontoid process

22551 Arthrodesis, anterior interbody, including disc space preparation, discectomy, osteophytectomy and decompression of spinal cord and/or nerve roots; cervical below C2

+ 22552 cervical below C2, each additional interspace (List separately in addition to code for separate procedure)

22554 Arthrodesis, anterior interbody technique, including minimal discectomy to prepare interspace (other than for decompression); cervical below C2

22556 thoracic

22558 lumbar

+ 22585 each additional interspace (List separately in addition to code for primary procedure)

22586 Arthrodesis, pre-sacral interbody technique, including disc space preparation, discectomy, with posterior instrumentation, with image guidance, includes bone graft when performed, L5-S1 interspace

Posterior, Posterolateral or Lateral Transverse Process Technique

22590 Arthrodesis, posterior technique, craniocervical (occiput-C2)

22595 Arthrodesis, posterior technique, atlas-axis (C1-C2)

22600 Arthrodesis, posterior or posterolateral technique, single level; cervical below C2 segment

22610 thoracic (with lateral transverse technique, when performed)

22612 lumbar (with lateral transverse technique, when performed)

+ 22614 each additional vertebral segment (List separately in addition to code for primary procedure)

22630 Arthrodesis, posterior interbody technique, including laminectomy and/or discectomy to prepare interspace (other than for decompression), single interspace; lumbar

+ 22632 each additional interspace (List separately in addition to code for primary procedure)

22633 Arthrodesis, combined posterior or posterolateral technique with posterior interbody technique including laminectomy and/or discectomy sufficient to prepare interspace (other than for decompression), single interspace and segment; lumbar

+ 22634 each additional interspace and segment (List separately in addition to code for primary procedure)

Spine Deformity (eg, Scoliosis, Kyphosis)

22800 Arthrodesis, posterior, for spinal deformity, with or without cast; up to 6 vertebral segments

22802 7 to 12 vertebral segments

22804 13 or more vertebral segments

22808 Arthrodesis, anterior, for spinal deformity, with or without cast; 2 to 3 vertebral segments

22810 4 to 7 vertebral segments

22812 8 or more vertebral segments

22818 Kyphectomy, circumferential exposure of spine and resection of vertebral segment(s) (including body and posterior elements); single or 2 segments

22819 3 or more segments

Exploration

22830 Exploration of spinal fusion

Spinal Instrumentation

Coding Atlas

Spinal instrumentation can add stability to vertebrae that are injured or diseased. The instrumentation is classified in the CPT code set as segmental or non-segmental. In either type, the instrumentation is designed to support the span of vertebrae it traverses, and either type is fixed to vertebrae at each end. Segmental instrumentation has at least one additional attachment somewhere along the expanse. The number of vertebral segments spanned contributes to code selection, as does the placement of the instrumentation, ie, anteriorly or posteriorly.

+ 22840 Posterior non-segmental instrumentation (eg, Harrington rod technique, pedicle fixation across 1 interspace, atlantoaxial transarticular screw fixation, sublaminar wiring at C1, facet screw fixation) (List separately in addition to code for primary procedure)

+ 22841 Internal spinal fixation by wiring of spinous processes (List separately in addition to code for primary procedure)

FIGURE 2-19. Atlas and Axis

The atlas is the topmost vertebra. Together with the axis, it forms the atlanto-occipital (atlantoaxial) joint, which connects the head to the spine. The atlas has no vertebral body, rather it is ring-shaped. The atlas carries the weight of the head and pivots from its position around the peg (dens), also documented as the odontoid process of the axis.

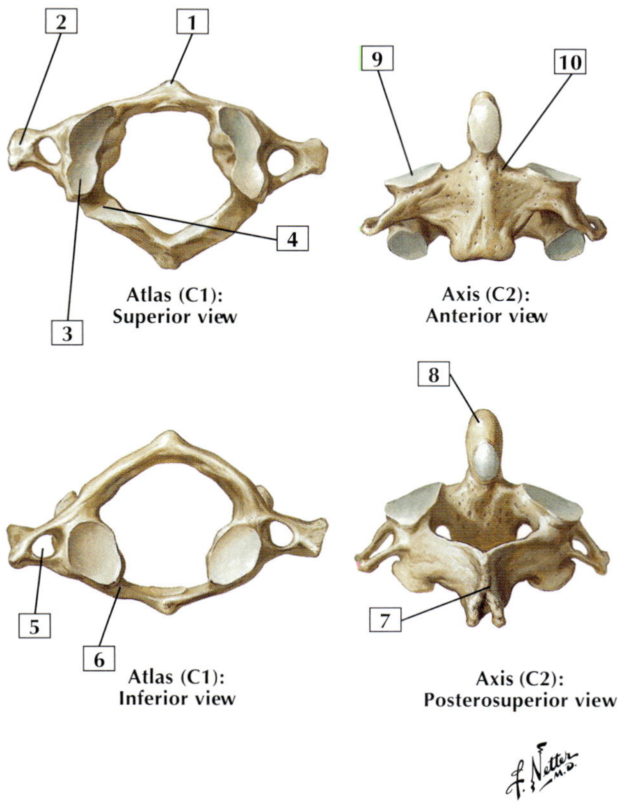

1. Anterior tubercle
2. Transverse process
3. Superior articular surface of lateral mass for occipital condyle
4. Groove for vertebral artery
5. Transverse foramen
6. Anterior arch
7. Spinous process
8. Dens
9. Superior articular facet for atlas
10. Pedicle

Comment: The 1st cervical vertebra is the atlas. It is named after the Greek god Atlas, who is often depicted with the world on his shoulders. The atlas has no body or spine but is made of anterior and posterior arches. The transverse processes contain a foramen that transmits the vertebral vessels.

The 2nd cervical vertebra is the axis. Its most characteristic feature is the dens (odontoid process). The dens articulates with the anterior arch of the atlas, providing a pivot about which the atlas and head can rotate.

A blow to the top of the head may fracture the atlas (across the anterior or posterior arch; called a Jefferson fracture). Fractures of the axis often involve the dens.

+ 22842 Posterior segmental instrumentation (eg, pedicle fixation, dual rods with multiple hooks and sublaminar wires); 3 to 6 vertebral segments (List separately in addition to code for primary procedure)

+ 22843 7 to 12 vertebral segments (List separately in addition to code for primary procedure)

+ 22844 13 or more vertebral segments (List separately in addition to code for primary procedure)

+ 22845 Anterior instrumentation; 2 to 3 vertebral segments (List separately in addition to code for primary procedure)

+ 22846 4 to 7 vertebral segments (List separately in addition to code for primary procedure)

+ 22847 8 or more vertebral segments (List separately in addition to code for primary procedure)

+ 22848 Pelvic fixation (attachment of caudal end of instrumentation to pelvic bony structures) other than sacrum (List separately in addition to code for primary procedure)

22849 Reinsertion of spinal fixation device

22850 Removal of posterior nonsegmental instrumentation (eg, Harrington rod)

+ 22851 Application of intervertebral biomechanical device(s) (eg, synthetic cage(s), methylmethacrylate) to vertebral defect or interspace (List separately in addition to code for primary procedure)

22852 Removal of posterior segmental instrumentation

22855 Removal of anterior instrumentation

22856 Total disc arthroplasty (artificial disc), anterior approach, including discectomy with end plate preparation (includes osteophytectomy for nerve root or spinal cord decompression and microdissection); single interspace, cervical

#+ 22858 second level, cervical (List separately in addition to code for primary procedure)

22857 Total disc arthroplasty (artificial disc), anterior approach, including discectomy to prepare interspace (other than for decompression), single interspace, lumbar

22858 Code is out of numerical sequence. See 22840-22865

22861 Revision including replacement of total disc arthroplasty (artificial disc), anterior approach, single interspace; cervical

22862 lumbar

22864 Removal of total disc arthroplasty (artificial disc), anterior approach, single interspace; cervical

22865 lumbar

Abdomen

Excision

Coding Atlas

Size and **tumor** origin play a role in code selection for excision of soft tissue tumors. The entire resection is measured, not the diameter of the lesion, to determine the excision size. Excision of a tumor originating in the integument, eg, **melanoma**, is reported using Integumentary System excision codes.

22900 Excision, tumor, soft tissue of abdominal wall, subfascial (eg, intramuscular); less than 5 cm

22901 5 cm or greater

22902 Excision, tumor, soft tissue of abdominal wall, subcutaneous; less than 3 cm

22903 3 cm or greater

22904 Radical resection of tumor (eg, sarcoma), soft tissue of abdominal wall; less than 5 cm

22905 5 cm or greater

Shoulder

Incision

Coding Atlas

An **arthrotomy** may also be called a **synosteotomy**. Both describe an incision into the joint capsule, which may be performed for **diagnostic** or **therapeutic** reasons. The joint capsule is a fluid-filled, fibrous sac that seals the joint space and provides lubrication for moving bones.

23000 Removal of subdeltoid calcareous deposits, open

23020 Capsular contracture release (eg, Sever type procedure)

23030 Incision and drainage, shoulder area; deep abscess or hematoma

23031 infected bursa

23035 Incision, bone cortex (eg, osteomyelitis or bone abscess), shoulder area

23040 Arthrotomy, glenohumeral joint, including exploration, drainage, or removal of foreign body

23044 Arthrotomy, acromioclavicular, sternoclavicular joint, including exploration, drainage, or removal of foreign body

Excision

Coding Atlas

Sequestrectomy is the surgical removal of a sequestrum, or a fragment of bone that has separated from healthy bone as a result of disease or injury. In **acromioplasty**, a small piece of the bone's surface (acromion) is excised. In some cases, this is done to smooth rough edges or growths on a bone near a joint.

23065 Biopsy, soft tissue of shoulder area; superficial

23066 deep

23071 Code is out of numerical sequence. See 23065-23220

23073 Code is out of numerical sequence. See 23065-23220

23075 Excision, tumor, soft tissue of shoulder area, subcutaneous; less than 3 cm

23071 3 cm or greater

23076 Excision, tumor, soft tissue of shoulder area, subfascial (eg, intramuscular); less than 5 cm

23073 5 cm or greater

23077 Radical resection of tumor (eg, sarcoma), soft tissue of shoulder area; less than 5 cm

23078 5 cm or greater

23100 Arthrotomy, glenohumeral joint, including biopsy

23101 Arthrotomy, acromioclavicular joint or sternoclavicular joint, including biopsy and/or excision of torn cartilage

23105 Arthrotomy; glenohumeral joint, with synovectomy, with or without biopsy

23106 sternoclavicular joint, with synovectomy, with or without biopsy

23107 Arthrotomy, glenohumeral joint, with joint exploration, with or without removal of loose or foreign body

FIGURE 2-20. Anterior Abdominal Wall

The **anterior** abdominal wall forms a flexible barrier that protects internal organs and contains muscles that assist with upper body movement. Several types of **fascia** support the abdomen, including Camper's fascia, fatty and superficial; deep fibrous Scarpa's fascia; linea alba, a fibrous layer along the abdominal midline; transversalis fascia, a barrier between the transverse abdominal muscle and **extraperitoneal** fascia; and linea semilunaris, a narrow fascia along the rectus abdominus muscle.

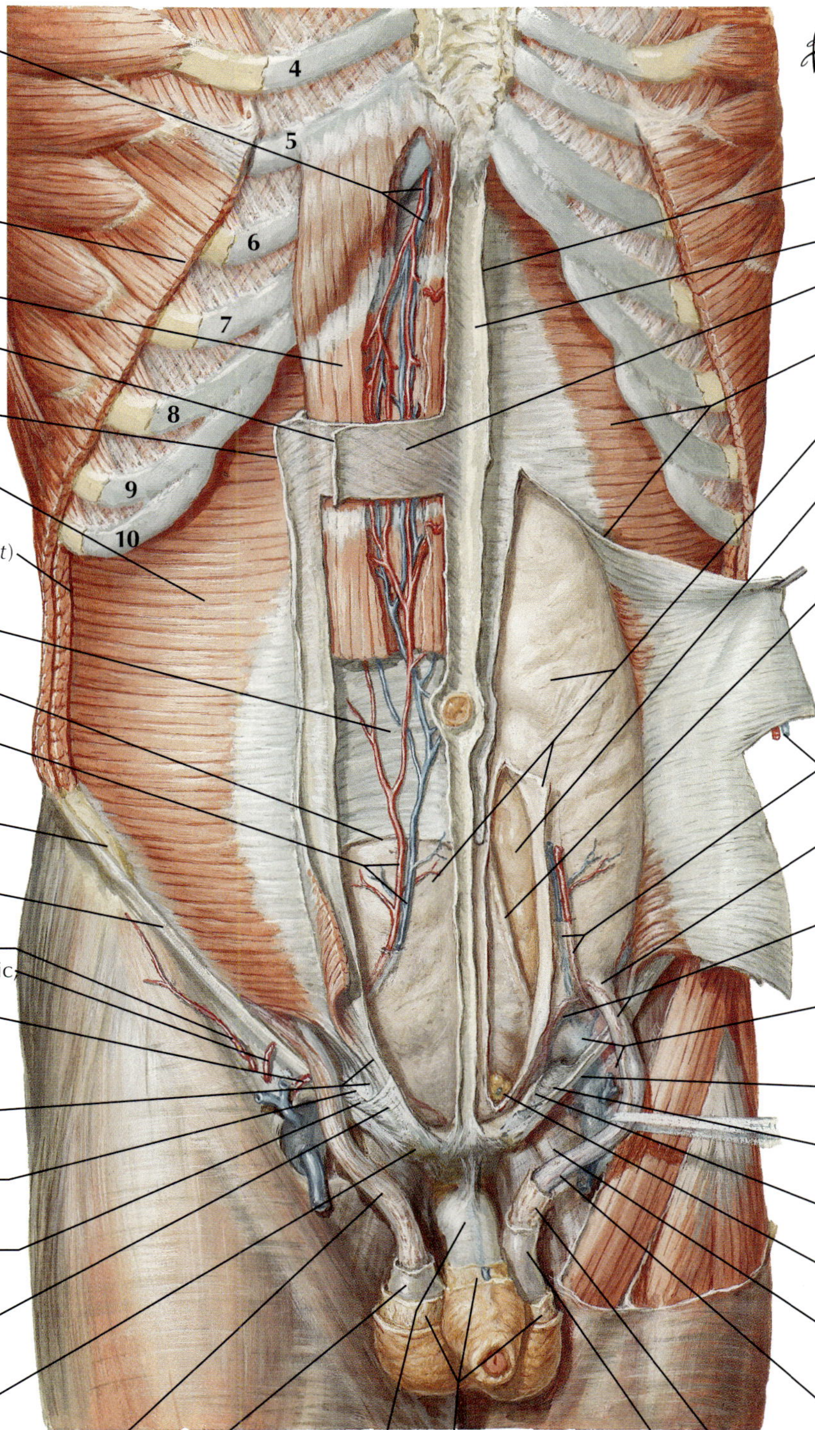

FIGURE 2-21. Shoulder Girdle

The shoulder girdle contains multiple joints. The major joint is the glenohumeral joint (GHJ), articulating the head of the humerus in the glenoid fossa of the scapula. The sternoclavicular (SC) joint stabilizes the clavicle by joining it to the superior sternum. The scapulothoracic (ST) joint is a small attachment between the scapula and rib. The acromioclavicular (AC) joint connects the clavicle to the acromion, an extension of the scapula. Together, the joints of the shoulder provide the body's widest range of motion.

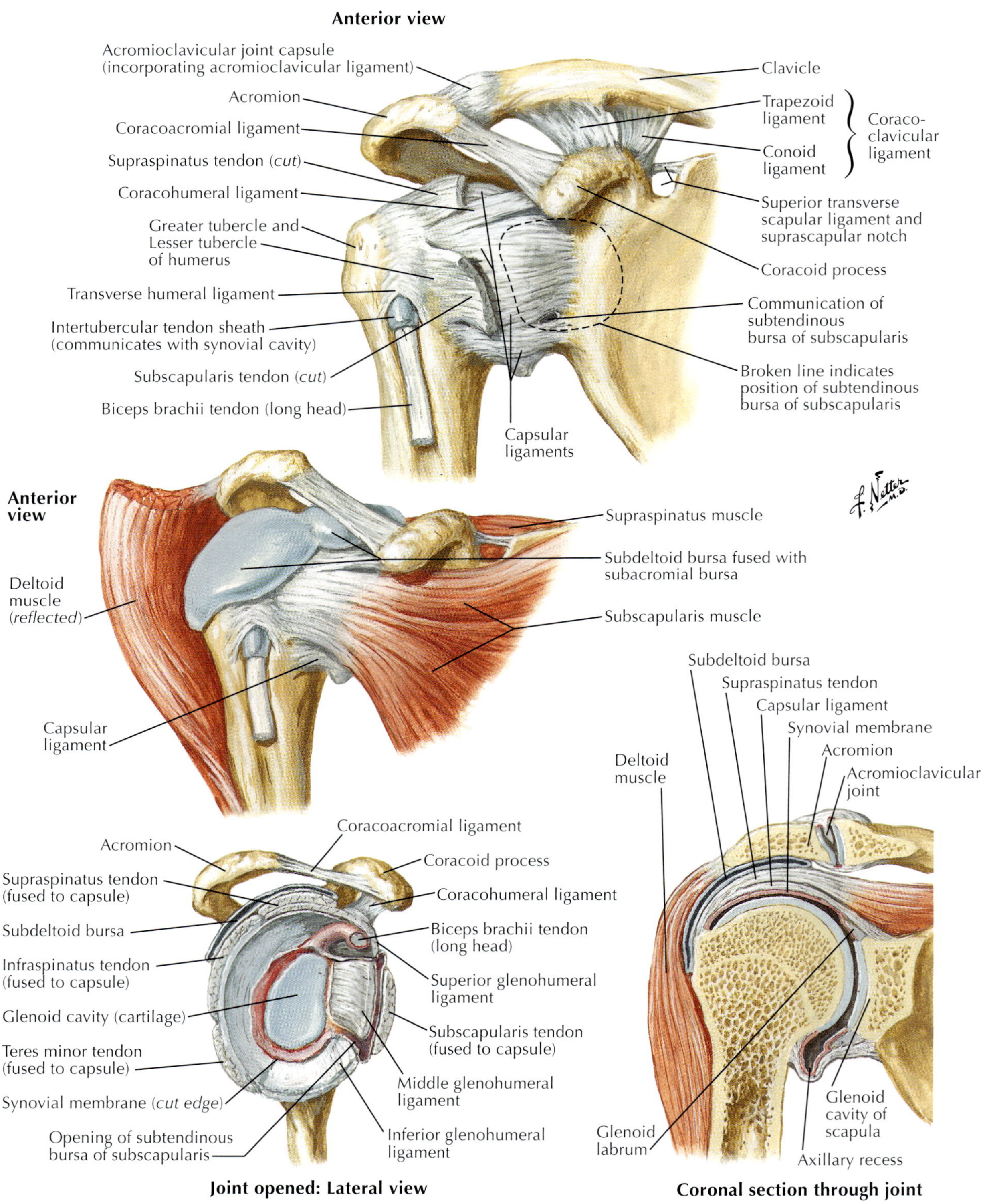

FIGURE 2-22. Muscles of the Shoulder

The muscles of the shoulder include very large mover muscles and small stabilizing muscles. The supraspinatus, infraspinatus, and teres minor protect the shoulder joint. The deltoid muscle, named for its triangular shape, covers the anterior, posterior, and lateral shoulder joint. The deltoid arises from the clavicle, acromion, and scapula and converges as a thick tendon into the humerus.

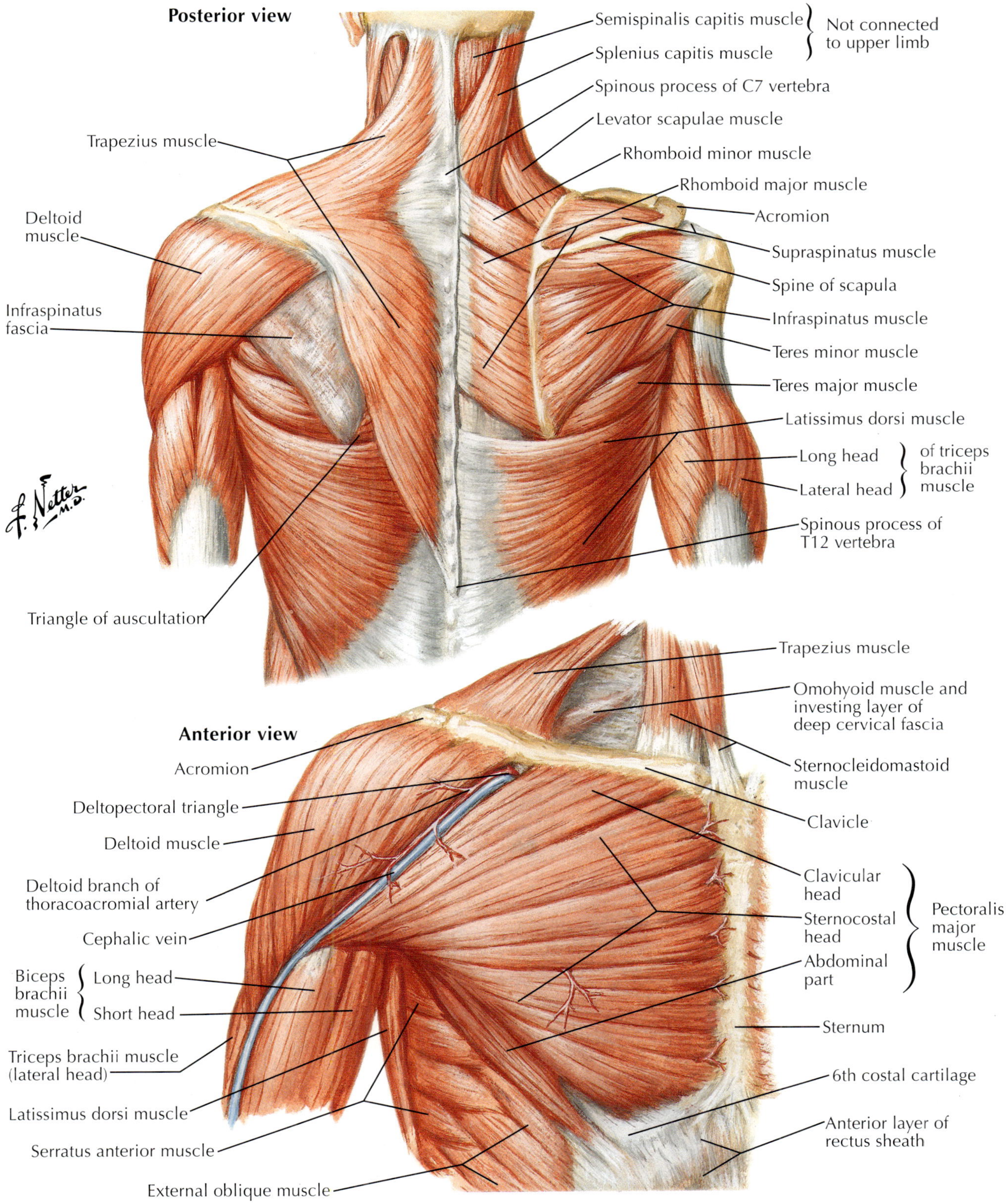

23120 Claviculectomy; partial

23125 total

23130 Acromioplasty or acromionectomy, partial, with or without coracoacromial ligament release

23140 Excision or curettage of bone cyst or benign tumor of clavicle or scapula;

23145 with autograft (includes obtaining graft)

23146 with allograft

23150 Excision or curettage of bone cyst or benign tumor of proximal humerus;

23155 with autograft (includes obtaining graft)

23156 with allograft

23170 Sequestrectomy (eg, for osteomyelitis or bone abscess), clavicle

23172 Sequestrectomy (eg, for osteomyelitis or bone abscess), scapula

23174 Sequestrectomy (eg, for osteomyelitis or bone abscess), humeral head to surgical neck

23180 Partial excision (craterization, saucerization, or diaphysectomy) bone (eg, osteomyelitis), clavicle

23182 Partial excision (craterization, saucerization, or diaphysectomy) bone (eg, osteomyelitis), scapula

23184 Partial excision (craterization, saucerization, or diaphysectomy) bone (eg, osteomyelitis), proximal humerus

23190 Ostectomy of scapula, partial (eg, superior medial angle)

23195 Resection, humeral head

23200 Radical resection of tumor; clavicle

23210 scapula

23220 Radical resection of tumor, proximal humerus

Introduction or Removal

Coding Atlas

Codes 23330 and 23333 are used to report removal of a **foreign body** resulting from trauma. Codes 23334 and 23335 are used to report the removal of previously placed hardware from the shoulder without a concurrent revision, also known as **arthroplasty**.

23330 Removal of foreign body, shoulder; subcutaneous

23333 deep (subfascial or intramuscular)

23334 Removal of prosthesis, includes debridement and synovectomy when performed; humeral **or** glenoid component

23335 humeral **and** glenoid components (eg, total shoulder)

23350 Injection procedure for shoulder arthrography or enhanced CT/MRI shoulder arthrography

Repair, Revision, and/or Reconstruction

Coding Atlas

In **hemiarthroplasty** of the shoulder, the head of the humerus bone is replaced. In total arthroplasty, both the head of the humerus (ball) and the glenoid (socket) are replaced. In the revision of a total arthroplasty, removal of existing hardware is inherent in the procedure and not reported separately.

23395 Muscle transfer, any type, shoulder or upper arm; single

23397 multiple

23400 Scapulopexy (eg, Sprengels deformity or for paralysis)

23405 Tenotomy, shoulder area; single tendon

23406 multiple tendons through same incision

23410 Repair of ruptured musculotendinous cuff (eg, rotator cuff) open; acute

23412 chronic

23415 Coracoacromial ligament release, with or without acromioplasty

23420 Reconstruction of complete shoulder (rotator) cuff avulsion, chronic (includes acromioplasty)

23430 Tenodesis of long tendon of biceps

23440 Resection or transplantation of long tendon of biceps

23450 Capsulorrhaphy, anterior; Putti-Platt procedure or Magnuson type operation

23455 with labral repair (eg, Bankart procedure)

23460 Capsulorrhaphy, anterior, any type; with bone block

23462 with coracoid process transfer

23465 Capsulorrhaphy, glenohumeral joint, posterior, with or without bone block

23466 Capsulorrhaphy, glenohumeral joint, any type multi-directional instability

23470 Arthroplasty, glenohumeral joint; hemiarthroplasty

23472 total shoulder (glenoid and proximal humeral replacement (eg, total shoulder))

23473 Revision of total shoulder arthroplasty, including allograft when performed; humeral **or** glenoid component

23474 humeral **and** glenoid component

23480 Osteotomy, clavicle, with or without internal fixation;

23485 with bone graft for nonunion or malunion (includes obtaining graft and/or necessary fixation)

⊙=Moderate sedation ✚=Add-on code ⊘=Modifier 51 exempt #=Resequenced code

FIGURE 2-23. Rotator Cuff

The humerus fits loosely into the shoulder joint and is held in place by a ring of muscles and tendons at its proximal head. This ring of muscles and tendons is called the rotator cuff. Tendons and muscles of the rotator cuff include the supraspinatus, intraspinatus, subscapularis, and teres minor. A rotator cuff tear can be an **acute** injury, a **chronic** condition, or an acute injury superimposed on a chronic condition.

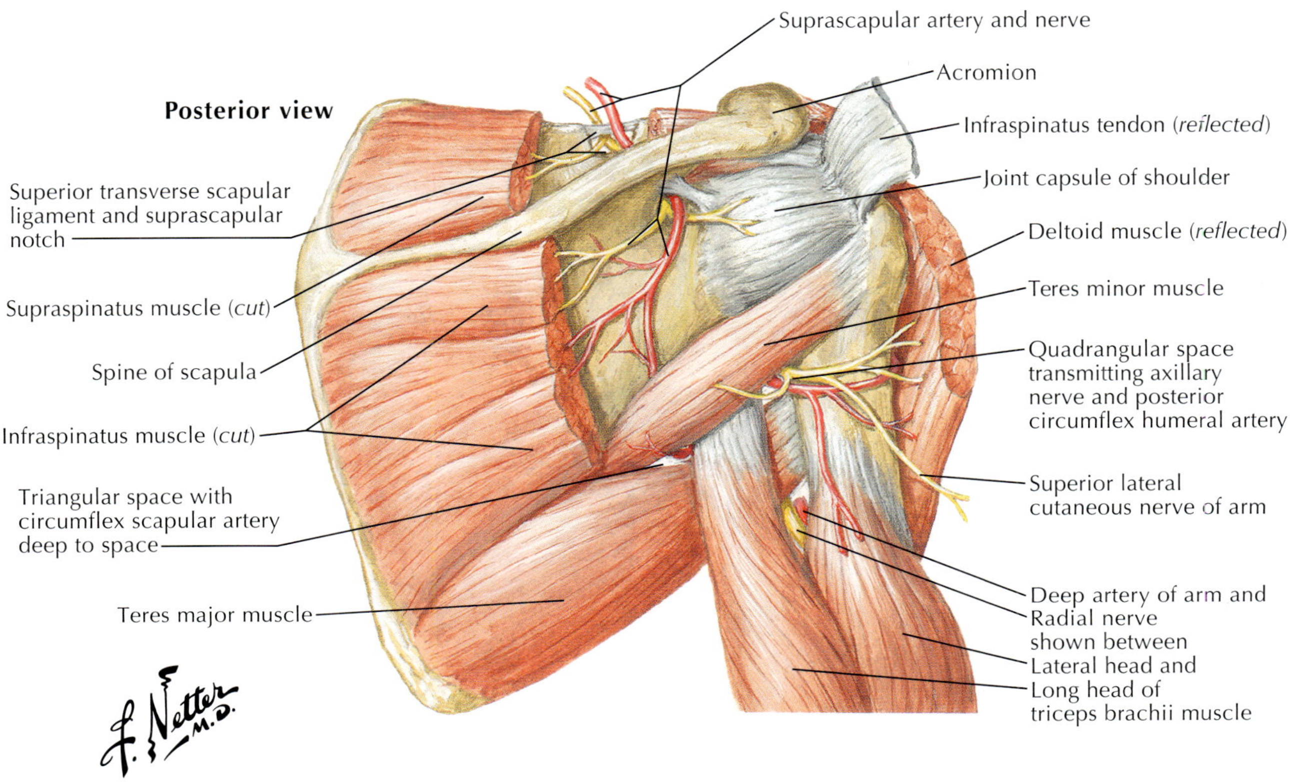

23490 Prophylactic treatment (nailing, pinning, plating or wiring) with or without methylmethacrylate; clavicle

23491 proximal humerus

Fracture and/or Dislocation

Coding Atlas

Bones can be characterized as **appendicular** or **axial**. Appendicular skeletal bones form the upper and lower extremities and provide locomotion and manipulation of objects. The axial skeleton contains bones of the head, neck, and trunk. Codes used to report fractures and dislocations of the shoulder are classified by the type of **reduction** and stabilization required. The type of fracture does not necessarily correspond to the type of treatment; a closed fracture may receive open treatment. Dislocations can occur in conjunction with fractures.

23500 Closed treatment of clavicular fracture; without manipulation

23505 with manipulation

23515 Open treatment of clavicular fracture, includes internal fixation, when performed

23520 Closed treatment of sternoclavicular dislocation; without manipulation

23525 with manipulation

23530 Open treatment of sternoclavicular dislocation, acute or chronic;

23532 with fascial graft (includes obtaining graft)

23540 Closed treatment of acromioclavicular dislocation; without manipulation

23545 with manipulation

23550 Open treatment of acromioclavicular dislocation, acute or chronic;

23552 with fascial graft (includes obtaining graft)

FIGURE 2-24. Bones of the Shoulder

The humeral head is more than twice the size of the glenoid socket into which it fits to form the glenohumeral joint. However, the glenoid cavity is augmented with a rim of fibrocartilage called the labrum that doubles the size of the socket. In a shoulder **dislocation**, the glenoid labrum is usually torn. A dislocated acromioclavicular (collar bone) joint is sometimes called a "separated shoulder."

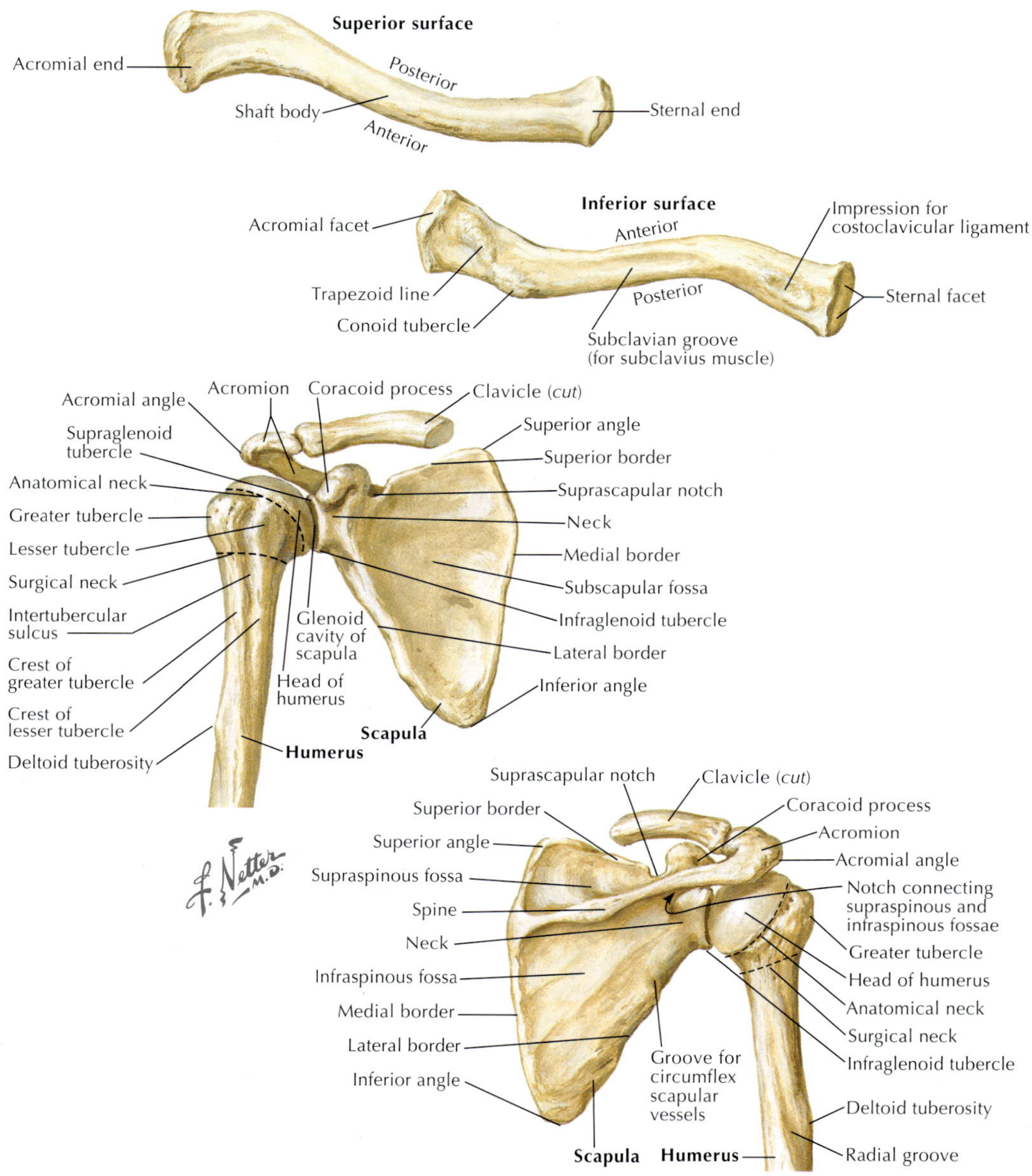

23570 Closed treatment of scapular fracture; without manipulation

23575 with manipulation, with or without skeletal traction (with or without shoulder joint involvement)

23585 Open treatment of scapular fracture (body, glenoid or acromion) includes internal fixation, when performed

23600 Closed treatment of proximal humeral (surgical or anatomical neck) fracture; without manipulation

23605 with manipulation, with or without skeletal traction

23615 Open treatment of proximal humeral (surgical or anatomical neck) fracture, includes internal fixation, when performed, includes repair of tuberosity(s), when performed;

23616 with proximal humeral prosthetic replacement

23620 Closed treatment of greater humeral tuberosity fracture; without manipulation

23625 with manipulation

23630 Open treatment of greater humeral tuberosity fracture, includes internal fixation, when performed

23650 Closed treatment of shoulder dislocation, with manipulation; without anesthesia

23655 requiring anesthesia

23660 Open treatment of acute shoulder dislocation

23665 Closed treatment of shoulder dislocation, with fracture of greater humeral tuberosity, with manipulation

23670 Open treatment of shoulder dislocation, with fracture of greater humeral tuberosity, includes internal fixation, when performed

23675 Closed treatment of shoulder dislocation, with surgical or anatomical neck fracture, with manipulation

23680 Open treatment of shoulder dislocation, with surgical or anatomical neck fracture, includes internal fixation, when performed

Manipulation

23700 Manipulation under anesthesia, shoulder joint, including application of fixation apparatus (dislocation excluded)

Arthrodesis

Coding Atlas

In glenohumeral **arthrodesis**, the joint is surgically fused and immobilized. Bone grafts may be placed to fix the joint; in other instances, hardware is placed.

23800 Arthrodesis, glenohumeral joint;

23802 with autogenous graft (includes obtaining graft)

Amputation

Coding Atlas

Amputation at the shoulder level is uncommon and usually due to **tumor** control or traumatic injury. **Disarticulation** of the shoulder includes surgical removal of the entire arm, severing at the glenohumeral joint. In a forequarter amputation, the scapula and all or part of the clavicle are also excised with surrounding soft tissue.

23900 Interthoracoscapular amputation (forequarter)

23920 Disarticulation of shoulder;

23921 secondary closure or scar revision

Humerus (Upper Arm) and Elbow

Incision

Coding Atlas

In **osteomyelitis**, inner bone may swell due to inflammation, and the swelling may reduce blood circulation. This limits the bone's access to antibodies and antibiotics, often making aggressive treatment necessary. In some cases, an incision through the skin and into the bone cortex allows for **irrigation and drainage** of the infection, as well as the **debridement** of any diseased bone and direct application of antibiotics.

23930 Incision and drainage, upper arm or elbow area; deep abscess or hematoma

23931 bursa

23935 Incision, deep, with opening of bone cortex (eg, for osteomyelitis or bone abscess), humerus or elbow

24000 Arthrotomy, elbow, including exploration, drainage, or removal of foreign body

24006 Arthrotomy of the elbow, with capsular excision for capsular release (separate procedure)

Excision

Coding Atlas

Size and **tumor** origin play a role in code selection for excision of soft tissue tumors. The entire resection is measured, not the diameter of the lesion itself, to determine the excision size. Excision of a tumor originating in the integument, eg, **melanoma**, is reported with Integumentary System excision codes.

24065 Biopsy, soft tissue of upper arm or elbow area; superficial

24066 deep (subfascial or intramuscular)

24071 Code is out of numerical sequence. See 24065-24155

24073 Code is out of numerical sequence. See 24065-24155

24075 Excision, tumor, soft tissue of upper arm or elbow area, subcutaneous; less than 3 cm

\# **24071** 3 cm or greater

FIGURE 2-25. Muscles of the Upper Arm

The biceps and triceps muscles of the upper arm work as antagonistic muscles to bend and straighten the elbow. Antagonistic muscles are muscles that work in opposition to each other, ie, when the triceps contract, the biceps are stretched and the elbow straightens. Conversely, when the biceps contract, the triceps are stretched and the elbow bends. It is because of this push-and-pull action that these and similarly paired muscles are called **antagonist muscles**.

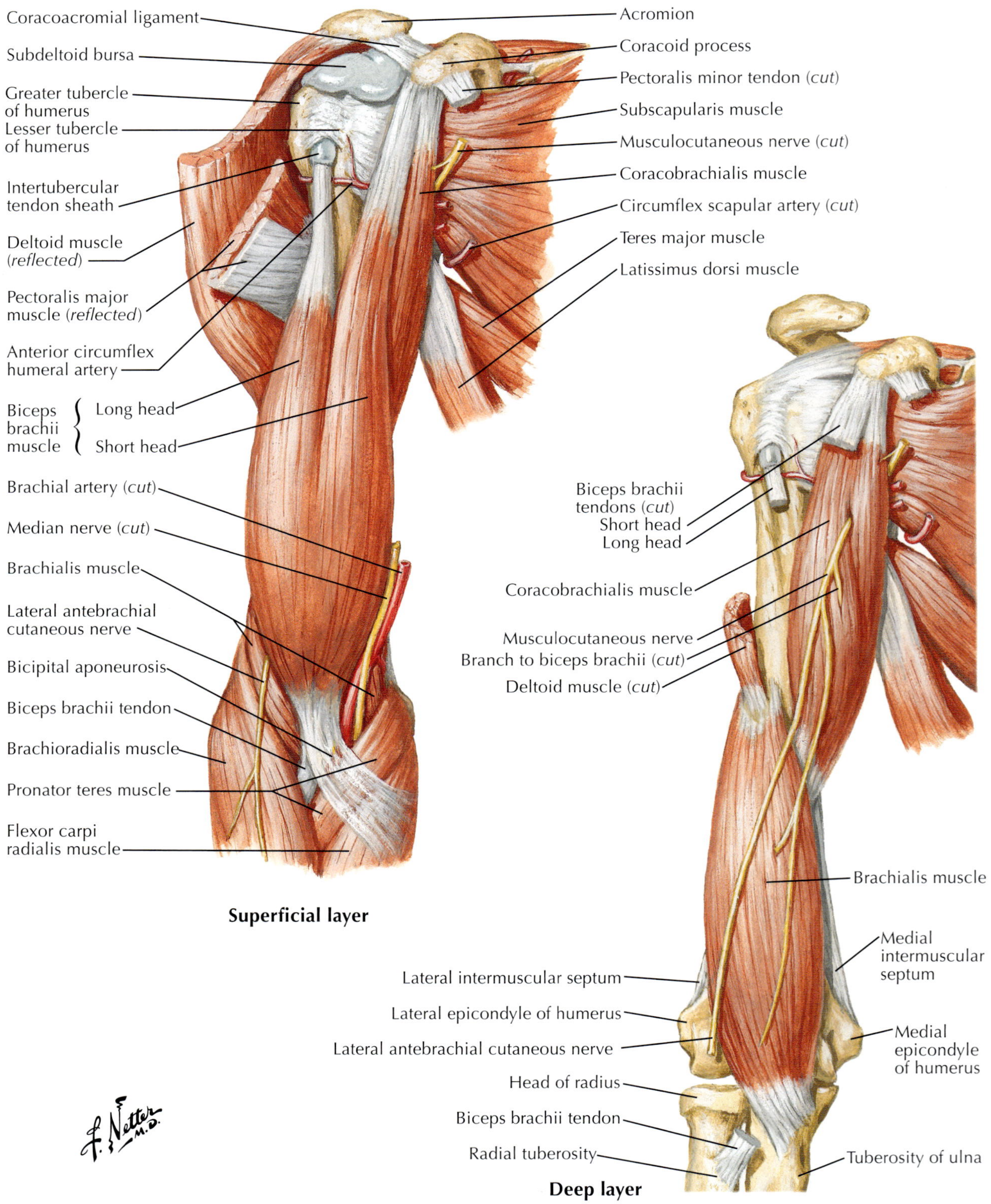

24076 Excision, tumor, soft tissue of upper arm or elbow area, subfascial (eg, intramuscular); less than 5 cm

24073 5 cm or greater

24077 Radical resection of tumor (eg, sarcoma), soft tissue of upper arm or elbow area; less than 5 cm

24079 5 cm or greater

24100 Arthrotomy, elbow; with synovial biopsy only

24101 with joint exploration, with or without biopsy, with or without removal of loose or foreign body

24102 with synovectomy

24105 Excision, olecranon bursa

24110 Excision or curettage of bone cyst or benign tumor, humerus;

24115 with autograft (includes obtaining graft)

24116 with allograft

24120 Excision or curettage of bone cyst or benign tumor of head or neck of radius or olecranon process;

24125 with autograft (includes obtaining graft)

24126 with allograft

24130 Excision, radial head

24134 Sequestrectomy (eg, for osteomyelitis or bone abscess), shaft or distal humerus

24136 Sequestrectomy (eg, for osteomyelitis or bone abscess), radial head or neck

24138 Sequestrectomy (eg, for osteomyelitis or bone abscess), olecranon process

24140 Partial excision (craterization, saucerization, or diaphysectomy) bone (eg, osteomyelitis), humerus

24145 Partial excision (craterization, saucerization, or diaphysectomy) bone (eg, osteomyelitis), radial head or neck

24147 Partial excision (craterization, saucerization, or diaphysectomy) bone (eg, osteomyelitis), olecranon process

24149 Radical resection of capsule, soft tissue, and heterotopic bone, elbow, with contracture release (separate procedure)

24150 Radical resection of tumor, shaft or distal humerus

24152 Radical resection of tumor, radial head or neck

24155 Resection of elbow joint (arthrectomy)

Introduction or Removal

Coding Atlas

When a contrast material is injected into any structure in the elbow as part of a separately reported radiographic study, the injection service is reported with code 24220. For arthrocentesis or needling of joint or bursa, code 20605 is used. For injection for tennis elbow, see code 20550.

24160 Removal of prosthesis, includes debridement and synovectomy when performed; humeral **and** ulnar components

24164 radial head

24200 Removal of foreign body, upper arm or elbow area; subcutaneous

24201 deep (subfascial or intramuscular)

24220 Injection procedure for elbow arthrography

Repair, Revision, and/or Reconstruction

Coding Atlas

The elbow is a joint of three bones: humerus, ulna, and radius. In total elbow arthroplasty, defective parts of the humerus and ulna are replaced with a hinged prosthesis.

24300 Manipulation, elbow, under anesthesia

24301 Muscle or tendon transfer, any type, upper arm or elbow, single (excluding 24320-24331)

24305 Tendon lengthening, upper arm or elbow, each tendon

24310 Tenotomy, open, elbow to shoulder, each tendon

24320 Tenoplasty, with muscle transfer, with or without free graft, elbow to shoulder, single (Seddon-Brookes type procedure)

24330 Flexor-plasty, elbow (eg, Steindler type advancement);

24331 with extensor advancement

24332 Tenolysis, triceps

24340 Tenodesis of biceps tendon at elbow (separate procedure)

24341 Repair, tendon or muscle, upper arm or elbow, each tendon or muscle, primary or secondary (excludes rotator cuff)

24342 Reinsertion of ruptured biceps or triceps tendon, distal, with or without tendon graft

24343 Repair lateral collateral ligament, elbow, with local tissue

FIGURE 2-26. Ligaments of the Elbow

Ligaments are dense regular connective tissues that connect bones to bones, usually around a joint. In the elbow, the ulnar collateral ligament (UCL) and the lateral collateral ligament (LCL) connect the humerus to the ulna and work to stabilize the elbow. The UCL, also called the medial collateral ligament, can become frayed, stretched, or torn while performing sports activities that involve throwing. This damage may lead to a total rupture of the UCL.

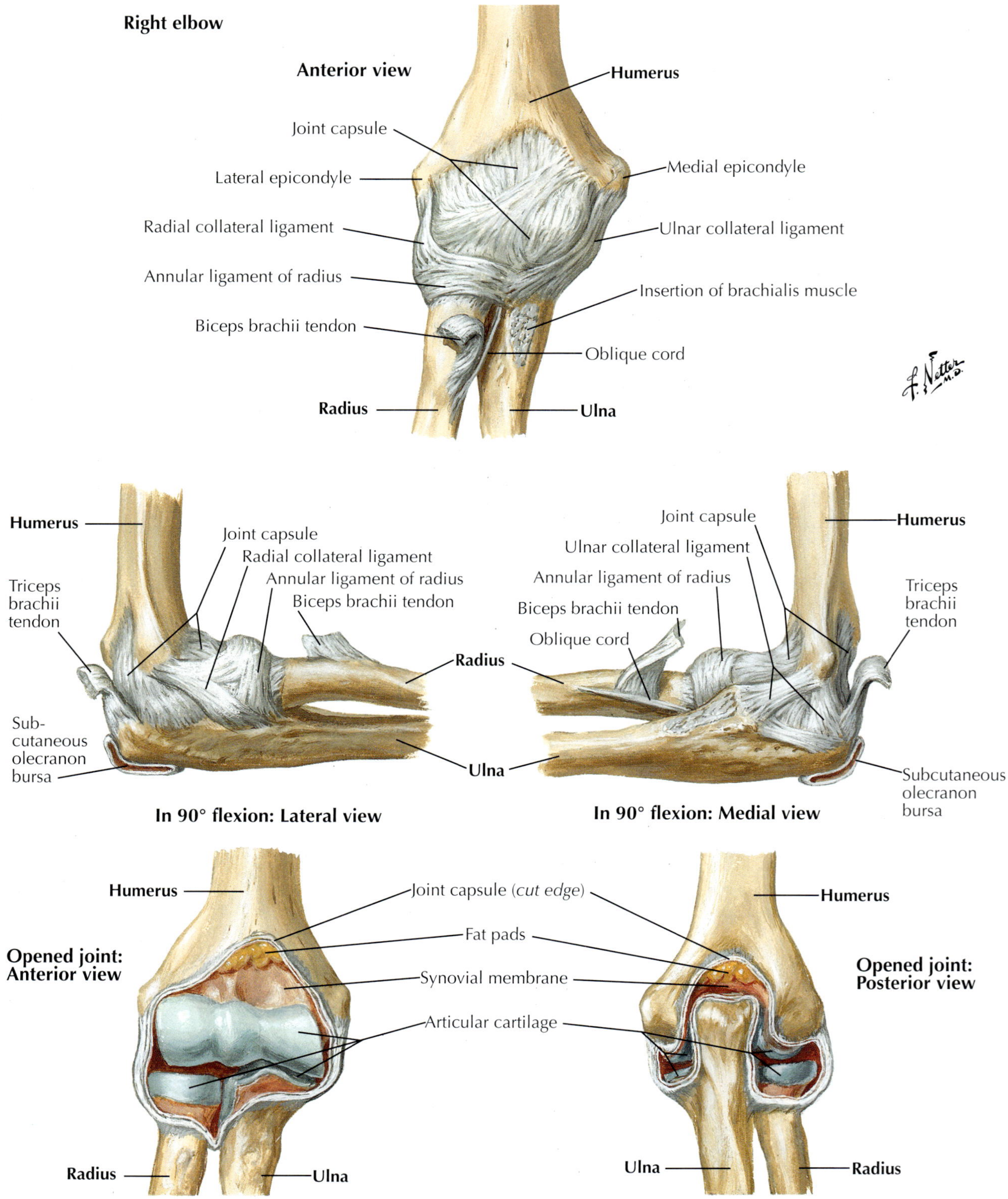

24344 Reconstruction lateral collateral ligament, elbow, with tendon graft (includes harvesting of graft)

24345 Repair medial collateral ligament, elbow, with local tissue

24346 Reconstruction medial collateral ligament, elbow, with tendon graft (includes harvesting of graft)

24357 Tenotomy, elbow, lateral or medial (eg epicondylitis, tennis elbow, golfer's elbow); percutaneous

24358 debridement, soft tissue and/or bone, open

24359 debridement, soft tissue and/or bone, open with tendon repair or reattachment

24360 Arthroplasty, elbow; with membrane (eg, fascial)

24361 with distal humeral prosthetic replacement

24362 with implant and fascia lata ligament reconstruction

24363 with distal humerus and proximal ulnar prosthetic replacement (eg, total elbow)

24365 Arthroplasty, radial head;

24366 with implant

24370 Revision of total elbow arthroplasty, including allograft when performed; humeral **or** ulnar component

24371 humeral **and** ulnar component

24400 Osteotomy, humerus, with or without internal fixation

24410 Multiple osteotomies with realignment on intramedullary rod, humeral shaft (Sofield type procedure)

24420 Osteoplasty, humerus (eg, shortening or lengthening) (excluding 64876)

24430 Repair of nonunion or malunion, humerus; without graft (eg, compression technique)

24435 with iliac or other autograft (includes obtaining graft)

24470 Hemiepiphyseal arrest (eg, cubitus varus or valgus, distal humerus)

24495 Decompression fasciotomy, forearm, with brachial artery exploration

24498 Prophylactic treatment (nailing, pinning, plating or wiring), with or without methylmethacrylate, humeral shaft

Fracture and/or Dislocation

Coding Atlas

Codes for reporting fractures and dislocations are classified by the type of **reduction** and stabilization required. The type of fracture does not necessarily correspond to the type of treatment; a closed fracture may receive open treatment. Dislocations can occur in conjunction with fractures. **Percutaneous skeletal fixation** describes the insertion of pins through the skin and into the bone fragments to secure the bones' positions. This is done without **direct visualization** of the bone. **Internal fixation** describes the application of pins, nails, or other hardware secured to the bone. **External fixation** describes multiple pins placed through bone cortex both proximal and distal to the fracture. The pins are attached to an external fixator.

24500 Closed treatment of humeral shaft fracture; without manipulation

24505 with manipulation, with or without skeletal traction

24515 Open treatment of humeral shaft fracture with plate/ screws, with or without cerclage

24516 Treatment of humeral shaft fracture, with insertion of intramedullary implant, with or without cerclage and/or locking screws

24530 Closed treatment of supracondylar or transcondylar humeral fracture, with or without intercondylar extension; without manipulation

24535 with manipulation, with or without skin or skeletal traction

24538 Percutaneous skeletal fixation of supracondylar or transcondylar humeral fracture, with or without intercondylar extension

24545 Open treatment of humeral supracondylar or transcondylar fracture, includes internal fixation, when performed; without intercondylar extension

24546 with intercondylar extension

24560 Closed treatment of humeral epicondylar fracture, medial or lateral; without manipulation

24565 with manipulation

24566 Percutaneous skeletal fixation of humeral epicondylar fracture, medial or lateral, with manipulation

24575 Open treatment of humeral epicondylar fracture, medial or lateral, includes internal fixation, when performed

24576 Closed treatment of humeral condylar fracture, medial or lateral; without manipulation

24577 with manipulation

FIGURE 2-27. Bones of the Elbow

The radius and ulna form the elbow joint along with the humerus. The radius, or radial bone, is located on the same side of the wrist as the thumb and **articulates** with the rounded capitulum of the humerus. It is shorter than the ulna but thicker. At its **proximal** end, the ulna's olecranon articulates with the **distal** humerus at the olecranon fossa.

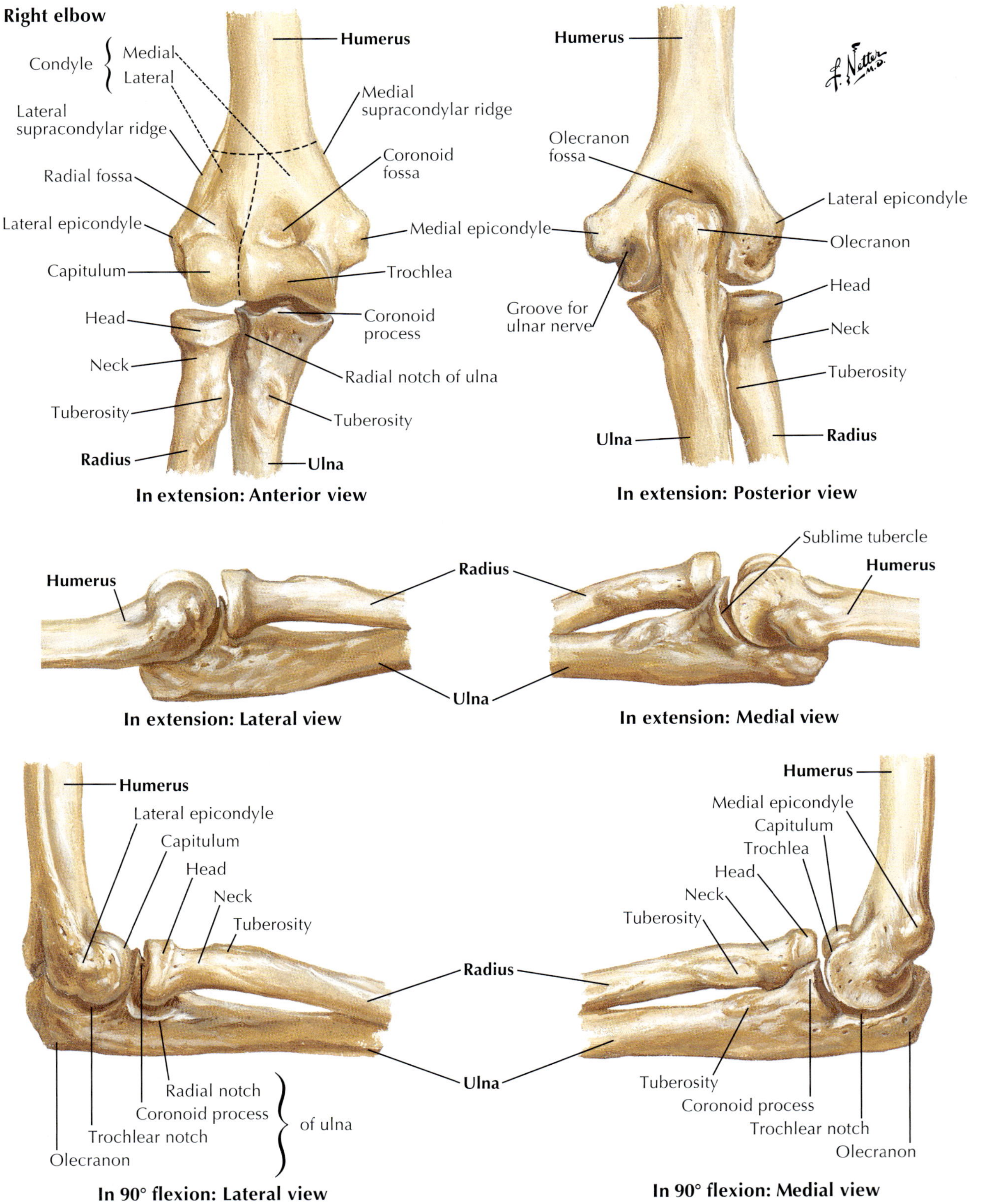

24579 Open treatment of humeral condylar fracture, medial or lateral, includes internal fixation, when performed

24582 Percutaneous skeletal fixation of humeral condylar fracture, medial or lateral, with manipulation

24586 Open treatment of periarticular fracture and/or dislocation of the elbow (fracture distal humerus and proximal ulna and/or proximal radius);

24587 with implant arthroplasty

24600 Treatment of closed elbow dislocation; without anesthesia

24605 requiring anesthesia

24615 Open treatment of acute or chronic elbow dislocation

24620 Closed treatment of Monteggia type of fracture dislocation at elbow (fracture proximal end of ulna with dislocation of radial head), with manipulation

24635 Open treatment of Monteggia type of fracture dislocation at elbow (fracture proximal end of ulna with dislocation of radial head), includes internal fixation, when performed

24640 Closed treatment of radial head subluxation in child, nursemaid elbow, with manipulation

24650 Closed treatment of radial head or neck fracture; without manipulation

24655 with manipulation

24665 Open treatment of radial head or neck fracture, includes internal fixation or radial head excision, when performed;

24666 with radial head prosthetic replacement

24670 Closed treatment of ulnar fracture, proximal end (eg, olecranon or coronoid process[es]); without manipulation

24675 with manipulation

24685 Open treatment of ulnar fracture, proximal end (eg, olecranon or coronoid process[es]), includes internal fixation, when performed

Arthrodesis

Coding Atlas

In elbow joint arthrodesis, the joint is surgically fused and immobilized. Bone grafts may be placed to fix the joint; otherwise, hardware is placed.

24800 Arthrodesis, elbow joint; local

24802 with autogenous graft (includes obtaining graft)

Amputation

Coding Atlas

A guillotine amputation creates a flat wound across the limb. It does not provide skin for adequate closure. Guillotine amputation is typically performed in emergent situations and is followed by wound monitoring for disease prior to a second surgery for revision and flap.

24900 Amputation, arm through humerus; with primary closure

24920 open, circular (guillotine)

24925 secondary closure or scar revision

24930 re-amputation

24931 with implant

24935 Stump elongation, upper extremity

24940 Cineplasty, upper extremity, complete procedure

Forearm and Wrist

Incision

Coding Atlas

Decompression fasciotomy treats compartment syndrome, a painful condition in which pressure within the fascia-bound muscle builds to potentially destructive levels. The pressure can restrict blood flow and prevent oxygen from reaching nerve and muscle cells. Compartments are groups of muscles bound by fascia. The forearm contains the flexor (anterior or volar) and extensor (posterior or dorsal) compartments. A third compartment, the "mobile wad," contains the brachioradialis, extensor carpi radialis, and extensor carpi radialis brevis muscles. Fasciotomy is an incision along the length of the fascia to release compression of the muscles within.

25000 Incision, extensor tendon sheath, wrist (eg, deQuervains disease)

25001 Incision, flexor tendon sheath, wrist (eg, flexor carpi radialis)

25020 Decompression fasciotomy, forearm and/or wrist, flexor OR extensor compartment; without debridement of nonviable muscle and/or nerve

25023 with debridement of nonviable muscle and/or nerve

25024 Decompression fasciotomy, forearm and/or wrist, flexor AND extensor compartment; without debridement of nonviable muscle and/or nerve

25025 with debridement of nonviable muscle and/or nerve

FIGURE 2-28. Muscles of the Forearm and Wrist

The forearm contains many muscles. Muscles in the forearm act as **extensors** and **flexors** of the wrist and fingers as well as **pronators** and **supinators** that turn the hand palm-up or palm-down. The brachioradialis muscle is a flexor of the elbow. The forearm is divided into two **fascial** compartments. The **posterior** compartment contains the **extensors** of the hands, and the **anterior** compartment contains the **flexors**.

Right forearm: Posterior (dorsal) view

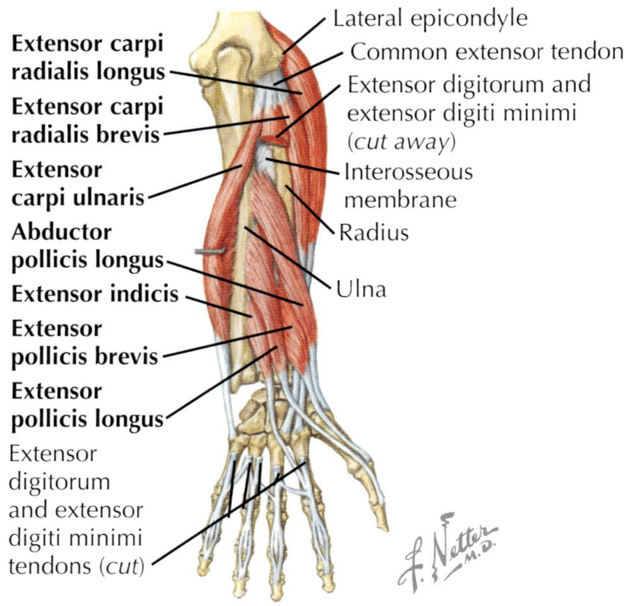

Posterior view

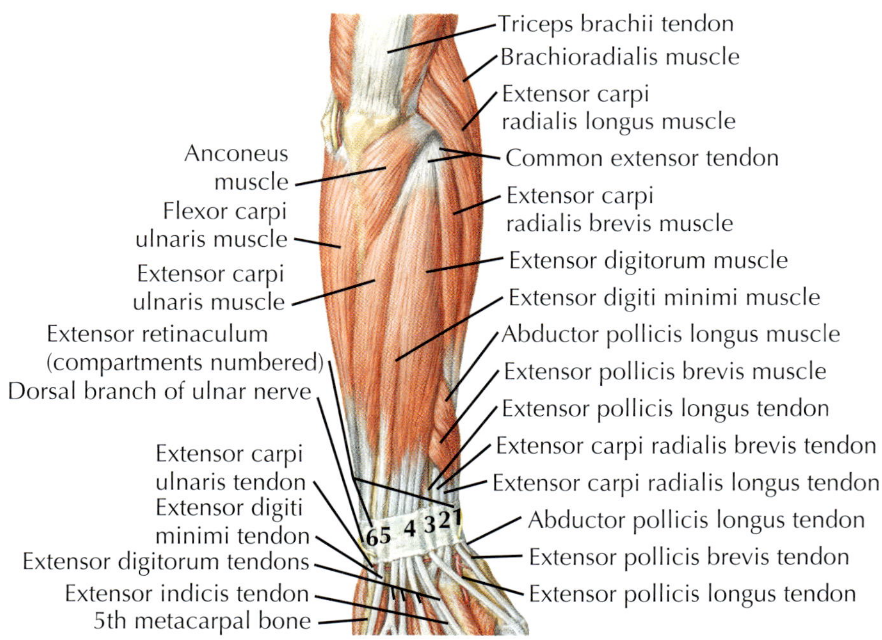

 ⊙=Moderate sedation ✚=Add-on code ⊘=Modifier 51 exempt #=Resequenced code

25028 Incision and drainage, forearm and/or wrist; deep abscess or hematoma

25031 bursa

25035 Incision, deep, bone cortex, forearm and/or wrist (eg, osteomyelitis or bone abscess)

25040 Arthrotomy, radiocarpal or midcarpal joint, with exploration, drainage, or removal of foreign body

Excision

Coding Atlas

Size and **tumor** origin play a role in code selection for excision of soft tissue tumors. The entire resection is measured, not the diameter of the lesion itself, to determine the excision size. Excision of a tumor originating in the integument, eg, **melanoma**, is reported with Integumentary System excision codes.

25065 Biopsy, soft tissue of forearm and/or wrist; superficial

25066 deep (subfascial or intramuscular)

25071 Code is out of numerical sequence. See 25065-25240

25073 Code is out of numerical sequence. See 25065-25240

25075 Excision, tumor, soft tissue of forearm and/or wrist area, subcutaneous; less than 3 cm

\# **25071** 3 cm or greater

25076 Excision, tumor, soft tissue of forearm and/or wrist area, subfascial (eg, intramuscular); less than 3 cm

\# **25073** 3 cm or greater

25077 Radical resection of tumor (eg, sarcoma), soft tissue of forearm and/or wrist area; less than 3 cm

25078 3 cm or greater

25085 Capsulotomy, wrist (eg, contracture)

25100 Arthrotomy, wrist joint; with biopsy

25101 with joint exploration, with or without biopsy, with or without removal of loose or foreign body

25105 with synovectomy

25107 Arthrotomy, distal radioulnar joint including repair of triangular cartilage, complex

25109 Excision of tendon, forearm and/or wrist, flexor or extensor, each

25110 Excision, lesion of tendon sheath, forearm and/or wrist

25111 Excision of ganglion, wrist (dorsal or volar); primary

25112 recurrent

25115 Radical excision of bursa, synovia of wrist, or forearm tendon sheaths (eg, tenosynovitis, fungus, Tbc, or other granulomas, rheumatoid arthritis); flexors

25116 extensors, with or without transposition of dorsal retinaculum

25118 Synovectomy, extensor tendon sheath, wrist, single compartment;

25119 with resection of distal ulna

25120 Excision or curettage of bone cyst or benign tumor of radius or ulna (excluding head or neck of radius and olecranon process);

25125 with autograft (includes obtaining graft)

25126 with allograft

25130 Excision or curettage of bone cyst or benign tumor of carpal bones;

25135 with autograft (includes obtaining graft)

25136 with allograft

25145 Sequestrectomy (eg, for osteomyelitis or bone abscess), forearm and/or wrist

25150 Partial excision (craterization, saucerization, or diaphysectomy) of bone (eg, for osteomyelitis); ulna

25151 radius

25170 Radical resection of tumor, radius or ulna

25210 Carpectomy; 1 bone

25215 all bones of proximal row

25230 Radial styloidectomy (separate procedure)

25240 Excision distal ulna partial or complete (eg, Darrach type or matched resection)

Introduction or Removal

Coding Atlas

A **foreign body** is an object that has become lodged in the body by accident. A **prosthesis** is an object that has been placed in the body to assume the role of a natural body part, eg, a joint or bone.

25246 Injection procedure for wrist arthrography

25248 Exploration with removal of deep foreign body, forearm or wrist

25250 Removal of wrist prosthesis; (separate procedure)

25251 complicated, including total wrist

25259 Manipulation, wrist, under anesthesia

Repair, Revision, and/or Reconstruction

Coding Atlas

Tenotomy is the surgical incision/division of a tendon. **Tenolysis** is a surgical procedure to remove adhesions that interfere with flexion of the fingers. **Tenodesis** is the surgical anchoring of a **tendon** to bone using a suture.

25260 Repair, tendon or muscle, flexor, forearm and/or wrist; primary, single, each tendon or muscle

25263 secondary, single, each tendon or muscle

25265 secondary, with free graft (includes obtaining graft), each tendon or muscle

25270 Repair, tendon or muscle, extensor, forearm and/or wrist; primary, single, each tendon or muscle

25272 secondary, single, each tendon or muscle

25274 secondary, with free graft (includes obtaining graft), each tendon or muscle

25275 Repair, tendon sheath, extensor, forearm and/or wrist, with free graft (includes obtaining graft) (eg, for extensor carpi ulnaris subluxation)

25280 Lengthening or shortening of flexor or extensor tendon, forearm and/or wrist, single, each tendon

25290 Tenotomy, open, flexor or extensor tendon, forearm and/or wrist, single, each tendon

25295 Tenolysis, flexor or extensor tendon, forearm and/or wrist, single, each tendon

25300 Tenodesis at wrist; flexors of fingers

25301 extensors of fingers

25310 Tendon transplantation or transfer, flexor or extensor, forearm and/or wrist, single; each tendon

25312 with tendon graft(s) (includes obtaining graft), each tendon

25315 Flexor origin slide (eg, for cerebral palsy, Volkmann contracture), forearm and/or wrist;

25316 with tendon(s) transfer

25320 Capsulorrhaphy or reconstruction, wrist, open (eg, capsulodesis, ligament repair, tendon transfer or graft) (includes synovectomy, capsulotomy and open reduction) for carpal instability

25332 Arthroplasty, wrist, with or without interposition, with or without external or internal fixation

25335 Centralization of wrist on ulna (eg, radial club hand)

25337 Reconstruction for stabilization of unstable distal ulna or distal radioulnar joint, secondary by soft tissue stabilization (eg, tendon transfer, tendon graft or weave, or tenodesis) with or without open reduction of distal radioulnar joint

25350 Osteotomy, radius; distal third

25355 middle or proximal third

25360 Osteotomy; ulna

25365 radius AND ulna

25370 Multiple osteotomies, with realignment on intramedullary rod (Sofield type procedure); radius OR ulna

25375 radius AND ulna

FIGURE 2-29. Flexor Tendons of the Wrist

Long tendon extensions of the **flexor** muscles of the forearm work together to produce flexion of the fingers of the hand. The flexor digitorum superficialis (FDS) and flexor digitorum profundus (FDP) tendons must pass through the carpal tunnel before entering the hand. Tendon sheaths act to lubricate the tendons with synovial fluid so that they glide smoothly.

Palmar view

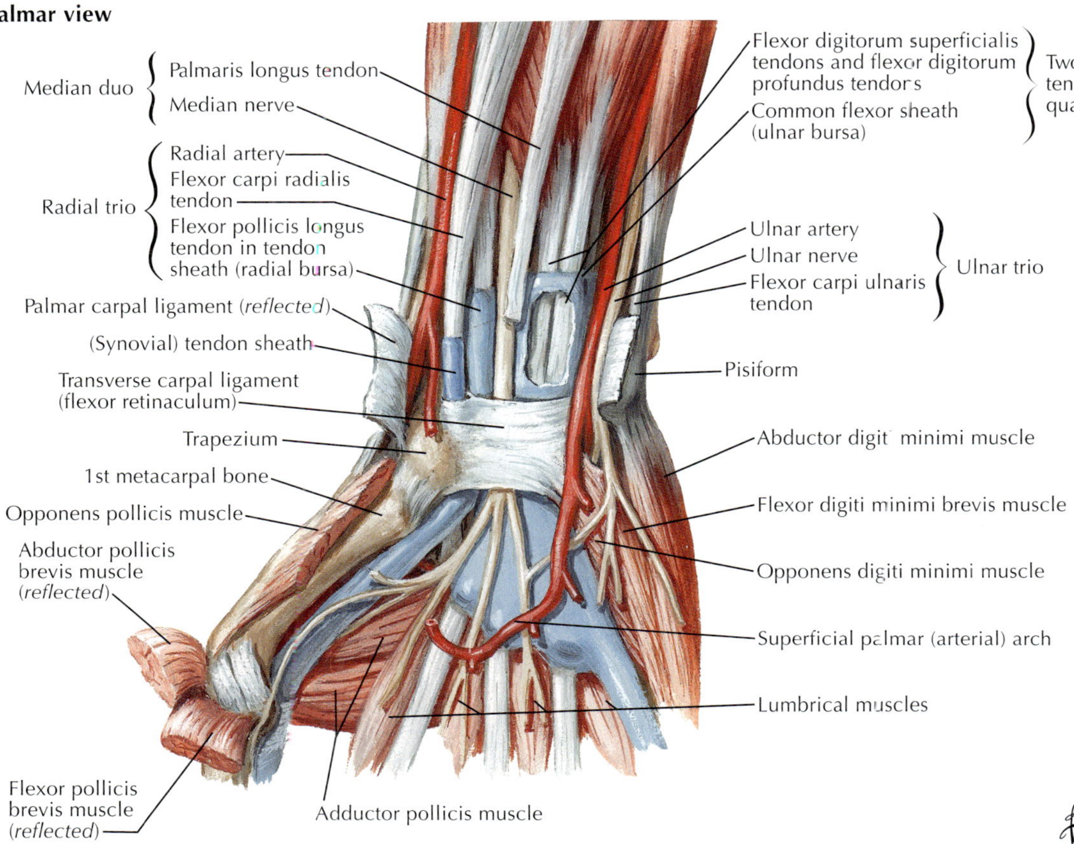

Transverse cross section of wrist demonstrating carpal tunnel

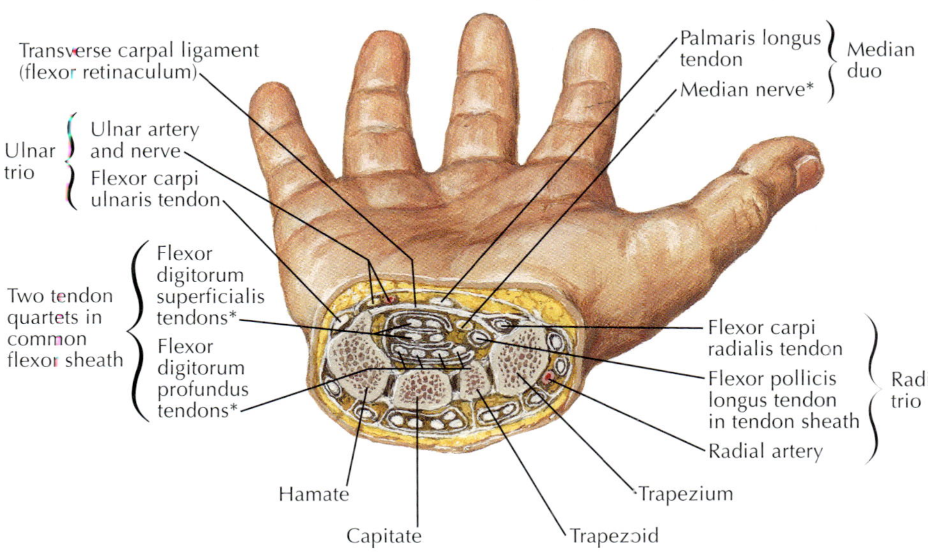

*Contents of carpal tunnel

25390 Osteoplasty, radius OR ulna; shortening

25391 lengthening with autograft

25392 Osteoplasty, radius AND ulna; shortening (excluding 64876)

25393 lengthening with autograft

25394 Osteoplasty, carpal bone, shortening

25400 Repair of nonunion or malunion, radius OR ulna; without graft (eg, compression technique)

25405 with autograft (includes obtaining graft)

25415 Repair of nonunion or malunion, radius AND ulna; without graft (eg, compression technique)

25420 with autograft (includes obtaining graft)

25425 Repair of defect with autograft; radius OR ulna

25426 radius AND ulna

25430 Insertion of vascular pedicle into carpal bone (eg, Hori procedure)

25431 Repair of nonunion of carpal bone (excluding carpal scaphoid (navicular)) (includes obtaining graft and necessary fixation), each bone

25440 Repair of nonunion, scaphoid carpal (navicular) bone, with or without radial styloidectomy (includes obtaining graft and necessary fixation)

25441 Arthroplasty with prosthetic replacement; distal radius

25442 distal ulna

25443 scaphoid carpal (navicular)

25444 lunate

25445 trapezium

25446 distal radius and partial or entire carpus (total wrist)

25447 Arthroplasty, interposition, intercarpal or carpometacarpal joints

25449 Revision of arthroplasty, including removal of implant, wrist joint

25450 Epiphyseal arrest by epiphysiodesis or stapling; distal radius OR ulna

25455 distal radius AND ulna

25490 Prophylactic treatment (nailing, pinning, plating or wiring) with or without methylmethacrylate; radius

25491 ulna

25492 radius AND ulna

Fracture and/or Dislocation

Coding Atlas

A Galeazzi fracture is a fracture of the radius with **dislocation** of the **distal** radioulnar joint and an intact ulna. Codes for fractures and dislocations are classified by the type of **reduction** and stabilization required. The type of fracture does not necessarily correspond to the type of treatment; a closed fracture may receive open treatment. Dislocations can occur in conjunction with fractures.

25500 Closed treatment of radial shaft fracture; without manipulation

25505 with manipulation

25515 Open treatment of radial shaft fracture, includes internal fixation, when performed

25520 Closed treatment of radial shaft fracture and closed treatment of dislocation of distal radioulnar joint (Galeazzi fracture/dislocation)

25525 Open treatment of radial shaft fracture, includes internal fixation, when performed, and closed treatment of distal radioulnar joint dislocation (Galeazzi fracture/dislocation), includes percutaneous skeletal fixation, when performed

25526 Open treatment of radial shaft fracture, includes internal fixation, when performed, and open treatment of distal radioulnar joint dislocation (Galeazzi fracture/dislocation), includes internal fixation, when performed, includes repair of triangular fibrocartilage complex

25530 Closed treatment of ulnar shaft fracture; without manipulation

25535 with manipulation

25545 Open treatment of ulnar shaft fracture, includes internal fixation, when performed

25560 Closed treatment of radial and ulnar shaft fractures; without manipulation

25565 with manipulation

25574 Open treatment of radial AND ulnar shaft fractures, with internal fixation, when performed; of radius OR ulna

25575 of radius AND ulna

25600 Closed treatment of distal radial fracture (eg, Colles or Smith type) or epiphyseal separation, includes closed treatment of fracture of ulnar styloid, when performed; without manipulation

25605 with manipulation

FIGURE 2-30. Carpal and Wrist Bones

The wrist contains eight carpal bones organized into two groups: **proximal** and **distal**. The proximal bones (scaphoid, lunate, triquetrum, and pisiform) have no **tendon** inserts, but instead move according to the mechanical forces of surrounding bones. The distal bones (trapezium, trapezoid, capitate, and hamate) are linked by **ligaments** to each other and to the five metacarpal bones, creating five carpometacarpal (CMC) joints. The CMC of the thumb is also called the trapezoid-metacarpal (TMC) joint.

A. Anterior (palmar) view of carpal bones

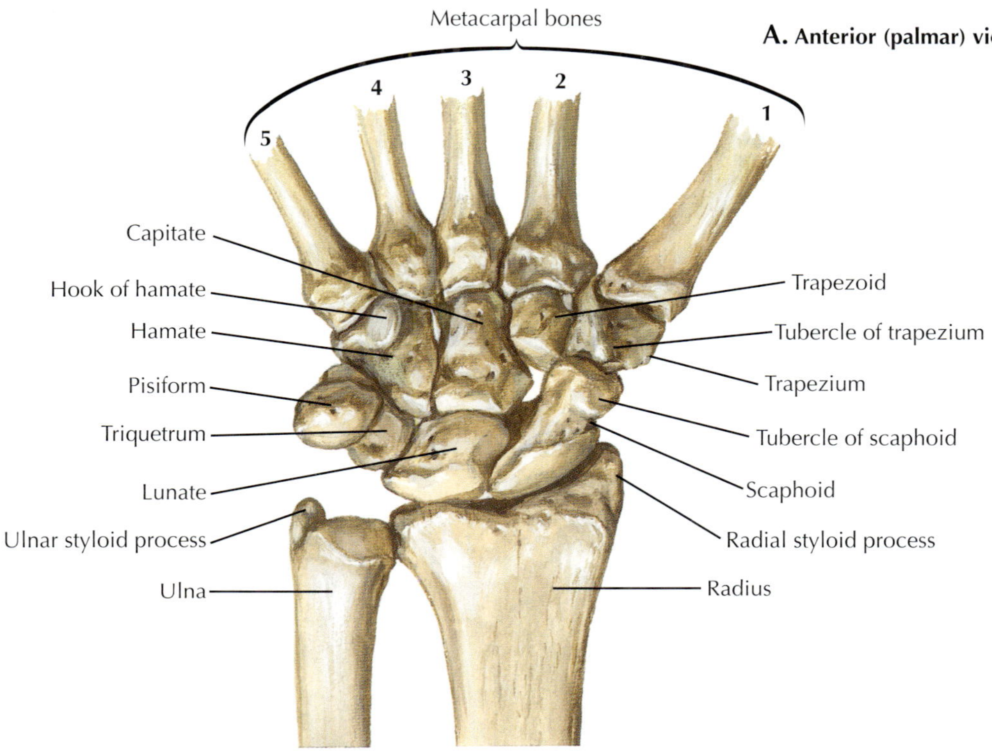

B. Coronal section: Dorsal view

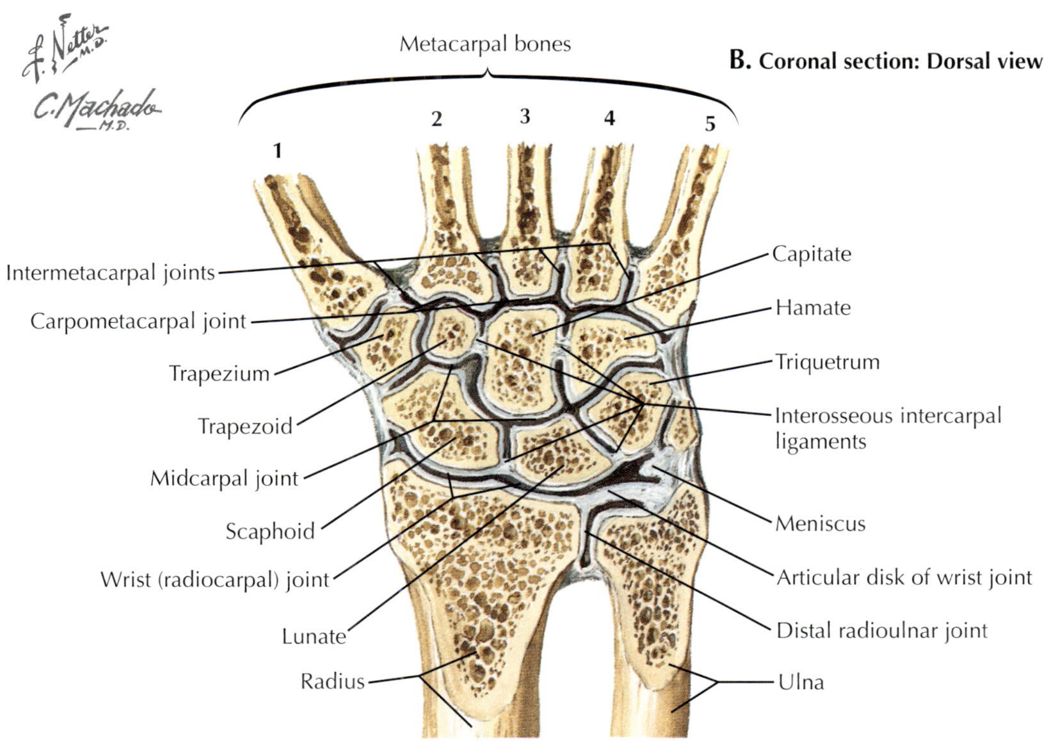

FIGURE 2-31. Colles Fracture

A Colles fracture, a fracture of the **distal** radius, is the most common fracture of the arm. It typically occurs when a person falls onto his or her outstretched arm. A Colles fracture is within an inch from the distal end of the radius. The fracture may extend into the wrist joint (**intra-articular**) or may include more than one break site (**comminuted**).

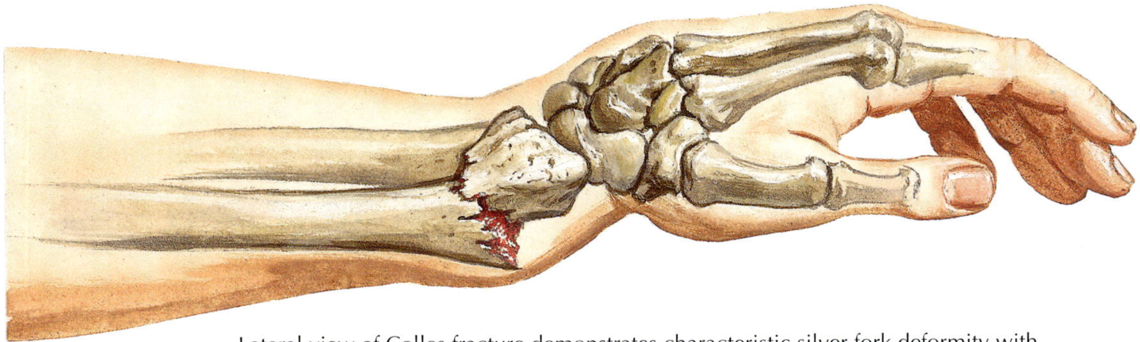

Lateral view of Colles fracture demonstrates characteristic silver fork deformity with dorsal and proximal displacement of distal fragment. Note dorsal instead of normal volar slope of articular surface of distal radius.

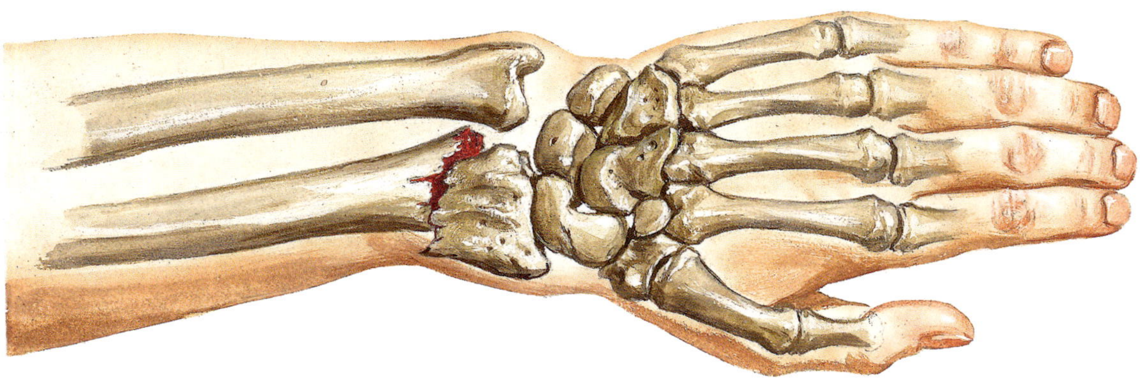

Dorsal view shows radial deviation of hand with ulnar prominence of styloid process of ulna and decrease or reverse of normal radial slope of articular surface of distal radius

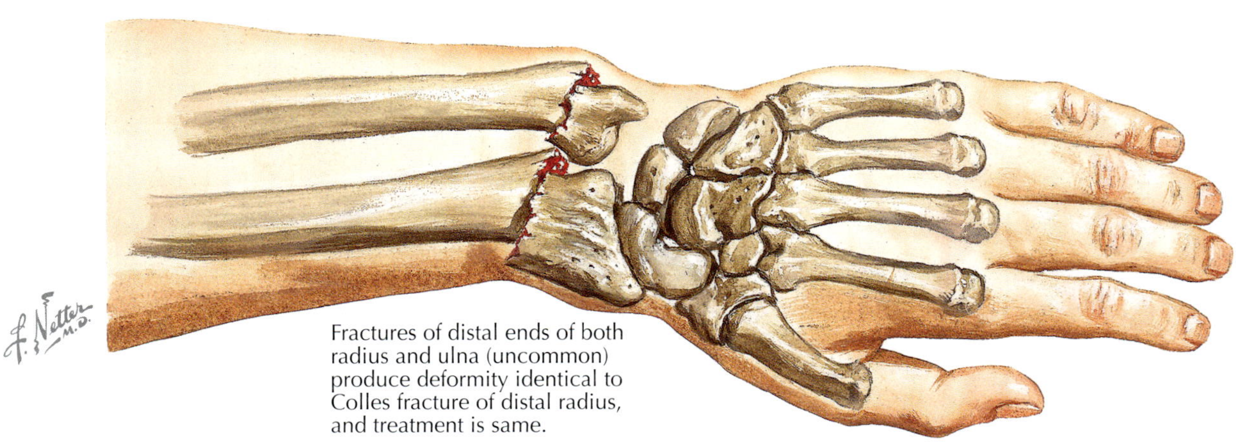

Fractures of distal ends of both radius and ulna (uncommon) produce deformity identical to Colles fracture of distal radius, and treatment is same.

25606 Percutaneous skeletal fixation of distal radial fracture or epiphyseal separation

25607 Open treatment of distal radial extra-articular fracture or epiphyseal separation, with internal fixation

25608 Open treatment of distal radial intra-articular fracture or epiphyseal separation; with internal fixation of 2 fragments

25609 with internal fixation of 3 or more fragments

25622 Closed treatment of carpal scaphoid (navicular) fracture; without manipulation

25624 with manipulation

25628 Open treatment of carpal scaphoid (navicular) fracture, includes internal fixation, when performed

25630 Closed treatment of carpal bone fracture (excluding carpal scaphoid [navicular]); without manipulation, each bone

25635 with manipulation, each bone

25645 Open treatment of carpal bone fracture (other than carpal scaphoid [navicular]), each bone

25650 Closed treatment of ulnar styloid fracture

25651 Percutaneous skeletal fixation of ulnar styloid fracture

25652 Open treatment of ulnar styloid fracture

25660 Closed treatment of radiocarpal or intercarpal dislocation, 1 or more bones, with manipulation

25670 Open treatment of radiocarpal or intercarpal dislocation, 1 or more bones

25671 Percutaneous skeletal fixation of distal radioulnar dislocation

25675 Closed treatment of distal radioulnar dislocation with manipulation

25676 Open treatment of distal radioulnar dislocation, acute or chronic

25680 Closed treatment of trans-scaphoperilunar type of fracture dislocation, with manipulation

25685 Open treatment of trans-scaphoperilunar type of fracture dislocation

25690 Closed treatment of lunate dislocation, with manipulation

25695 Open treatment of lunate dislocation

Arthrodesis

Coding Atlas

Wrist arthrodesis is typically performed to reduce pain in a patient with arthritic joints, eg, scapholunate advanced collapse (SLAC), a common pattern of degenerative arthritis. In SLAC, ligament injury is followed by collapse of the radial side of the wrist. Arthrodesis of the wrist may be complete (codes 25800-25810) or partial (codes 25820-25830).

25800 Arthrodesis, wrist; complete, without bone graft (includes radiocarpal and/or intercarpal and/or carpometacarpal joints)

25805 with sliding graft

25810 with iliac or other autograft (includes obtaining graft)

25820 Arthrodesis, wrist; limited, without bone graft (eg, intercarpal or radiocarpal)

25825 with autograft (includes obtaining graft)

25830 Arthrodesis, distal radioulnar joint with segmental resection of ulna, with or without bone graft (eg, Sauve-Kapandji procedure)

Amputation

Coding Atlas

In a Krukenberg procedure, the radius and ulna are separated, and a pincer-like grasp is created from the opposable bones that retain muscle attachments and are enclosed in skin. A guillotine amputation creates a flat wound across the limb. It does not provide skin for adequate closure. Guillotine amputation is typically performed in emergent situations and is followed by wound monitoring for disease prior to a second surgery for revision and flap.

25900 Amputation, forearm, through radius and ulna;

25905 open, circular (guillotine)

25907 secondary closure or scar revision

25909 re-amputation

25915 Krukenberg procedure

25920 Disarticulation through wrist;

25922 secondary closure or scar revision

25924 re-amputation

25927 Transmetacarpal amputation;

25929 secondary closure or scar revision

25931 re-amputation

FIGURE 2-32. Deep Palmar Soft Tissue

The palmar aponeurosis is a tough membrane overlying the **tendons** of the palm. Triangular in shape, it is narrow at the wrist and wider at its terminus at the base of the four fingers. The central portion of the palmar aponeurosis is thick and helps form the superficial palmar **fascia**. The **lateral** portion covers the muscles of the ball of the thumb.

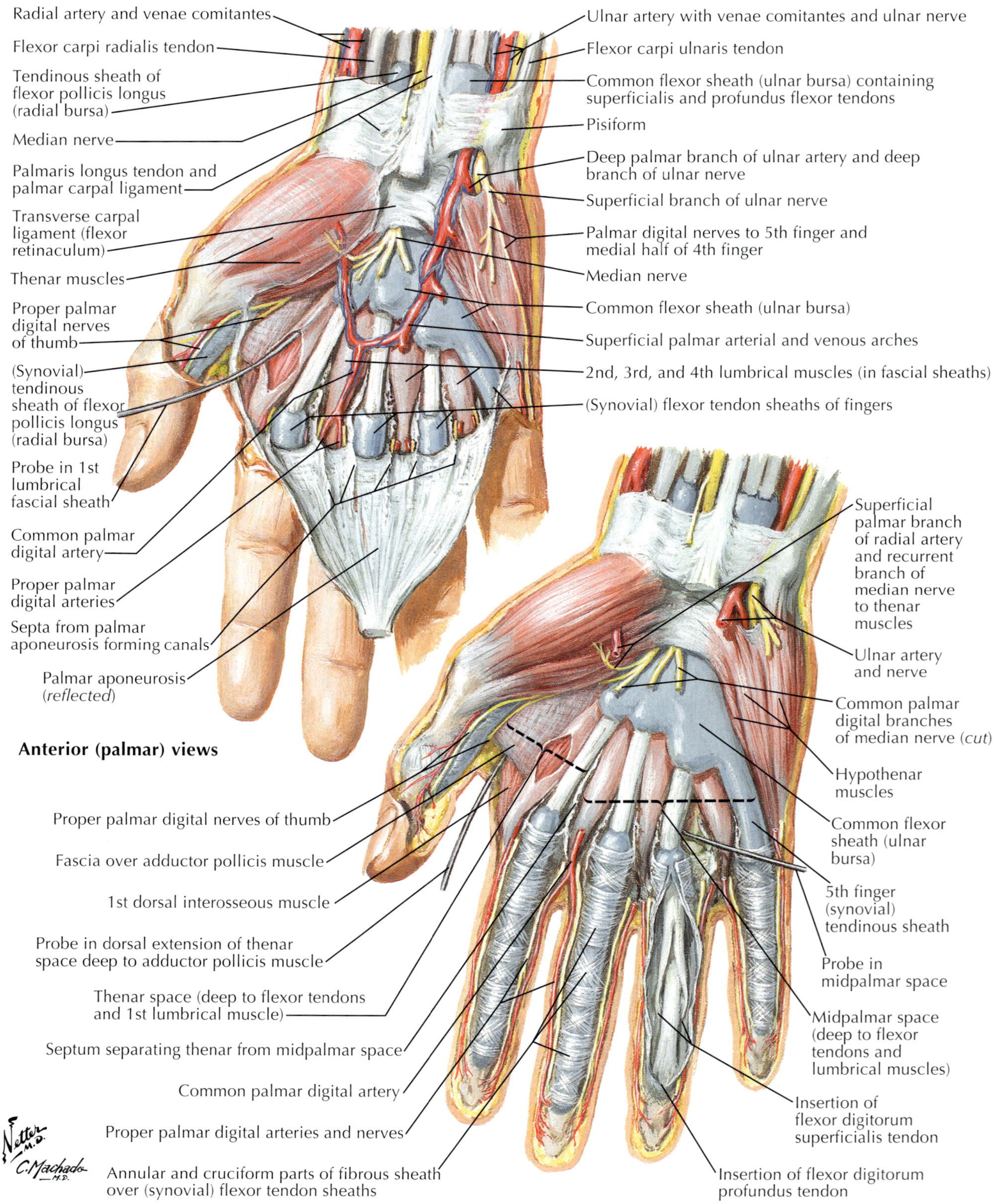

Hand and Fingers

Incision

Coding Atlas

A synovial joint is enclosed in a ligamentous capsule. **Arthrotomy** is a surgical incision into a joint capsule. Codes 26070-26080 are used to report arthrotomy with **foreign body** (FB) removal. Removal of an FB documented as embedded on the exterior of the joint capsule or described as an FB that may have penetrated the joint capsule does not qualify as arthrotomy.

26010 Drainage of finger abscess; simple

26011 complicated (eg, felon)

26020 Drainage of tendon sheath, digit and/or palm, each

26025 Drainage of palmar bursa; single, bursa

26030 multiple bursa

26034 Incision, bone cortex, hand or finger (eg, osteomyelitis or bone abscess)

26035 Decompression fingers and/or hand, injection injury (eg, grease gun)

26037 Decompressive fasciotomy, hand (excludes 26035)

26040 Fasciotomy, palmar (eg, Dupuytren's contracture); percutaneous

26045 open, partial

26055 Tendon sheath incision (eg, for trigger finger)

26060 Tenotomy, percutaneous, single, each digit

26070 Arthrotomy, with exploration, drainage, or removal of loose or foreign body; carpometacarpal joint

26075 metacarpophalangeal joint, each

26080 interphalangeal joint, each

Excision

Coding Atlas

Fasciectomy is excision of strips of **fascia**, usually as a treatment to relieve pressure in the underlying muscle or other soft tissue. This may be performed to treat Dupuytren's contracture. In **synovectomy**, all or part of the synovial membrane is surgically removed from the joint. Usually, the portion of synovium being removed is defective, causing pain or limiting range of motion. Ulnar superficialis slip resection (USSR), a surgical treatment for trigger finger, is reported with code 26170.

26100 Arthrotomy with biopsy; carpometacarpal joint, each

26105 metacarpophalangeal joint, each

26110 interphalangeal joint, each

26111 Code is out of numerical sequence. See 26100-26262

26113 Code is out of numerical sequence. See 26100-26262

26115 Excision, tumor or vascular malformation, soft tissue of hand or finger, subcutaneous; less than 1.5 cm

 # 26111 1.5 cm or greater

26116 Excision, tumor, soft tissue, or vascular malformation, of hand or finger, subfascial (eg, intramuscular); less than 1.5 cm

 # 26113 1.5 cm or greater

26117 Radical resection of tumor (eg, sarcoma), soft tissue of hand or finger; less than 3 cm

26118 3 cm or greater

26121 Fasciectomy, palm only, with or without Z-plasty, other local tissue rearrangement, or skin grafting (includes obtaining graft)

26123 Fasciectomy, partial palmar with release of single digit including proximal interphalangeal joint, with or without Z-plasty, other local tissue rearrangement, or skin grafting (includes obtaining graft);

✚ 26125 each additional digit (List separately in addition to code for primary procedure)

26130 Synovectomy, carpometacarpal joint

26135 Synovectomy, metacarpophalangeal joint including intrinsic release and extensor hood reconstruction, each digit

26140 Synovectomy, proximal interphalangeal joint, including extensor reconstruction, each interphalangeal joint

26145 Synovectomy, tendon sheath, radical (tenosynovectomy), flexor tendon, palm and/or finger, each tendon

26160 Excision of lesion of tendon sheath or joint capsule (eg, cyst, mucous cyst, or ganglion), hand or finger

26170 Excision of tendon, palm, flexor or extensor, single, each tendon

26180 Excision of tendon, finger, flexor or extensor, each tendon

26185 Sesamoidectomy, thumb or finger (separate procedure)

26200 Excision or curettage of bone cyst or benign tumor of metacarpal;

26205 with autograft (includes obtaining graft)

26210 Excision or curettage of bone cyst or benign tumor of proximal, middle, or distal phalanx of finger;

26215 with autograft (includes obtaining graft)

26230 Partial excision (craterization, saucerization, or diaphysectomy) bone (eg, osteomyelitis); metacarpal

26235 proximal or middle phalanx of finger

FIGURE 2-33. Intrinsic Muscles of the Hand

Muscles acting on the hand can be divided into two categories: **extrinsic** and **intrinsic**. Extrinsic muscles of the hand have their origins and the bulk of their muscle body on the forearm. A tendon on the extrinsic muscle crosses the wrist to act on bones in the hand. Intrinsic muscles are muscles originating in the hand.

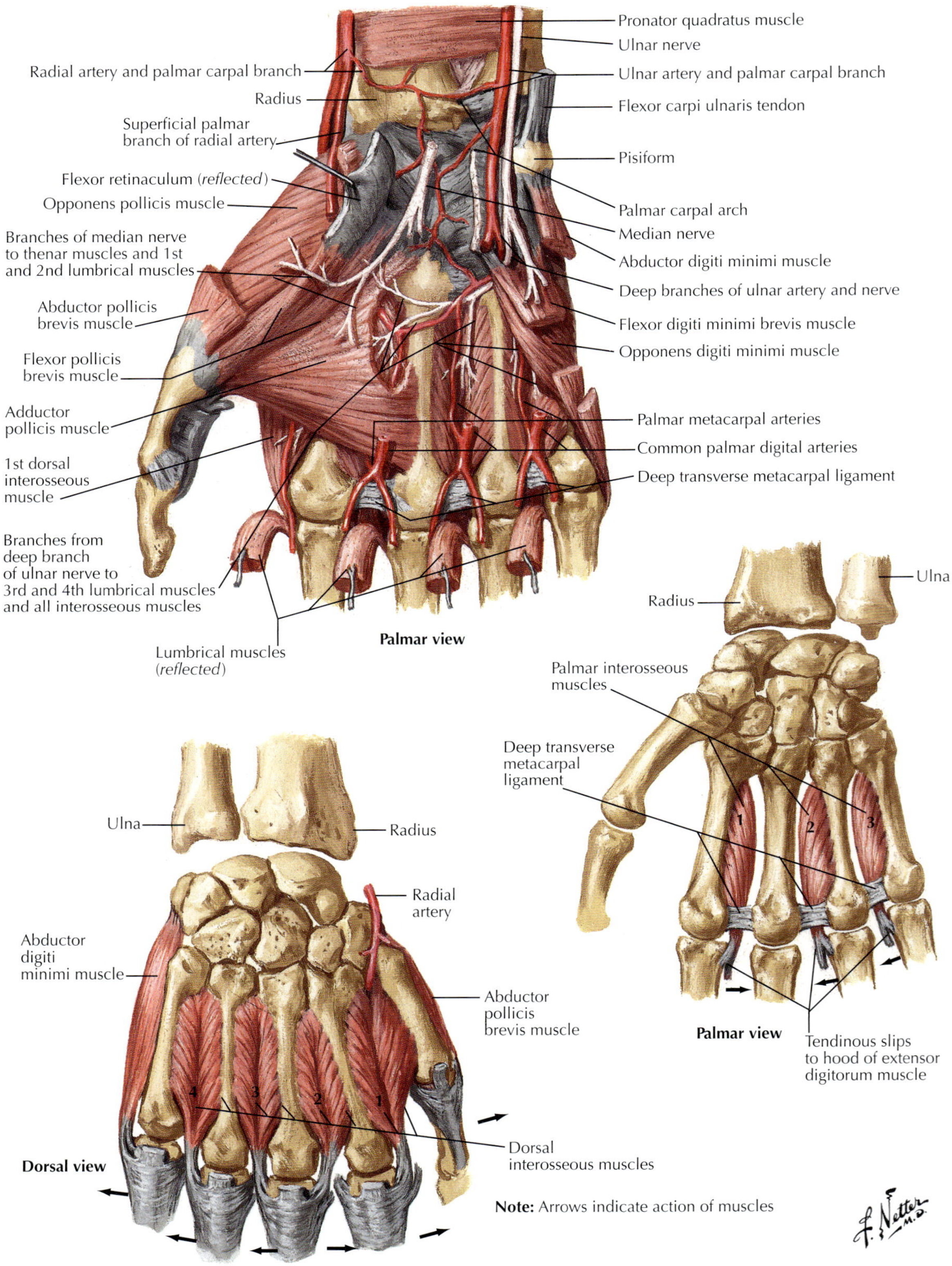

26236 distal phalanx of finger

26250 Radical resection of tumor, metacarpal

26260 Radical resection of tumor, proximal or middle phalanx of finger

26262 Radical resection of tumor, distal phalanx of finger

Introduction or Removal

26320 Removal of implant from finger or hand

Repair, Revision, and/or Reconstruction

Coding Atlas

Codes 26551-26554 are used to report toe-to-hand transfer with microvascular anastomosis. Code 26551 includes a partial skinning of the toe and an initial bone graft. Code 26556 is used to report a toe joint transfer with microvascular anastomosis.

26340 Manipulation, finger joint, under anesthesia, each joint

26341 Manipulation, palmar fascial cord (ie, Dupuytren's cord), post enzyme injection (eg, collagenase), single cord

26350 Repair or advancement, flexor tendon, not in zone 2 digital flexor tendon sheath (eg, no man's land); primary or secondary without free graft, each tendon

26352 secondary with free graft (includes obtaining graft), each tendon

26356 Repair or advancement, flexor tendon, in zone 2 digital flexor tendon sheath (eg, no man's land); primary, without free graft, each tendon

26357 secondary, without free graft, each tendon

26358 secondary, with free graft (includes obtaining graft), each tendon

26370 Repair or advancement of profundus tendon, with intact superficialis tendon; primary, each tendon

26372 secondary with free graft (includes obtaining graft), each tendon

26373 secondary without free graft, each tendon

26390 Excision flexor tendon, with implantation of synthetic rod for delayed tendon graft, hand or finger, each rod

26392 Removal of synthetic rod and insertion of flexor tendon graft, hand or finger (includes obtaining graft), each rod

26410 Repair, extensor tendon, hand, primary or secondary; without free graft, each tendon

26412 with free graft (includes obtaining graft), each tendon

26415 Excision of extensor tendon, with implantation of synthetic rod for delayed tendon graft, hand or finger, each rod

26416 Removal of synthetic rod and insertion of extensor tendon graft (includes obtaining graft), hand or finger, each rod

26418 Repair, extensor tendon, finger, primary or secondary; without free graft, each tendon

26420 with free graft (includes obtaining graft) each tendon

26426 Repair of extensor tendon, central slip, secondary (eg, boutonniere deformity); using local tissue(s), including lateral band(s), each finger

26428 with free graft (includes obtaining graft), each finger

26432 Closed treatment of distal extensor tendon insertion, with or without percutaneous pinning (eg, mallet finger)

26433 Repair of extensor tendon, distal insertion, primary or secondary; without graft (eg, mallet finger)

26434 with free graft (includes obtaining graft)

26437 Realignment of extensor tendon, hand, each tendon

26440 Tenolysis, flexor tendon; palm OR finger, each tendon

26442 palm AND finger, each tendon

26445 Tenolysis, extensor tendon, hand OR finger, each tendon

26449 Tenolysis, complex, extensor tendon, finger, including forearm, each tendon

26450 Tenotomy, flexor, palm, open, each tendon

26455 Tenotomy, flexor, finger, open, each tendon

26460 Tenotomy, extensor, hand or finger, open, each tendon

26471 Tenodesis; of proximal interphalangeal joint, each joint

26474 of distal joint, each joint

26476 Lengthening of tendon, extensor, hand or finger, each tendon

26477 Shortening of tendon, extensor, hand or finger, each tendon

26478 Lengthening of tendon, flexor, hand or finger, each tendon

26479 Shortening of tendon, flexor, hand or finger, each tendon

26480 Transfer or transplant of tendon, carpometacarpal area or dorsum of hand; without free graft, each tendon

26483 with free tendon graft (includes obtaining graft), each tendon

26485 Transfer or transplant of tendon, palmar; without free tendon graft, each tendon

26489 with free tendon graft (includes obtaining graft), each tendon

26490 Opponensplasty; superficialis tendon transfer type, each tendon

FIGURE 2-34. Ligaments of the Fingers

Ligaments are tough, fibrous bands. Most **ligaments** in the hand stabilize articulating joints, eg, the collateral ligaments. A syndesmotic ligament binds two bones together, eg, the deep transverse metacarpal ligaments of the hand, without creating an articulating joint.

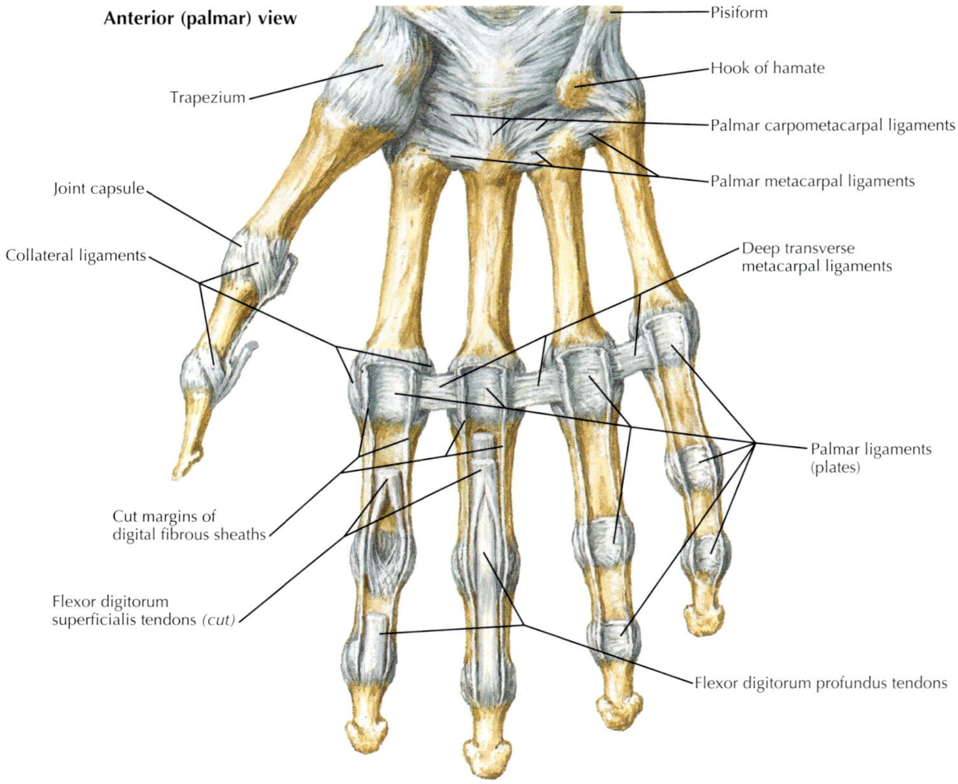

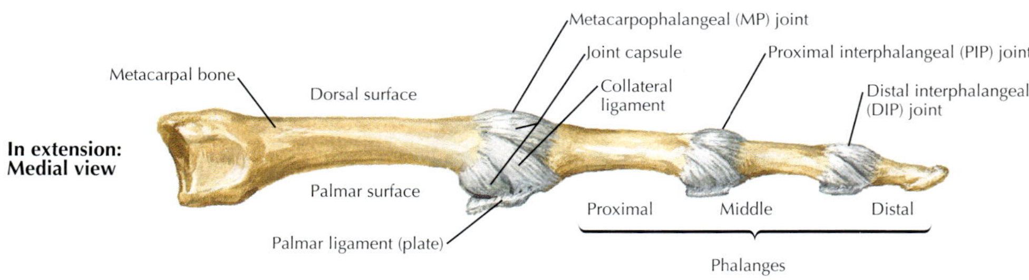

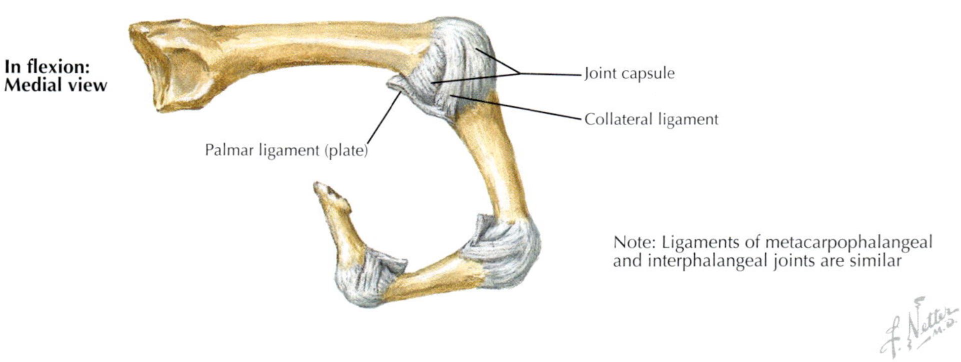

FIGURE 2-35. Flexor and Extensor Tendons of the Finger

Many **extensor** and **flexor** tendons of the fingers are **extrinsic**. The extensor tendons insert at the sagittal bands, the bases of the middle and distal phalanges, and an attachment at the base of the proximal phalanx. The paired action of **flexion** and **extension** keeps digits moving smoothly. Extensor tendon injuries occur when the finger is cut or crushed.

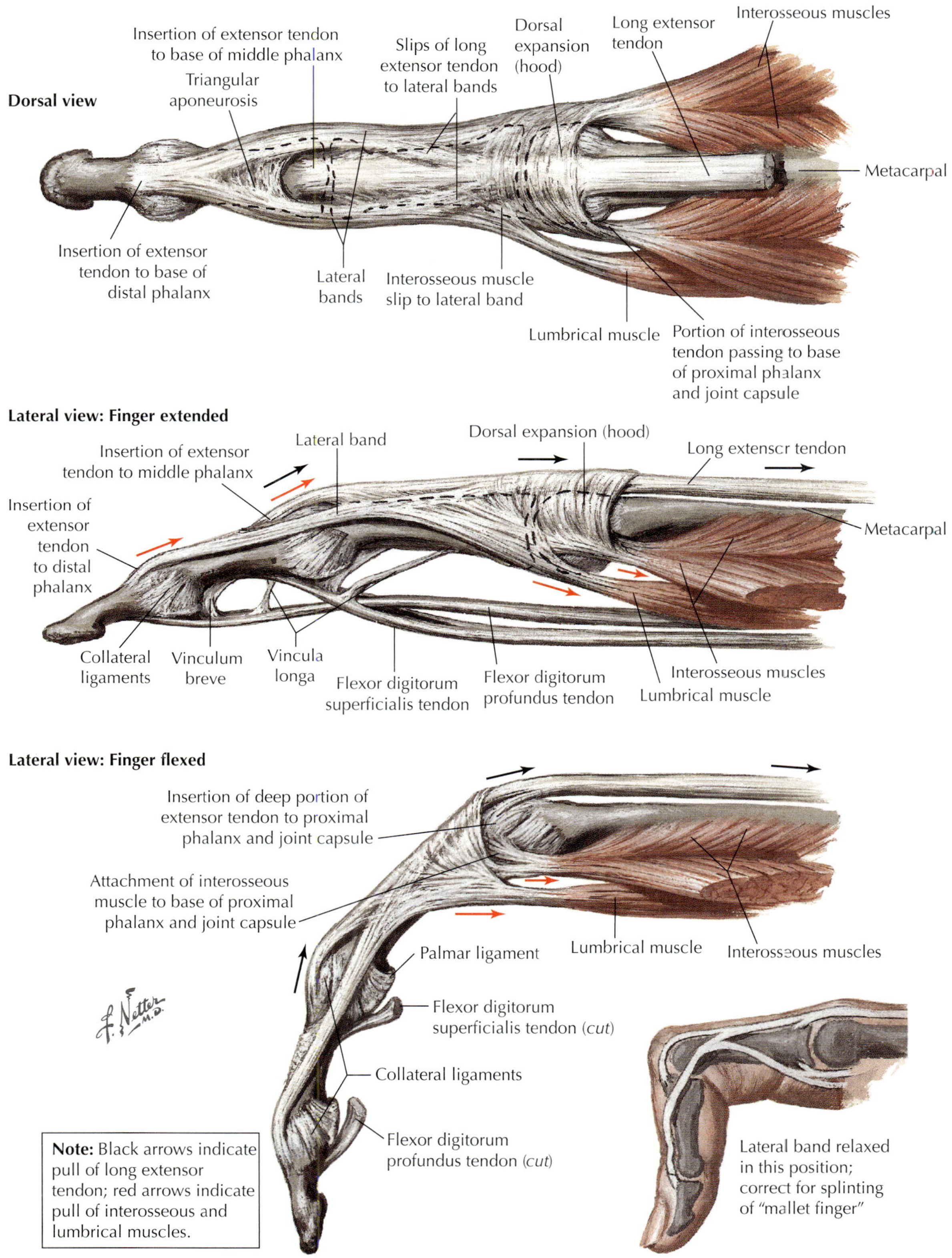

26492 tendon transfer with graft (includes obtaining graft), each tendon

26494 hypothenar muscle transfer

26496 other methods

26497 Transfer of tendon to restore intrinsic function; ring and small finger

26498 all 4 fingers

26499 Correction claw finger, other methods

26500 Reconstruction of tendon pulley, each tendon; with local tissues (separate procedure)

26502 with tendon or fascial graft (includes obtaining graft) (separate procedure)

26508 Release of thenar muscle(s) (eg, thumb contracture)

26510 Cross intrinsic transfer, each tendon

26516 Capsulodesis, metacarpophalangeal joint; single digit

26517 2 digits

26518 3 or 4 digits

26520 Capsulectomy or capsulotomy; metacarpophalangeal joint, each joint

26525 interphalangeal joint, each joint

26530 Arthroplasty, metacarpophalangeal joint; each joint

26531 with prosthetic implant, each joint

26535 Arthroplasty, interphalangeal joint; each joint

26536 with prosthetic implant, each joint

26540 Repair of collateral ligament, metacarpophalangeal or interphalangeal joint

26541 Reconstruction, collateral ligament, metacarpophalangeal joint, single; with tendon or fascial graft (includes obtaining graft)

26542 with local tissue (eg, adductor advancement)

26545 Reconstruction, collateral ligament, interphalangeal joint, single, including graft, each joint

26546 Repair non-union, metacarpal or phalanx (includes obtaining bone graft with or without external or internal fixation)

26548 Repair and reconstruction, finger, volar plate, interphalangeal joint

26550 Pollicization of a digit

26551 Transfer, toe-to-hand with microvascular anastomosis; great toe wrap-around with bone graft

26553 other than great toe, single

26554 other than great toe, double

26555 Transfer, finger to another position without microvascular anastomosis

26556 Transfer, free toe joint, with microvascular anastomosis

26560 Repair of syndactyly (web finger) each web space; with skin flaps

26561 with skin flaps and grafts

26562 complex (eg, involving bone, nails)

26565 Osteotomy; metacarpal, each

26567 phalanx of finger, each

26568 Osteoplasty, lengthening, metacarpal or phalanx

26580 Repair cleft hand

26587 Reconstruction of polydactylous digit, soft tissue and bone

26590 Repair macrodactylia, each digit

26591 Repair, intrinsic muscles of hand, each muscle

26593 Release, intrinsic muscles of hand, each muscle

26596 Excision of constricting ring of finger, with multiple Z-plasties

Fracture and/or Dislocation

Coding Atlas

Codes for fractures and dislocations are classified by the type of reduction and stabilization required. The type of fracture does not necessarily correspond to the type of treatment; a closed fracture may receive open treatment. Dislocations can occur in conjunction with fractures.

26600 Closed treatment of metacarpal fracture, single; without manipulation, each bone

26605 with manipulation, each bone

26607 Closed treatment of metacarpal fracture, with manipulation, with external fixation, each bone

26608 Percutaneous skeletal fixation of metacarpal fracture, each bone

26615 Open treatment of metacarpal fracture, single, includes internal fixation, when performed, each bone

26641 Closed treatment of carpometacarpal dislocation, thumb, with manipulation

26645 Closed treatment of carpometacarpal fracture dislocation, thumb (Bennett fracture), with manipulation

26650 Percutaneous skeletal fixation of carpometacarpal fracture dislocation, thumb (Bennett fracture), with manipulation

26665 Open treatment of carpometacarpal fracture dislocation, thumb (Bennett fracture), includes internal fixation, when performed

FIGURE 2-36. Bones of the Wrist and Hand

Five long, thin metacarpal bones of the palm extend to each digit of the hand. Each metacarpal is numbered, with "1" being the thumb and "5" being the pinky finger. The distal end of the metacarpal is rounded to form an oval joint with the phalanges. Each finger contains three phalanges: **proximal**, middle, and **distal**. The thumb contains only a proximal and distal phalanx.

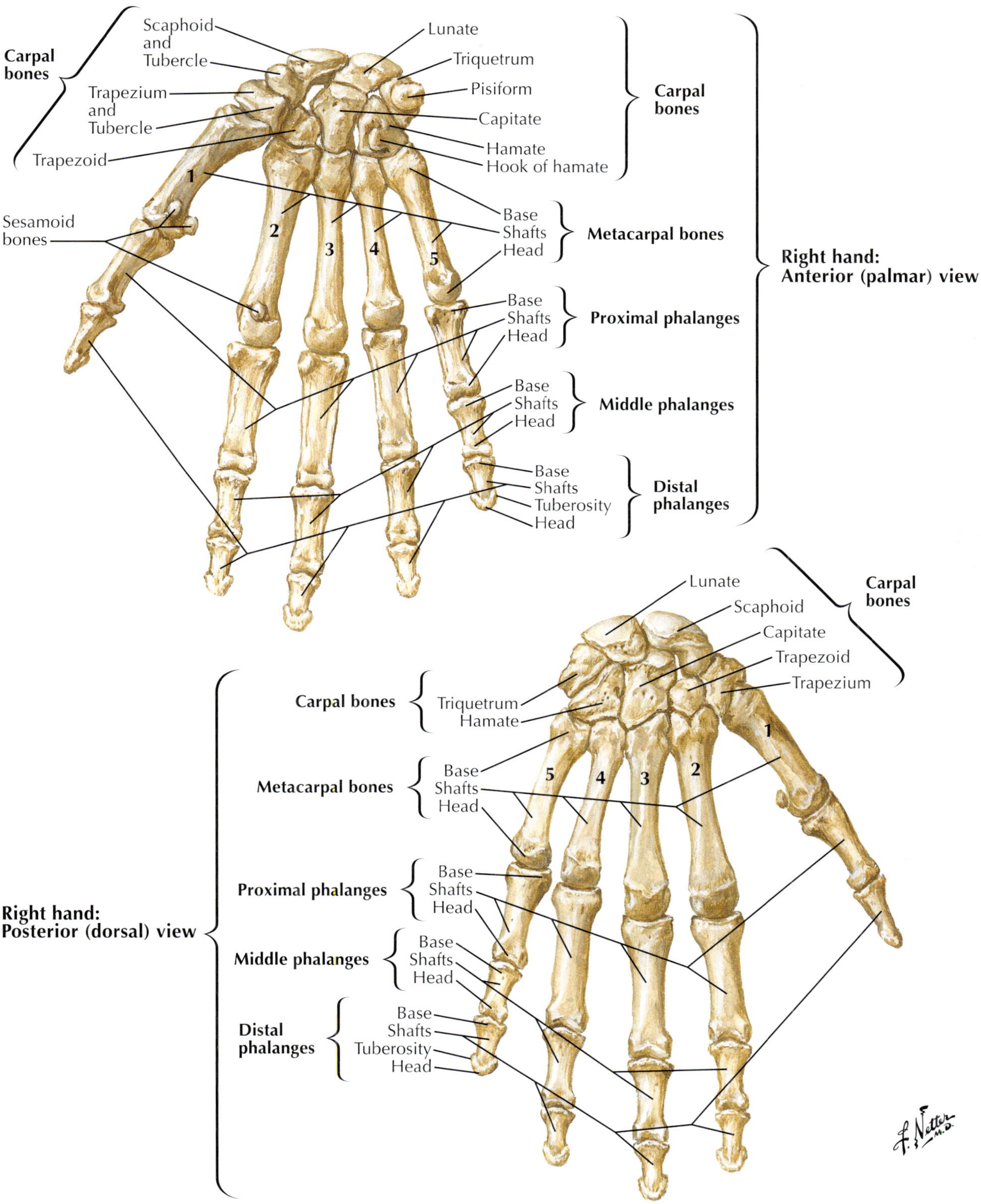

26670 Closed treatment of carpometacarpal dislocation, other than thumb, with manipulation, each joint; without anesthesia

26675 requiring anesthesia

26676 Percutaneous skeletal fixation of carpometacarpal dislocation, other than thumb, with manipulation, each joint

26685 Open treatment of carpometacarpal dislocation, other than thumb; includes internal fixation, when performed, each joint

26686 complex, multiple, or delayed reduction

26700 Closed treatment of metacarpophalangeal dislocation, single, with manipulation; without anesthesia

26705 requiring anesthesia

26706 Percutaneous skeletal fixation of metacarpophalangeal dislocation, single, with manipulation

26715 Open treatment of metacarpophalangeal dislocation, single, includes internal fixation, when performed

26720 Closed treatment of phalangeal shaft fracture, proximal or middle phalanx, finger or thumb; without manipulation, each

26725 with manipulation, with or without skin or skeletal traction, each

26727 Percutaneous skeletal fixation of unstable phalangeal shaft fracture, proximal or middle phalanx, finger or thumb, with manipulation, each

26735 Open treatment of phalangeal shaft fracture, proximal or middle phalanx, finger or thumb, includes internal fixation, when performed, each

26740 Closed treatment of articular fracture, involving metacarpophalangeal or interphalangeal joint; without manipulation, each

26742 with manipulation, each

26746 Open treatment of articular fracture, involving metacarpophalangeal or interphalangeal joint, includes internal fixation, when performed, each

26750 Closed treatment of distal phalangeal fracture, finger or thumb; without manipulation, each

26755 with manipulation, each

26756 Percutaneous skeletal fixation of distal phalangeal fracture, finger or thumb, each

26765 Open treatment of distal phalangeal fracture, finger or thumb, includes internal fixation, when performed, each

26770 Closed treatment of interphalangeal joint dislocation, single, with manipulation; without anesthesia

26775 requiring anesthesia

26776 Percutaneous skeletal fixation of interphalangeal joint dislocation, single, with manipulation

26785 Open treatment of interphalangeal joint dislocation, includes internal fixation, when performed, single

Arthrodesis

Coding Atlas

In **arthrodesis**, the joint is surgically fused and immobilized. Bone **grafts** may be placed to fix the joint; otherwise, hardware is placed. Code choice is based on the joint(s) treated.

26820 **Fusion** in opposition, thumb, with **autogenous** graft (includes obtaining graft)

26841 **Arthrodesis**, carpometacarpal joint, thumb, with or without **internal fixation**;

26842 with **autograft** (includes obtaining graft)

26843 Arthrodesis, carpometacarpal joint, digit, other than thumb, each;

26844 with autograft (includes obtaining graft)

26850 Arthrodesis, metacarpophalangeal joint, with or without internal fixation;

26852 with autograft (includes obtaining graft)

26860 Arthrodesis, interphalangeal joint, with or without internal fixation;

✚ **26861** each additional interphalangeal joint (List separately in addition to code for primary procedure)

26862 with autograft (includes obtaining graft)

✚ **26863** with autograft (includes obtaining graft), each additional joint (List separately in addition to code for primary procedure)

Amputation

Coding Atlas

Soft tissue and bone are excised in amputation. In some cases, a flap may be required to cover the defect created. Codes 26951 and 26952 are used to report complete or partial amputation of a finger/thumb.

26910 Amputation, metacarpal, with finger or thumb (ray amputation), single, with or without **interosseous** transfer

26951 Amputation, finger or thumb, primary or secondary, any joint or phalanx, single, including **neurectomies**; with direct closure

26952 with local advancement **flaps** (V-Y, hood)

Pelvis and Hip Joint

Incision

Coding Atlas

Decompression fasciotomy (code 27027) is performed to relieve **compartment syndrome** (CS), a condition in which pressure builds within a muscle bound by fascia. CS causes pressure and **ischemia** in the tissues within the compartment and can lead to tissue **necrosis**.

26990 Incision and drainage, pelvis or hip joint area; deep abscess or hematoma

26991 infected bursa

26992 Incision, bone cortex, pelvis and/or hip joint (eg, osteomyelitis or bone abscess)

27000 Tenotomy, adductor of hip, percutaneous (separate procedure)

27001 Tenotomy, adductor of hip, open

27003 Tenotomy, adductor, subcutaneous, open, with obturator neurectomy

27005 Tenotomy, hip flexor(s), open (separate procedure)

27006 Tenotomy, abductors and/or extensor(s) of hip, open (separate procedure)

27025 Fasciotomy, hip or thigh, any type

27027 Decompression fasciotomy(ies), pelvic (buttock) compartment(s) (eg, gluteus medius-minimus, gluteus maximus, iliopsoas, and/or tensor fascia lata muscle), unilateral

27030 Arthrotomy, hip, with drainage (eg, infection)

27033 Arthrotomy, hip, including exploration or removal of loose or foreign body

27035 Denervation, hip joint, intrapelvic or extrapelvic intra-articular branches of sciatic, femoral, or obturator nerves

27036 Capsulectomy or capsulotomy, hip, with or without excision of heterotopic bone, with release of hip flexor muscles (ie, gluteus medius, gluteus minimus, tensor fascia latae, rectus femoris, sartorius, iliopsoas)

Excision

Coding Atlas

Size and **tumor** origin play a role in code selection for excision of soft tissue tumors. The entire resection is measured, not the diameter of the lesion itself, to determine the excision size. Excision of a tumor originating in the integument, eg, **melanoma**, is reported with Integumentary System excision codes.

27040 Biopsy, soft tissue of pelvis and hip area; superficial

27041 deep, subfascial or intramuscular

27043 Code is out of numerical sequence. See 27040-27080

27045 Code is out of numerical sequence. See 27040-27080

27047 Excision, tumor, soft tissue of pelvis and hip area, subcutaneous; less than 3 cm

27043 3 cm or greater

27048 Excision, tumor, soft tissue of pelvis and hip area, subfascial (eg, intramuscular); less than 5 cm

27045 5 cm or greater

27049 Radical resection of tumor (eg, sarcoma), soft tissue of pelvis and hip area; less than 5 cm

27059 5 cm or greater

27050 Arthrotomy, with biopsy; sacroiliac joint

27052 hip joint

27054 Arthrotomy with synovectomy, hip joint

27057 Decompression fasciotomy(ies), pelvic (buttock) compartment(s) (eg, gluteus medius-minimus, gluteus maximus, iliopsoas, and/or tensor fascia lata muscle) with debridement of nonviable muscle, unilateral

27059 Code is out of numerical sequence. See 27040-27080

27060 Excision; ischial bursa

27062 trochanteric bursa or calcification

27065 Excision of bone cyst or benign tumor, wing of ilium, symphysis pubis, or greater trochanter of femur; superficial, includes autograft, when performed

27066 deep (subfascial), includes autograft, when performed

27067 with autograft requiring separate incision

27070 Partial excision, wing of ilium, symphysis pubis, or greater trochanter of femur, (craterization, saucerization) (eg, osteomyelitis or bone abscess); superficial

27071 deep (subfascial or intramuscular)

27075 Radical resection of tumor; wing of ilium, 1 pubic or ischial ramus or symphysis pubis

27076 ilium, including acetabulum, both pubic rami, or ischium and acetabulum

FIGURE 2-37. Hip Joint

The hip joint secures the femur head to the pelvic acetabulum, connecting the **axial skeleton** to the lower extremity. This synovial ball-and-socket joint is weight-bearing. The bony pelvis is formed by the fusion of ilium, ischium, and pubis, creating the right and left hip bone (os coxae). The head, neck, and greater and lesser trochanters of the femur are considered part of the hip joint.

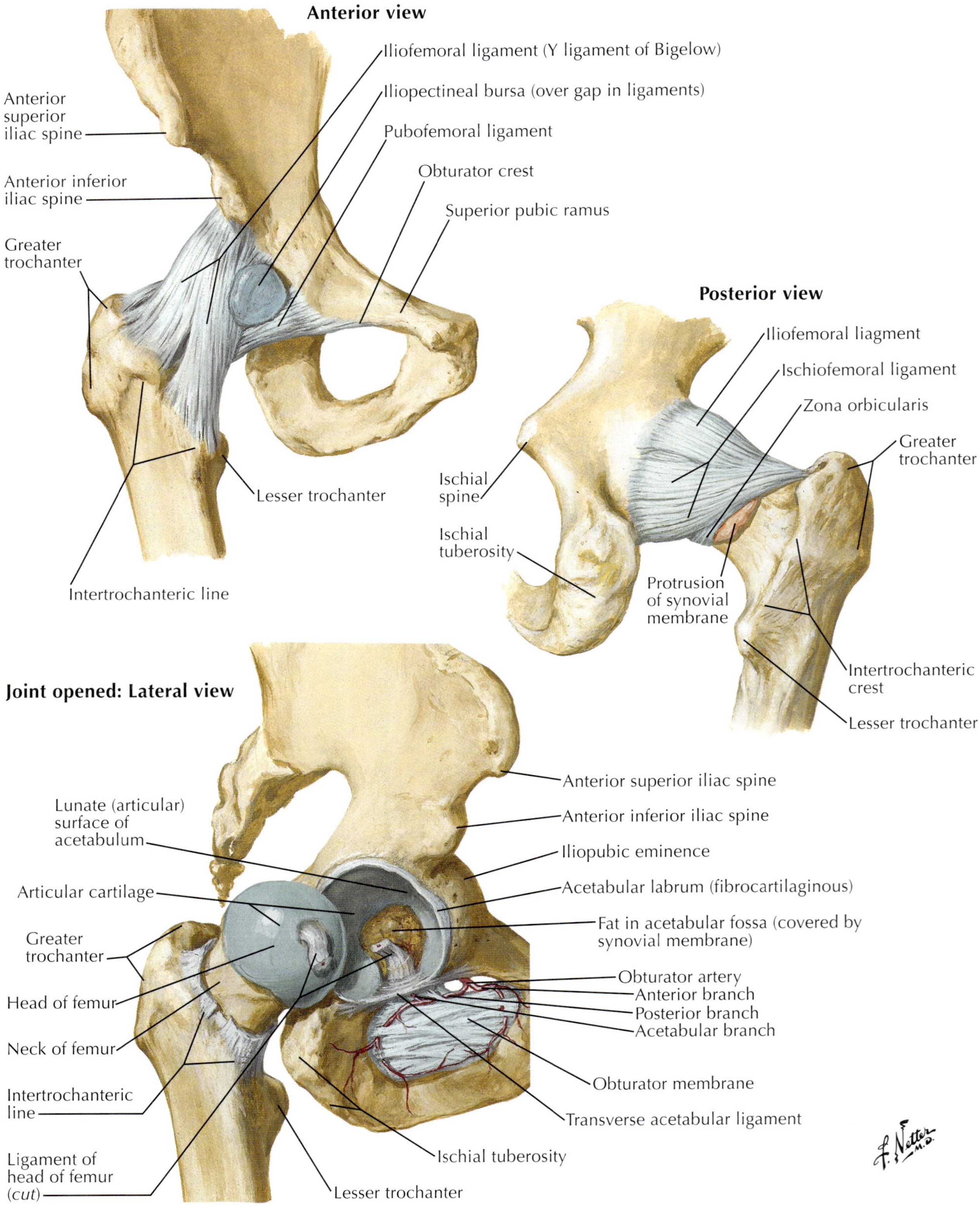

FIGURE 2-38. Muscles of the Hip

Many hip muscles stabilize the hip joint and provide its movement and strength. The muscles fall into four groups based on their location: anterior, posterior, adductor, and abductor. **Anterior** muscles flex the thigh at the hip and include iliopsoas and quadriceps. **Posterior** muscles straighten the thigh at the hip. These include gluteus maximus and hamstrings. The **adductor** group includes groin muscles. The **abductors** are on the **lateral** side of the thigh.

Superficial dissection

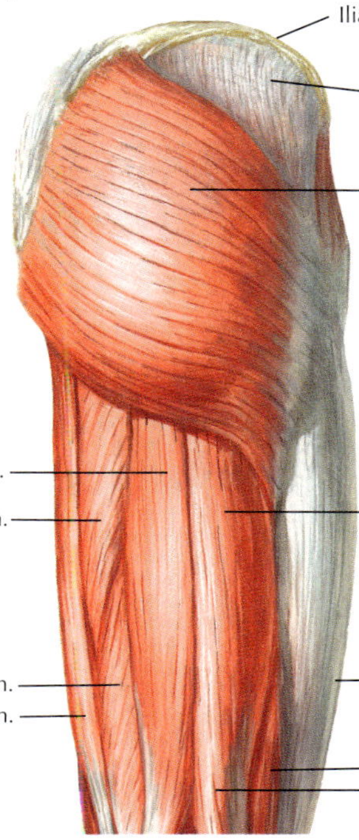

Deep dissection

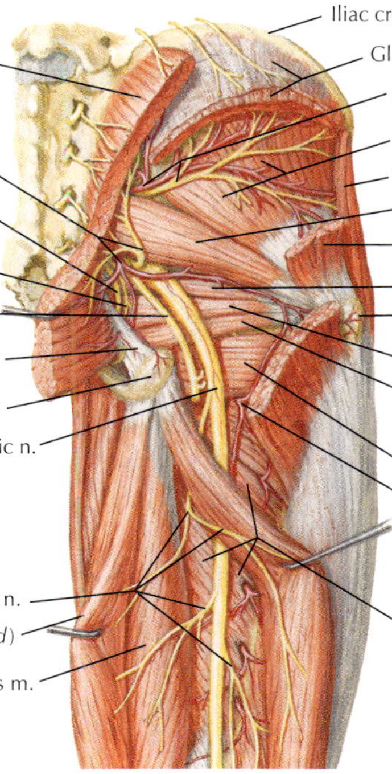

27077 innominate bone, total

27078 ischial tuberosity and greater trochanter of femur

27080 Coccygectomy, primary

Introduction or Removal

Coding Atlas

A **foreign body** is an object that has become lodged in the body by accident. A **prosthesis** is an object that has been placed in the body to assume the role of a natural body part, eg, a joint prosthesis.

27086 Removal of foreign body, pelvis or hip; subcutaneous tissue

27087 deep (subfascial or intramuscular)

27090 Removal of hip prosthesis; (separate procedure)

27091 complicated, including total hip prosthesis, methylmethacrylate with or without insertion of spacer

27093 Injection procedure for hip arthrography; without anesthesia

27095 with anesthesia

27096 Injection procedure for sacroiliac joint, anesthetic/steroid, with image guidance (fluoroscopy or CT) including arthrography when performed

Repair, Revision, and/or Reconstruction

Coding Atlas

In a **unipolar** hemiarthroplasty, there is an **articulation** between the prosthetic head and the **native** acetabulum. In **bipolar** hemiarthroplasty, the **prosthetic** head has a component that is an artificial acetabulum cup, however, no work is done on the native acetabulum. In a total hip arthroplasty, the native acetabulum is sculpted to fit a prosthetic cup. **Hemiarthroplasty**, which is reported using code 27125, should not be considered when listing the code for a partial hip replacement that is the result of traumatic hip fracture. For prosthesis placed following hip fracture, see code 27238.

27097 Release or recession, hamstring, proximal

27098 Transfer, adductor to ischium

27100 Transfer external oblique muscle to greater trochanter including fascial or tendon extension (graft)

27105 Transfer paraspinal muscle to hip (includes fascial or tendon extension graft)

27110 Transfer iliopsoas; to greater trochanter of femur

27111 to femoral neck

27120 Acetabuloplasty; (eg, Whitman, Colonna, Haygroves, or cup type)

27122 resection, femoral head (eg, Girdlestone procedure)

27125 Hemiarthroplasty, hip, partial (eg, femoral stem prosthesis, bipolar arthroplasty)

27130 Arthroplasty, acetabular and proximal femoral prosthetic replacement (total hip arthroplasty), with or without autograft or allograft

27132 Conversion of previous hip surgery to total hip arthroplasty, with or without autograft or allograft

27134 Revision of total hip arthroplasty; both components, with or without autograft or allograft

27137 acetabular component only, with or without autograft or allograft

27138 femoral component only, with or without allograft

27140 Osteotomy and transfer of greater trochanter of femur (separate procedure)

27146 Osteotomy, iliac, acetabular or innominate bone;

27147 with open reduction of hip

27151 with femoral osteotomy

27156 with femoral osteotomy and with open reduction of hip

27158 Osteotomy, pelvis, bilateral (eg, congenital malformation)

27161 Osteotomy, femoral neck (separate procedure)

27165 Osteotomy, intertrochanteric or subtrochanteric including internal or external fixation and/or cast

27170 Bone graft, femoral head, neck, intertrochanteric or subtrochanteric area (includes obtaining bone graft)

27175 Treatment of slipped femoral epiphysis; by traction, without reduction

27176 by single or multiple pinning, in situ

27177 Open treatment of slipped femoral epiphysis; single or multiple pinning or bone graft (includes obtaining graft)

27178 closed manipulation with single or multiple pinning

27179 osteoplasty of femoral neck (Heyman type procedure)

27181 osteotomy and internal fixation

27185 Epiphyseal arrest by epiphysiodesis or stapling, greater trochanter of femur

27187 Prophylactic treatment (nailing, pinning, plating or wiring) with or without methylmethacrylate, femoral neck and proximal femur

FIGURE 2-39. Pelvic Fracture With No Pelvic Ring Disruption

The ilium, ischium, and pubis form the **pelvic ring** with the sacrum. Fractures that are through the bone of the ring are documented as "with pelvic ring disruption." This type of fracture greatly affects the stability of the pelvis. Nondisplaced fractures that do not interrupt the pelvic ring may be effectively treated with bed rest and pain management.

Avulsions

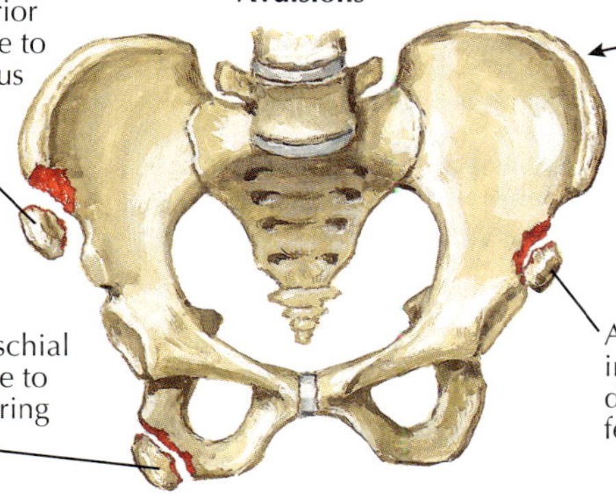

Fracture of iliac wing

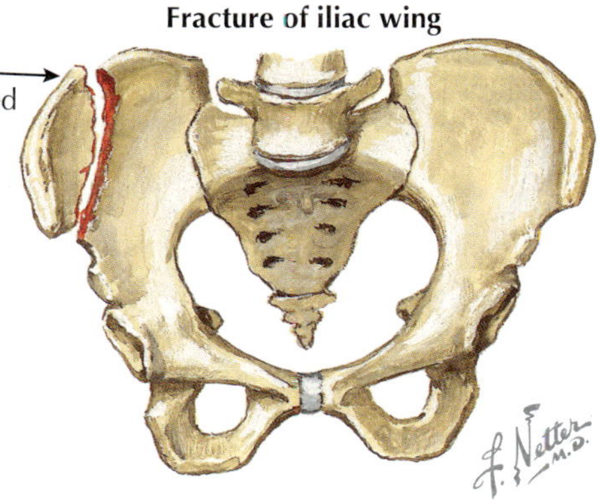

Fracture of one pubic or ischial ramus

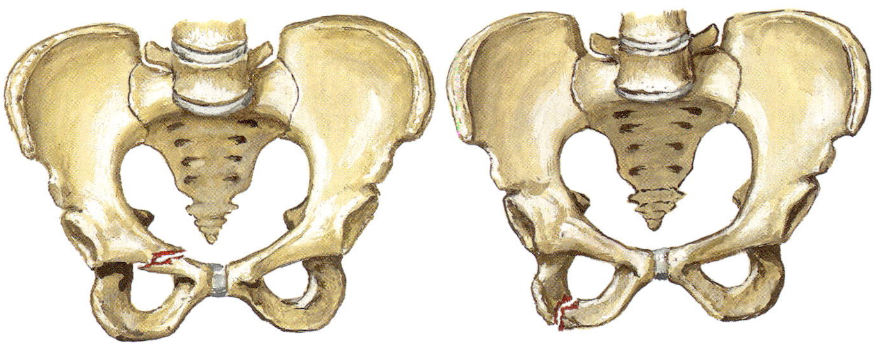

Isolated fracture of one pubic or ischial ramus requires only bed rest until pain diminishes, followed by limited activity for 4–5 weeks, provided there is no visceral or vascular injury.

Fractures of sacrum

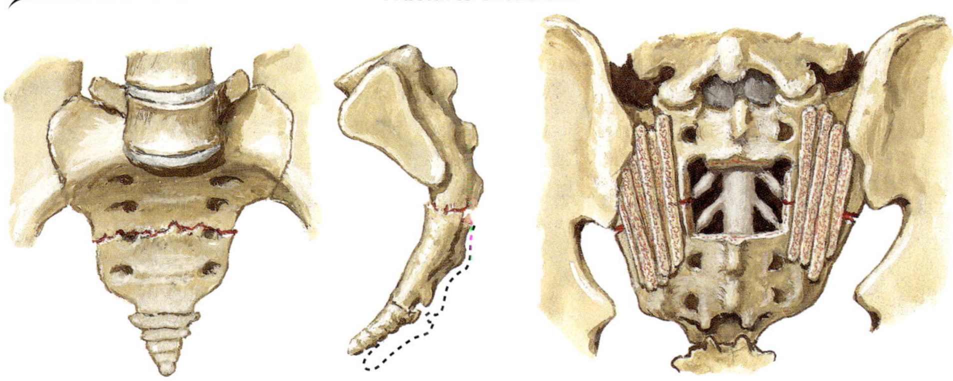

Impacted transverse fracture that is minimally displaced is most common type. Conservative treatment sufficient unless there is nerve injury.

Sacral laminectomy and bone grafts from ilium used for sharply angulated fractures with nerve injury.

Fracture of coccyx

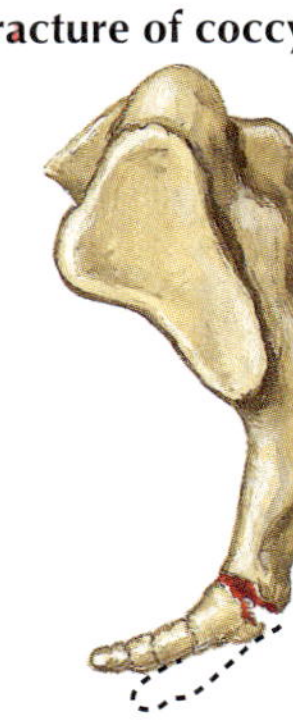

Fracture usually requires no treatment other than care in sitting; inflatable ring helpful. Pain may persist for long time.

Fracture and/or Dislocation

Coding Atlas

Percutaneous skeletal fixation describes pins that are inserted through the skin and into the bone fragments to secure the bones' position. This is done without **direct visualization** of the bone. **Internal fixation** describes the application of pins, nails, or other hardware secured to the bone. **External fixation** describes multiple pins placed through bone cortex both proximal and distal to the fracture. The pins are attached to an external fixator.

27193 Closed treatment of pelvic ring fracture, dislocation, diastasis or subluxation; without manipulation

27194 with manipulation, requiring more than local anesthesia

27200 Closed treatment of coccygeal fracture

27202 Open treatment of coccygeal fracture

27215 Open treatment of iliac spine(s), tuberosity avulsion, or iliac wing fracture(s), unilateral, for pelvic bone fracture patterns that do not disrupt the pelvic ring, includes internal fixation, when performed

27216 Percutaneous skeletal fixation of posterior pelvic bone fracture and/or dislocation, for fracture patterns that disrupt the pelvic ring, unilateral (includes ipsilateral ilium, sacroiliac joint and/or sacrum)

27217 Open treatment of anterior pelvic bone fracture and/or dislocation for fracture patterns that disrupt the pelvic ring, unilateral, includes internal fixation, when performed (includes pubic symphysis and/or ipsilateral superior/inferior rami)

27218 Open treatment of posterior pelvic bone fracture and/or dislocation, for fracture patterns that disrupt the pelvic ring, unilateral, includes internal fixation, when performed (includes ipsilateral ilium, sacroiliac joint and/or sacrum)

27220 Closed treatment of acetabulum (hip socket) fracture(s); without manipulation

27222 with manipulation, with or without skeletal traction

27226 Open treatment of posterior or anterior acetabular wall fracture, with internal fixation

27227 Open treatment of acetabular fracture(s) involving anterior or posterior (one) column, or a fracture running transversely across the acetabulum, with internal fixation

27228 Open treatment of acetabular fracture(s) involving anterior and posterior (two) columns, includes T-fracture and both column fracture with complete articular detachment, or single column or transverse fracture with associated acetabular wall fracture, with internal fixation

27230 Closed treatment of femoral fracture, proximal end, neck; without manipulation

27232 with manipulation, with or without skeletal traction

27235 Percutaneous skeletal fixation of femoral fracture, proximal end, neck

27236 Open treatment of femoral fracture, proximal end, neck, internal fixation or prosthetic replacement

27238 Closed treatment of intertrochanteric, peritrochanteric, or subtrochanteric femoral fracture; without manipulation

27240 with manipulation, with or without skin or skeletal traction

27244 Treatment of intertrochanteric, peritrochanteric, or subtrochanteric femoral fracture; with plate/screw type implant, with or without cerclage

27245 with intramedullary implant, with or without interlocking screws and/or cerclage

27246 Closed treatment of greater trochanteric fracture, without manipulation

27248 Open treatment of greater trochanteric fracture, includes internal fixation, when performed

27250 Closed treatment of hip dislocation, traumatic; without anesthesia

27252 requiring anesthesia

27253 Open treatment of hip dislocation, traumatic, without internal fixation

27254 Open treatment of hip dislocation, traumatic, with acetabular wall and femoral head fracture, with or without internal or external fixation

27256 Treatment of spontaneous hip dislocation (developmental, including congenital or pathological), by abduction, splint or traction; without anesthesia, without manipulation

27257 with manipulation, requiring anesthesia

27258 Open treatment of spontaneous hip dislocation (developmental, including congenital or pathological), replacement of femoral head in acetabulum (including tenotomy, etc);

27259 with femoral shaft shortening

27265 Closed treatment of post hip arthroplasty dislocation; without anesthesia

27266 requiring regional or general anesthesia

27267 Closed treatment of femoral fracture, proximal end, head; without manipulation

27268 with manipulation

27269 Open treatment of femoral fracture, proximal end, head, includes internal fixation, when performed

FIGURE 2-40. Femur

The femur is the longest and strongest bone in the body and extends from hip to knee. It is a very vascular bone, and fracture may result in blood loss requiring transfusion. Fractures of the head, neck, trochanteric, or subtrochanteric portion of the femur are reported with codes in the Hip subsection within the CPT code set. Fractures of more **distal** portions of the femur are reported with codes from the Femur (Thigh Region) and Knee Joint subsection.

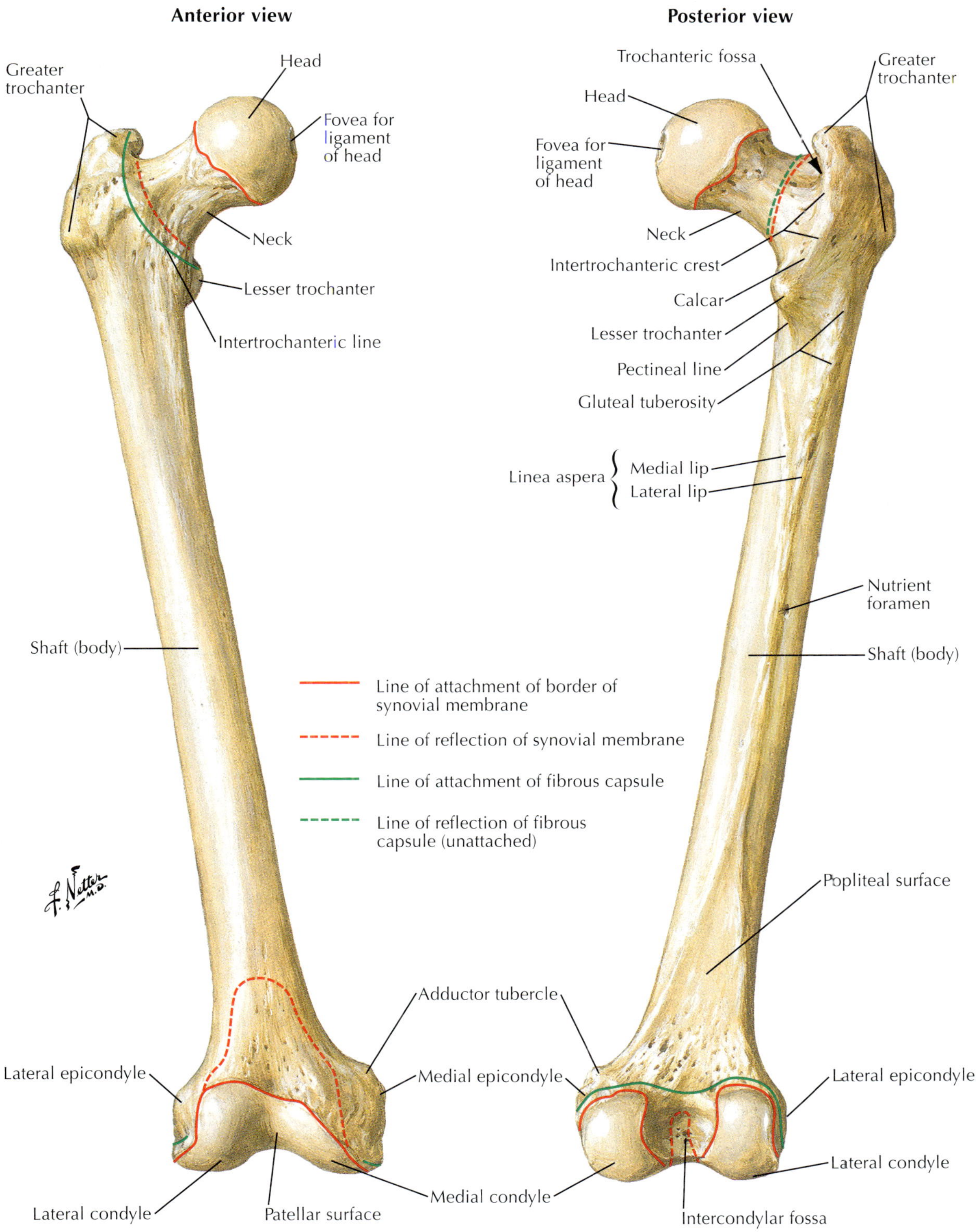

Manipulation

27275 Manipulation, hip joint, requiring general anesthesia

Arthrodesis

Coding Atlas

Sacroiliac joint **arthrodesis** is joint **fusion** of the iliac bone to the sacrum. This procedure may be performed as part of the treatment for sacral **tumor**, infection, injury associated with **pelvic ring** fracture, or to correct a spinal deformity.

27279 Arthrodesis, sacroiliac joint, percutaneous or minimally invasive (indirect visualization), with image guidance, includes obtaining bone graft when performed, and placement of transfixing device

27280 Arthrodesis, open, sacroiliac joint, including obtaining bone graft, including instrumentation, when performed

27282 Arthrodesis, symphysis pubis (including obtaining graft)

27284 Arthrodesis, hip joint (including obtaining graft);

27286 with subtrochanteric osteotomy

Amputation

Coding Atlas

In a hindquarter amputation, the lower extremity is excised with the inclusion of the hip joint and a portion of the pelvis. In the **disarticulation** of the hip, the femur and everything distal to the femur is excised.

27290 Interpelviabdominal amputation (hindquarter amputation)

27295 Disarticulation of hip

Femur (Thigh Region) and Knee Joint

Incision

Coding Atlas

A joint is completely enclosed in a ligamentous capsule. **Arthrotomy** is a surgical incision into a joint capsule. Code 27310 is used to report arthrotomy with **foreign body** (FB) removal. Removal of an FB documented as embedded on the exterior of the joint capsule or described as an FB that may have penetrated the joint capsule does not qualify as arthrotomy. Documentation must state that the joint capsule has been surgically opened.

27301 Incision and drainage, deep abscess, bursa, or hematoma, thigh or knee region

27303 Incision, deep, with opening of bone cortex, femur or knee (eg, osteomyelitis or bone abscess)

27305 Fasciotomy, iliotibial (tenotomy), open

27306 Tenotomy, percutaneous, adductor or hamstring; single tendon (separate procedure)

27307 multiple tendons

27310 Arthrotomy, knee, with exploration, drainage, or removal of foreign body (eg, infection)

Excision

Coding Atlas

Biopsy, which is described using code 27323, involves tissue from above the superficial **fascia** and beneath subcutaneous tissue, usually in the layer of fat over the fascia. Size and **tumor** origin play a role in code selection for excision of soft tissue tumors of the thigh. The entire resection is measured, not the diameter of the lesion itself, to determine the excision size. Excision of a tumor originating in the integument, eg, **melanoma**, is reported with Integumentary System excision codes.

27323 Biopsy, soft tissue of thigh or knee area; superficial

27324 deep (subfascial or intramuscular)

27325 Neurectomy, hamstring muscle

27326 Neurectomy, popliteal (gastrocnemius)

27327 Excision, tumor, soft tissue of thigh or knee area, subcutaneous; less than 3 cm

27337 3 cm or greater

27328 Excision, tumor, soft tissue of thigh or knee area, subfascial (eg, intramuscular); less than 5 cm

27329 Code is out of numerical sequence. See 27323-27365

27339 5 cm or greater

27330 Arthrotomy, knee; with synovial biopsy only

27331 including joint exploration, biopsy, or removal of loose or foreign bodies

27332 Arthrotomy, with excision of semilunar cartilage (meniscectomy) knee; medial OR lateral

27333 medial AND lateral

27334 Arthrotomy, with synovectomy, knee; anterior OR posterior

27335 anterior AND posterior including popliteal area

27337 Code is out of numerical sequence. See 27323-27365

27339 Code is out of numerical sequence. See 27323-27365

FIGURE 2-41. Knee Joint

The knee is a hinge formed by the connection of three joints. The femur's medial and lateral condyles **articulate** with the tibia's medial and lateral condyles, and the third joint is between the patella and the femur. The patella protects the knee from its position **anterior** to the knee joint and slides up and down as the leg moves.

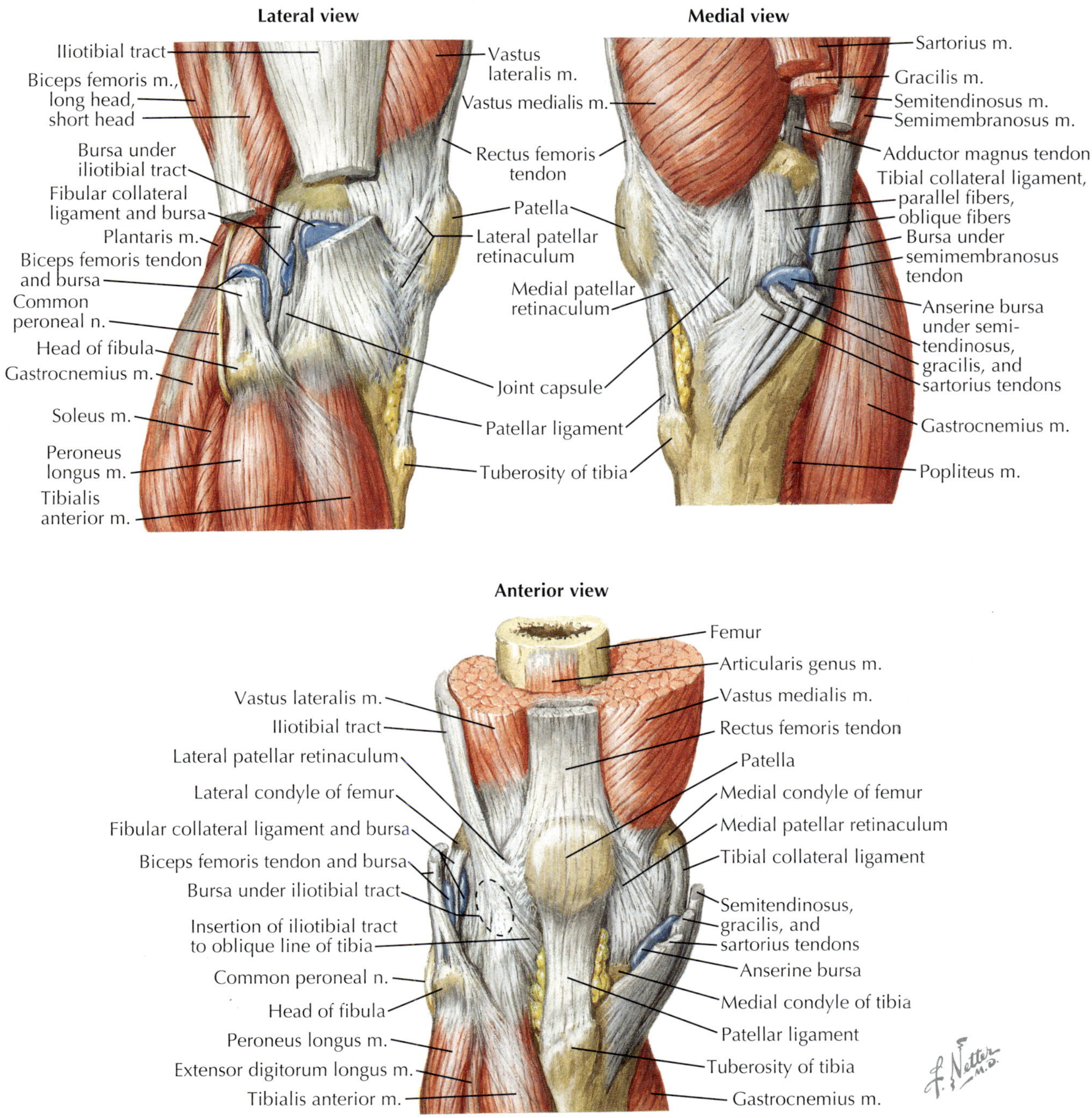

FIGURE 2-42. Interior of the Knee

The knee has three compartments: medial, lateral, and patello-femoral. The **medial** compartment is the area of joint contact between the femur and tibia on the inside of the knee (eg, right side of left knee and left side of right knee). The **lateral** compartment is the outside (eg, left side of left knee and right side of right knee). The patello-femoral compartment is the area at which the patella articulates with the femur.

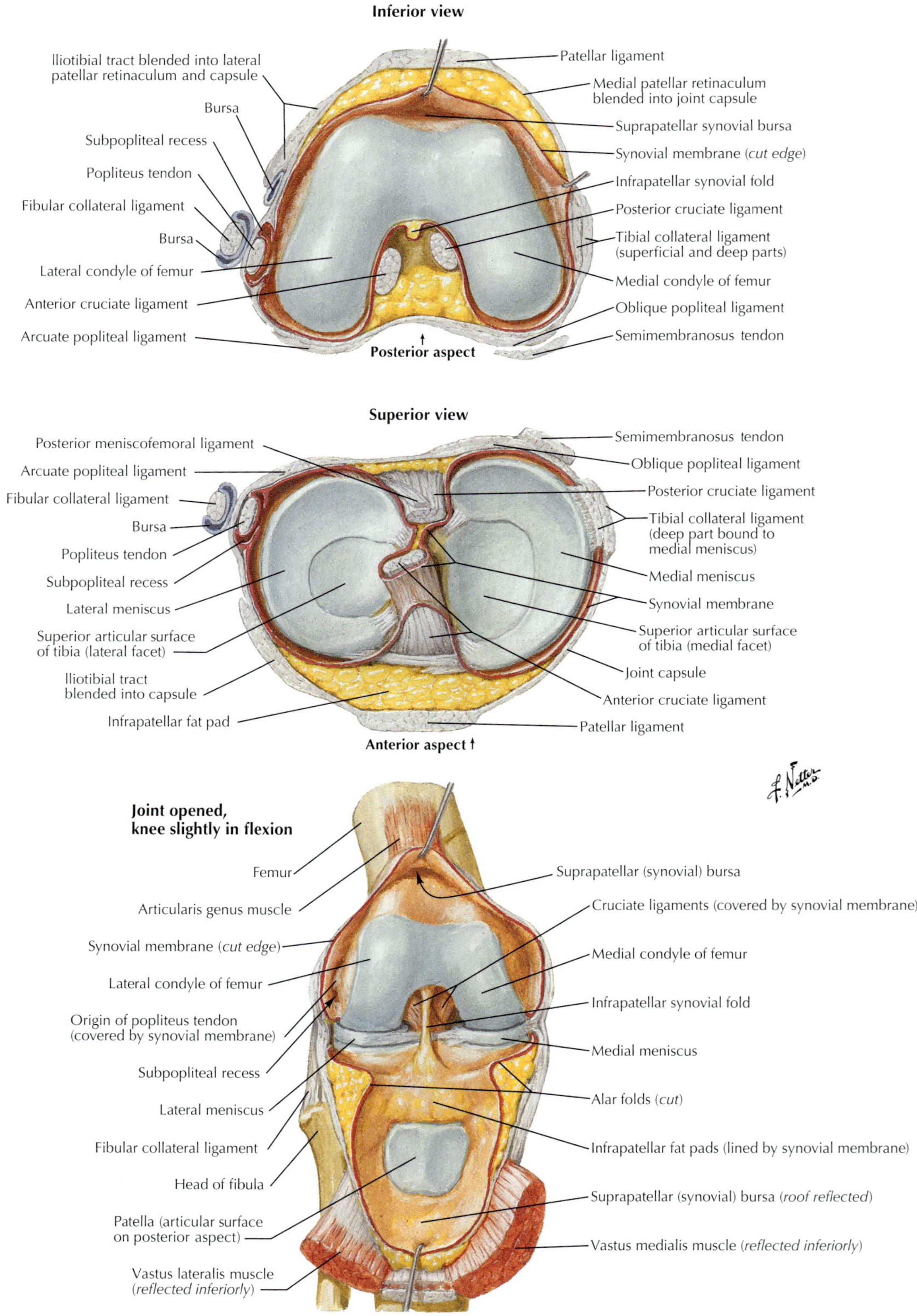

27340 Excision, prepatellar bursa

27345 Excision of synovial cyst of popliteal space (eg, Baker's cyst)

27347 Excision of lesion of meniscus or capsule (eg, cyst, ganglion), knee

27350 Patellectomy or hemipatellectomy

27355 Excision or curettage of bone cyst or benign tumor of femur;

27356 with allograft

27357 with autograft (includes obtaining graft)

✚ **27358** with internal fixation (List in addition to code for primary procedure)

27360 Partial excision (craterization, saucerization, or diaphysectomy) bone, femur, proximal tibia and/or fibula (eg, osteomyelitis or bone abscess)

27329 Radical resection of tumor (eg, sarcoma), soft tissue of thigh or knee area; less than 5 cm

27364 5 cm or greater

27365 Radical resection of tumor, femur or knee

Introduction or Removal

Coding Atlas

Foreign body (FB) removal is reported using code 27372 when the FB is in muscle or deep fascia or in soft tissue adjacent to the knee capsule. Code 27372 does not include arthrotomy; see code 27331.

27370 Injection of contrast for knee arthrography

27372 Removal of foreign body, deep, thigh region or knee area

Repair, Revision, and/or Reconstruction

Coding Atlas

In arthroplasty, the native joint surface(s) are replaced with prosthetic parts. In revision arthroplasty, an existing prosthesis is replaced with a new component. In some cases, infection requires that an existing prosthesis be removed; however, a new prosthesis is not placed until weeks later when the infection has been eliminated.

27380 Suture of infrapatellar tendon; primary

27381 secondary reconstruction, including fascial or tendon graft

27385 Suture of quadriceps or hamstring muscle rupture; primary

27386 secondary reconstruction, including fascial or tendon graft

27390 Tenotomy, open, hamstring, knee to hip; single tendon

27391 multiple tendons, 1 leg

27392 multiple tendons, bilateral

27393 Lengthening of hamstring tendon; single tendon

27394 multiple tendons, 1 leg

27395 multiple tendons, bilateral

27396 Transplant or transfer (with muscle redirection or rerouting), thigh (eg, extensor to flexor); single tendon

27397 multiple tendons

27400 Transfer, tendon or muscle, hamstrings to femur (eg, Egger's type procedure)

27403 Arthrotomy with meniscus repair, knee

27405 Repair, primary, torn ligament and/or capsule, knee; collateral

27407 cruciate

27409 collateral and cruciate ligaments

27412 Autologous chondrocyte implantation, knee

27415 Osteochondral allograft, knee, open

27416 Osteochondral autograft(s), knee, open (eg, mosaicplasty) (includes harvesting of autograft[s])

27418 Anterior tibial tubercleplasty (eg, Maquet type procedure)

27420 Reconstruction of dislocating patella; (eg, Hauser type procedure)

27422 with extensor realignment and/or muscle advancement or release (eg, Campbell, Goldwaite type procedure)

27424 with patellectomy

27425 Lateral retinacular release, open

27427 Ligamentous reconstruction (augmentation), knee; extra-articular

27428 intra-articular (open)

27429 intra-articular (open) and extra-articular

27430 Quadricepsplasty (eg, Bennett or Thompson type)

27435 Capsulotomy, posterior capsular release, knee

27437 Arthroplasty, patella; without prosthesis

27438 with prosthesis

27440 Arthroplasty, knee, tibial plateau;

27441 with debridement and partial synovectomy

27442 Arthroplasty, femoral condyles or tibial plateau(s), knee;

27443 with debridement and partial synovectomy

FIGURE 2-43. Ligaments of the Knee

Stability to the knee joint is provided by the medial collateral ligament (MCL), posterior cruciate ligament (PCL), and anterior cruciate ligament (ACL). The MCL and LCL limit sideways motion, and the PCL and ACL control the front and back motion of the knee. The MCL is also called the tibial collateral ligament.

Right knee in flexion: Anterior view

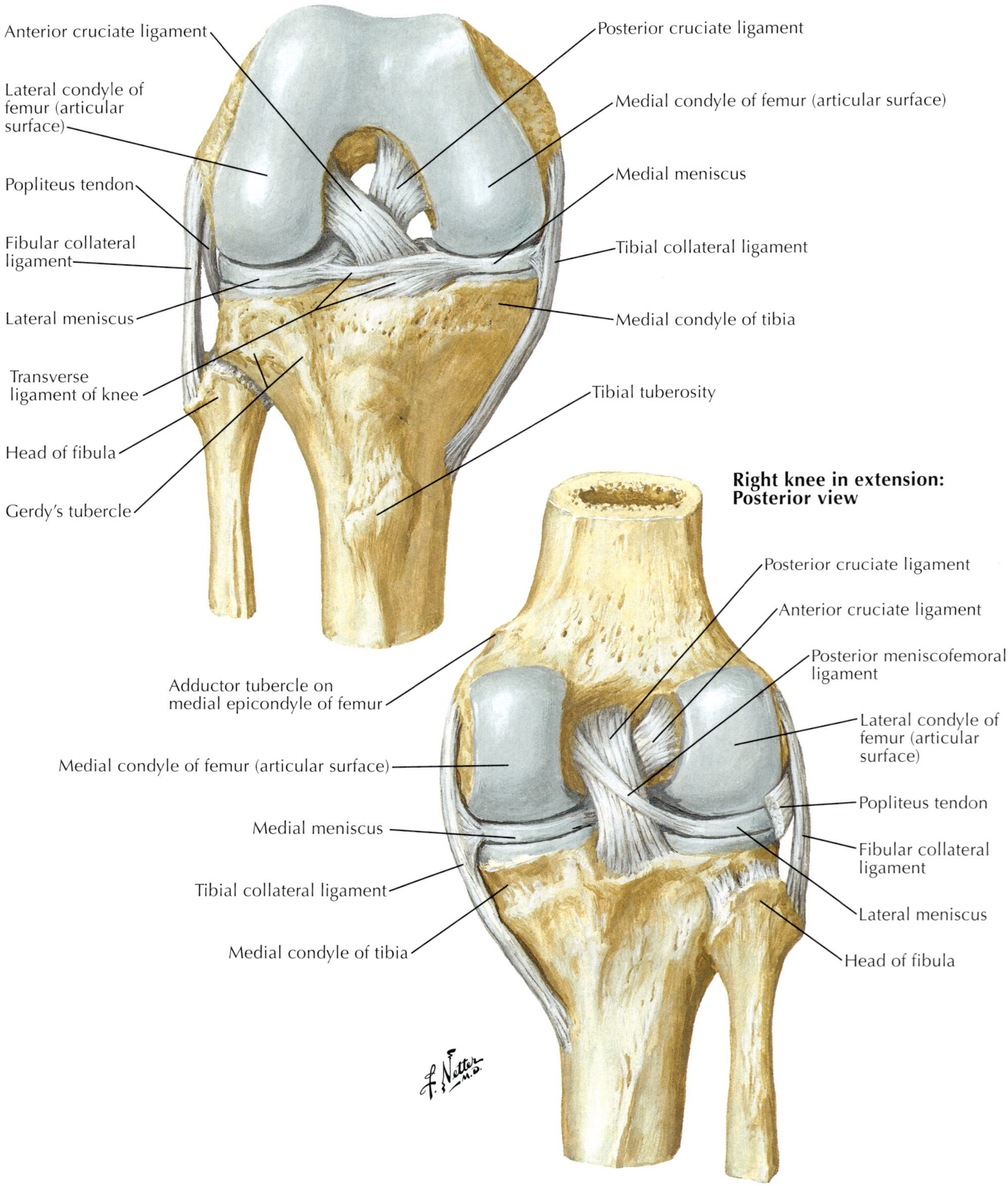

27445 Arthroplasty, knee, hinge prosthesis (eg, Walldius type)

27446 Arthroplasty, knee, condyle and plateau; medial OR lateral compartment

27447 medial AND lateral compartments with or without patella resurfacing (total knee arthroplasty)

27448 Osteotomy, femur, shaft or supracondylar; without fixation

27450 with fixation

27454 Osteotomy, multiple, with realignment on intramedullary rod, femoral shaft (eg, Sofield type procedure)

27455 Osteotomy, proximal tibia, including fibular excision or osteotomy (includes correction of genu varus [bowleg] or genu valgus [knock-knee]); before epiphyseal closure

27457 after epiphyseal closure

27465 Osteoplasty, femur; shortening (excluding 64876)

27466 lengthening

27468 combined, lengthening and shortening with femoral segment transfer

27470 Repair, nonunion or malunion, femur, distal to head and neck; without graft (eg, compression technique)

27472 with iliac or other autogenous bone graft (includes obtaining graft)

27475 Arrest, epiphyseal, any method (eg, epiphysiodesis); distal femur

27477 tibia and fibula, proximal

27479 combined distal femur, proximal tibia and fibula

27485 Arrest, hemiepiphyseal, distal femur or proximal tibia or fibula (eg, genu varus or valgus)

27486 Revision of total knee arthroplasty, with or without allograft; 1 component

27487 femoral and entire tibial component

27488 Removal of prosthesis, including total knee prosthesis, methylmethacrylate with or without insertion of spacer, knee

27495 Prophylactic treatment (nailing, pinning, plating, or wiring) with or without methylmethacrylate, femur

27496 Decompression fasciotomy, thigh and/or knee, 1 compartment (flexor or extensor or adductor);

27497 with debridement of nonviable muscle and/or nerve

27498 Decompression fasciotomy, thigh and/or knee, multiple compartments;

27499 with debridement of nonviable muscle and/or nerve

Fracture and/or Dislocation

Coding Atlas

Closed treatment of a fracture occurs when the fracture site is not surgically opened and directly viewed. In closed treatment, the physician may provide traction, manipulation, or no reduction at all. Open treatment of a fracture occurs when the fracture site is surgically opened and viewed. Internal fixation may be applied. Open treatment may be applied to open or closed fractures; conversely, closed treatment may be applied to open or closed fractures.

27500 Closed treatment of femoral shaft fracture, without manipulation

27501 Closed treatment of supracondylar or transcondylar femoral fracture with or without intercondylar extension, without manipulation

27502 Closed treatment of femoral shaft fracture, with manipulation, with or without skin or skeletal traction

27503 Closed treatment of supracondylar or transcondylar femoral fracture with or without intercondylar extension, with manipulation, with or without skin or skeletal traction

27506 Open treatment of femoral shaft fracture, with or without external fixation, with insertion of intramedullary implant, with or without cerclage and/or locking screws

27507 Open treatment of femoral shaft fracture with plate/screws, with or without cerclage

27508 Closed treatment of femoral fracture, distal end, medial or lateral condyle, without manipulation

27509 Percutaneous skeletal fixation of femoral fracture, distal end, medial or lateral condyle, or supracondylar or transcondylar, with or without intercondylar extension, or distal femoral epiphyseal separation

27510 Closed treatment of femoral fracture, distal end, medial or lateral condyle, with manipulation

27511 Open treatment of femoral supracondylar or transcondylar fracture without intercondylar extension, includes internal fixation, when performed

27513 Open treatment of femoral supracondylar or transcondylar fracture with intercondylar extension, includes internal fixation, when performed

27514 Open treatment of femoral fracture, distal end, medial or lateral condyle, includes internal fixation, when performed

27516 Closed treatment of distal femoral epiphyseal separation; without manipulation

27517 with manipulation, with or without skin or skeletal traction

FIGURE 2-44. Fracture of the Patella

The patella protects the knee joint from its **subcutaneous** position **anterior** to the femur and tibia. This position also makes it prone to fracture, as it often takes full impact in a fall. If the fracture is not **displaced** and the **extensor** mechanism is intact, the fractured patella may simply be immobilized with a cast. Minimally displaced fractures may be treated with **reduction** and casting. Other fractures require surgical treatment to restore extensor function. Note: Tools, implants, and/or equipment depicted in the illustration may be outdated but the procedural approach is valid.

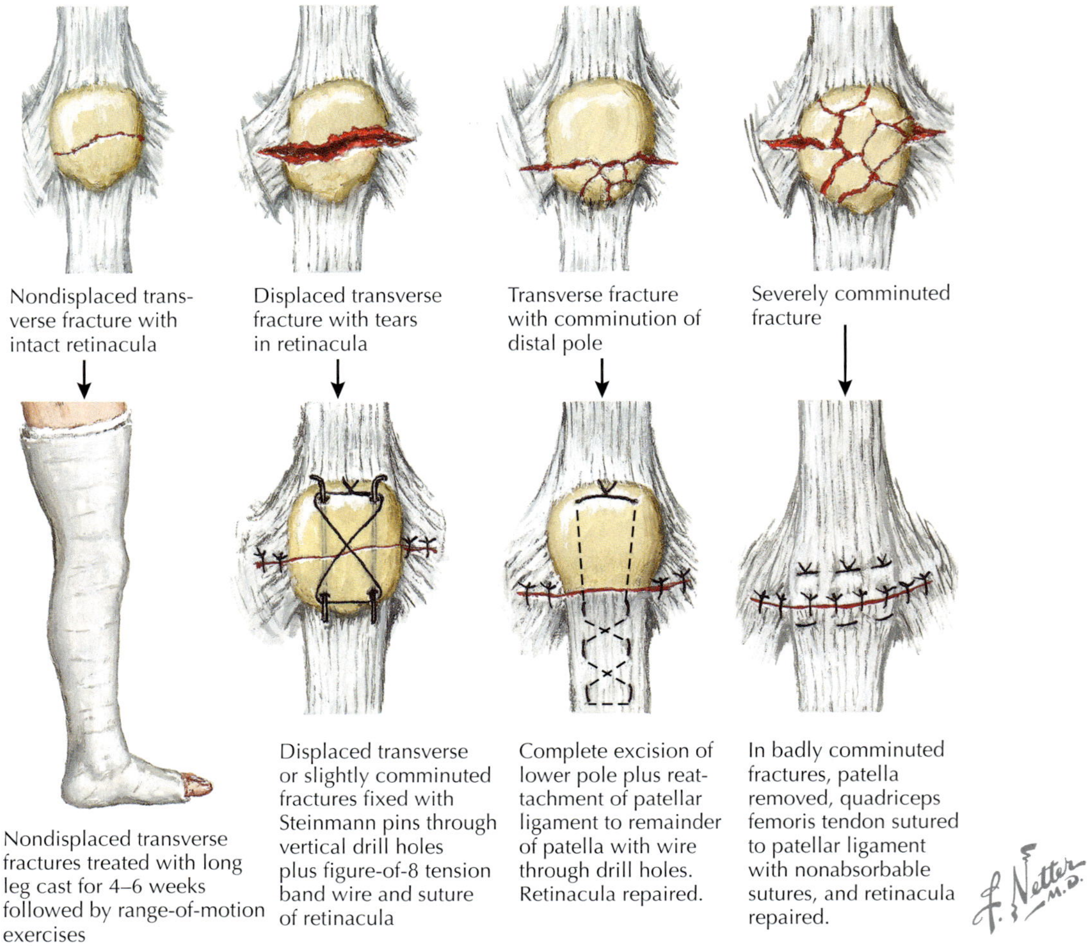

27519 Open treatment of distal femoral epiphyseal separation, includes internal fixation, when performed

27520 Closed treatment of patellar fracture, without manipulation

27524 Open treatment of patellar fracture, with internal fixation and/or partial or complete **patellectomy** and soft tissue repair

27530 Closed treatment of tibial fracture, proximal (plateau); without manipulation

27532 with or without manipulation, with skeletal traction

27535 Open treatment of tibial fracture, proximal (plateau); unicondylar, includes internal fixation, when performed

27536 bicondylar, with or without internal fixation

27538 Closed treatment of intercondylar spine(s) and/or tuberosity fracture(s) of knee, with or without manipulation

27540 Open treatment of intercondylar spine(s) and/or tuberosity fracture(s) of the knee, includes internal fixation, when performed

27550 Closed treatment of knee dislocation; without anesthesia

27552 requiring anesthesia

27556 Open treatment of knee dislocation, includes internal fixation, when performed; without primary ligamentous repair or augmentation/reconstruction

27557 with primary ligamentous repair

27558 with primary ligamentous repair, with augmentation/reconstruction

27560 Closed treatment of patellar dislocation, without anesthesia

27562 requiring anesthesia

27566 Open treatment of patellar dislocation, with or without partial or total patellectomy

Manipulation

27570 Manipulation of knee joint under general anesthesia (includes application of traction or other fixation devices)

Arthrodesis

27580 Arthrodesis, knee, any technique

Amputation

Coding Atlas

A guillotine amputation creates a flat wound across the limb. It does not provide skin for adequate closure. Guillotine amputation is typically performed in emergent situations and is followed by wound monitoring for disease prior to a second surgery for revision and flap.

27590 Amputation, thigh, through femur, any level;

27591 immediate fitting technique including first cast

27592 open, circular (guillotine)

27594 secondary closure or scar revision

27596 re-amputation

27598 Disarticulation at knee

Leg (Tibia and Fibula) and Ankle Joint

Incision

Coding Atlas

A synovial joint is completely enclosed in a ligamentous capsule. Arthrotomy is a surgical incision into a joint capsule. Codes 27610 and 27612 are used to report ankle arthrotomy. Removal of a foreign body (FB) documented as embedded on the exterior of the joint capsule or described as an FB that may have penetrated the joint capsule does not qualify as arthrotomy.

27600 Decompression fasciotomy, leg; anterior and/or lateral compartments only

27601 posterior compartment(s) only

27602 anterior and/or lateral, and posterior compartment(s)

27603 Incision and drainage, leg or ankle; deep abscess or hematoma

27604 infected bursa

27605 Tenotomy, percutaneous, Achilles tendon (separate procedure); local anesthesia

27606 general anesthesia

27607 Incision (eg, osteomyelitis or bone abscess), leg or ankle

27610 Arthrotomy, ankle, including exploration, drainage, or removal of foreign body

27612 Arthrotomy, posterior capsular release, ankle, with or without Achilles tendon lengthening

Excision

Coding Atlas

Excisions of soft tissue lesions above the fascia that require wide margins that extend into the subfascia are reported using subfascial codes. Radical resection of soft tissue tumor is generally due to soft tissue sarcoma. Do not use the radical resection codes in the Musculoskeletal section to report deep excision of skin tumors. Instead, use codes from the Integumentary System subsection.

27613 Biopsy, soft tissue of leg or ankle area; superficial

27614 deep (subfascial or intramuscular)

27615 Radical resection of tumor (eg, sarcoma), soft tissue of leg or ankle area; less than 5 cm

27616 5 cm or greater

27618 Excision, tumor, soft tissue of leg or ankle area, subcutaneous; less than 3 cm

\# **27632** 3 cm or greater

27619 Excision, tumor, soft tissue of leg or ankle area, subfascial (eg, intramuscular); less than 5 cm

\# **27634** 5 cm or greater

27620 Arthrotomy, ankle, with joint exploration, with or without biopsy, with or without removal of loose or foreign body

27625 Arthrotomy, with synovectomy, ankle;

27626 including tenosynovectomy

27630 Excision of lesion of tendon sheath or capsule (eg, cyst or ganglion), leg and/or ankle

27632 Code is out of numerical sequence. See 27613-27647

27634 Code is out of numerical sequence. See 27613-27647

FIGURE 2-45. Decompression Fasciotomy

Surgical therapy for **compartment syndrome** (CS) is fasciotomy. In **fasciotomy**, the skin is incised down to the **fascia** surrounding the compartment that is compressed. The incision is long in order to provide relief along the length of the muscle compartment. The goal is to release pressure within the compartment where tissue has swelled and, in turn, restore blood **perfusion** to the muscle tissue and reduce **ischemia**. Note: Tools, implants, and/or equipment depicted in the illustration may be outdated but the procedural approach is valid.

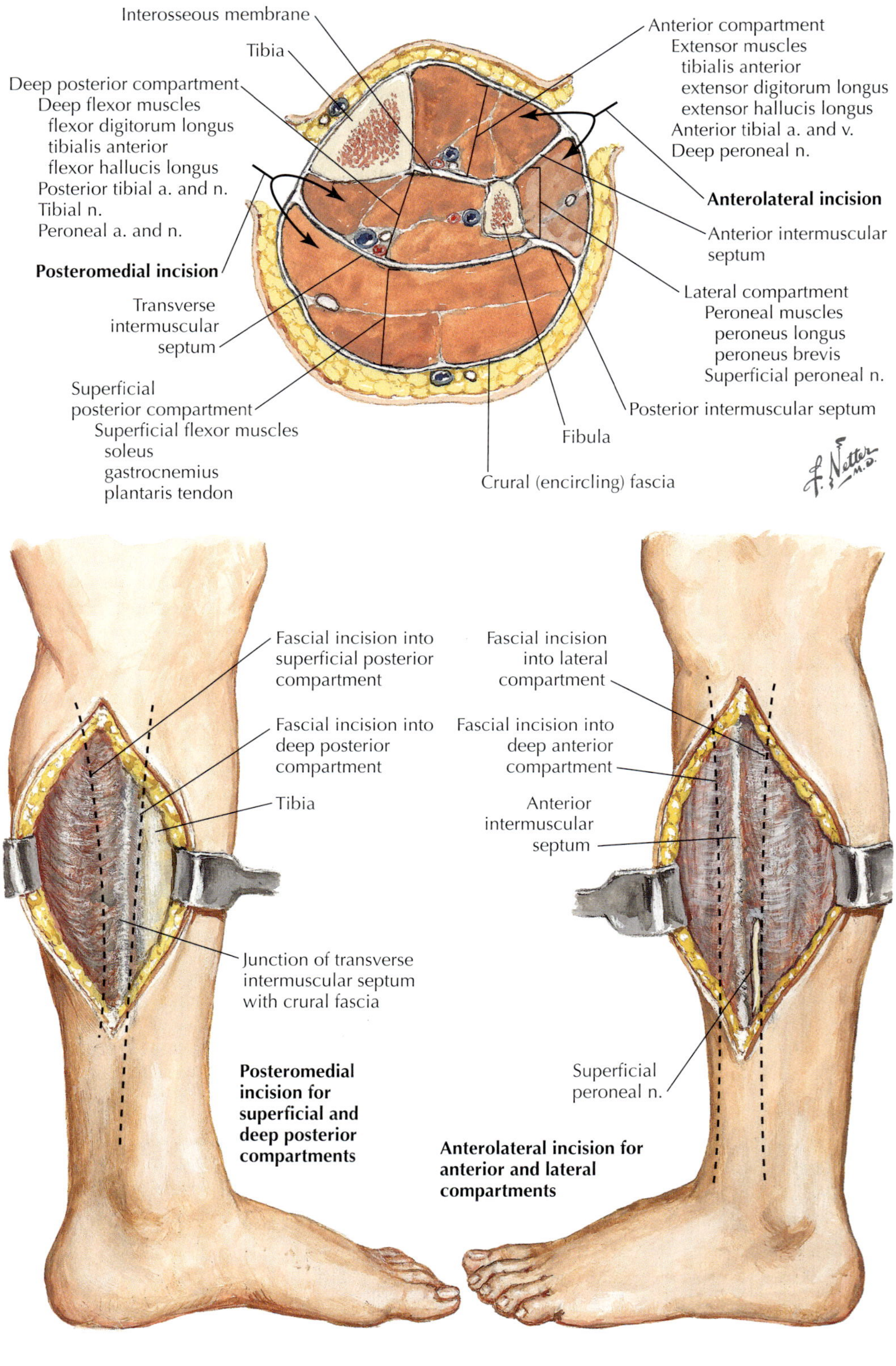

27635 Excision or curettage of bone cyst or benign tumor, tibia or fibula;

27637 with autograft (includes obtaining graft)

27638 with allograft

27640 Partial excision (craterization, saucerization, or diaphysectomy), bone (eg, osteomyelitis); tibia

27641 fibula

27645 Radical resection of tumor; tibia

27646 fibula

27647 talus or calcaneus

Introduction or Removal

27648 Injection procedure for ankle arthrography

Repair, Revision, and/or Reconstruction

Coding Atlas

Tenolysis is surgical removal of adhesions on a **tendon**. **Osteoplasty** is surgical modification of bone. **Epiphysiodesis** is the reversible surgical fusion of the epiphyseal plate to forestall growth in a child who has one leg that is longer than the other and needs to wait until the other leg grows to the same length.

27650 Repair, primary, open or percutaneous, ruptured Achilles tendon;

27652 with graft (includes obtaining graft)

27654 Repair, secondary, Achilles tendon, with or without graft

27656 Repair, fascial defect of leg

27658 Repair, flexor tendon, leg; primary, without graft, each tendon

27659 secondary, with or without graft, each tendon

27664 Repair, extensor tendon, leg; primary, without graft, each tendon

27665 secondary, with or without graft, each tendon

27675 Repair, dislocating peroneal tendons; without fibular osteotomy

27676 with fibular osteotomy

27680 Tenolysis, flexor or extensor tendon, leg and/or ankle; single, each tendon

27681 multiple tendons (through separate incision[s])

27685 Lengthening or shortening of tendon, leg or ankle; single tendon (separate procedure)

27686 multiple tendons (through same incision), each

27687 Gastrocnemius recession (eg, Strayer procedure)

27690 Transfer or transplant of single tendon (with muscle redirection or rerouting); superficial (eg, anterior tibial extensors into midfoot)

27691 deep (eg, anterior tibial or posterior tibial through interosseous space, flexor digitorum longus, flexor hallucis longus, or peroneal tendon to midfoot or hindfoot)

✚ **27692** each additional tendon (List separately in addition to code for primary procedure)

27695 Repair, primary, disrupted ligament, ankle; collateral

27696 both collateral ligaments

27698 Repair, secondary, disrupted ligament, ankle, collateral (eg, Watson-Jones procedure)

27700 Arthroplasty, ankle;

27702 with implant (total ankle)

27703 revision, total ankle

27704 Removal of ankle implant

27705 Osteotomy; tibia

27707 fibula

27709 tibia and fibula

27712 multiple, with realignment on intramedullary rod (eg, Sofield type procedure)

27715 Osteoplasty, tibia and fibula, lengthening or shortening

27720 Repair of nonunion or malunion, tibia; without graft, (eg, compression technique)

27722 with sliding graft

27724 with iliac or other autograft (includes obtaining graft)

27725 by synostosis, with fibula, any method

27726 Repair of fibula nonunion and/or malunion with internal fixation

27727 Repair of congenital pseudarthrosis, tibia

27730 Arrest, epiphyseal (epiphysiodesis), open; distal tibia

27732 distal fibula

27734 distal tibia and fibula

27740 Arrest, epiphyseal (epiphysiodesis), any method, combined, proximal and distal tibia and fibula;

27742 and distal femur

27745 Prophylactic treatment (nailing, pinning, plating or wiring) with or without methylmethacrylate, tibia

FIGURE 2-46. Muscles of the Leg

Like the hands, the feet are animated by **tendons** attached to muscles of the adjacent limb (**extrinsic**); they do not rely on their own **intrinsic** muscle groups. In the anterior lower leg, the tibialis anterior, extensor digitorum longus, and extensor halluces longus provide **dorsal** extension to the ankle joint and toes. The calf muscles of the lower leg, ie, gastrocnemius and soleus, merge into the Achilles tendon at the base of the calf muscle. The Achilles tendon inserts into the calcaneus.

Superficial Dissection: Anterior View

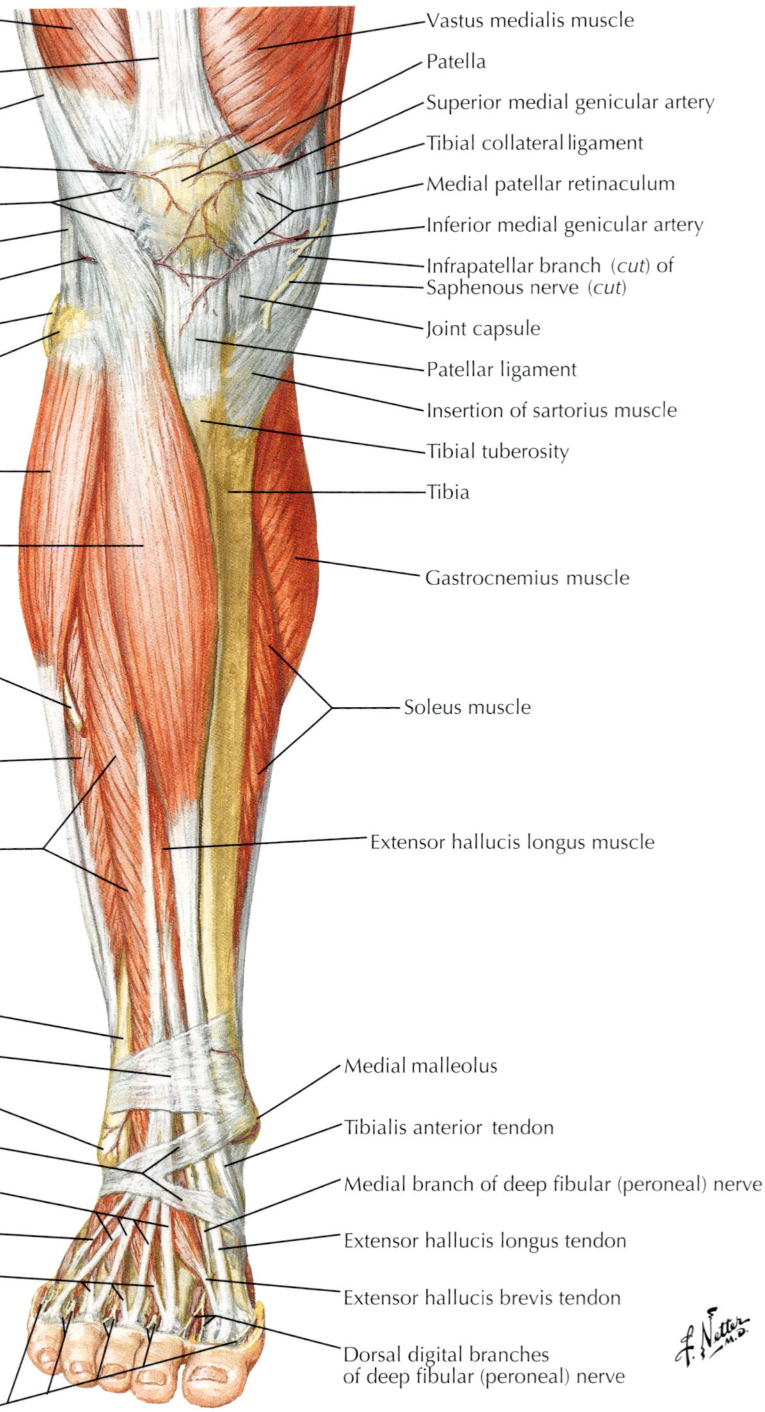

Continued on next page

FIGURE 2-46. Muscles of the Leg *(continued)*

Lateral View

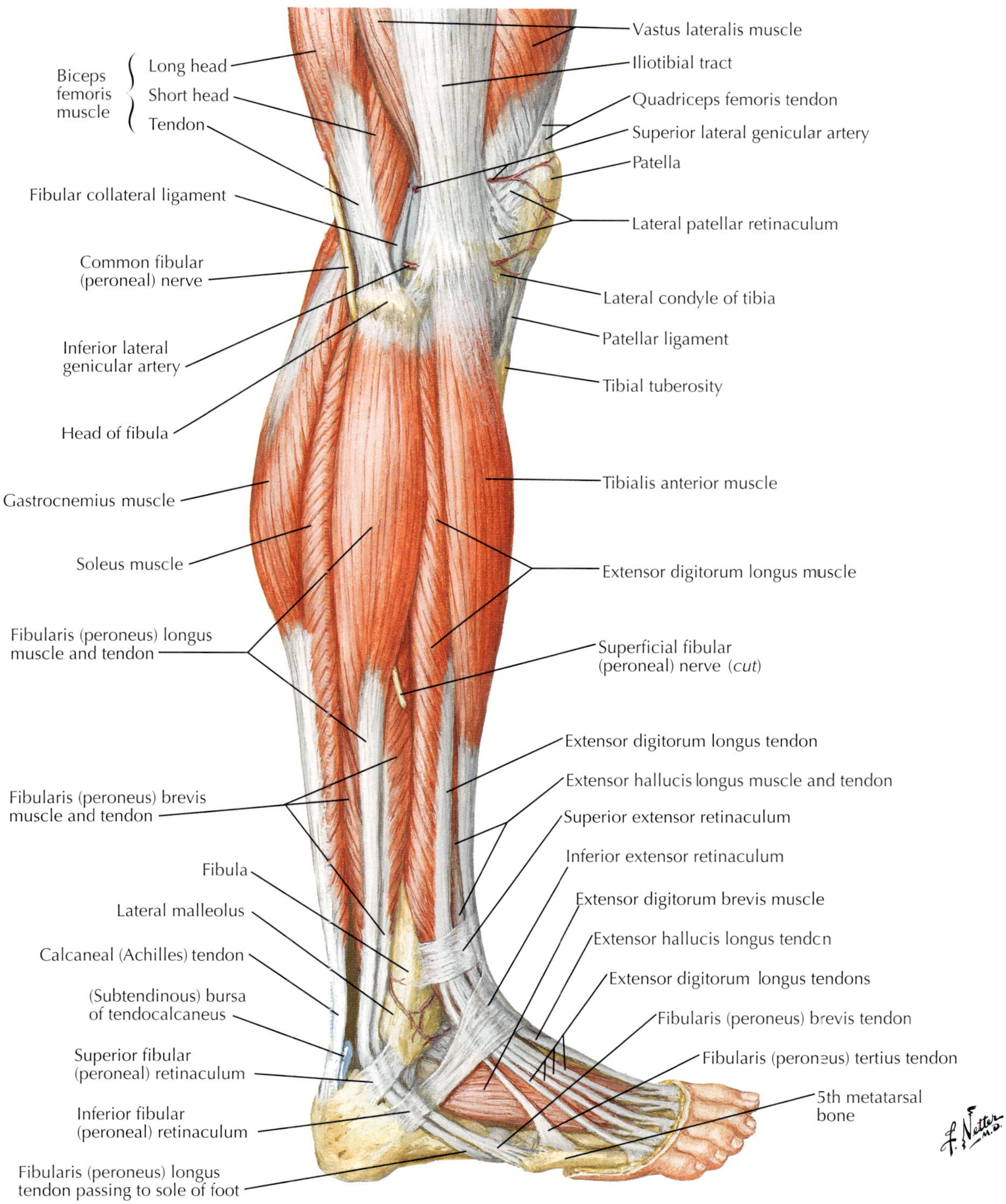

FIGURE 2-47. Tibia and Fibula

The fibula connects to the tibia by means of an **articulation** and with **ligaments**. Only the tibia articulates in the knee joint itself, though both bones articulate at the talus to form the ankle joint. The tibia carries body weight, while the smaller, thinner fibula does not. The anterior tibia lies close to the skin surface and is referred to as the shin bone.

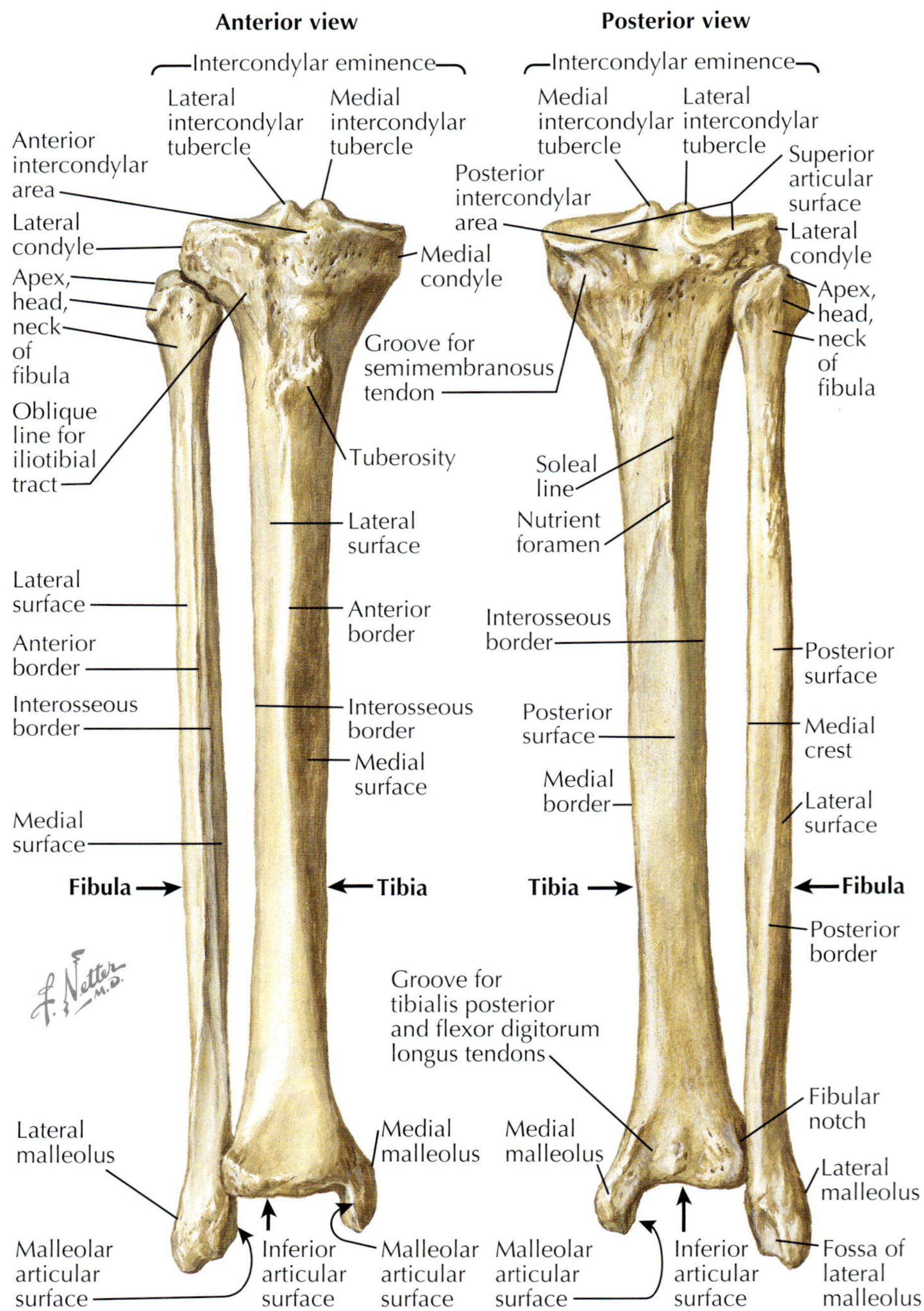

Fracture and/or Dislocation

Coding Atlas

The tibia is the most commonly fractured long bone. Sports and motor vehicle accidents account for many of these fractures. Because the skin over the anterior and medial tibia is thin, tibial fractures are often open fractures. Fibula fractures usually occur in conjunction with tibia fractures.

27750 Closed treatment of tibial shaft fracture (with or without fibular fracture); without manipulation

27752 with manipulation, with or without skeletal traction

27756 Percutaneous skeletal fixation of tibial shaft fracture (with or without fibular fracture) (eg, pins or screws)

27758 Open treatment of tibial shaft fracture (with or without fibular fracture), with plate/screws, with or without cerclage

27759 Treatment of tibial shaft fracture (with or without fibular fracture) by intramedullary implant, with or without interlocking screws and/or cerclage

27760 Closed treatment of medial malleolus fracture; without manipulation

27762 with manipulation, with or without skin or skeletal traction

27766 Open treatment of medial malleolus fracture, includes internal fixation, when performed

27767 Closed treatment of posterior malleolus fracture; without manipulation

27768 with manipulation

27769 Open treatment of posterior malleolus fracture, includes internal fixation, when performed

27780 Closed treatment of proximal fibula or shaft fracture; without manipulation

27781 with manipulation

27784 Open treatment of proximal fibula or shaft fracture, includes internal fixation, when performed

27786 Closed treatment of distal fibular fracture (lateral malleolus); without manipulation

27788 with manipulation

27792 Open treatment of distal fibular fracture (lateral malleolus), includes internal fixation, when performed

27808 Closed treatment of bimalleolar ankle fracture (eg, lateral and medial malleoli, or lateral and posterior malleoli or medial and posterior malleoli); without manipulation

27810 with manipulation

27814 Open treatment of bimalleolar ankle fracture (eg, lateral and medial malleoli, or lateral and posterior malleoli, or medial and posterior malleoli), includes internal fixation, when performed

27816 Closed treatment of trimalleolar ankle fracture; without manipulation

27818 with manipulation

27822 Open treatment of trimalleolar ankle fracture, includes internal fixation, when performed, medial and/or lateral malleolus; without fixation of posterior lip

27823 with fixation of posterior lip

27824 Closed treatment of fracture of weight bearing articular portion of distal tibia (eg, pilon or tibial plafond), with or without anesthesia; without manipulation

27825 with skeletal traction and/or requiring manipulation

27826 Open treatment of fracture of weight bearing articular surface/portion of distal tibia (eg, pilon or tibial plafond), with internal fixation, when performed; of fibula only

27827 of tibia only

27828 of both tibia and fibula

27829 Open treatment of distal tibiofibular joint (syndesmosis) disruption, includes internal fixation, when performed

27830 Closed treatment of proximal tibiofibular joint dislocation; without anesthesia

27831 requiring anesthesia

27832 Open treatment of proximal tibiofibular joint dislocation, includes internal fixation, when performed, or with excision of proximal fibula

27840 Closed treatment of ankle dislocation; without anesthesia

27842 requiring anesthesia, with or without percutaneous skeletal fixation

27846 Open treatment of ankle dislocation, with or without percutaneous skeletal fixation; without repair or internal fixation

27848 with repair or internal or external fixation

Manipulation

27860 Manipulation of ankle under general anesthesia (includes application of traction or other fixation apparatus)

FIGURE 2-48. Ligaments and Tendons of the Ankle and Foot

Tendons emerge from muscle to connect to bone. When the muscle contracts, the tendon pulls the bone and causes it to move. Muscle action is affected when a tendon is injured. **Ligaments** provide stability by connecting bone to bone. An ankle sprain occurs when ligaments are torn or stretched. In the ankle, the **lateral** ligaments are the most common sites of a sprain, as the outer ankle turns under, injuring the **anterior** talofibular ligament (ATFL) and/or calcaneofibular ligament (CFL).

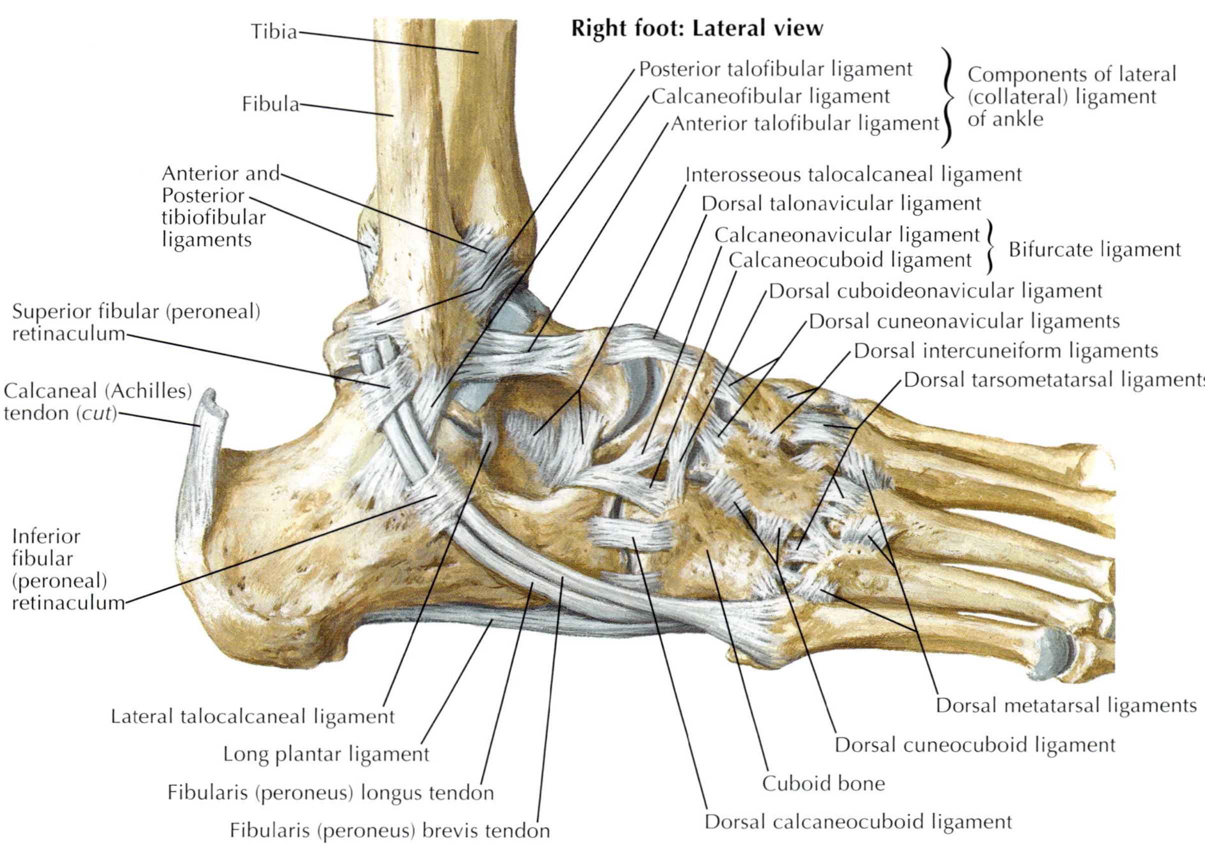

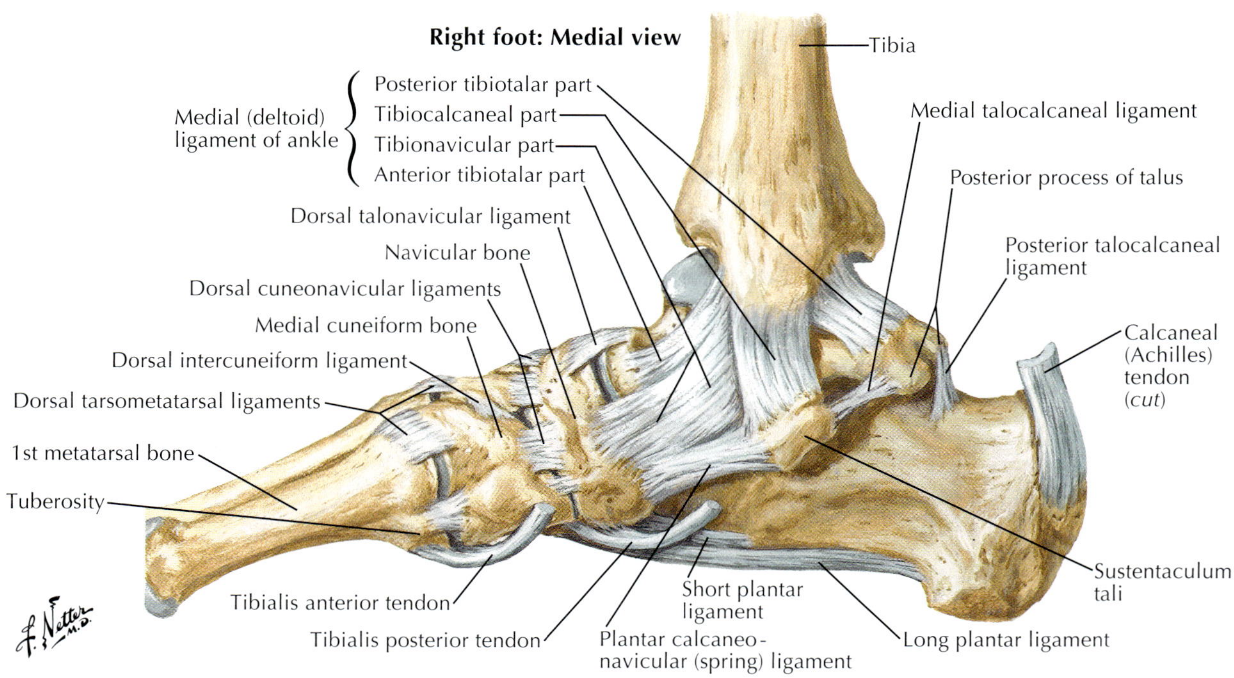

Arthrodesis

Coding Atlas

In **arthrodesis**, the joint is surgically fused and immobilized. Bone grafts may be placed to fix the joint; otherwise, hardware is placed. Code selection is based on the joint(s) treated.

27870 Arthrodesis, ankle, open

27871 Arthrodesis, tibiofibular joint, proximal or distal

Amputation

Coding Atlas

A guillotine amputation creates a flat wound across the limb. It does not provide skin for adequate closure. Guillotine amputation is typically performed in emergent situations and is followed by wound monitoring for disease prior to a second surgery for revision and **flap**.

27880 Amputation, leg, through tibia and fibula;

27881 with immediate fitting technique including application of first cast

27882 open, circular (guillotine)

27884 secondary closure or scar revision

27886 re-amputation

27888 Amputation, ankle, through malleoli of tibia and fibula (eg, Syme, Pirogoff type procedures), with plastic closure and resection of nerves

27889 Ankle disarticulation

Other Procedures

Coding Atlas

If **compartment syndrome** (CS) is not treated, blood flow to muscle tissue is compromised and **necrosis** results. These codes are used to report **decompression** fasciotomy with **debridement** of necrotic or otherwise **nonviable** tissues within the compartment.

27892 Decompression fasciotomy, leg; anterior and/or lateral compartments only, with debridement of nonviable muscle and/or nerve

27893 posterior compartment(s) only, with debridement of nonviable muscle and/or nerve

27894 anterior and/or lateral, and posterior compartment(s), with debridement of nonviable muscle and/or nerve

Foot and Toes

Incision

Coding Atlas

A synovial joint is completely enclosed in a ligamentous capsule. **Arthrotomy** is a surgical incision into a joint capsule. Codes 28020-28024 are used to report arthrotomy with **foreign body** (FB) removal, exploration, or drainage. Removal of an FB documented as embedded on the exterior of the joint capsule or described as an FB that may have penetrated the joint capsule does not qualify as arthrotomy. Documentation must state that the joint capsule has been surgically opened. **Extra-articular** refers to tissue outside of the joint capsule.

28001 Incision and drainage, bursa, foot

28002 Incision and drainage below fascia, with or without tendon sheath involvement, foot; single bursal space

28003 multiple areas

28005 Incision, bone cortex (eg, osteomyelitis or bone abscess), foot

28008 Fasciotomy, foot and/or toe

28010 Tenotomy, percutaneous, toe; single tendon

28011 multiple tendons

28020 Arthrotomy, including exploration, drainage, or removal of loose or foreign body; intertarsal or tarsometatarsal joint

28022 metatarsophalangeal joint

28024 interphalangeal joint

28035 Release, tarsal tunnel (posterior tibial nerve decompression)

Excision

Coding Atlas

Size and **tumor** origin play a role in code selection for reporting excision of soft tissue tumors. The entire resection is measured, not the diameter of the lesion itself, to determine the excision size. Excision of a tumor originating in the integument, eg, **melanoma**, is reported using Integumentary Excision codes. In **arthrotomy**, the joint capsule is entered.

28039 Code is out of numerical sequence. See 28043-28175

28041 Code is out of numerical sequence. See 28043-28175

FIGURE 2-49. Soft Tissue of the Foot

In addition to 26 bones, the foot has more than 100 muscles, **tendons**, and **ligaments**. The **extensor** muscles and tendons help to raise and extend the toes, an essential part of precision locomotion. The **flexor** muscles and tendons bend the toes in flexion.

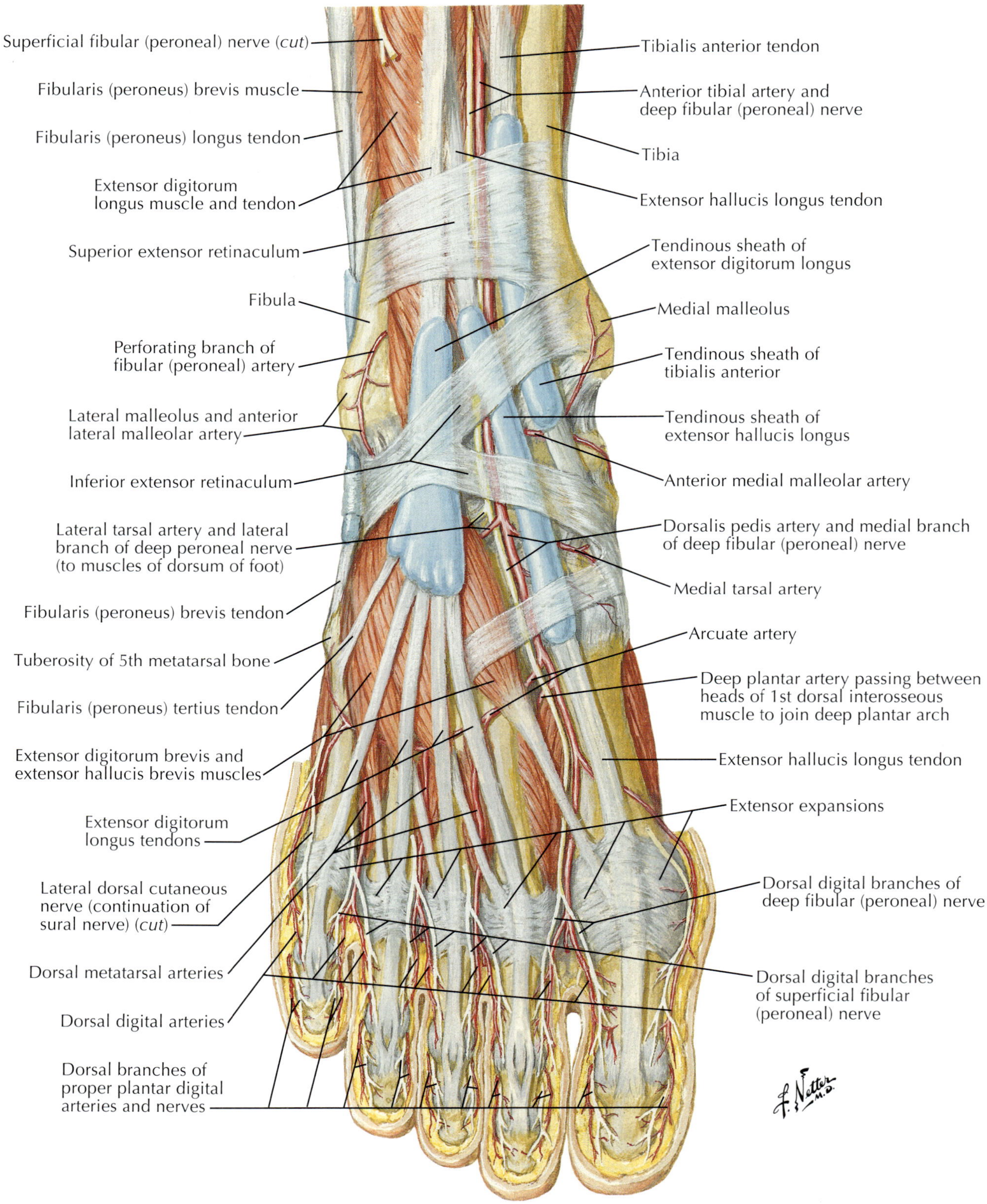

28043 Excision, tumor, soft tissue of foot or toe, subcutaneous; less than 1.5 cm

28039 1.5 cm or greater

28045 Excision, tumor, soft tissue of foot or toe, subfascial (eg, intramuscular); less than 1.5 cm

28041 1.5 cm or greater

28046 Radical resection of tumor (eg, sarcoma), soft tissue of foot or toe; less than 3 cm

28047 3 cm or greater

28050 Arthrotomy with biopsy; intertarsal or tarsometatarsal joint

28052 metatarsophalangeal joint

28054 interphalangeal joint

28055 Neurectomy, intrinsic musculature of foot

28060 Fasciectomy, plantar fascia; partial (separate procedure)

28062 radical (separate procedure)

28070 Synovectomy; intertarsal or tarsometatarsal joint, each

28072 metatarsophalangeal joint, each

28080 Excision, interdigital (Morton) neuroma, single, each

28086 Synovectomy, tendon sheath, foot; flexor

28088 extensor

28090 Excision of lesion, tendon, tendon sheath, or capsule (including synovectomy) (eg, cyst or ganglion); foot

28092 toe(s), each

28100 Excision or curettage of bone cyst or benign tumor, talus or calcaneus;

28102 with iliac or other autograft (includes obtaining graft)

28103 with allograft

28104 Excision or curettage of bone cyst or benign tumor, tarsal or metatarsal, except talus or calcaneus;

28106 with iliac or other autograft (includes obtaining graft)

28107 with allograft

28108 Excision or curettage of bone cyst or benign tumor, phalanges of foot

28110 Ostectomy, partial excision, fifth metatarsal head (bunionette) (separate procedure)

28111 Ostectomy, complete excision; first metatarsal head

28112 other metatarsal head (second, third or fourth)

28113 fifth metatarsal head

28114 all metatarsal heads, with partial proximal phalangectomy, excluding first metatarsal (eg, Clayton type procedure)

28116 Ostectomy, excision of tarsal coalition

28118 Ostectomy, calcaneus;

28119 for spur, with or without plantar fascial release

28120 Partial excision (craterization, saucerization, sequestrectomy, or diaphysectomy) bone (eg, osteomyelitis or bossing); talus or calcaneus

28122 tarsal or metatarsal bone, except talus or calcaneus

28124 phalanx of toe

28126 Resection, partial or complete, phalangeal base, each toe

28130 Talectomy (astragalectomy)

28140 Metatarsectomy

28150 Phalangectomy, toe, each toe

28153 Resection, condyle(s), distal end of phalanx, each toe

28160 Hemiphalangectomy or interphalangeal joint excision, toe, proximal end of phalanx, each

28171 Radical resection of tumor tarsal (except talus or calcaneus)

28173 metatarsal

28175 phalanx of toe

Introduction or Removal

Coding Atlas

Codes 28190-28193 are used to report removal of a **foreign body** that is the result of recent or past trauma. These codes should not be used to report removal of **prosthesis**.

28190 Removal of foreign body, foot; subcutaneous

28192 deep

28193 complicated

Repair, Revision, and/or Reconstruction

Coding Atlas

A **hallux valgus** is a bunion, or forefoot deformity, in which there is a **lateral** deviation in the great toe. This deformity is usually acquired (extrinsic factor, such as the types of shoes worn) and more frequently seen in women as a result of genetic predisposition (intrinsic factor). The goal of surgery for hallux valgus is correction of the defect, which may be accomplished by **osteotomy**, resection **arthroplasty**, or **arthrodesis**.

28200 Repair, tendon, flexor, foot; primary or secondary, without free graft, each tendon

28202 secondary with free graft, each tendon (includes obtaining graft)

28208 Repair, tendon, extensor, foot; primary or secondary, each tendon

28210 secondary with free graft, each tendon (includes obtaining graft)

28220 Tenolysis, flexor, foot; single tendon

28222 multiple tendons

28225 Tenolysis, extensor, foot; single tendon

28226 multiple tendons

28230 Tenotomy, open, tendon flexor; foot, single or multiple tendon(s) (separate procedure)

28232 toe, single tendon (separate procedure)

28234 Tenotomy, open, extensor, foot or toe, each tendon

28238 Reconstruction (advancement), posterior tibial tendon with excision of accessory tarsal navicular bone (eg, Kidner type procedure)

28240 Tenotomy, lengthening, or release, abductor hallucis muscle

28250 Division of plantar fascia and muscle (eg, Steindler stripping) (separate procedure)

28260 Capsulotomy, midfoot; medial release only (separate procedure)

28261 with tendon lengthening

28262 extensive, including posterior talotibial capsulotomy and tendon(s) lengthening (eg, resistant clubfoot deformity)

28264 Capsulotomy, midtarsal (eg, Heyman type procedure)

28270 Capsulotomy; metatarsophalangeal joint, with or without tenorrhaphy, each joint (separate procedure)

28272 interphalangeal joint, each joint (separate procedure)

28280 Syndactylization, toes (eg, webbing or Kelikian type procedure)

28285 Correction, hammertoe (eg, interphalangeal fusion, partial or total phalangectomy)

28286 Correction, cock-up fifth toe, with plastic skin closure (eg, Ruiz-Mora type procedure)

28288 Ostectomy, partial, exostectomy or condylectomy, metatarsal head, each metatarsal head

28289 Hallux rigidus correction with cheilectomy, debridement and capsular release of the first metatarsophalangeal joint

28290 Correction, hallux valgus (bunion), with or without sesamoidectomy; simple exostectomy (eg, Silver type procedure)

28292 Keller, McBride, or Mayo type procedure

28293 resection of joint with implant

28294 with tendon transplants (eg, Joplin type procedure)

28296 with metatarsal osteotomy (eg, Mitchell, Chevron, or concentric type procedures)

28297 Lapidus-type procedure

28298 by phalanx osteotomy

28299 by double osteotomy

28300 Osteotomy; calcaneus (eg, Dwyer or Chambers type procedure), with or without internal fixation

28302 talus

28304 Osteotomy, tarsal bones, other than calcaneus or talus;

28305 with autograft (includes obtaining graft) (eg, Fowler type)

28306 Osteotomy, with or without lengthening, shortening or angular correction, metatarsal; first metatarsal

28307 first metatarsal with autograft (other than first toe)

28308 other than first metatarsal, each

28309 multiple (eg, Swanson type cavus foot procedure)

28310 Osteotomy, shortening, angular or rotational correction; proximal phalanx, first toe (separate procedure)

28312 other phalanges, any toe

28313 Reconstruction, angular deformity of toe, soft tissue procedures only (eg, overlapping second toe, fifth toe, curly toes)

28315 Sesamoidectomy, first toe (separate procedure)

28320 Repair, nonunion or malunion; tarsal bones

28322 metatarsal, with or without bone graft (includes obtaining graft)

28340 Reconstruction, toe, macrodactyly; soft tissue resection

28341 requiring bone resection

28344 Reconstruction, toe(s); polydactyly

28345 syndactyly, with or without skin graft(s), each web

28360 Reconstruction, cleft foot

FIGURE 2-50. Correction of Toe Deformities

Toe-joint deformities are commonly corrected with surgery that may involve the bone, **tendons**, or **ligaments**, or a combination of those structures. In **hallux valgus**, the joint at the base of the big toe is deformed, causing a painful outward (**lateral**) bowing. The first metatarsal becomes prominent in the **medial foot**, creating what is commonly called a **bunion**. Note: Tools, implants, and/or equipment depicted in the illustration may be outdated but the procedural approach is valid.

Hyperextension deformity of great toe

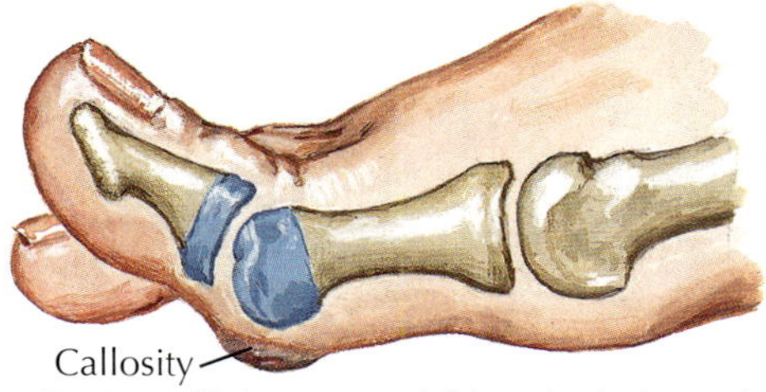

Portion of joint resected (blue-shaded areas)

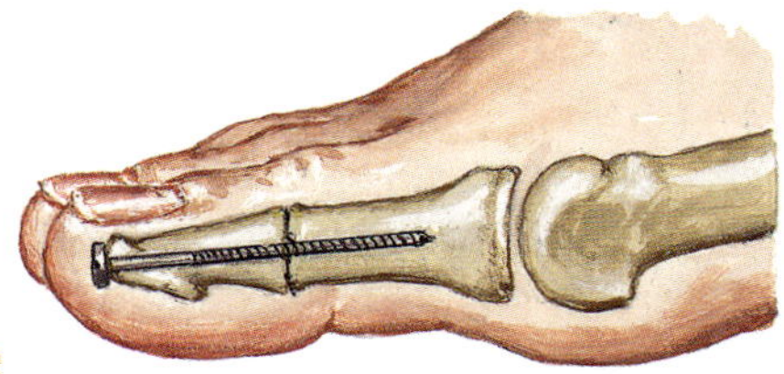

Toe straightened; joint fused and fixed with screw. Callosity heals.

Cock-up deformity of lesser toe (metatarsophalangeal joint satisfactory)

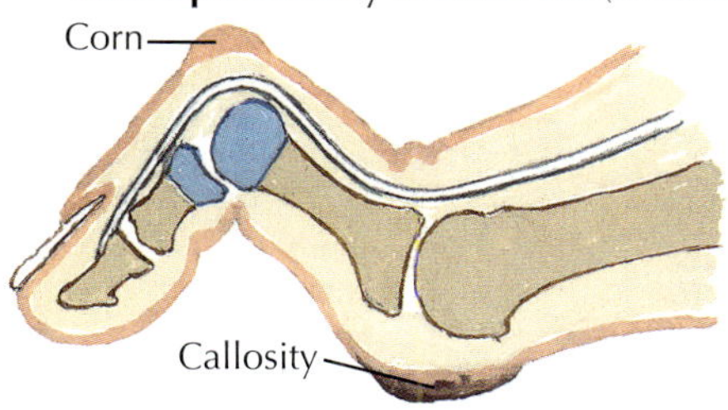

Portion of proximal interphalangeal joint resected (blue-shaded areas)

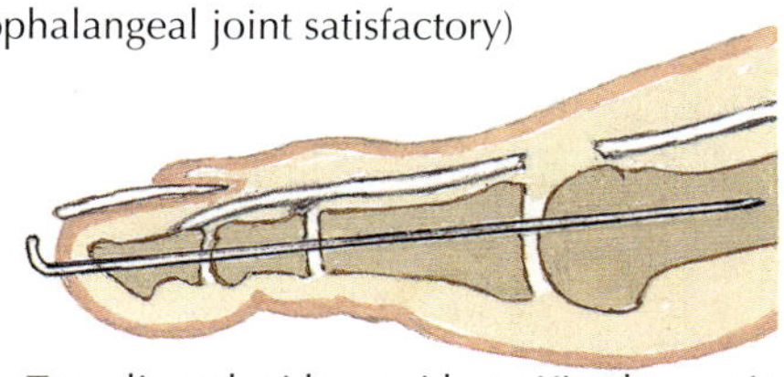

Toe aligned with or without Kirschner wire. Extensor tenotomy over metatarsophalangeal joint. Callosity and corn heal.

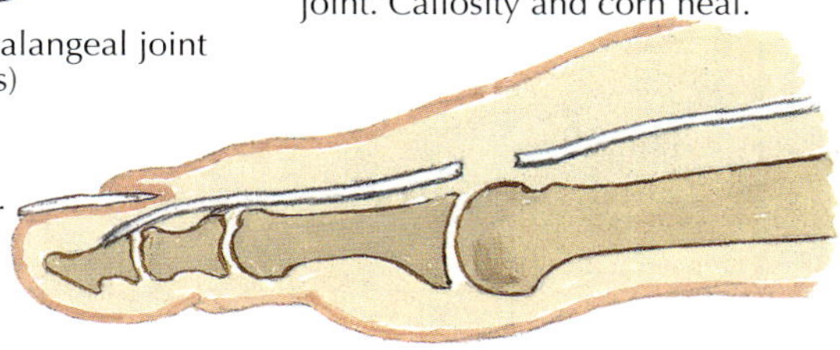

In very mild cases, transcutaneous extensor tenotomy without bone resection followed by manipulative alignment may suffice.

Keller operation for hallux valgus with bunion (other toes satisfactory)

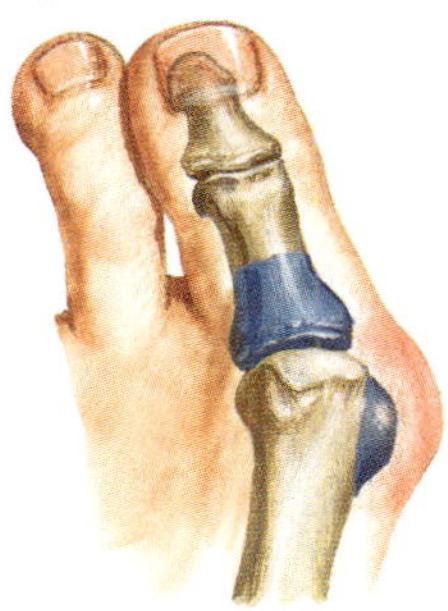

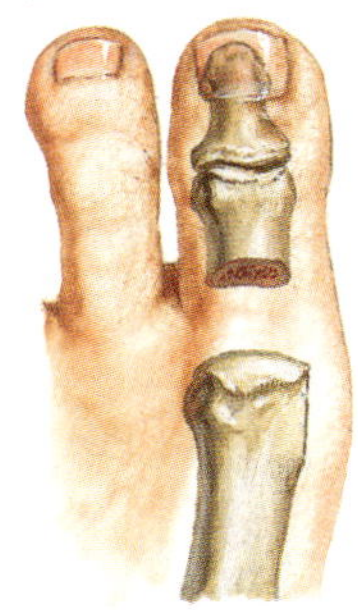

About half of proximal phalanx and exostosis resected (shown in blue) and toe straightened

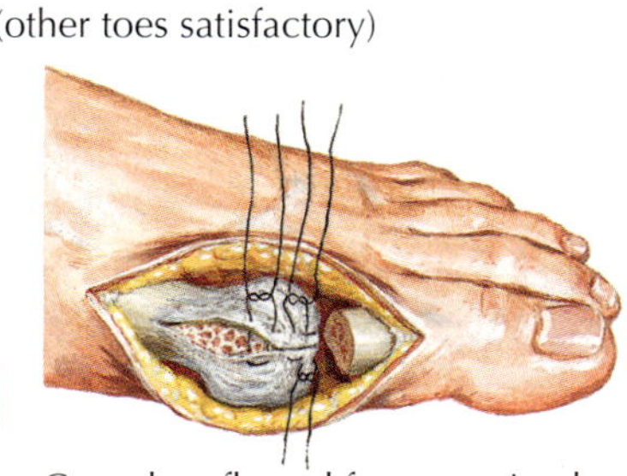

Capsule reflected from proximal phalanx interposed into joint and sutured over raw area of metatarsal head (pin fixation may be used if necessary)

Swanson flexible implant resection arthroplasty for great toe

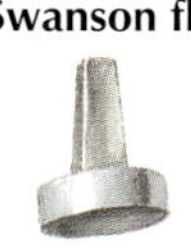

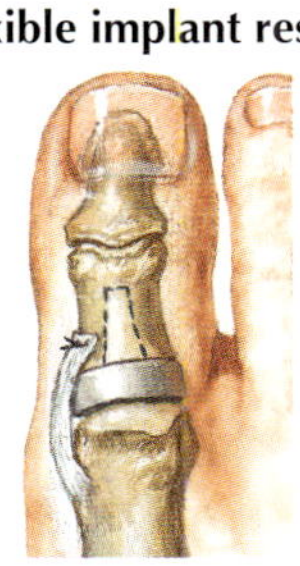

Base of proximal phalanx and exostosis resected. Medullary canal prepared and single-stemmed implant inserted. Capsular flap sutured to proximal phalanx.

FIGURE 2-51. Bones of the Foot

The foot contains 26 bones (plus two tiny sesamoid bones): 7 tarsal, 5 metatarsal, and 14 phalanges. The foot is divided into hindfoot, midfoot, and forefoot. The hindfoot contains two tarsal bones (calcaneus and talus). The midfoot contains the balance of the tarsal bones (three cuneiform, one navicular, and one cuboid). The forefoot contains the metatarsals and phalanges. The sesamoid bones are embedded in the muscles of the forefoot connected to the tendons.

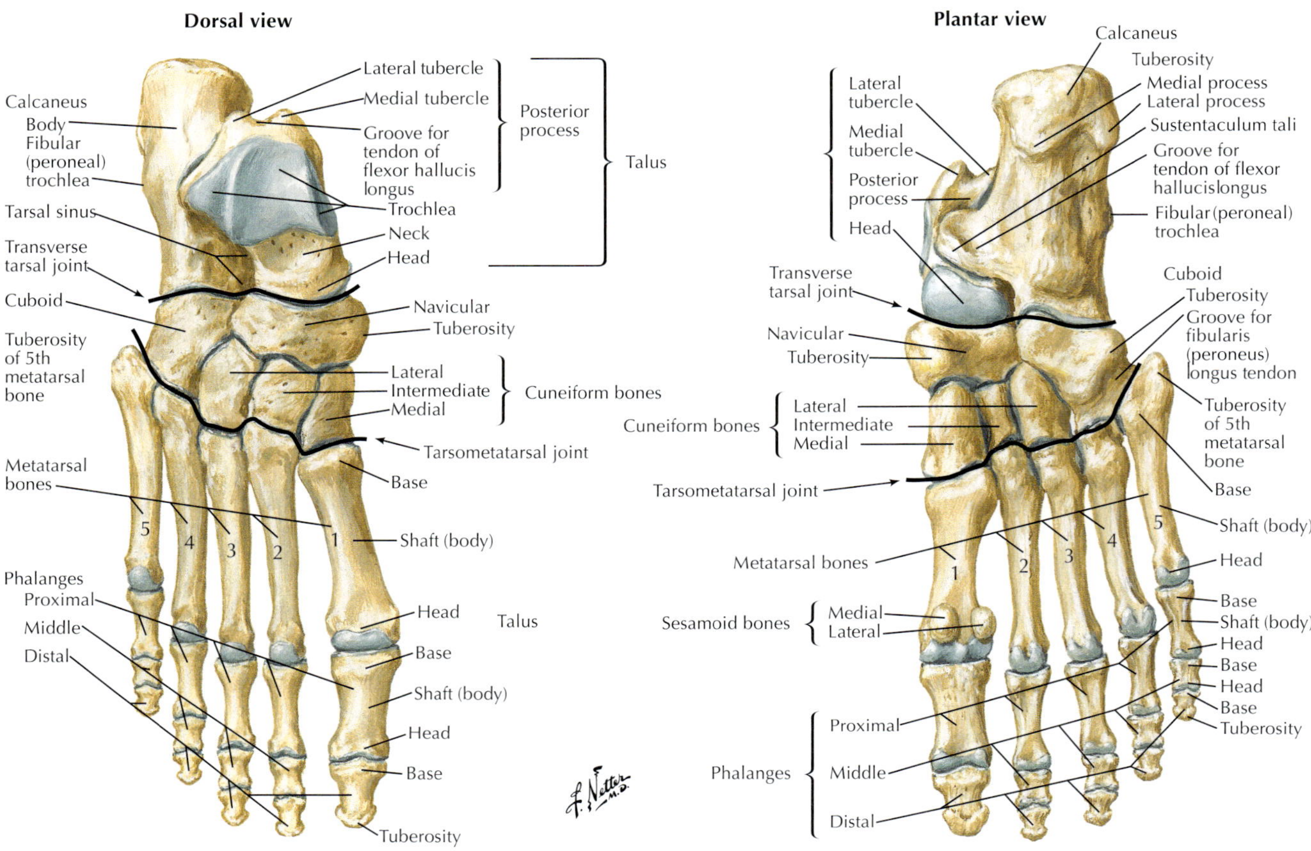

Continued on next page

Fracture and/or Dislocation

Coding Atlas

Percutaneous skeletal fixation describes the insertion of pins through the skin and into the bone fragments to secure the bones' position. This is done without **direct visualization** of the bone. **Internal fixation** describes the application of pins, nails, or other hardware secured to the bone. **External fixation** describes multiple pins placed through bone cortex both **proximal** and **distal** to the fracture. The pins are attached to an external fixator.

28400 Closed treatment of calcaneal fracture; without manipulation

28405 with manipulation

28406 Percutaneous skeletal fixation of calcaneal fracture, with manipulation

28415 Open treatment of calcaneal fracture, includes internal fixation, when performed;

28420 with primary iliac or other autogenous bone graft (includes obtaining graft)

28430 Closed treatment of talus fracture; without manipulation

28435 with manipulation

28436 Percutaneous skeletal fixation of talus fracture, with manipulation

28445 Open treatment of talus fracture, includes internal fixation, when performed

28446 Open osteochondral autograft, talus (includes obtaining graft[s])

FIGURE 2-51. Bones of the Foot *(continued)*

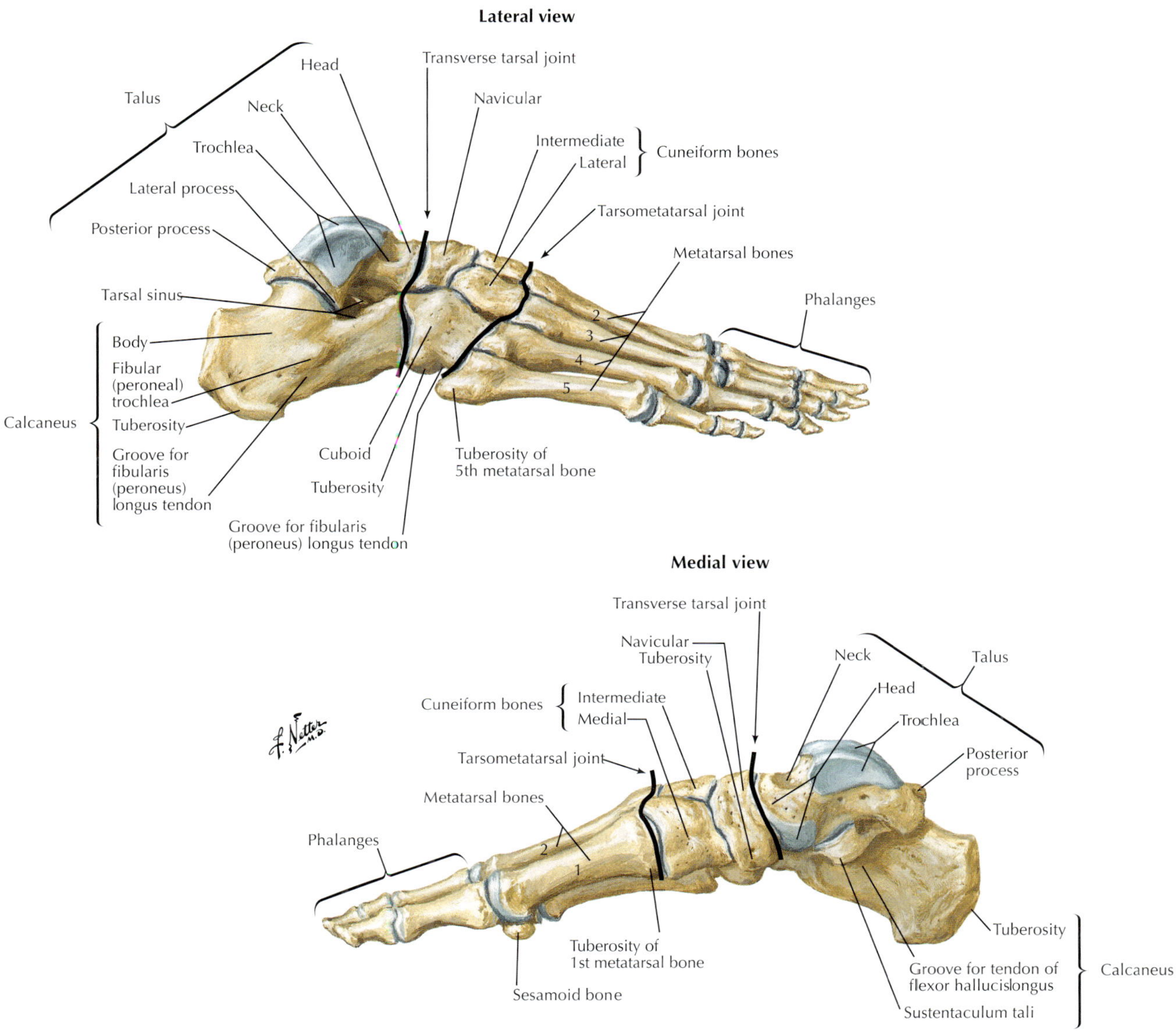

28450 Treatment of tarsal bone fracture (except talus and calcaneus); without manipulation, each

28455 with manipulation, each

28456 Percutaneous skeletal fixation of tarsal bone fracture (except talus and calcaneus), with manipulation, each

28465 Open treatment of tarsal bone fracture (except talus and calcaneus), includes internal fixation, when performed, each

28470 Closed treatment of metatarsal fracture; without manipulation, each

28475 with manipulation, each

28476 Percutaneous skeletal fixation of metatarsal fracture, with manipulation, each

28485 Open treatment of metatarsal fracture, includes internal fixation, when performed, each

28490 Closed treatment of fracture great toe, phalanx or phalanges; without manipulation

28495 with manipulation

28496 Percutaneous skeletal fixation of fracture great toe, phalanx or phalanges, with manipulation

28505 Open treatment of fracture, great toe, phalanx or phalanges, includes internal fixation, when performed

28510 Closed treatment of fracture, phalanx or phalanges, other than great toe; without manipulation, each

28515 with manipulation, each

28525 Open treatment of fracture, phalanx or phalanges, other than great toe, includes internal fixation, when performed, each

28530 Closed treatment of sesamoid fracture

28531 Open treatment of sesamoid fracture, with or without internal fixation

28540 Closed treatment of tarsal bone dislocation, other than talotarsal; without anesthesia

28545 requiring anesthesia

28546 Percutaneous skeletal fixation of tarsal bone dislocation, other than talotarsal, with manipulation

28555 Open treatment of tarsal bone dislocation, includes internal fixation, when performed

28570 Closed treatment of talotarsal joint dislocation; without anesthesia

28575 requiring anesthesia

28576 Percutaneous skeletal fixation of talotarsal joint dislocation, with manipulation

28585 Open treatment of talotarsal joint dislocation, includes internal fixation, when performed

28600 Closed treatment of tarsometatarsal joint dislocation; without anesthesia

28605 requiring anesthesia

28606 Percutaneous skeletal fixation of tarsometatarsal joint dislocation, with manipulation

28615 Open treatment of tarsometatarsal joint dislocation, includes internal fixation, when performed

28630 Closed treatment of metatarsophalangeal joint dislocation; without anesthesia

28635 requiring anesthesia

28636 Percutaneous skeletal fixation of metatarsophalangeal joint dislocation, with manipulation

28645 Open treatment of metatarsophalangeal joint dislocation, includes internal fixation, when performed

28660 Closed treatment of interphalangeal joint dislocation; without anesthesia

28665 requiring anesthesia

28666 Percutaneous skeletal fixation of interphalangeal joint dislocation, with manipulation

28675 Open treatment of interphalangeal joint dislocation, includes internal fixation, when performed

Arthrodesis

Coding Atlas

In arthrodesis, a joint is surgically fused or immobilized. Bone grafts may be placed to fix the joint; otherwise, hardware is placed.

28705 Arthrodesis; pantalar

28715 triple

28725 subtalar

28730 Arthrodesis, midtarsal or tarsometatarsal, multiple or transverse;

28735 with osteotomy (eg, flatfoot correction)

28737 Arthrodesis, with tendon lengthening and advancement, midtarsal, tarsal navicular-cuneiform (eg, Miller type procedure)

28740 Arthrodesis, midtarsal or tarsometatarsal, single joint

28750 Arthrodesis, great toe; metatarsophalangeal joint

28755 interphalangeal joint

28760 Arthrodesis, with extensor hallucis longus transfer to first metatarsal neck, great toe, interphalangeal joint (eg, Jones type procedure)

Amputation

Coding Atlas

In a midtarsal amputation, the midfoot is amputated between the calcaneous and cuboid bones and the talus and navicular bones. In transmetatarsal amputation, all toes are excised at the level of the metatarsals. Toe amputation is coded according to the level of joint amputated.

28800 Amputation, foot; midtarsal (eg, Chopart type procedure)

28805 transmetatarsal

28810 Amputation, metatarsal, with toe, single

28820 Amputation, toe; metatarsophalangeal joint

28825 interphalangeal joint

Other Procedures

28890 Extracorporeal shock wave, high energy, performed by a physician or other qualified health care professional, requiring anesthesia other than local, including ultrasound guidance, involving the plantar fascia

FIGURE 2-52. Amputation of the Foot

A partial foot amputation (PFA) may be performed to eliminate diseased tissue and preserve as much healthy foot as possible. CPT code selection is based on the level of amputation as defined by the bones removed, from midfoot amputations to amputations that involve removal of only the distal phalange. Note: Tools, implants, and/or equipment depicted in the illustration may be outdated but the procedural approach is valid.

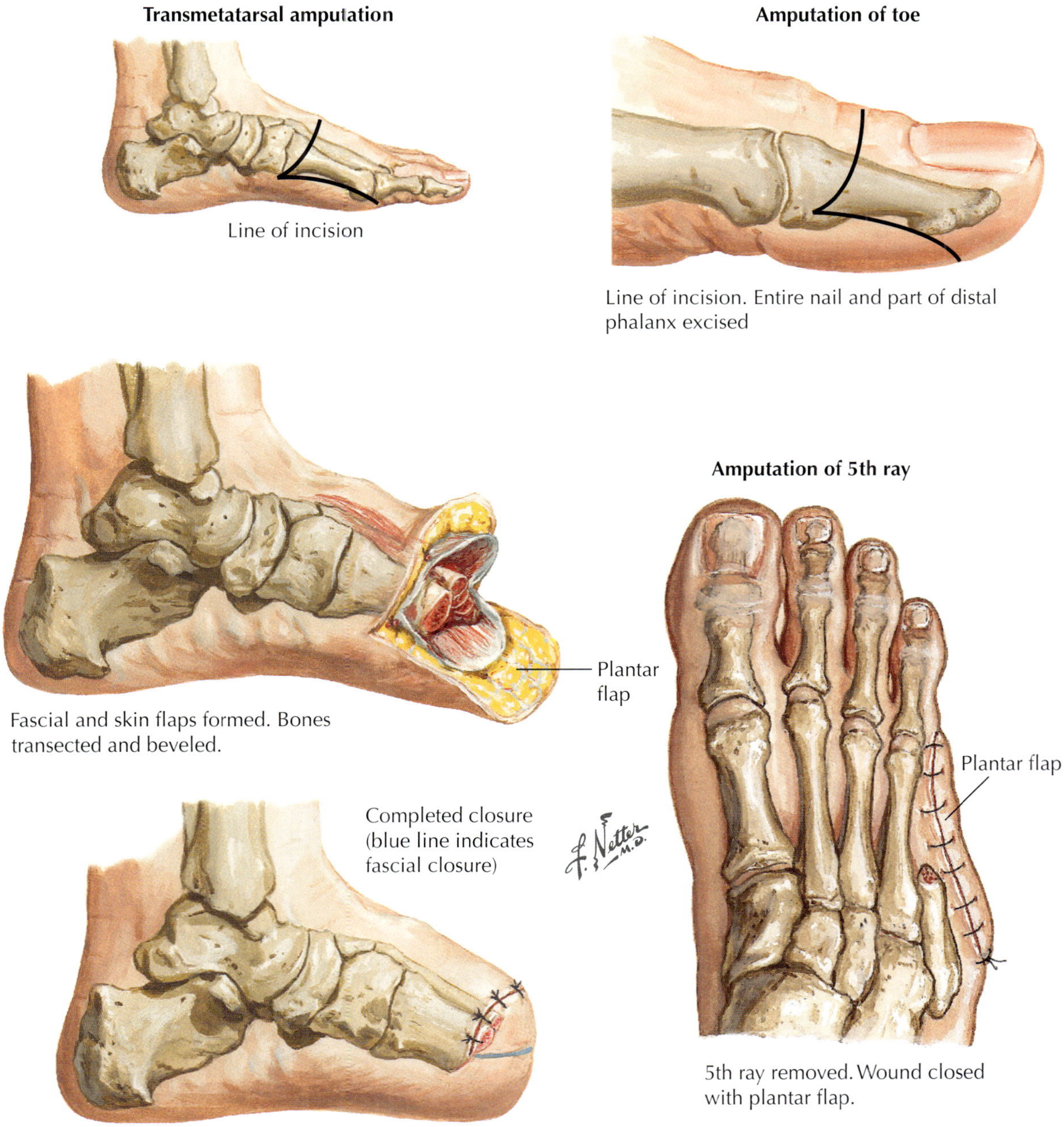

FIGURE 2-53. Velpeau Shoulder Strapping

Velpeau shoulder strapping or Velpeau sling, is a shoulder bandage that relieves the forearm of weight bearing during the healing process. It keeps the capus, elbow, and shoulder joints in a flexed position. This sling virtually eliminates **abduction** and **rotation** and is often applied to sprains and dislocations. Note: Tools, implants, and/or equipment depicted in the illustration may be outdated but the procedural approach is valid.

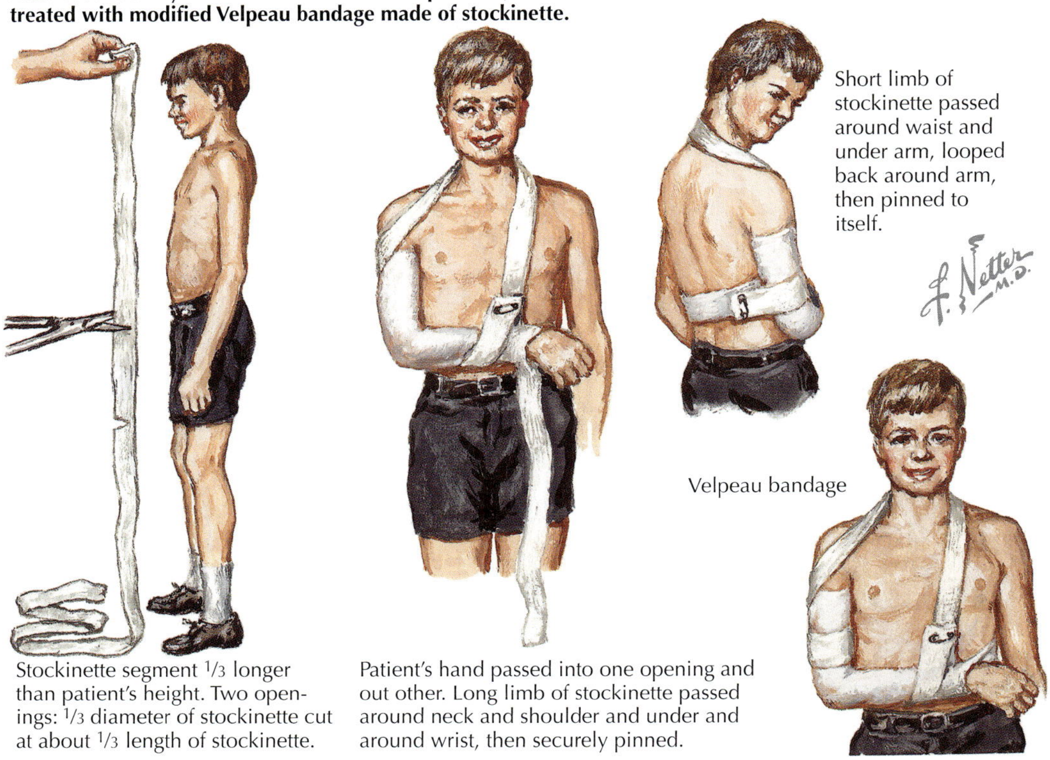

Application of Casts and Strapping

Body and Upper Extremity

Coding Atlas

When a fracture, dislocation, or other injury requires **casting** or **strapping**, the initial cast, strap, or splint is included in the initial service. Codes for casting, **splinting**, and strapping procedures are reported only when these procedures are performed as a replacement procedure or if no restorative procedure was performed as part of the initial treatment.

Casts

29000 Application of halo type body cast (see 20661-20663 for insertion)

29010 Application of Risser jacket, localizer, body; only

29015 including head

29035 Application of body cast, shoulder to hips;

29040 including head, Minerva type

29044 including 1 thigh

29046 including both thighs

29049 Application, cast; figure-of-eight

29055 shoulder spica

29058 plaster Velpeau

29065 shoulder to hand (long arm)

29075 elbow to finger (short arm)

29085 hand and lower forearm (gauntlet)

29086 finger (eg, contracture)

Splints

29105 Application of long arm splint (shoulder to hand)

29125 Application of short arm splint (forearm to hand); static

29126 dynamic

29130 Application of finger splint; static

29131 dynamic

Strapping—Any Age

29200 Strapping; thorax

29240 shoulder (eg, Velpeau)

29260 elbow or wrist

29280 hand or finger

Lower Extremity

Coding Atlas

When a fracture, dislocation, or other injury requires casting or strapping, the initial cast, strap, or splint is included in the initial service. Codes for a casting, splinting, and strapping procedure are reported only when the procedure is performed as a replacement procedure or if no restorative procedure was performed as part of the initial treatment.

Casts

29305 Application of hip spica cast; 1 leg

29325 1 and one-half spica or both legs

29345 Application of long leg cast (thigh to toes);

29355 walker or ambulatory type

29358 Application of long leg cast brace

29365 Application of cylinder cast (thigh to ankle)

29405 Application of short leg cast (below knee to toes);

29425 walking or ambulatory type

29435 Application of patellar tendon bearing (PTB) cast

29440 Adding walker to previously applied cast

29445 Application of rigid total contact leg cast

29450 Application of clubfoot cast with molding or manipulation, long or short leg

Splints

29505 Application of long leg splint (thigh to ankle or toes)

29515 Application of short leg splint (calf to foot)

Strapping—Any Age

29520 Strapping; hip

29530 knee

29540 ankle and/or foot

29550 toes

29580 Unna boot

29581 Application of multi-layer compression system; leg (below knee), including ankle and foot

29582 thigh and leg, including ankle and foot, when performed

29583 upper arm and forearm

29584 upper arm, forearm, hand, and fingers

Removal or Repair

Coding Atlas

Removal of a cast is included in the services during which the cast is applied. These codes are used to report removing, windowing, or wedging of the cast by someone other than the physician who applied the cast.

29700 Removal or bivalving; gauntlet, boot or body cast

29705 full arm or full leg cast

29710 shoulder or hip spica, Minerva, or Risser jacket, etc.

29720 Repair of spica, body cast or jacket

29730 Windowing of cast

29740 Wedging of cast (except clubfoot casts)

29750 Wedging of clubfoot cast

FIGURE 2-54. Arthroscopic Approach

In **arthroscopy**, two or more small incisions are made into the joint capsule and a small endoscope is inserted into the joint. Exploration and/or repair is performed without **direct visualization**. Instead, a camera is used to transmit images to a video screen or into an eyepiece. The small incision size reduces recovery time and causes less trauma to the surgical site. Note: Tools, implants, and/or equipment depicted in the illustration may be outdated but the procedural approach is valid.

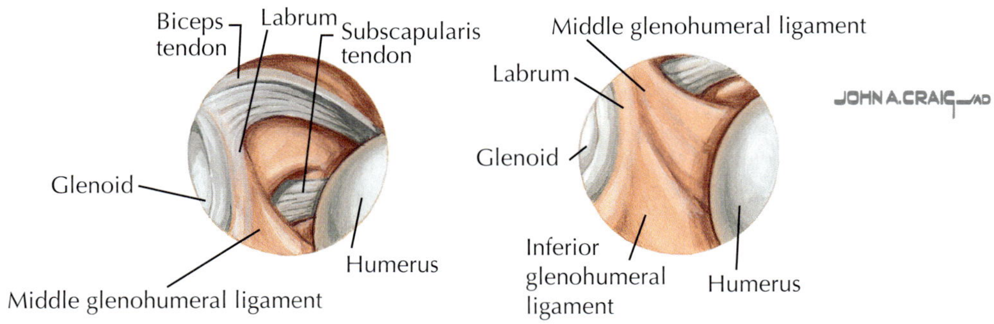

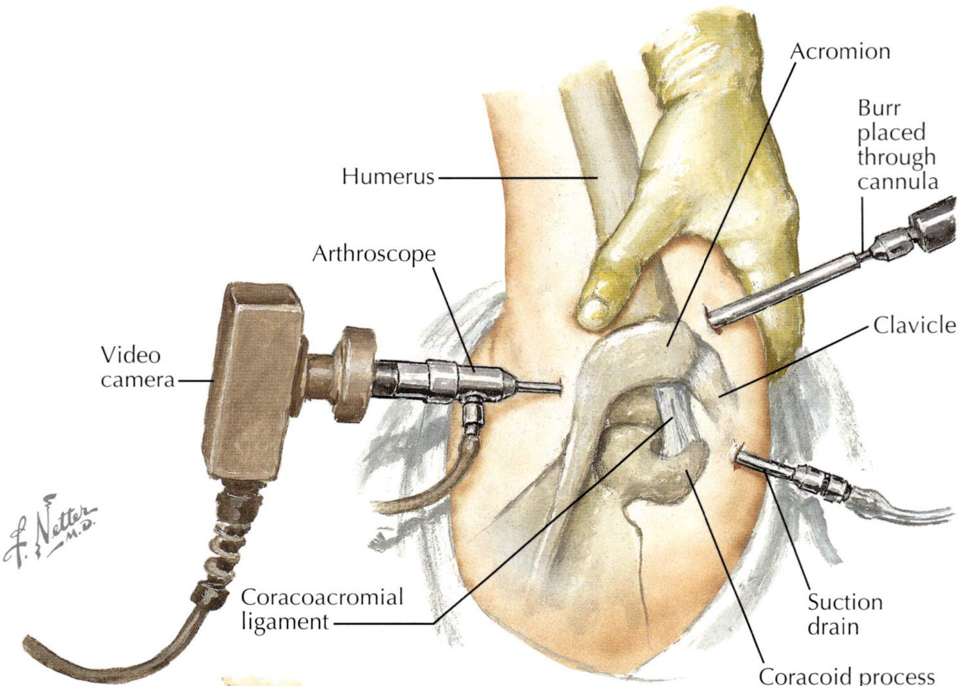

Arthroscope introduced just below posterior angle of acromion, suction drain and burr passed through cannulas via anterior incisions.

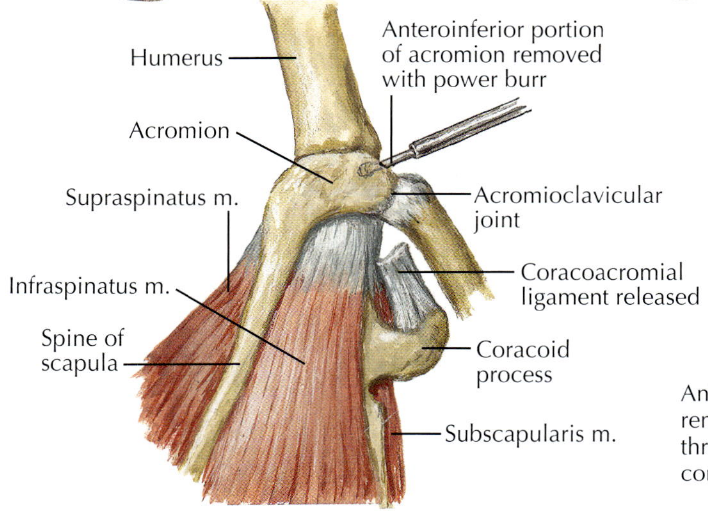

Anteroinferior portion of acromion removed with power burr passed through cannula, thus releasing coracoacromial ligament.

Endoscopy/Arthroscopy

Coding Atlas

For many procedures of the large joints, arthroscopy is performed more frequently than an open arthrotomy. Injuries to smaller joints are increasingly being diagnosed/treated with arthroscopic approaches. The number of portals made to access the joint does not affect code selection.

29800 Arthroscopy, temporomandibular joint, diagnostic, with or without synovial biopsy (separate procedure)

29804 Arthroscopy, temporomandibular joint, surgical

29805 Arthroscopy, shoulder, diagnostic, with or without synovial biopsy (separate procedure)

29806 Arthroscopy, shoulder, surgical; capsulorrhaphy

29807 repair of SLAP lesion

29819 with removal of loose body or foreign body

29820 synovectomy, partial

29821 synovectomy, complete

29822 debridement, limited

29823 debridement, extensive

29824 distal claviculectomy including distal articular surface (Mumford procedure)

29825 with lysis and resection of adhesions, with or without manipulation

✚ **29826** decompression of subacromial space with partial acromioplasty, with coracoacromial ligament (ie, arch) release, when performed (List separately in addition to code for primary procedure)

29827 with rotator cuff repair

29828 biceps tenodesis

29830 Arthroscopy, elbow, diagnostic, with or without synovial biopsy (separate procedure)

29834 Arthroscopy, elbow, surgical; with removal of loose body or foreign body

29835 synovectomy, partial

29836 synovectomy, complete

29837 debridement, limited

29838 debridement, extensive

29840 Arthroscopy, wrist, diagnostic, with or without synovial biopsy (separate procedure)

29843 Arthroscopy, wrist, surgical; for infection, lavage and drainage

29844 synovectomy, partial

29845 synovectomy, complete

29846 excision and/or repair of triangular fibrocartilage and/or joint debridement

29847 internal fixation for fracture or instability

29848 Endoscopy, wrist, surgical, with release of transverse carpal ligament

29850 Arthroscopically aided treatment of intercondylar spine(s) and/or tuberosity fracture(s) of the knee, with or without manipulation; without internal or external fixation (includes arthroscopy)

29851 with internal or external fixation (includes arthroscopy)

29855 Arthroscopically aided treatment of tibial fracture, proximal (plateau); unicondylar, includes internal fixation, when performed (includes arthroscopy)

29856 bicondylar, includes internal fixation, when performed (includes arthroscopy)

29860 Arthroscopy, hip, diagnostic with or without synovial biopsy (separate procedure)

29861 Arthroscopy, hip, surgical; with removal of loose body or foreign body

29862 with debridement/shaving of articular cartilage (chondroplasty), abrasion arthroplasty, and/or resection of labrum

29863 with synovectomy

29914 with femoroplasty (ie, treatment of cam lesion)

29915 with acetabuloplasty (ie, treatment of pincer lesion)

29916 with labral repair

29866 Arthroscopy, knee, surgical; osteochondral autograft(s) (eg, mosaicplasty) (includes harvesting of the autograft[s])

29867 osteochondral allograft (eg, mosaicplasty)

29868 meniscal transplantation (includes arthrotomy for meniscal insertion), medial or lateral

29870 Arthroscopy, knee, diagnostic, with or without synovial biopsy (separate procedure)

29871 Arthroscopy, knee, surgical; for infection, lavage and drainage

29873 with lateral release

29874 for removal of loose body or foreign body (eg, osteochondritis dissecans fragmentation, chondral fragmentation)

29875 synovectomy, limited (eg, plica or shelf resection) (separate procedure)

29876 synovectomy, major, 2 or more compartments (eg, medial or lateral)

29877 debridement/shaving of articular cartilage (chondroplasty)

FIGURE 2-55. Knee Arthroscopy

In arthroscopic surgery, the knee is divided into three compartments: medial, lateral, and patellofemoral. Attention to documented compartments scoped during arthroscopy is essential to proper coding. For example, if a **foreign body** (FB) is removed from the medial compartment during another arthroscopic procedure within the medial compartment, removal of the FB would be considered as part of the larger procedure. However, if the FB is removed arthroscopically from the **lateral** compartment during a **medial** compartment arthroscopic procedure, FB removal may be reported separately. Note: Tools, implants, and/or equipment depicted in the illustration may be outdated but the procedural approach is valid.

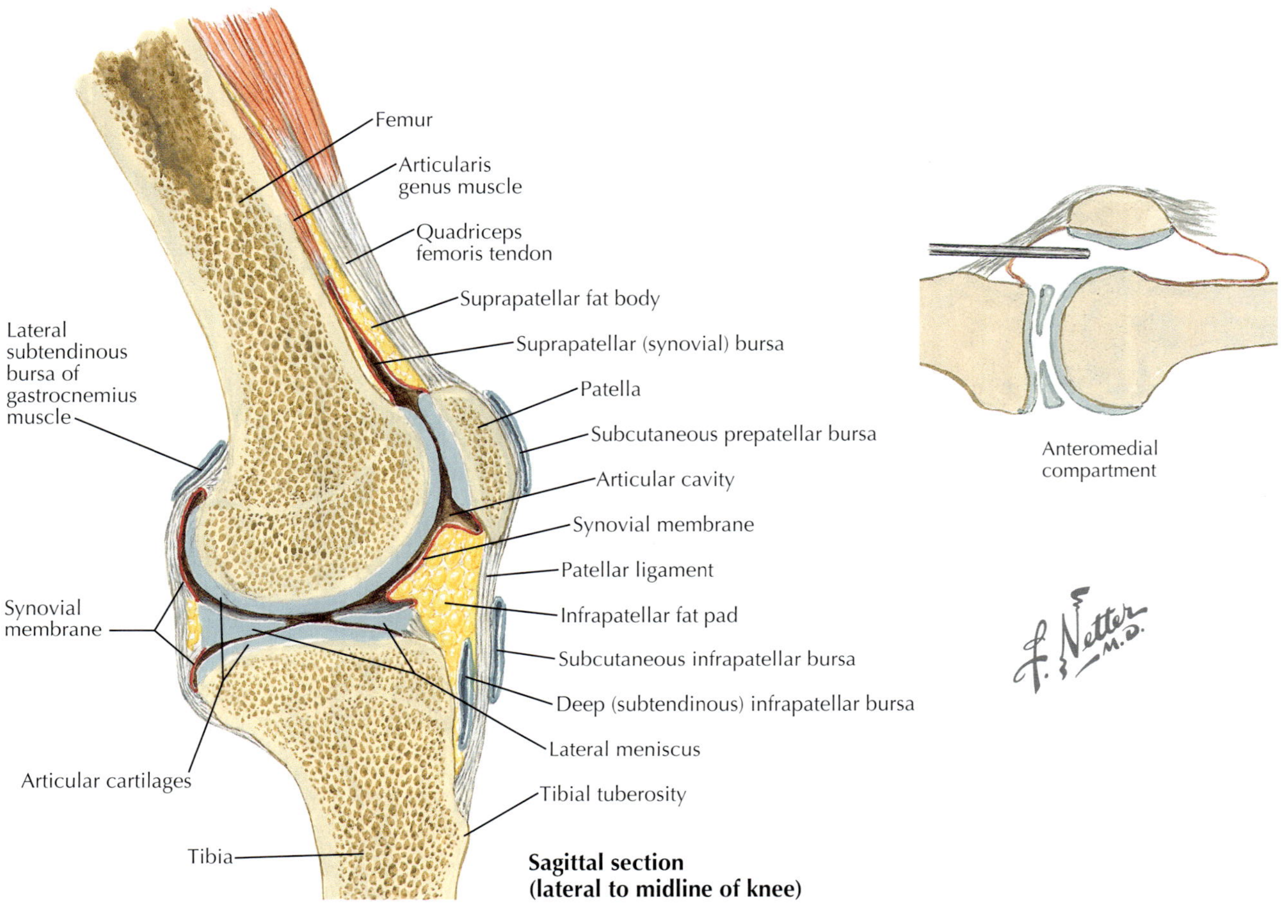

Sagittal section (lateral to midline of knee)

29879 abrasion arthroplasty (includes chondroplasty where necessary) or multiple drilling or microfracture

29880 with meniscectomy (medial AND lateral, including any meniscal shaving) including debridement/shaving of articular cartilage (chondroplasty), same or separate compartment(s), when performed

29881 with meniscectomy (medial OR lateral, including any meniscal shaving) including debridement/shaving of articular cartilage (chondroplasty), same or separate compartment(s), when performed

29882 with meniscus repair (medial OR lateral)

29883 with meniscus repair (medial AND lateral)

29884 with lysis of adhesions, with or without manipulation (separate procedure)

29885 drilling for osteochondritis dissecans with bone grafting, with or without internal fixation (including debridement of base of lesion)

29886 drilling for intact osteochondritis dissecans lesion

29887 drilling for intact osteochondritis dissecans lesion with internal fixation

29888 Arthroscopically aided anterior cruciate ligament repair/augmentation or reconstruction

29889 Arthroscopically aided posterior cruciate ligament repair/augmentation or reconstruction

29891 Arthroscopy, ankle, surgical, excision of osteochondral defect of talus and/or tibia, including drilling of the defect

29892 Arthroscopically aided repair of large osteochondritis dissecans lesion, talar dome fracture, or tibial plafond fracture, with or without internal fixation (includes arthroscopy)

29893 Endoscopic plantar fasciotomy

29894 Arthroscopy, ankle (tibiotalar and fibulotalar joints), surgical; with removal of loose body or foreign body

29895 synovectomy, partial

29897 debridement, limited

29898 debridement, extensive

29899 with ankle arthrodesis

29900 Arthroscopy, metacarpophalangeal joint, diagnostic, includes synovial biopsy

29901 Arthroscopy, metacarpophalangeal joint, surgical; with debridement

29902 with reduction of displaced ulnar collateral ligament (eg, Stenar lesion)

29904 Arthroscopy, subtalar joint, surgical; with removal of loose body or foreign body

29905 with synovectomy

29906 with debridement

29907 with subtalar arthrodesis

29914 Code is out of numerical sequence. See 29800-29999

29915 Code is out of numerical sequence. See 29800-29999

29916 Code is out of numerical sequence. See 29800-29999

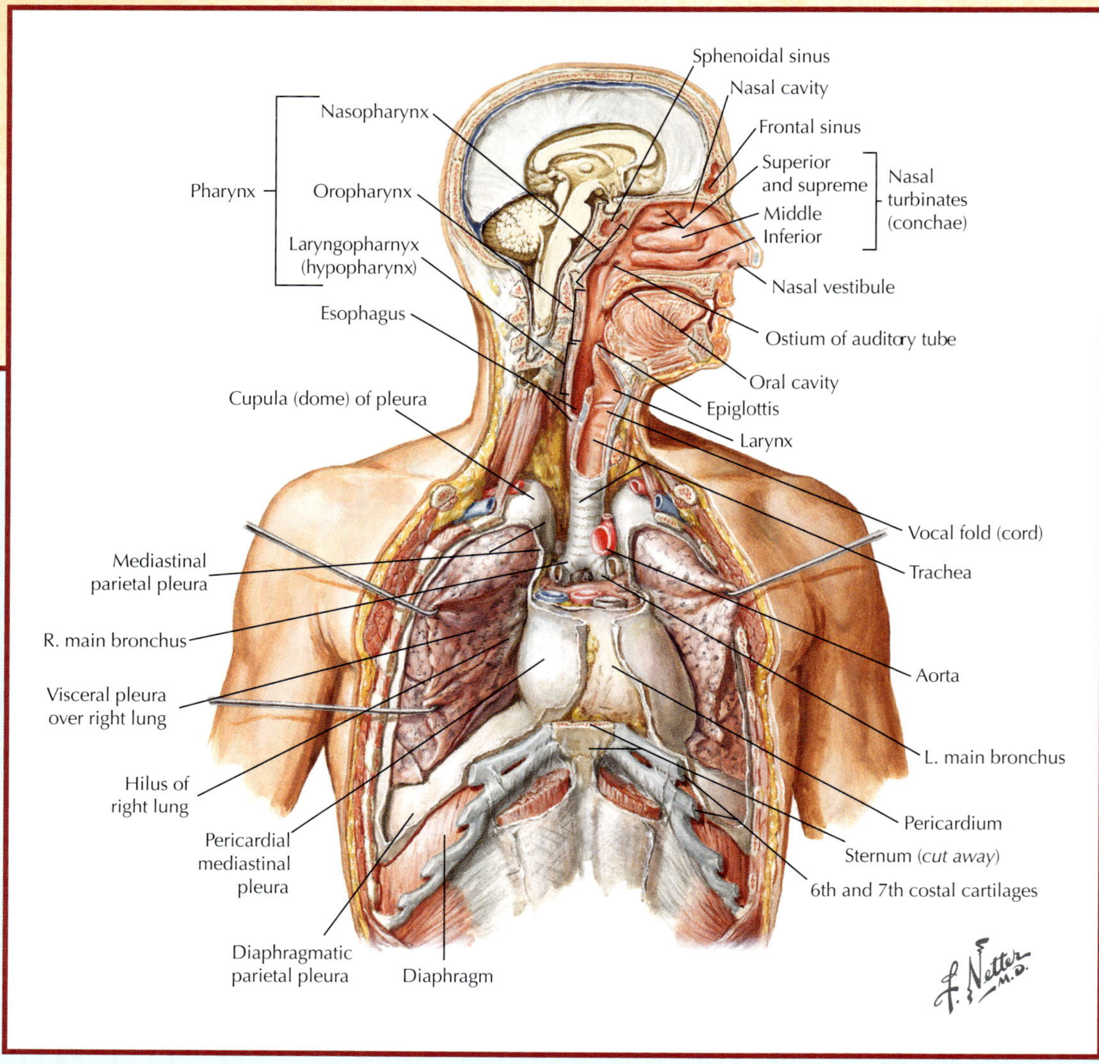
Sphenoidal sinus
Nasal cavity
Frontal sinus
Superior
and supreme
Middle
Inferior
Nasal
turbinates
(conchae)
Nasal vestibule
Ostium of auditory tube
Oral cavity
Epiglottis
Larynx
Vocal fold (cord)
Trachea
Aorta
L. main bronchus
Pericardium
Sternum (cut away)
6th and 7th costal cartilages
Pharynx
Nasopharynx
Oropharynx
Laryngopharnyx
(hypopharynx)
Esophagus
Cupula (dome) of pleura
Mediastinal
parietal pleura
R. main bronchus
Visceral pleura
over right lung
Hilus of
right lung
Pericardial
mediastinal
pleura
Diaphragmatic
parietal pleura
Diaphragm
F. Netter M.D.

◆ CHAPTER 3 ◆

Respiratory System

In simplest terms, oxygen is required at the cellular level in order to produce energy from the food that we consume; this is similar to a fire needing oxygen in order to burn. The respiratory system transports oxygen from outside the body to the bloodstream, which carries it to individual cells throughout the body. The bloodstream also picks up an important waste product of energy production, carbon dioxide, and carries it back to the respiratory system. Each **inspiration** (breath in) delivers oxygen-rich air, and each **expiration** (breath out) removes carbon dioxide and other gaseous waste products from the body.

Air is drawn in through the nose or mouth and, as it travels, it is moistened and warmed in the nasal cavity. Surrounding the nose are four paired sinuses: maxillary, frontal, sphenoid, and ethmoid. The sinuses are a bony framework covered in mucous membrane. Sinuses generate mucus that drains into the nasal structure through openings called **ostia**. **Cilia** on the surface of the **epithelium** of the sinuses and nose filter particles from incoming air. Mucus manufactured in the nose and sinuses collects what has been deposited on cilia, and movement of cilia transports the mucus toward the pharynx.

The pathways for air inhaled through the nose and mouth converge at the pharynx, which is divided into three parts: the nasopharynx, behind the nose and sinuses and above the soft palate; the oropharynx, behind the tongue and above the epiglottis; and the laryngopharynx, above the laryngeal inlet. The oropharynx is a conduit shared by digestive and respiratory systems. At the base of the oropharynx is the epiglottis, which serves as a valve to close the trachea during swallowing so that matter does not enter the lung.

The trachea connects to the right and left main bronchus. These divide and subdivide like inverted trees. Small, branching bronchioles further divide into alveoli, microscopic air sacs responsible for air exchange.

The lungs are dense with bronchi, bronchioles, and alveoli and also with a vascular system; air exchange is dependent on this system. Tiny capillaries wrap around the alveoli to make gas exchange efficient.

The lungs expand greatly during inspiration. To reduce friction in the thorax during inspiration and expiration, the lungs are lined in pleural membranes: the inner visceral pleura and outer parietal pleura. Between these membranes is lubricating fluid that allows the lungs to easily slide within the thorax. The lungs are not mirror images of one another. The right lung has three lobes, while the left lung has two because it shares space with the heart.

The respiratory system also houses the apparatus for sound production: the larynx. During expiration, air passes through the larynx, which contains vibratory cords that produce sound.

There are a significant number of respiratory disorders that are treated surgically. Because of its prominence on the face, the nose is often the site of impact in an injury. The septum dividing the nasal passages, the paired nasal bones, and local cartilage are all easily damaged. Inflammation can cause hyperplasia in the sinuses, which can impede function. The lungs must be a closed system in order to operate properly and, like a balloon being blown up, will fail to inflate if there is a route for air to escape. This condition is called **pneumothorax** and can be treated surgically.

The proliferation of **lumens** in the lower respiratory system and network of cavities in the upper respiratory system are conducive to **endoscopic** approach. The codes for reporting this approach are integrated throughout the Respiratory System code set.

Nose

Incision

Coding Atlas

The nose, sinus, and larynx form the upper respiratory tract, while the trachea, bronchi, and lungs form the lower respiratory tract. A **hematoma** is a pocket of blood between two structures. An **abscess** is a pocket of pus that forms as the result of an infection. The nasal **septum** is the tissue that divides the nose into two nostrils. Trauma to the nose can lead to the formation of a hematoma. To treat the hematoma or abscess, the tissue within the nasal canal that is overlying the defect is incised and the defect is removed.

30000 Drainage abscess or hematoma, nasal, internal approach

30020 Drainage abscess or hematoma, nasal septum

Excision

Coding Atlas

For an **intranasal** approach, an incision is made within the nostril or nasal cavity. An external approach occurs when the skin of the nose is incised to access the nostril or nasal cavity. **Submucous** resection of the inferior turbinate describes the removal of **concha** bone with preservation of the mucosa covering it.

30100 Biopsy, intranasal

30110 Excision, nasal polyp(s), simple

30115 Excision, nasal polyp(s), extensive

30117 Excision or destruction (eg, laser), intranasal lesion; internal approach

30118 external approach (lateral rhinotomy)

30120 Excision or surgical planing of skin of nose for rhinophyma

30124 Excision dermoid cyst, nose; simple, skin, subcutaneous

30125 complex, under bone or cartilage

30130 Excision inferior turbinate, partial or complete, any method

30140 Submucous resection inferior turbinate, partial or complete, any method

30150 Rhinectomy; partial

30160 total

Introduction

Coding Atlas

In displacement therapy, saline solution displaces infected sinus discharge, eg, pus, using pressure flow and suction. A nasal septal button typically is secured over a hole in the nasal **septum**.

30200 Injection into turbinate(s), therapeutic

30210 Displacement therapy (Proetz type)

30220 Insertion, nasal septal prosthesis (button)

Removal of Foreign Body

Coding Atlas

A nasal **foreign body** (NFB) is an **organic** or **inorganic** material that has been forced into the nasal cavity during trauma or placed in the nose where it inadvertently became lodged. An NFB differs from a **prosthesis**, which is implanted by a health care professional. NFBs may be removed using an **intranasal** approach or they may require a skin incision through the **lateral** nose and into the nostril or nasal cavity. Code 30300 is used to report removal of an NFB under **direct visualization** using forceps.

30300 Removal foreign body, intranasal; office type procedure

30310 requiring general anesthesia

30320 by lateral rhinotomy

Repair

Coding Atlas

Rhinoplasty is a type of surgery that changes the appearance and functionality of the nose by changing its skin, cartilage, bone, and lining. A rhinoplasty may be the first surgery performed on the nose (**primary**) or it may be performed after a previous surgery (**secondary**), indicating a follow-up surgery to revise previous work. Many rhinoplasties are **cosmetic**, but some are performed to reverse the effects of trauma or a previous surgical procedure, or to repair a **congenital** deformity.

30400 Rhinoplasty, primary; lateral and alar cartilages and/or elevation of nasal tip

30410 complete, external parts including bony pyramid, lateral and alar cartilages, and/or elevation of nasal tip

30420 including major septal repair

FIGURE 3-1. Nasal Examination and Polyps

The external nose is only part of the nasal anatomy. The nasal cavity continues behind the nostrils above the palate and is filled with conchae (**turbinates**) that extend from the **lateral** nasal walls toward the nasal **septum**. The conchae are composed of spiral-shaped bone covered with mucous membrane. Inhaled air passes through the conchae en route to the lungs. Sinuses, **eustachian tubes**, and **nasolacrimal ducts** all drain into the nasal cavity; any blockage in this area can be disruptive or inflammatory. Note: Tools, implants, and/or equipment depicted in the illustration may be outdated but the procedural approach is valid.

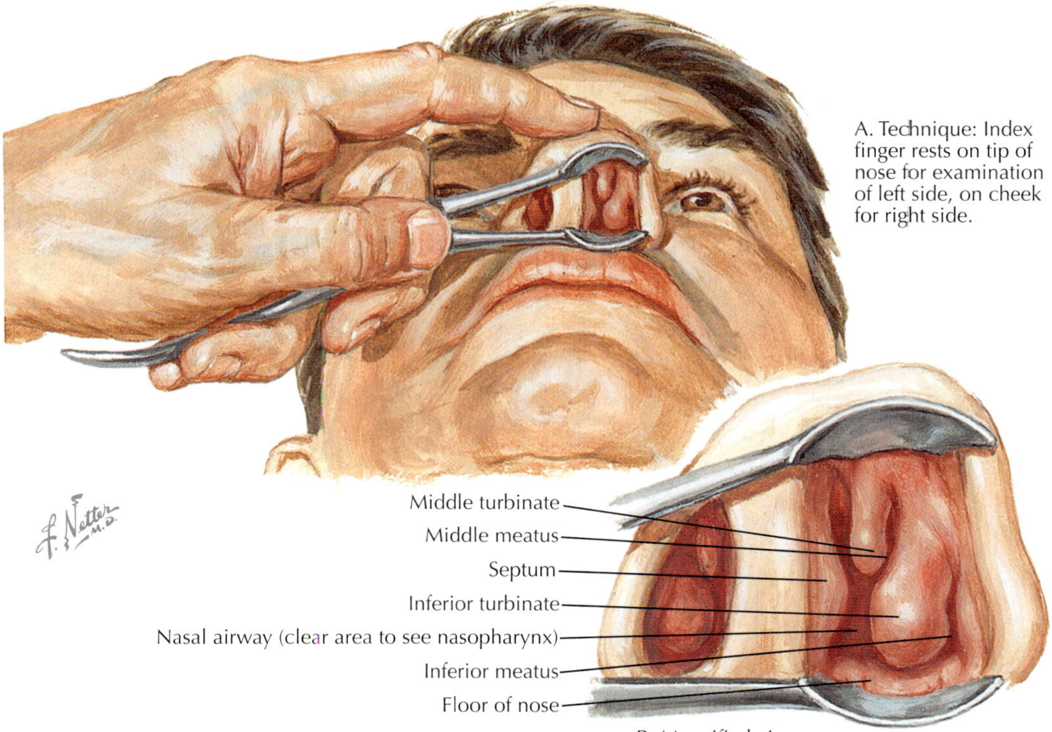

Anatomy of the Nose

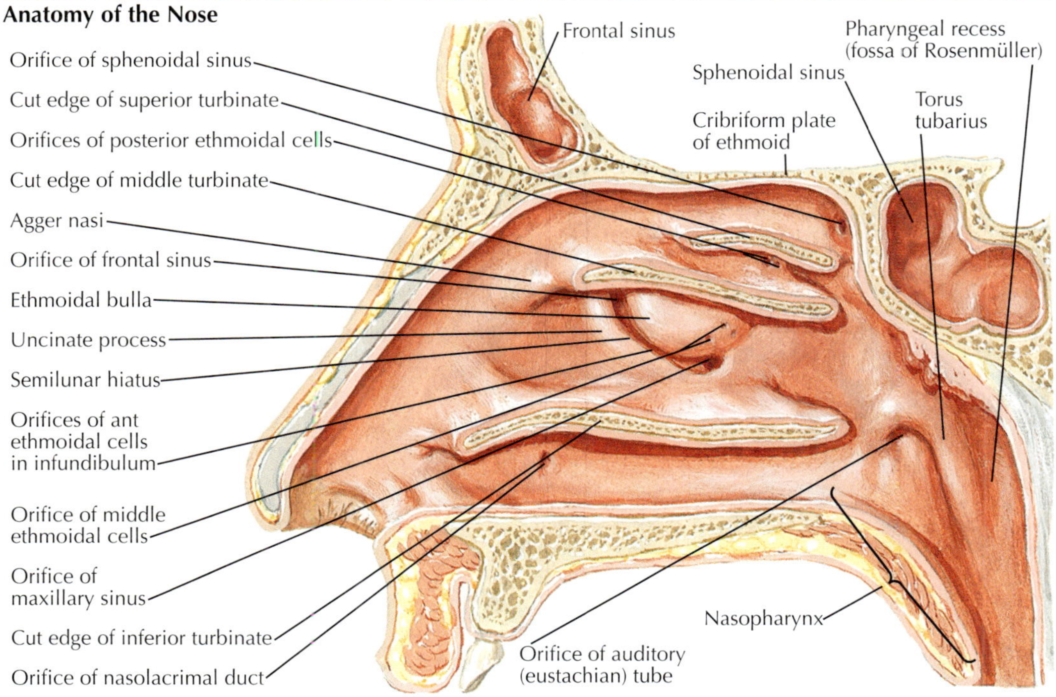

FIGURE 3-2. The Nose

Paired nasal bones begin at the frontal bone of the forehead and end at the top third of the nasal prominence. **Cartilage** supports the remaining two-thirds of the nose. The midline nasal septum is also primarily cartilage, with ethmoid bone located posteriorly. The nose and nasal cavity are highly **innervated** and **vascularized**.

Anterolateral view

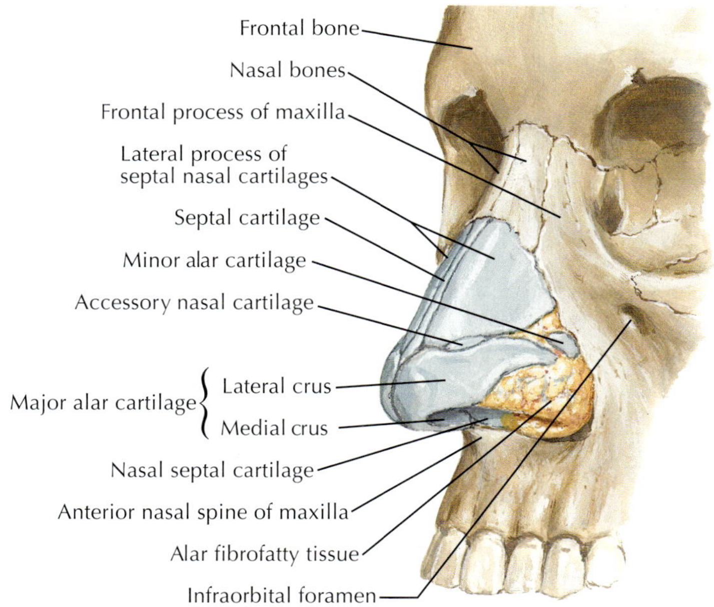

Inferior view

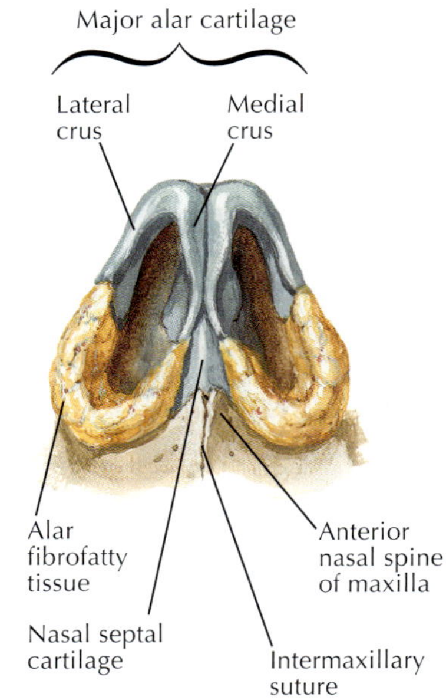

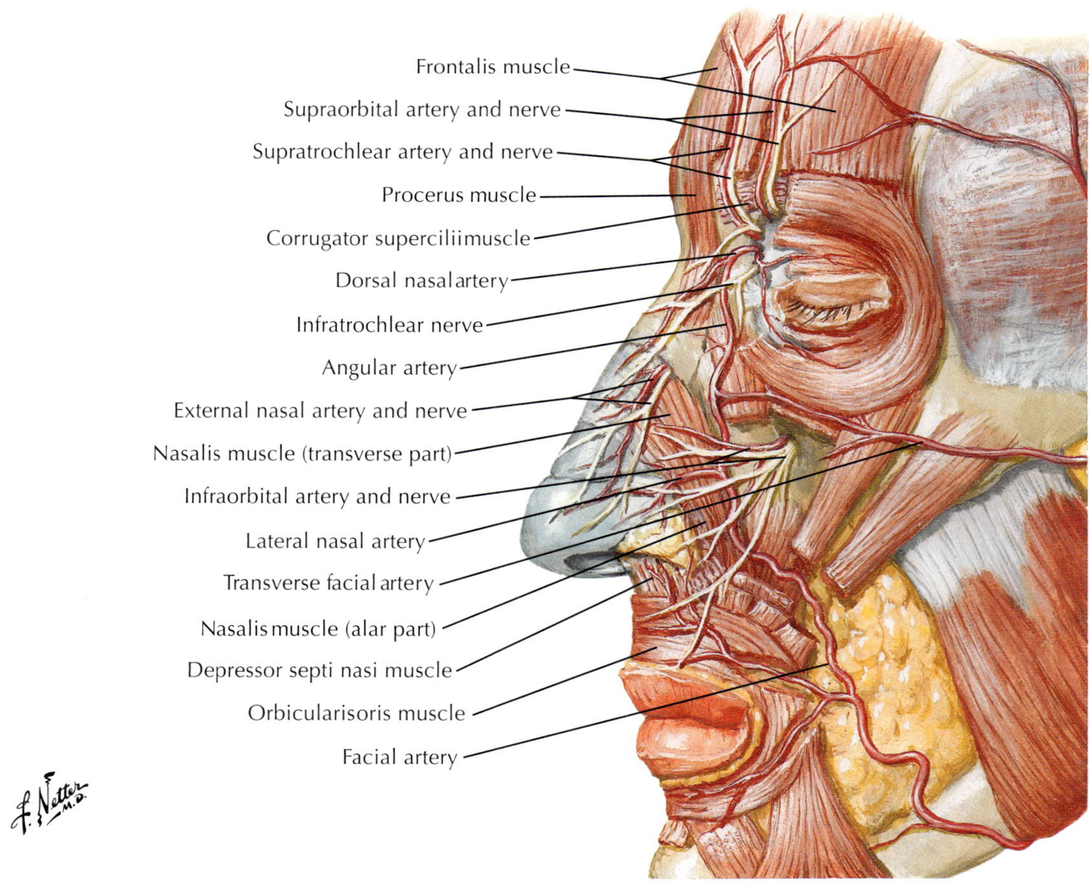

30430 Rhinoplasty, secondary; minor revision (small amount of nasal tip work)

30435 intermediate revision (bony work with osteotomies)

30450 major revision (nasal tip work and osteotomies)

30460 Rhinoplasty for nasal deformity secondary to congenital cleft lip and/or palate, including columellar lengthening; tip only

30462 tip, septum, osteotomies

30465 Repair of nasal vestibular stenosis (eg, spreader grafting, lateral nasal wall reconstruction)

30520 Septoplasty or submucous resection, with or without cartilage scoring, contouring or replacement with graft

30540 Repair choanal atresia; intranasal

30545 transpalatine

30560 Lysis intranasal synechia

30580 Repair fistula; oromaxillary (combine with 31030 if antrotomy is included)

30600 oronasal

30620 Septal or other intranasal dermatoplasty (does not include obtaining graft)

30630 Repair nasal septal perforations

Destruction

Coding Atlas

Superficial turbinate reduction involves treatment of only the surface layer of the turbinates. **Intramural** or **submucosal** ablation involves deeper tissue and the piercing of the surface mucosa of the turbinate to deliver the **ablation** device. **Radiofrequency** ablation is a common intramural ablation method. For ablation of the middle or superior concha/turbinates, an unlisted nasal procedure is reported using code 30999.

30801 Ablation, soft tissue of inferior turbinates, unilateral or bilateral, any method (eg, electrocautery, radiofrequency ablation, or tissue volume reduction); superficial

30802 intramural (ie, submucosal)

Other Procedures

Coding Atlas

Anterior nosebleeds occur in the front of the nose and typically are treated with nasal tampons and/or **cautery**. **Posterior** nose bleeds of the nasal vestibule are treated with cautery and/or an inflated balloon catheter.

30901 Control nasal hemorrhage, anterior, simple (limited cautery and/or packing) any method

30903 Control nasal hemorrhage, anterior, complex (extensive cautery and/or packing) any method

30905 Control nasal hemorrhage, posterior, with posterior nasal packs and/or cautery, any method; initial

30906 subsequent

30915 Ligation arteries; ethmoidal

30920 internal maxillary artery transantral

30930 Fracture nasal inferior turbinate(s), therapeutic

Accessory Sinuses

Incision

Coding Atlas

Sinus blockage is a common cause for sinus surgery. The **ostiomeatal complex** (OMC) is often the target for sinus surgery, as this area is easily impeded by **hypertrophy**, chronic inflammation, or swelling. The OMC includes tissues between the middle concha (**turbinate**) and the orbital bone. **Concha bullosa** is a common abnormality in which the bone in a **concha** contains an air-filled pocket. If the air pocket significantly increases the size of the concha, it may lead to a blocked pathway.

31000 Lavage by cannulation; maxillary sinus (antrum puncture or natural ostium)

31002 sphenoid sinus

31020 Sinusotomy, maxillary (antrotomy); intranasal

31030 radical (Caldwell-Luc) without removal of antrochoanal polyps

31032 radical (Caldwell-Luc) with removal of antrochoanal polyps

31040 Pterygomaxillary fossa surgery, any approach

31050 Sinusotomy, sphenoid, with or without biopsy;

31051 with mucosal stripping or removal of polyp(s)

31070 Sinusotomy frontal; external, simple (trephine operation)

31075 transorbital, unilateral (for mucocele or osteoma, Lynch type)

31080 obliterative without osteoplastic flap, brow incision (includes ablation)

31081 obliterative, without osteoplastic flap, coronal incision (includes ablation)

31084 obliterative, with osteoplastic flap, brow incision

31085 obliterative, with osteoplastic flap, coronal incision

FIGURE 3-3. The Paranasal Sinuses

There are four sets of paired, epithelium-lined sinuses: maxillary (**posterior** to cheeks); frontal (posterior to eyebrows); ethmoid (between the eyes); and sphenoid (behind the nose). Each sinus communicates with the nasal cavity through an **ostium**, or small orifice, through which mucus can drain. The sinus cavities are named according to bones within which the sinuses lie. The maxillary sinuses are also called maxillary **antra**.

Coronal section

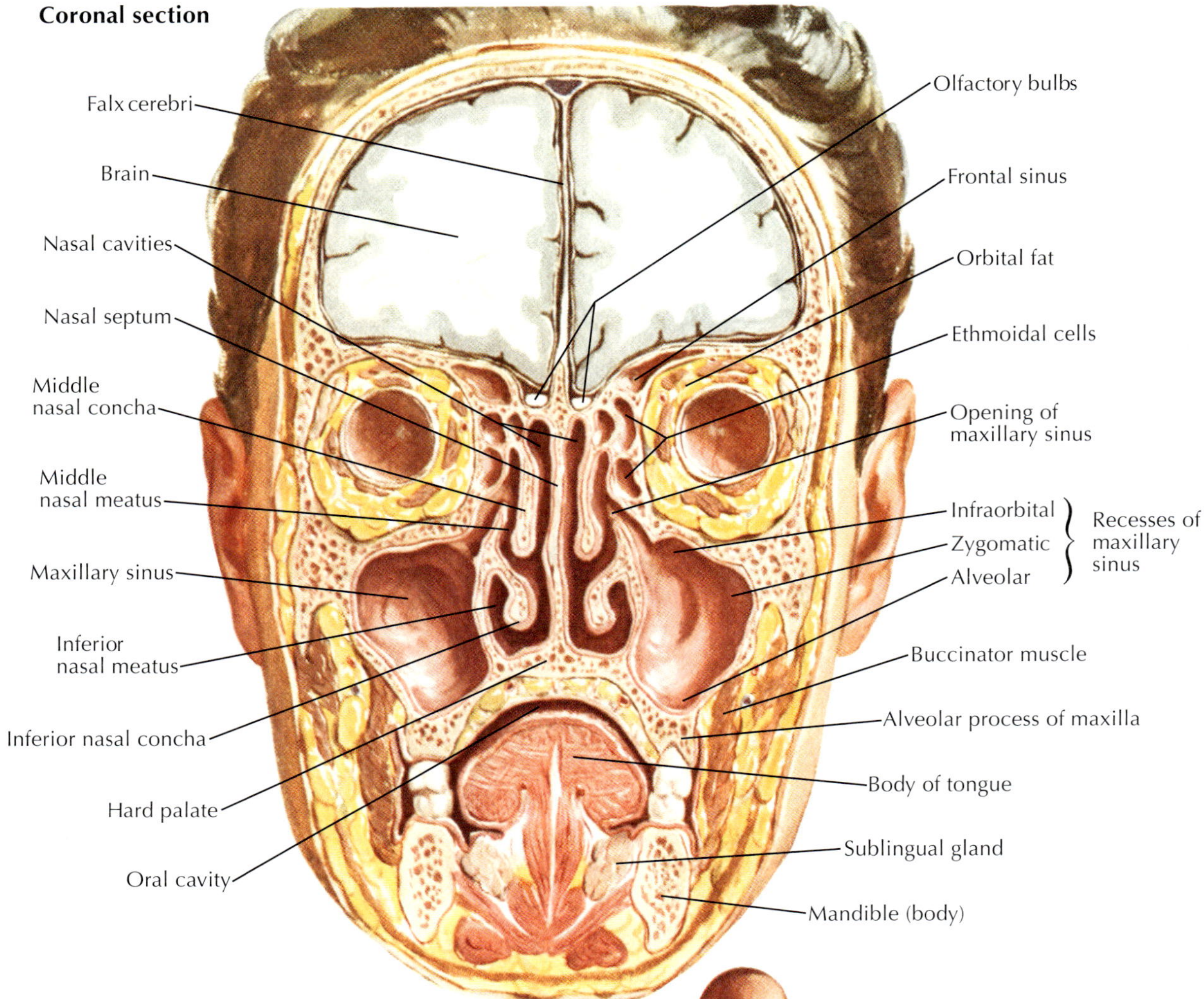

Horizontal section

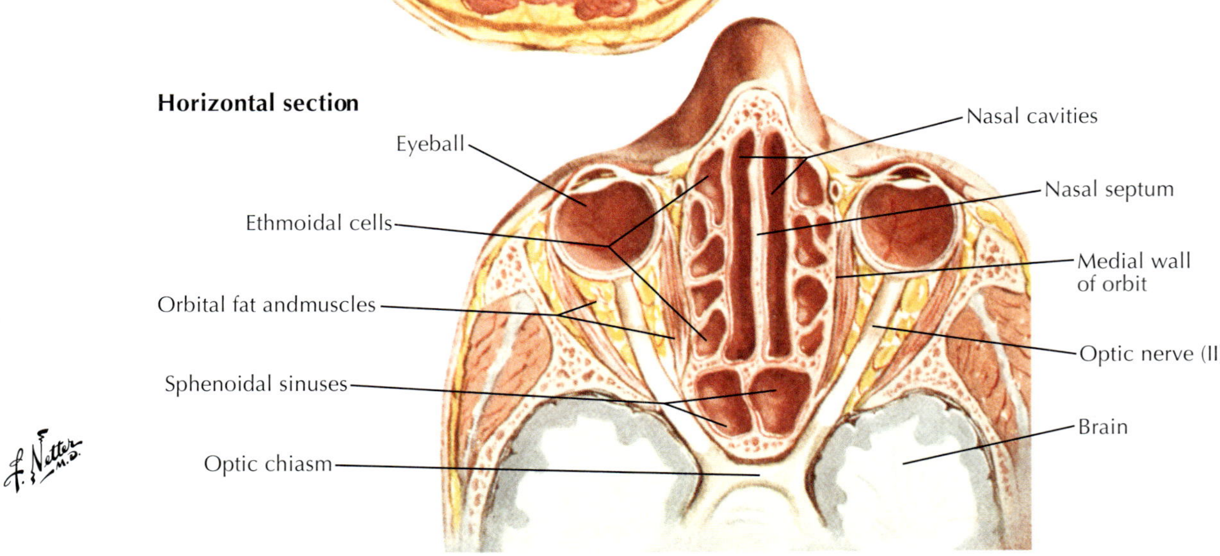

31086 nonobliterative, with osteoplastic flap, brow incision

31087 nonobliterative, with osteoplastic flap, coronal incision

31090 Sinusotomy, unilateral, 3 or more paranasal sinuses (frontal, maxillary, ethmoid, sphenoid)

Excision

Coding Atlas

Maxillary and ethmoidal sinus excisions are performed to remove **tumors**, diseased **granulomatous** tissue, or fungal infection. Open approaches to sinus surgery are varied. In a Caldwell-Luc (CWL) approach, the maxillary sinus is entered through an **intraoral** incision above the upper gum line. In an **intranasal** approach, an incision is made with **direct visualization** of the sinus incision site through the nostril. In an **extranasal** approach, an incision of the skin overlying the nostril opens the nasal cavity for **direct visualization**.

31200 Ethmoidectomy; intranasal, anterior

31201 intranasal, total

31205 extranasal, total

31225 Maxillectomy; without orbital exenteration

31230 with orbital exenteration (en bloc)

Endoscopy

Coding Atlas

Functional endoscopic sinus surgery (FESS) may be noted when a physician uses an endoscope to access the patient's nasal sinuses in order to remove diseased tissue and bone, with a goal of opening passageways, improving drainage, or promoting healthy tissue growth. FESS is reported according to site. For example, code 31254 is used to report FESS with anterior **ethmoidectomy**. Codes in the range 31295-31297 are used to describe **dilation** of sinus **ostia** by displacement of tissue using any method, including codes for reporting any **fluoroscopy** performed.

31231 Nasal endoscopy, diagnostic, unilateral or bilateral (separate procedure)

31233 Nasal/sinus endoscopy, diagnostic with maxillary sinusoscopy (via inferior meatus or canine fossa puncture)

31235 Nasal/sinus endoscopy, diagnostic with sphenoid sinusoscopy (via puncture of sphenoidal face or cannulation of ostium)

31237 Nasal/sinus endoscopy, surgical; with biopsy, polypectomy or debridement (separate procedure)

31238 with control of nasal hemorrhage

31239 with dacryocystorhinostomy

31240 with concha bullosa resection

31254 Nasal/sinus endoscopy, surgical; with ethmoidectomy, partial (anterior)

31255 with ethmoidectomy, total (anterior and posterior)

31256 Nasal/sinus endoscopy, surgical, with maxillary antrostomy;

31267 with removal of tissue from maxillary sinus

31276 Nasal/sinus endoscopy, surgical with frontal sinus exploration, with or without removal of tissue from frontal sinus

31287 Nasal/sinus endoscopy, surgical, with sphenoidotomy;

31288 with removal of tissue from the sphenoid sinus

31290 Nasal/sinus endoscopy, surgical, with repair of cerebrospinal fluid leak; ethmoid region

31291 sphenoid region

31292 Nasal/sinus endoscopy, surgical; with medial or inferior orbital wall decompression

31293 with medial orbital wall and inferior orbital wall decompression

31294 with optic nerve decompression

31295 Nasal/sinus endoscopy, surgical; with dilation of maxillary sinus ostium (eg, balloon dilation), transnasal or via canine fossa

31296 with dilation of frontal sinus ostium (eg, balloon dilation)

31297 with dilation of sphenoid sinus ostium (eg, balloon dilation)

FIGURE 3-4. The Larynx and Trachea

The larynx is **superior** to the trachea in the **anterior** neck. The epiglottis is the laryngeal cartilage responsible for protecting the respiratory system from **aspiration** of food and drink; it does this by closing off the respiratory tract during swallowing. The larynx also houses the vocal cords; during **expiration** of breath, air is forced through the vocal cords to produce sounds. The thyroid and its **cartilage** are adjacent to the larynx. Procedures on the thyroid gland appear in the Endocrine section of the CPT code set.

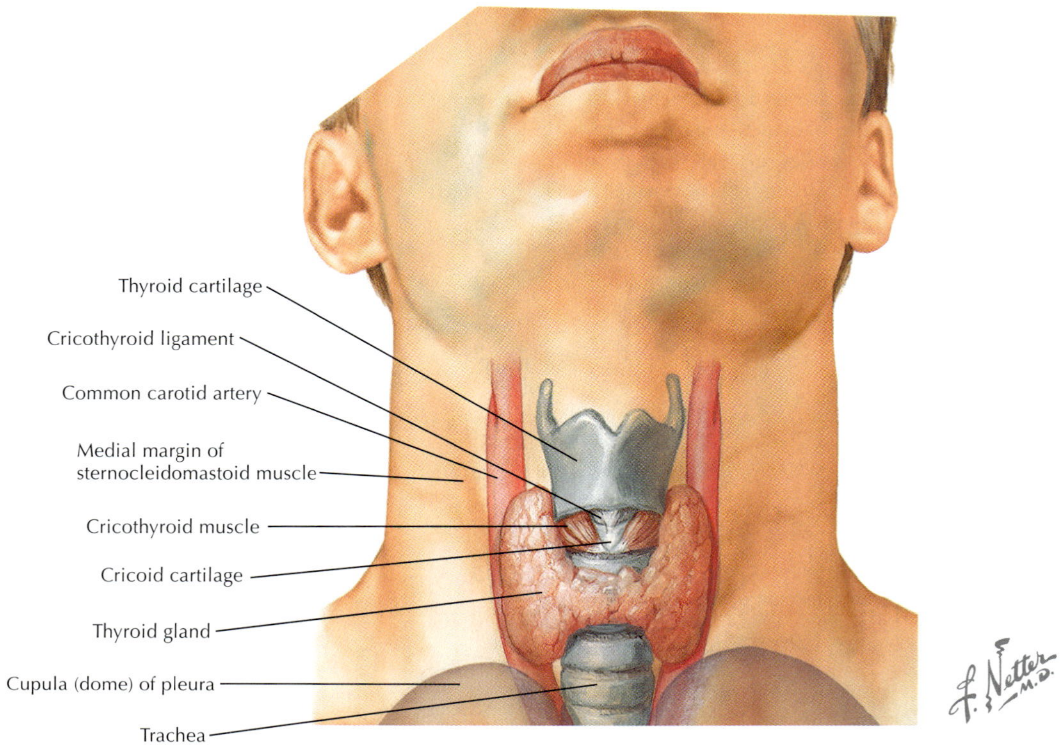

Larynx

Excision

Coding Atlas

Cordectomy is the surgical removal of the vocal cord. **Laryngectomy** is removal of the larynx, and **pharyngolaryngectomy** (PL) is surgical excision of the larynx along with the tissue at the back of the throat. **Arytenoidectomy** is performed to treat vocal cord paralysis by enlarging the laryngeal cavity across which the vocal cords stretch.

31300 Laryngotomy (thyrotomy, laryngofissure); with removal of tumor or laryngocele, cordectomy

31320 diagnostic

31360 Laryngectomy; total, without radical neck dissection

31365 total, with radical neck dissection

31367 subtotal supraglottic, without radical neck dissection

31368 subtotal supraglottic, with radical neck dissection

31370 Partial laryngectomy (hemilaryngectomy); horizontal

31375 laterovertical

31380 anterovertical

31382 antero-latero-vertical

31390 Pharyngolaryngectomy, with radical neck dissection; without reconstruction

31395 with reconstruction

31400 Arytenoidectomy or arytenoidopexy, external approach

(For endoscopic arytenoidectomy, use 31560)

31420 Epiglottidectomy

FIGURE 3-5. Radical Neck Dissection

Radical neck dissection (RND) includes the removal of all lymph nodes including submental, submandibular, and jugular, together with the **ipsilateral** spinal accessory nerve (SAN), sternocleidomastoid muscle (SCM), and internal jugular vein (IJV). RND is considered a **unilateral** procedure. Any **midline** nodes are considered ipsilateral. Note: Tools, implants, and/or equipment depicted in the illustration may be outdated but the procedural approach is valid.

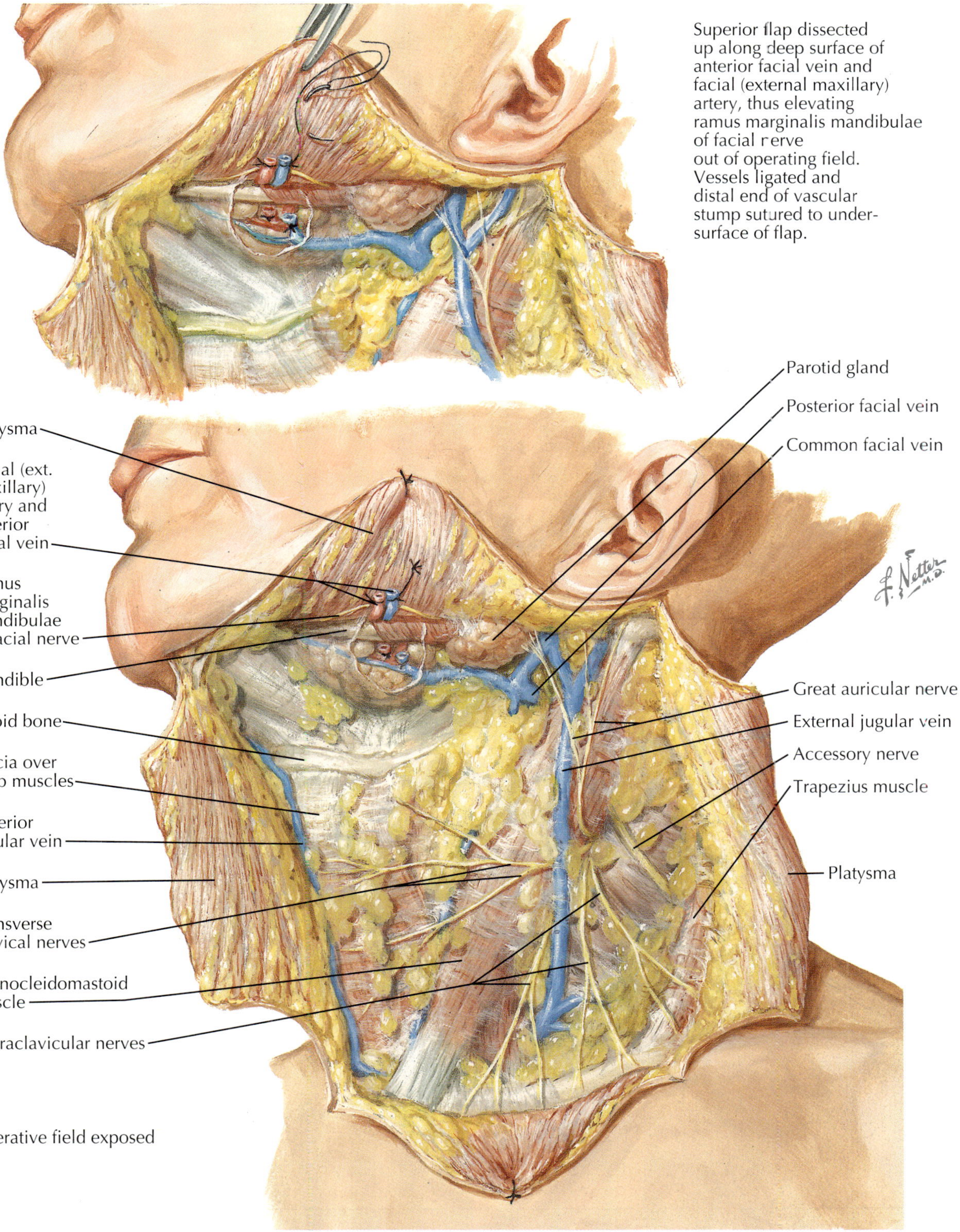

Operative field exposed

Introduction

Coding Atlas

Code 31500 can be used to report stand-alone emergent or semi-emergent endotracheal intubation such as rapid sequence intubation with use of either a flexible or rigid endoscope. Code 31502 is used to report complex changing of a tracheotomy tube that requires reestablishing a fistula tract that has not yet been permanently formed.

⊘ **31500** Intubation, endotracheal, emergency procedure

31502 Tracheotomy tube change prior to establishment of fistula tract

Endoscopy

Coding Atlas

In indirect laryngoscopy, a small mirror is held at the back of the patient's throat and the physician shines a light on the mirror to view the larynx. In direct laryngoscopy, a laryngoscope is placed in the patient's throat. The scope may be flexible or stiff. The physician is able to see deep into the throat and may be able to manipulate tools through the scope to remove tissue for biopsy or to remove a foreign body from the larynx. In fiberoptic laryngoscopy, a flexible endoscope allows the physician to view an image of the larynx.

31505 Laryngoscopy, indirect; diagnostic (separate procedure)

31510 with biopsy

31511 with removal of foreign body

31512 with removal of lesion

31513 with vocal cord injection

31515 Laryngoscopy direct, with or without tracheoscopy; for aspiration

31520 diagnostic, newborn

31525 diagnostic, except newborn

31526 diagnostic, with operating microscope or telescope

31527 with insertion of obturator

31528 with dilation, initial

31529 with dilation, subsequent

31530 Laryngoscopy, direct, operative, with foreign body removal;

31531 with operating microscope or telescope

31535 Laryngoscopy, direct, operative, with biopsy;

31536 with operating microscope or telescope

31540 Laryngoscopy, direct, operative, with excision of tumor and/or stripping of vocal cords or epiglottis;

31541 with operating microscope or telescope

31545 Laryngoscopy, direct, operative, with operating microscope or telescope, with submucosal removal of non-neoplastic lesion(s) of vocal cord; reconstruction with local tissue flap(s)

31546 reconstruction with graft(s) (includes obtaining autograft)

31560 Laryngoscopy, direct, operative, with arytenoidectomy;

31561 with operating microscope or telescope

31570 Laryngoscopy, direct, with injection into vocal cord(s), therapeutic;

31571 with operating microscope or telescope

31575 Laryngoscopy, flexible fiberoptic; diagnostic

31576 with biopsy

31577 with removal of foreign body

31578 with removal of lesion

31579 Laryngoscopy, flexible or rigid fiberoptic, with stroboscopy

Repair

Coding Atlas

Codes in the range 31580-31590 are used to report open procedures that include incision into the skin of the neck to access the larynx. For endoscopic approach to laryngoplasty, see codes 31545-31546.

31580 Laryngoplasty; for laryngeal web, 2-stage, with keel insertion and removal

31582 for laryngeal stenosis, with graft or core mold, including tracheotomy

31584 with open reduction of fracture

31587 Laryngoplasty, cricoid split

31588 Laryngoplasty, not otherwise specified (eg, for burns, reconstruction after partial laryngectomy)

31590 Laryngeal reinnervation by neuromuscular pedicle

FIGURE 3-6. The Larynx

Thyroid cartilage forms the Adam's apple, and cricoid cartilage forms the **inferior** wall of the larynx. Bilateral arytenoid cartilage are important because they affect the tension of the vocal cords. The **posterior** cricoarytenoid muscles separate the vocal cords for normal breathing. If these muscles become paralyzed, eg, as a result of **bilateral** injury of the recurrent laryngeal nerve, the result is difficulty when breathing.

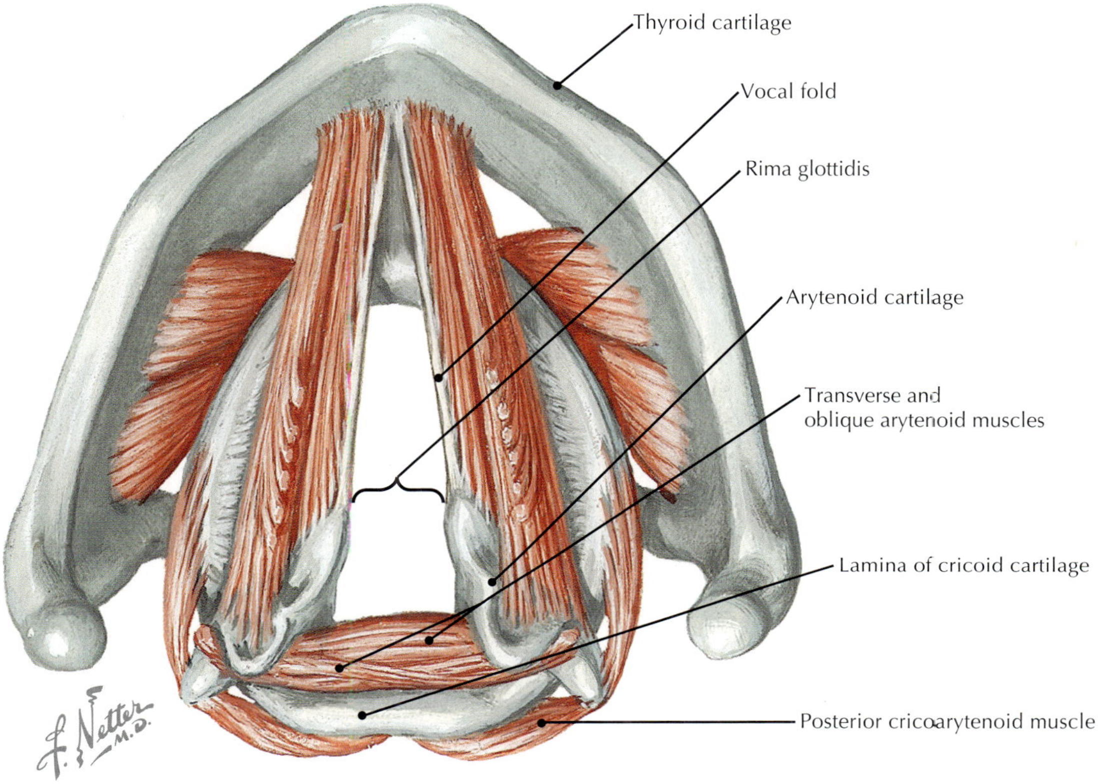

FIGURE 3-7. The Trachea and Pharynx

The pharynx communicates with the esophagus, nasal cavity, middle ear, and larynx. It is divided into three anatomical sites: nasopharynx, oropharynx, and laryngopharynx. The trachea, or windpipe, is composed of about 20 rings of tough **cartilage** and is lined in **mucosa**. At its base, it divides into the right and left bronchus. A **posterior** view of the pharynx can be seen in Figure 5-6.

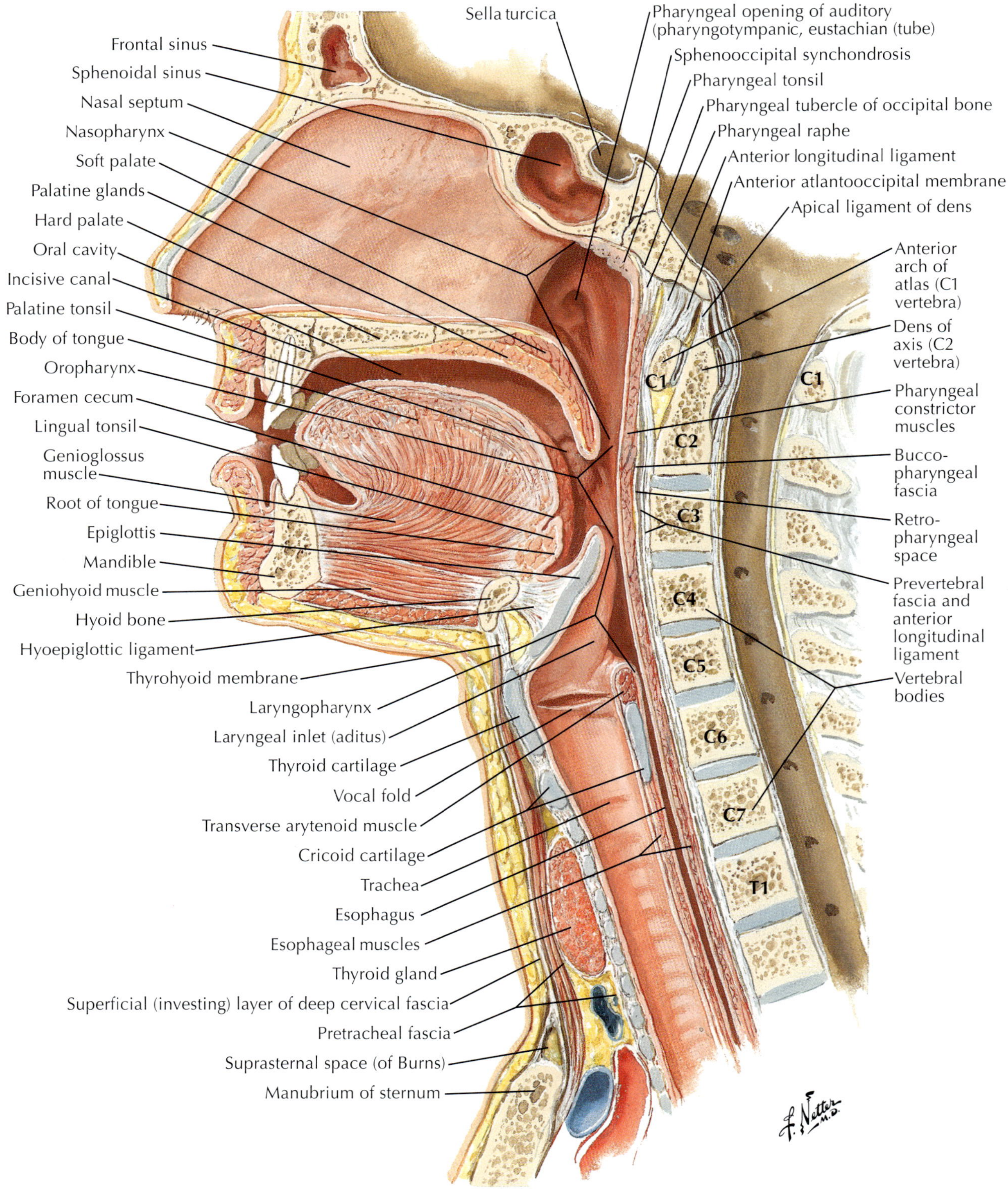

Destruction

31595 Section recurrent laryngeal nerve, therapeutic (separate procedure), unilateral

Trachea and Bronchi

Incision

Coding Atlas

Tracheostomies are often performed for transient conditions when patients require ventilation. When the patient recovers, the ventilator is removed and the tracheostomy is closed. Some patients require permanent tracheostomies and may be fitted with a laryngeal speech prosthesis.

31600 Tracheostomy, planned (separate procedure);

31601 younger than 2 years

31603 Tracheostomy, emergency procedure; transtracheal

31605 cricothyroid membrane

31610 Tracheostomy, fenestration procedure with skin flaps

31611 Construction of tracheoesophageal fistula and subsequent insertion of an alaryngeal speech prosthesis (eg, voice button, Blom-Singer prosthesis)

31612 Tracheal puncture, percutaneous with transtracheal aspiration and/or injection

31613 Tracheostoma revision; simple, without flap rotation

31614 complex, with flap rotation

Endoscopy

Coding Atlas

Fiducial markers (code 31626) are placed prior to excisional surgery or radiation therapy to mark the site(s) targeted for treatment. Computer-assisted, image-guided navigation (code 31627) is typically performed in a planning phase during which software reconstructs three-dimensional images of lesions that are targeted for sampling. This is often called navigational bronchoscopy.

⊙ 31615 Tracheobronchoscopy through established tracheostomy incision

⊙+ 31620 Endobronchial ultrasound (EBUS) during bronchoscopic diagnostic or therapeutic intervention(s) (List separately in addition to code for primary procedure[s])

⊙ 31622 Bronchoscopy, rigid or flexible, including fluoroscopic guidance, when performed; diagnostic, with cell washing, when performed (separate procedure)

⊙ 31623 with brushing or protected brushings

⊙ 31624 with bronchial alveolar lavage

⊙ 31625 with bronchial or endobronchial biopsy(s), single or multiple sites

⊙ 31626 with placement of fiducial markers, single or multiple

⊙+ 31627 with computer-assisted, image-guided navigation (List separately in addition to code for primary procedure[s])

⊙ 31628 with transbronchial lung biopsy(s), single lobe

⊙ 31629 with transbronchial needle aspiration biopsy(s), trachea, main stem and/or lobar bronchus(i)

31630 with tracheal/bronchial dilation or closed reduction of fracture

31631 with placement of tracheal stent(s) (includes tracheal/bronchial dilation as required)

+ 31632 with transbronchial lung biopsy(s), each additional lobe (List separately in addition to code for primary procedure)

+ 31633 with transbronchial needle aspiration biopsy(s), each additional lobe (List separately in addition to code for primary procedure)

⊙ 31634 with balloon occlusion, with assessment of air leak, with administration of occlusive substance (eg, fibrin glue), if performed

⊙ 31635 with removal of foreign body

31636 with placement of bronchial stent(s) (includes tracheal/bronchial dilation as required), initial bronchus

+ 31637 each additional major bronchus stented (List separately in addition to code for primary procedure)

31638 with revision of tracheal or bronchial stent inserted at previous session (includes tracheal/bronchial dilation as required)

31640 with excision of tumor

31641 with destruction of tumor or relief of stenosis by any method other than excision (eg, laser therapy, cryotherapy)

31643 with placement of catheter(s) for intracavitary radioelement application

⊙ 31645 with therapeutic aspiration of tracheobronchial tree, initial (eg, drainage of lung abscess)

⊙ 31646 with therapeutic aspiration of tracheobronchial tree, subsequent

⊙ 31647 with balloon occlusion, when performed, assessment of air leak, airway sizing, and insertion of bronchial valve(s), initial lobe

#⊙+ 31651 with balloon occlusion, when performed, assessment of air leak, airway sizing, and insertion of bronchial valve(s), each additional lobe (List separately in addition to code for primary procedure[s])

FIGURE 3-8. Tracheostomy

A **tracheostomy** is either a planned or emergency procedure. A planned tracheostomy occurs when a patient with compromised health is already in a health care setting and requires breathing assistance. An emergency tracheostomy occurs when a person's respiration is suddenly blocked and health care professionals must quickly open an airway. A tracheostomy may be **percutaneous** or **open**. Figure 3-8 shows an open tracheostomy. Note: Tools, implants, and/or equipment depicted in the illustration may be outdated but the procedural approach is valid.

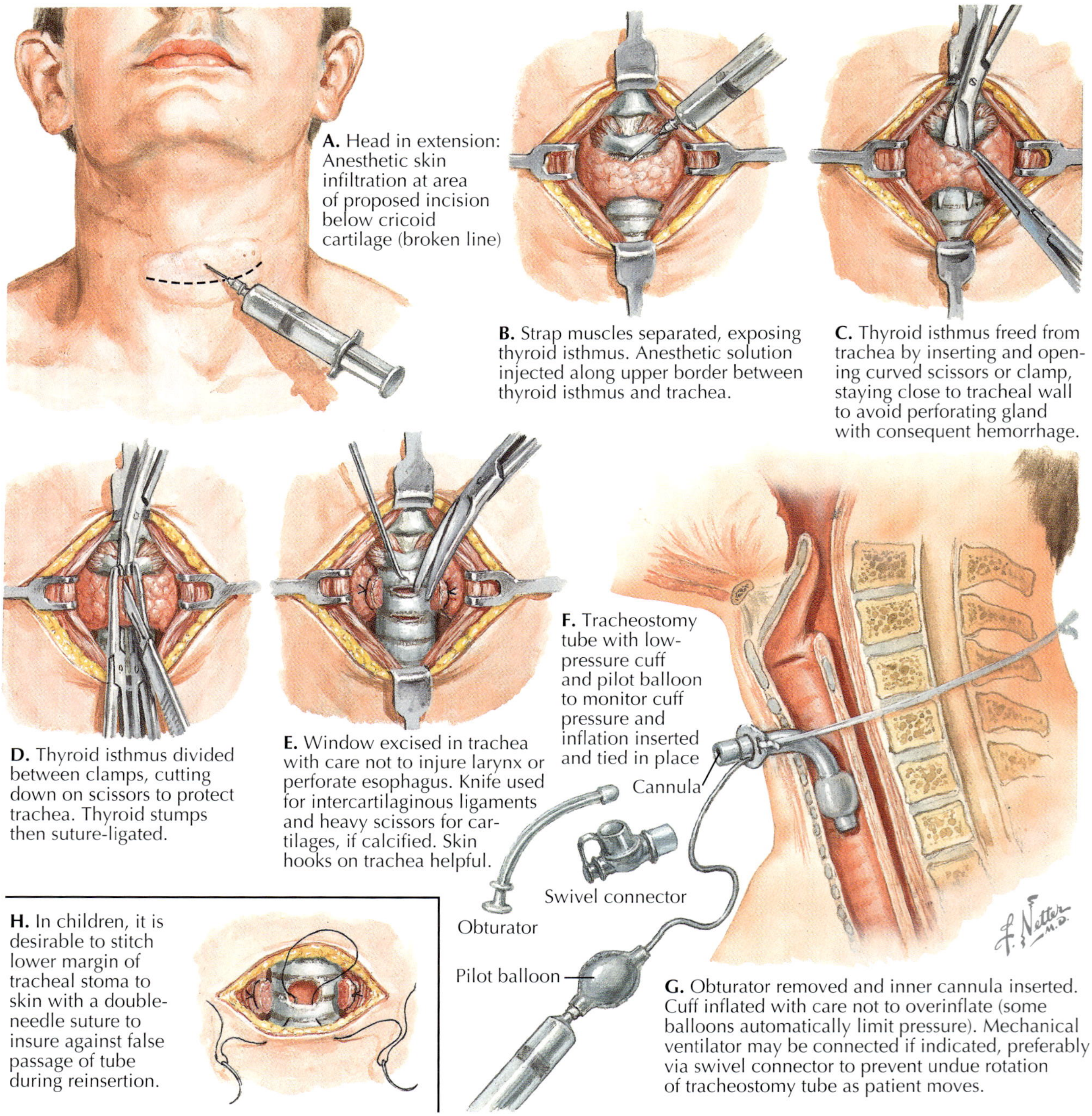

A. Head in extension: Anesthetic skin infiltration at area of proposed incision below cricoid cartilage (broken line)

B. Strap muscles separated, exposing thyroid isthmus. Anesthetic solution injected along upper border between thyroid isthmus and trachea.

C. Thyroid isthmus freed from trachea by inserting and opening curved scissors or clamp, staying close to tracheal wall to avoid perforating gland with consequent hemorrhage.

D. Thyroid isthmus divided between clamps, cutting down on scissors to protect trachea. Thyroid stumps then suture-ligated.

E. Window excised in trachea with care not to injure larynx or perforate esophagus. Knife used for intercartilaginous ligaments and heavy scissors for cartilages, if calcified. Skin hooks on trachea helpful.

F. Tracheostomy tube with low-pressure cuff and pilot balloon to monitor cuff pressure and inflation inserted and tied in place

G. Obturator removed and inner cannula inserted. Cuff inflated with care not to overinflate (some balloons automatically limit pressure). Mechanical ventilator may be connected if indicated, preferably via swivel connector to prevent undue rotation of tracheostomy tube as patient moves.

H. In children, it is desirable to stitch lower margin of tracheal stoma to skin with a double-needle suture to insure against false passage of tube during reinsertion.

⊙ **31648** with removal of bronchial valve(s), initial lobe

⊙✚ **31649** with removal of bronchial valve(s), each additional lobe (List separately in addition to code for primary procedure)

31651 Code is out of numerical sequence. See 31615-31649

Bronchial Thermoplasty

Coding Atlas

Bronchial **thermoplasty** is a bronchoscopic procedure in which **radiofrequency ablation** shrinks the airway smooth muscle of a severely asthmatic patient. It is intended to open the bronchial airways.

⊙ **31660** Bronchoscopy, rigid or flexible, including fluoroscopic guidance, when performed; with bronchial thermoplasty, 1 lobe

⊙ **31661** with bronchial thermoplasty, 2 or more lobes

Introduction

Coding Atlas

Nasotracheal refers to an approach through the nose, along the pharynx to the trachea. **Tracheobronchial** refers to an approach beyond the trachea and into a main bronchus. **Percutaneous** transtracheal refers to an approach through the skin and into the trachea.

31717 Catheterization with bronchial brush biopsy

31720 Catheter aspiration (separate procedure); nasotracheal

⊙ **31725** tracheobronchial with fiberscope, bedside

31730 Transtracheal (percutaneous) introduction of needle wire dilator/stent or indwelling tube for oxygen therapy

Excision, Repair

Coding Atlas

The cervical trachea is usually defined as the portion that is above the arch of the aorta, while the thoracic trachea is between the arch of the aorta and the carina.

31750 Tracheoplasty; cervical

31755 tracheopharyngeal fistulization, each stage

31760 intrathoracic

31766 Carinal reconstruction

31770 Bronchoplasty; graft repair

31775 excision stenosis and anastomosis

31780 Excision tracheal stenosis and anastomosis; cervical

31781 cervicothoracic

31785 Excision of tracheal tumor or carcinoma; cervical

31786 thoracic

31800 Suture of tracheal wound or injury; cervical

31805 intrathoracic

31820 Surgical closure tracheostomy or fistula; without plastic repair

31825 with plastic repair

31830 Revision of tracheostomy scar

FIGURE 3-9. Bronchi

The anatomical site at which the trachea branches into the right and left bronchus is known as the carina. Just as the right and left lungs are different, the right and left bronchi differ, too. The right main bronchus has three secondary branches, and the left has two.

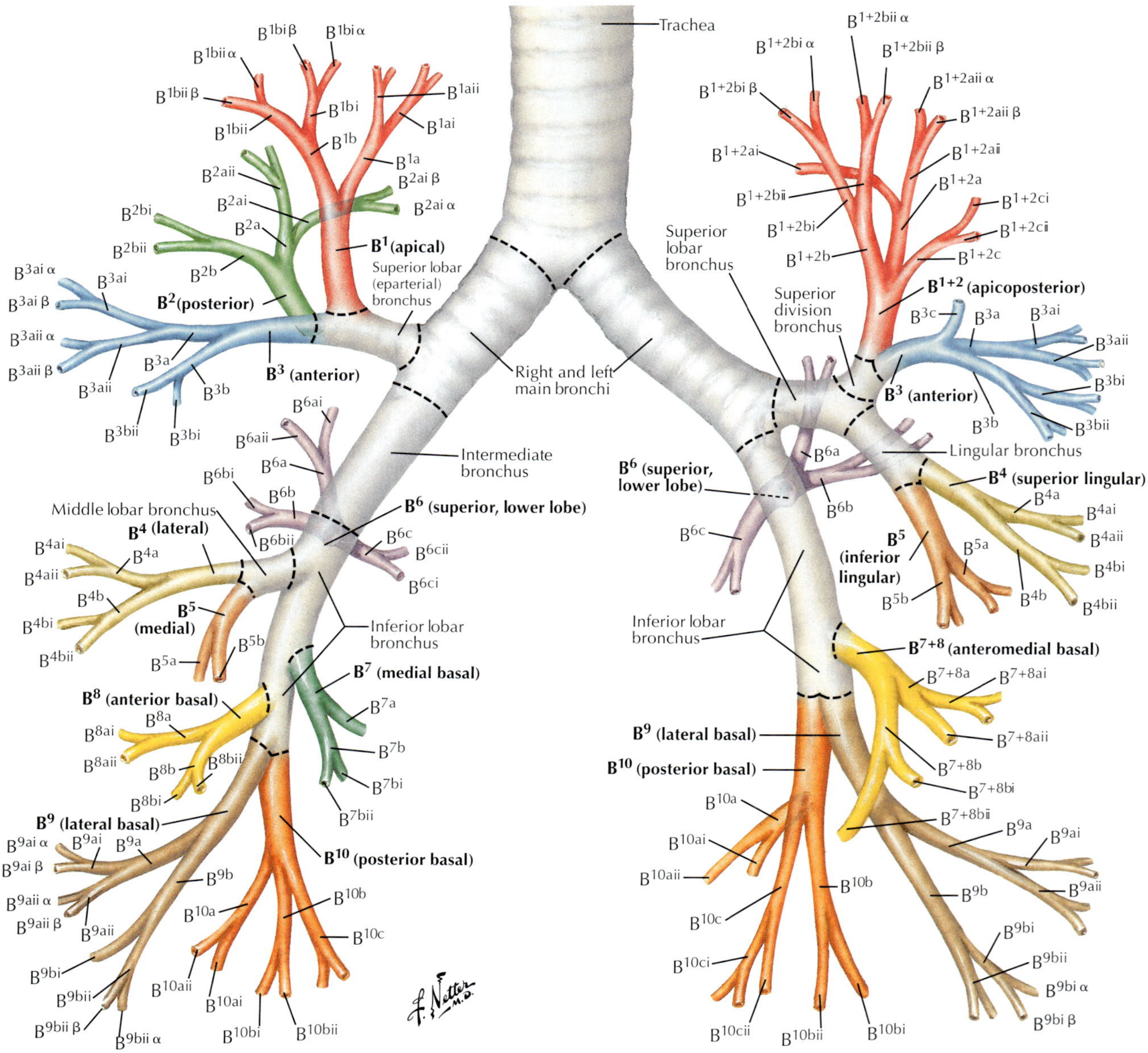

Nomenclature in common usage for bronchopulmonary segments is that of Jackson and Huber, and segmental bronchi are named accordingly. Ikeda proposed nomenclature forbronchial subdivisions as far as 6th generation. For simplification on this illustration, only some bronchial subdivisions are labeled as far as 5th or 6th generation. Segmental bronchi (B) are numbered from 1 to 10 in each lung, corresponding to pulmonary segments. In left lung, B^1 and B^2 are combined as are B^7 and B^8. Subsegmental, or 4th order, bronchi are indicated by addition of lower-case letters a, b, or c when an additional branch is present. Fifth order bronchi are designated by Roman numerals i (anterior) or ii (posterior) and 6th order bronchi by Greek letters α or β. Several texts use alternate numbers (as proposed by Boyden) for segmental bronchi.

Variations of standard bronchial pattern shown here are common, especially in peripheral airways.

Lungs and Pleura

Incision

Coding Atlas

A **thoracotomy** is a surgical incision through the skin, between the ribs, and into the pleural space of the thorax to access or expose the lung. A thoracotomy may be **diagnostic** or **therapeutic** in nature. **Empyema** is a pocket of pus inside the pleural cavity. Intrapleural **pneumonolysis** is the separation of the visceral and parietal layers of the pleura.

32035 Thoracostomy; with rib resection for empyema

32036 with open flap drainage for empyema

32096 Thoracotomy, with diagnostic biopsy(ies) of lung infiltrate(s) (eg, wedge, incisional), unilateral

32097 Thoracotomy, with diagnostic biopsy(ies) of lung nodule(s) or mass(es) (eg, wedge, incisional), unilateral

32098 Thoracotomy, with biopsy(ies) of pleura

32100 Thoracotomy; with exploration

32110 with control of traumatic hemorrhage and/or repair of lung tear

32120 for postoperative complications

32124 with open intrapleural pneumonolysis

32140 with cyst(s) removal, includes pleural procedure when performed

32141 with resection-plication of bullae, includes any pleural procedure when performed

32150 with removal of intrapleural foreign body or fibrin deposit

32151 with removal of intrapulmonary foreign body

32160 with cardiac massage

32200 Pneumonostomy, with open drainage of abscess or cyst

32215 Pleural scarification for repeat pneumothorax

32220 Decortication, pulmonary (separate procedure); total

32225 partial

Excision/Resection

Coding Atlas

The thoracic cavity is lined with a continuous sheet of **endothelial** tissue called the pleura. **Biopsies** of the pleural cavity or lung may be accomplished using a **percutaneous** thoracoscopic or open (**thoracotomy**) approach. If biopsies are collected and examined by pathology intraoperatively during a larger procedure, the collection of the specimen is considered inherent to the larger procedure.

32310 Pleurectomy, parietal (separate procedure)

32320 Decortication and parietal pleurectomy

32400 Biopsy, pleura; percutaneous needle

⊙ **32405** Biopsy, lung or mediastinum, percutaneous needle

Removal

Coding Atlas

Add-on code 32507 is used to report a situation in which a **wedge resection** is performed and intraoperative findings from that encounter lead to a more extensive procedure at the same location. In this case, what was a **therapeutic** wedge resection is reclassified as **diagnostic** (code 32507), and the diagnostic resection is reported in addition to the more extensive procedure.

32440 Removal of lung, pneumonectomy;

32442 with resection of segment of trachea followed by broncho-tracheal anastomosis (sleeve pneumonectomy)

32445 extrapleural

32480 Removal of lung, other than pneumonectomy; single lobe (lobectomy)

32482 2 lobes (bilobectomy)

32484 single segment (segmentectomy)

32486 with circumferential resection of segment of bronchus followed by broncho-bronchial anastomosis (sleeve lobectomy)

32488 with all remaining lung following previous removal of a portion of lung (completion pneumonectomy)

32491 with resection-plication of emphysematous lung(s) (bullous or non-bullous) for lung volume reduction, sternal split or transthoracic approach, includes any pleural procedure, when performed

FIGURE 3-10. The Thoracic Cavity

The lungs are covered by the **visceral** pleura, which forms two complete **fissures** in the right lung and one complete fissure in the left lung. This effectively separates each lung lobe. The diaphragm is a sheet of muscle stretching across the base of the ribcage. The diaphragm contracts during **inspiration** and expands during **expiration**.

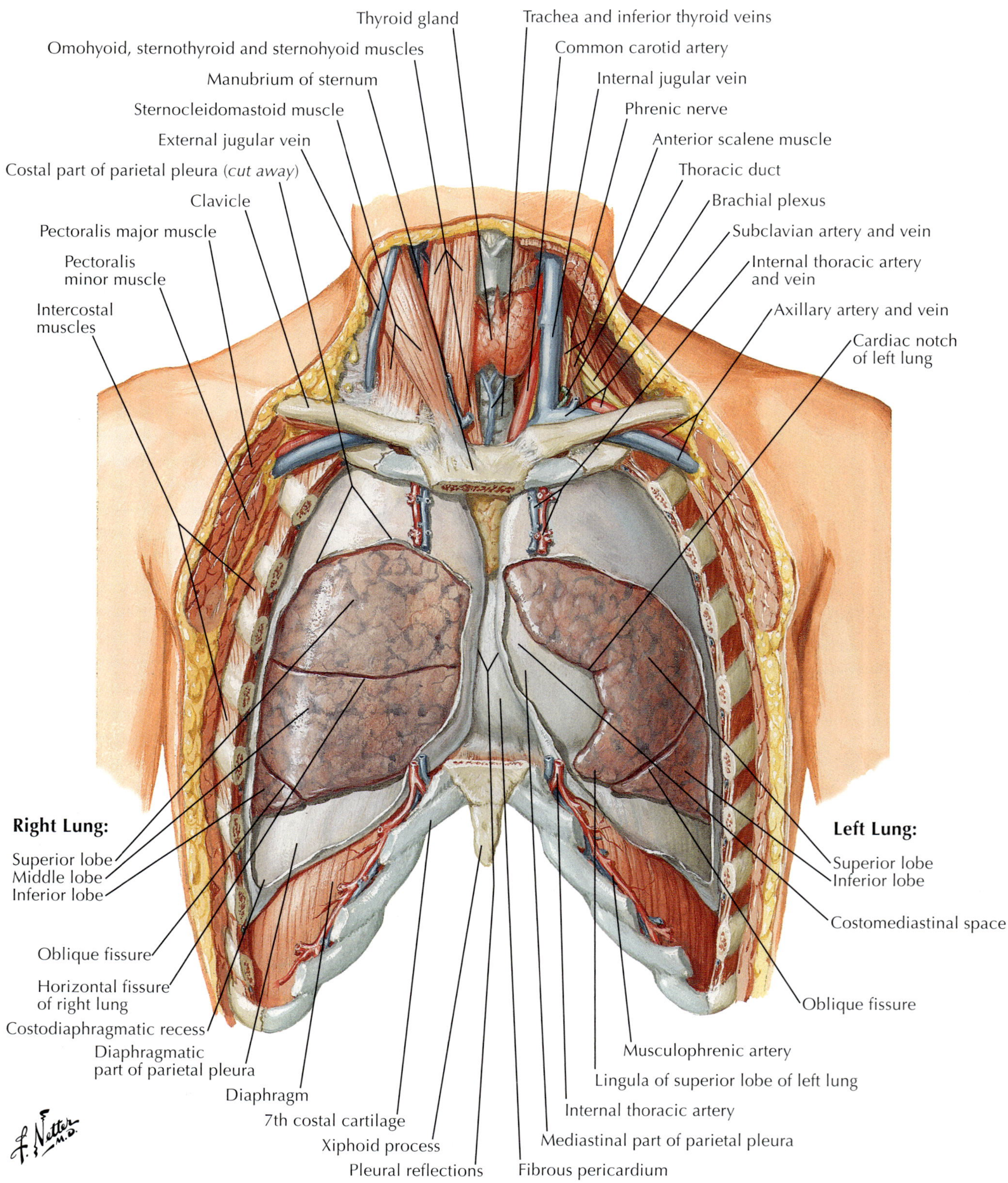

+ 32501 Resection and repair of portion of bronchus (bronchoplasty) when performed at time of lobectomy or segmentectomy (List separately in addition to code for primary procedure)

32503 Resection of apical lung tumor (eg, Pancoast tumor), including chest wall resection, rib(s) resection(s), neurovascular dissection, when performed; without chest wall reconstruction(s)

32504 with chest wall reconstruction

32505 Thoracotomy; with therapeutic wedge resection (eg, mass, nodule), initial

+ 32506 with therapeutic wedge resection (eg, mass or nodule), each additional resection, ipsilateral (List separately in addition to code for primary procedure)

+ 32507 with diagnostic wedge resection followed by anatomic lung resection (List separately in addition to code for primary procedure)

32540 Extrapleural enucleation of empyema (empyemectomy)

Introduction and Removal

Coding Atlas

In order to determine whether a physician performed **thoracentesis** or **thoracostomy**, documentation regarding the technique used should be considered, not the size of the drain placed. Use of thoracostomy codes indicates that an open, **cutdown** incision was made in the skin overlying the space between the ribs to access the lung. In thoracentesis, a **percutaneous** needle or catheter technique is used to place a drain.

⊙ 32550 Insertion of indwelling tunneled pleural catheter with cuff

⊙ 32551 Tube thoracostomy, includes connection to drainage system (eg, water seal), when performed, open (separate procedure)

32552 Removal of indwelling tunneled pleural catheter with cuff

⊙ 32553 Placement of interstitial device(s) for radiation therapy guidance (eg, fiducial markers, dosimeter), percutaneous, intra-thoracic, single or multiple

32554 Thoracentesis, needle or catheter, aspiration of the pleural space; without imaging guidance

32555 with imaging guidance

32556 Pleural drainage, percutaneous, with insertion of indwelling catheter; without imaging guidance

32557 with imaging guidance

Destruction

Coding Atlas

Pleurodesis describes instillation of an agent into the pleural space to get the visceral pleura to stick to the **parietal** pleura and prevent the lungs from collapsing. **Fibrinolysis** is the installation of an agent into the pleural space to free up an entrapped lung.

32560 Instillation, via chest tube/catheter, agent for pleurodesis (eg, talc for recurrent or persistent pneumothorax)

32561 Instillation(s), via chest tube/catheter, agent for fibrinolysis (eg, fibrinolytic agent for break up of multiloculated effusion); initial day

32562 subsequent day

Thoracoscopy

Coding Atlas

Thoracoscopy, or video-assisted thoracic surgery (VATS), refers to minimally invasive thoracic surgery that is performed using endoscopes and one or multiple small incisions. It is similar to **laparoscopic** surgery.

32601 Thoracoscopy, diagnostic (separate procedure); lungs, pericardial sac, mediastinal or pleural space, without biopsy

32604 pericardial sac, with biopsy

32606 mediastinal space, with biopsy

32607 Thoracoscopy; with diagnostic biopsy(ies) of lung infiltrate(s) (eg, wedge, incisional), unilateral

32608 with diagnostic biopsy(ies) of lung nodule(s) or mass(es) (eg, wedge, incisional), unilateral

32609 with biopsy(ies) of pleura

32650 Thoracoscopy, surgical; with pleurodesis (eg, mechanical or chemical)

32651 with partial pulmonary decortication

32652 with total pulmonary decortication, including intrapleural pneumonolysis

32653 with removal of intrapleural foreign body or fibrin deposit

32654 with control of traumatic hemorrhage

32655 with resection-plication of bullae, includes any pleural procedure when performed

32656 with parietal pleurectomy

32658 with removal of clot or foreign body from pericardial sac

FIGURE 3-11. Bronchopulmonary Segments

From the main bronchus on each side, the lungs subdivide further. Each segment has its own name and its own pulmonary arterial branch, and each is anatomically discrete. This means that a single segment can be surgically removed without affecting the blood supply to neighboring segments. The left lung has eight segments, and the right lung has 10 segments.

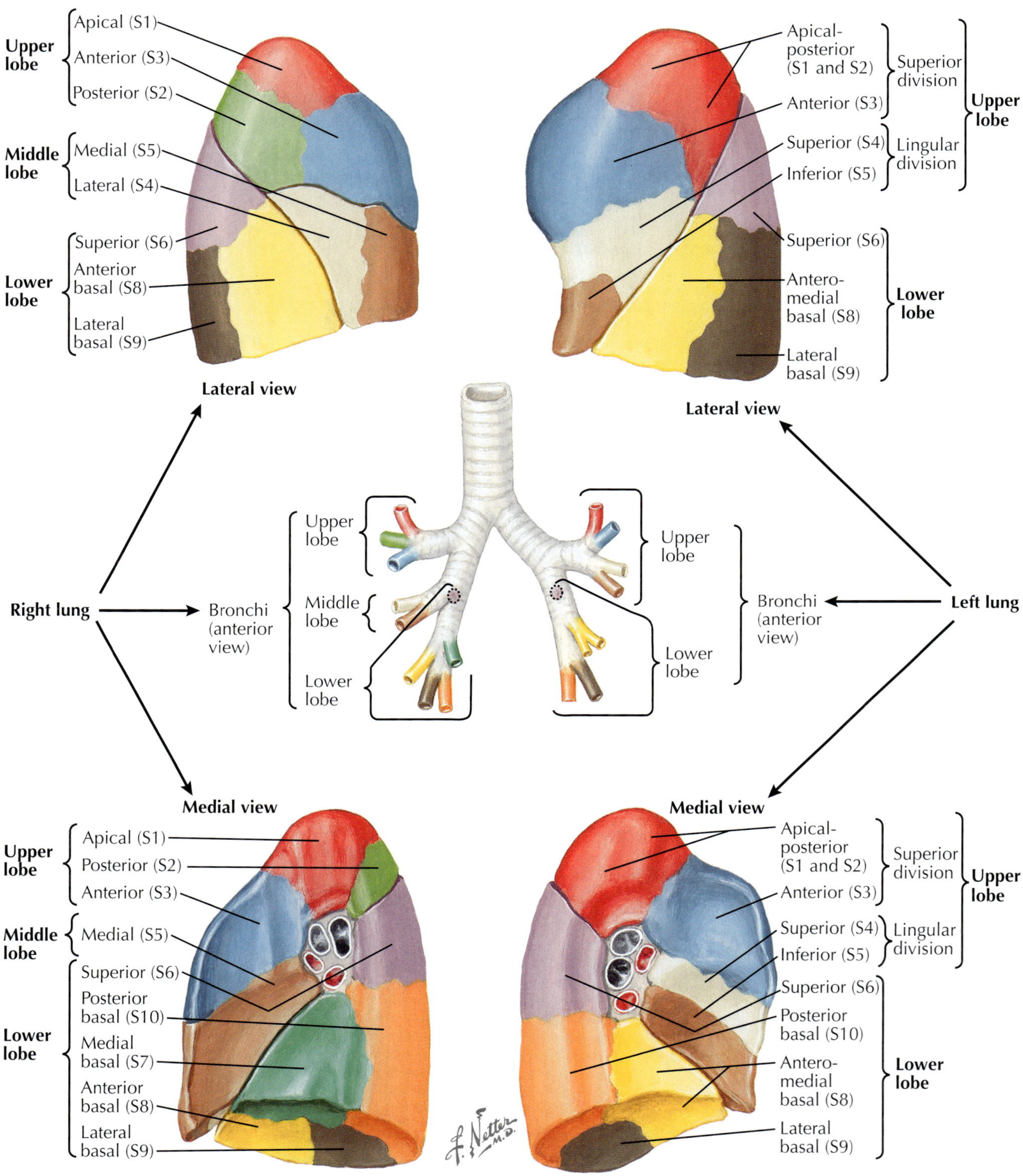

32659 with creation of pericardial window or partial resection of pericardial sac for drainage

32661 with excision of pericardial cyst, tumor, or mass

32662 with excision of mediastinal cyst, tumor, or mass

32663 with lobectomy (single lobe)

32664 with thoracic sympathectomy

32665 with esophagomyotomy (Heller type)

32666 with therapeutic wedge resection (eg, mass, nodule), initial unilateral

+ 32667 with therapeutic wedge resection (eg, mass or nodule), each additional resection, ipsilateral (List separately in addition to code for primary procedure)

+ 32668 with diagnostic wedge resection followed by anatomic lung resection (List separately in addition to code for primary procedure)

32669 with removal of a single lung segment (segmentectomy)

32670 with removal of two lobes (bilobectomy)

32671 with removal of lung (pneumonectomy)

32672 with resection-plication for emphysematous lung (bullous or non-bullous) for lung volume reduction (LVRS), unilateral includes any pleural procedure, when performed

32673 with resection of thymus, unilateral or bilateral

+ 32674 with mediastinal and regional lymphadenectomy (List separately in addition to code for primary procedure)

Stereotactic Radiation Therapy

Coding Atlas

Tumor delineation involves determination of tumor borders to identify their volume and relationship to nearby structures and to validate the target prior to treatment. Tumor delineation is reported once per the entire course of treatment.

32701 Thoracic target(s) delineation for stereotactic body radiation therapy (SRS/SBRT), (photon or particle beam), entire course of treatment

Repair

Coding Atlas

A bronchiopleural fistula is an abnormal passageway that develops between the bronchus and the pleura as a complication of lung surgery, infection, pneumothorax, chemotherapy, or radiation therapy. The problem with a bronchial or bronchiopleural fistula is that air escapes from the bronchus into the pleural cavity and may reduce lung capacity or lead to lung collapse.

32800 Repair lung hernia through chest wall

32810 Closure of chest wall following open flap drainage for empyema (Clagett type procedure)

32815 Open closure of major bronchial fistula

32820 Major reconstruction, chest wall (posttraumatic)

Lung Transplantation

Coding Atlas

A lung transplant can be divided into three elements: procurement of the donor lung from a cadaver; preparation of the donor lung for transplantation; and transplant of the donor lung into the patient. Allograft indicates the donor tissue is from the same species and a single or double lung may be transplanted. The procedure may require cardiopulmonary bypass.

32850 Donor pneumonectomy(s) (including cold preservation), from cadaver donor

32851 Lung transplant, single; without cardiopulmonary bypass

32852 with cardiopulmonary bypass

32853 Lung transplant, double (bilateral sequential or en bloc); without cardiopulmonary bypass

32854 with cardiopulmonary bypass

32855 Backbench standard preparation of cadaver donor lung allograft prior to transplantation, including dissection of allograft from surrounding soft tissues to prepare pulmonary venous/atrial cuff, pulmonary artery, and bronchus; unilateral

32856 bilateral

FIGURE 3-12. **Chest Tube Placement**

In **thoracentesis**, a needle or catheter is inserted into the lung to treat an **abscess**, **hemothorax**, **pleural effusion**, **pneumothorax**, or **empyema**. In some cases, imaging guidance is used to place the needle or catheter. Accumulated air or fluid is removed from the pleural space by syringe or catheter aspiration; if removed via suction drainage, codes from the code set 32556-32557 are used. Note: Tools, implants, and/or equipment depicted in the illustration may be outdated but the procedural approach is valid.

Preferred sites
1. For pneumothorax (2nd or 3rd interspace at midclavicular line)
2. For hemothorax (5th interspace at midaxillary line)

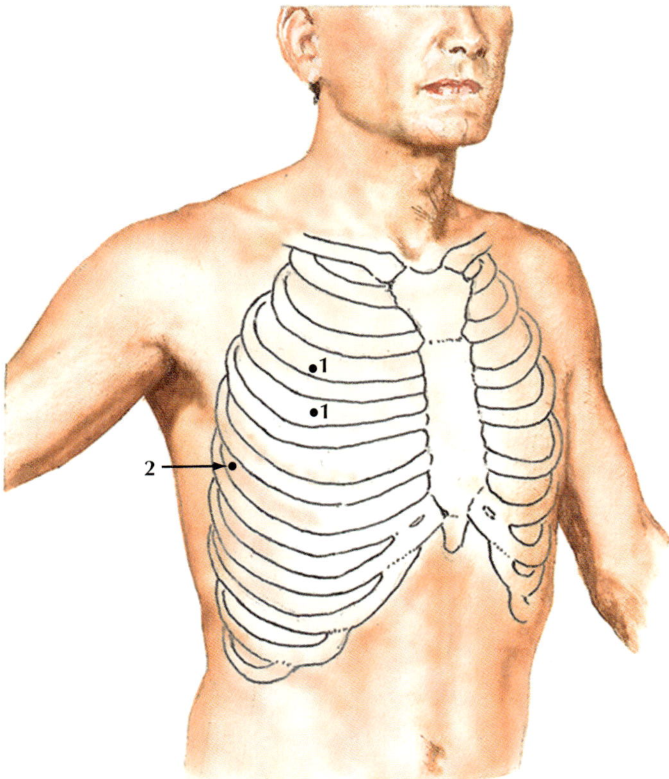

A. Trocar and cannula pushed through intercostal space

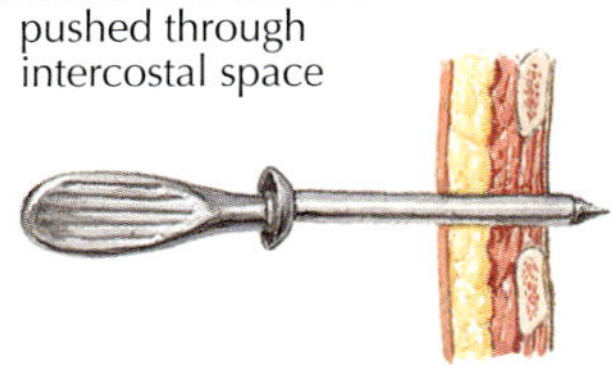

B. Trocar withdrawn; tube passed into chest through cannula

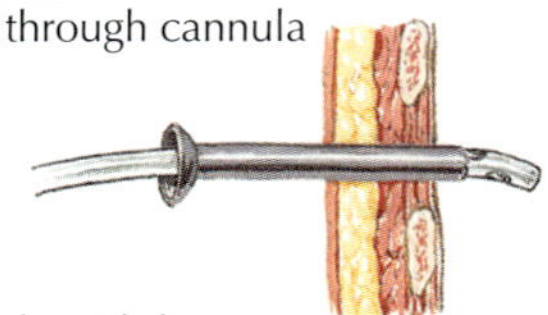

C. Cannula withdrawn; tube connected to underwater seal (with suction if indicated)

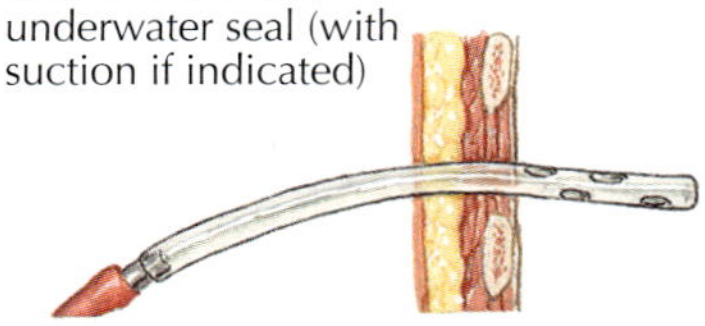

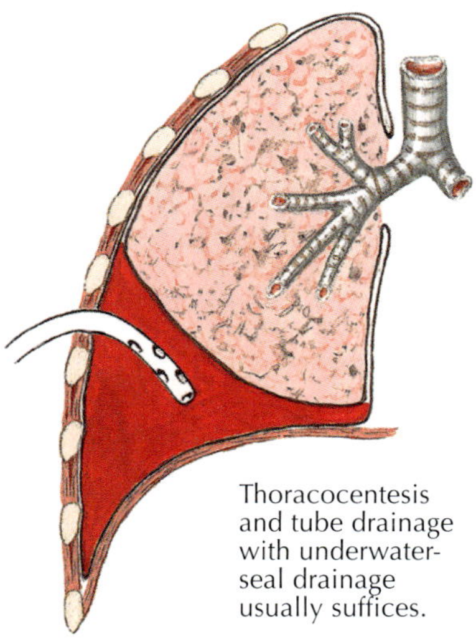

Thoracocentesis and tube drainage with underwater-seal drainage usually suffices.

D. Intercostal space is pierced above rib to avoid damage to neurovascular bundle lying in costal groove

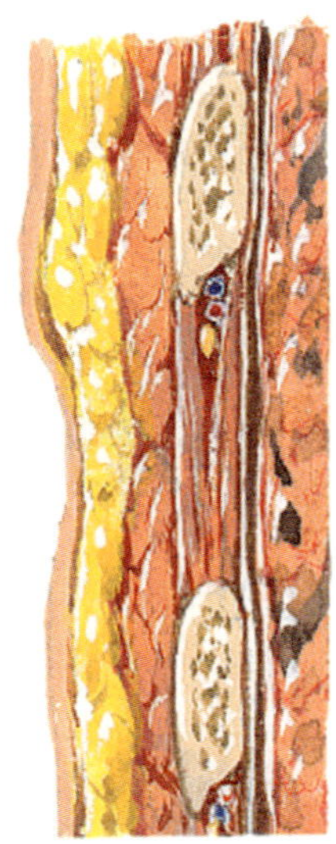

Surgical Collapse Therapy; Thoracoplasty

Coding Atlas

Thoracoplasty is the surgical removal of portions of the ribs to effect change on the lungs. **Pneumolysis** is the removal of **adhesions** in the pleural space.

32900 Resection of ribs, extrapleural, all stages

32905 Thoracoplasty, Schede type or extrapleural (all stages);

32906 with closure of bronchopleural fistula

32940 Pneumonolysis, extraperiosteal, including filling or packing procedures

32960 Pneumothorax, therapeutic, intrapleural injection of air

Other Procedures

Coding Atlas

In **percutaneous** ablation therapy of the lung, a **radiofrequency** (RF) ablation needle is inserted through a small incision between the ribs. RF power is used to heat a lung lesion to destroy it.

32997 Total lung lavage (unilateral)

32998 Ablation therapy for reduction or eradication of 1 or more pulmonary tumor(s) including pleura or chest wall when involved by tumor extension, percutaneous, radiofrequency, unilateral

FIGURE 3-13. Topography of the Lung

The location of the **thoracotomy** or **thoracentesis** site in the lung is often documented according to anatomical hallmarks including numbered ribs or vertebrae. Ribs and vertebrae also provide landmarks for physicians when locating anatomical sites. For example, the carina (juncture of bronchi and trachea) is usually found at the level of the fifth thoracic vertebra, although it is occasionally found up to two vertebrae higher or lower.

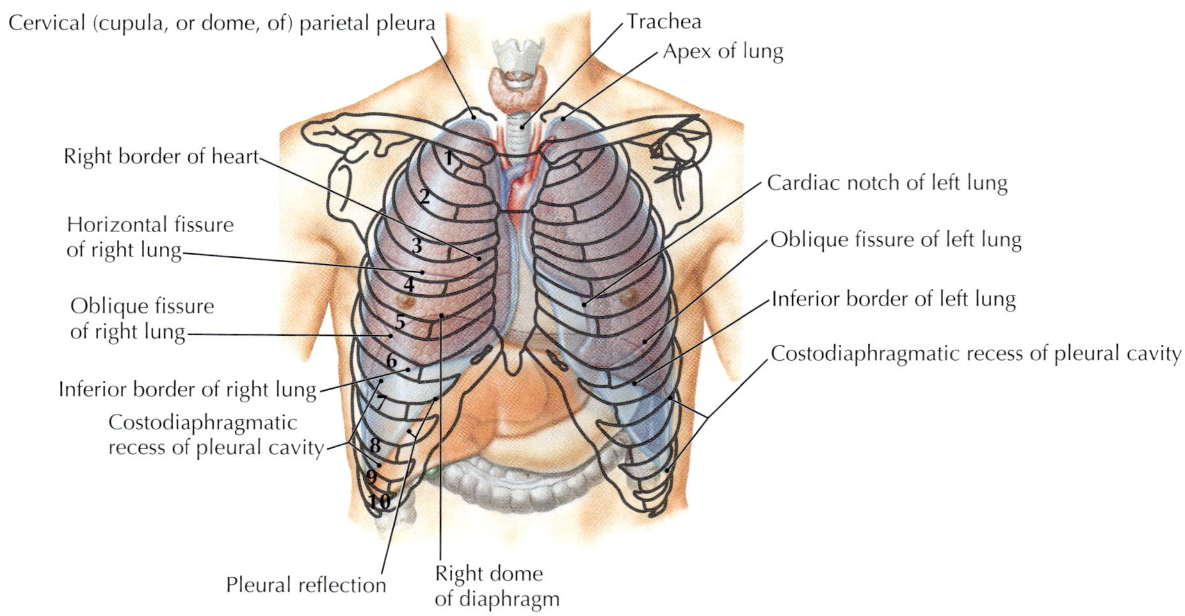

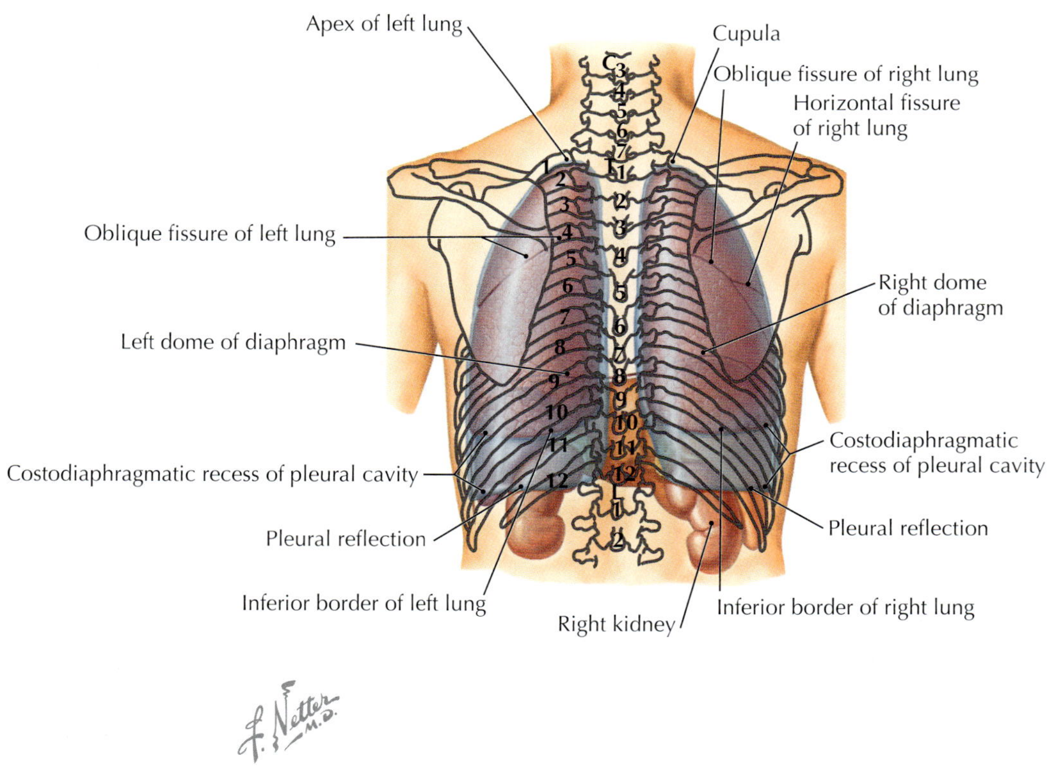

FIGURE 3-14. Lymph Nodes of the Lung

The paired hila are formed where a main bronchus and associated pulmonary veins and arteries enter the lungs. Because swelling in local lymph nodes can displace these two structures and because the bronchus and vessels are visible on X ray, these two structures take on clinical importance. When the hilar lymph nodes swell (usually **unilaterally**), they displace the hila, and the patient is said to have hilar **adenopathy**.

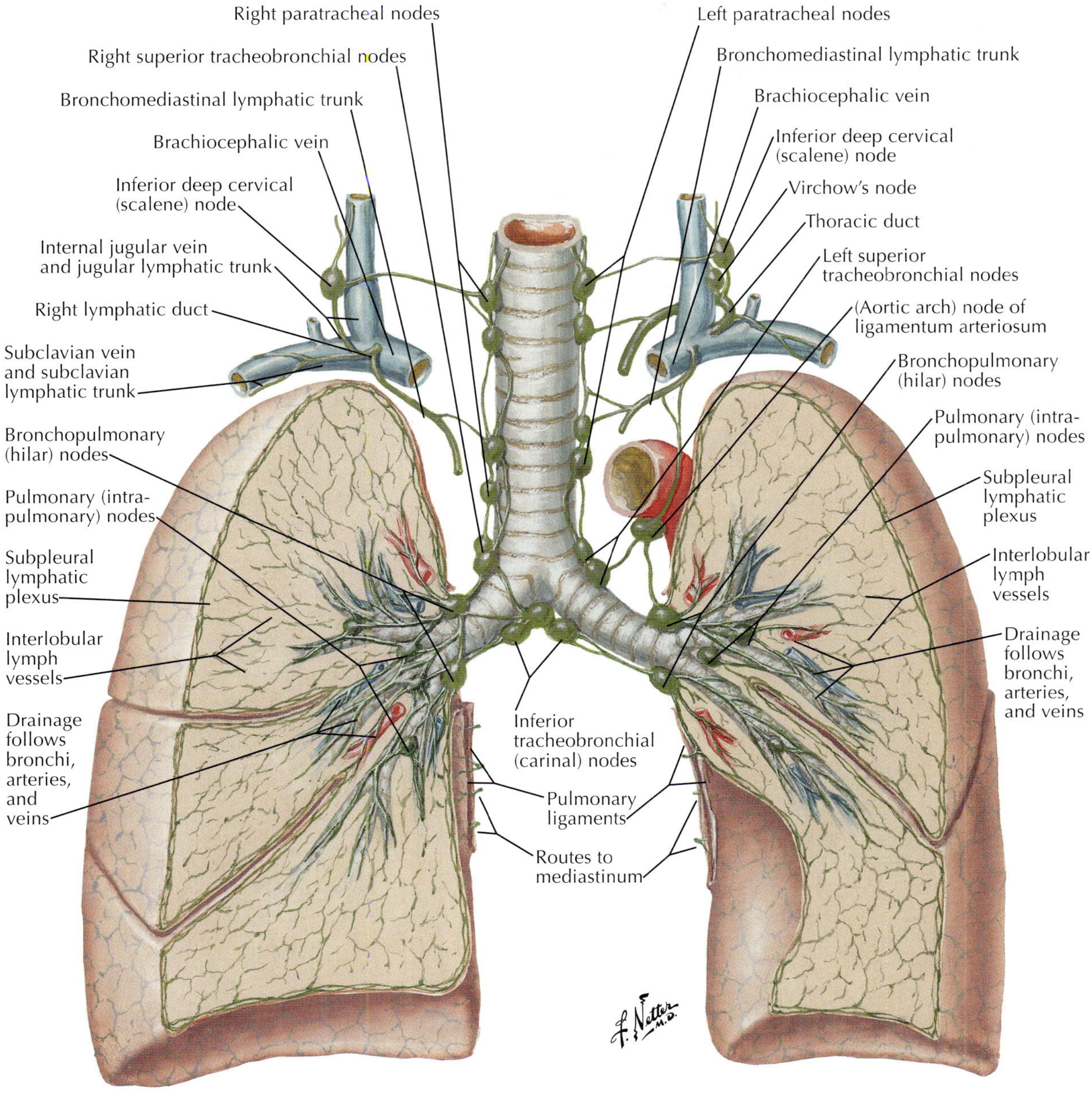

Drainage routes

Right lung: All lobes drain to pulmonary and bronchopulmonary (hilar) nodes, then to inferior tracheobronchial (carinal) nodes, right superior tracheobronchial nodes, and right paratracheal nodes on way to brachiocephalic vein via bronchomediastinal lymphatic trunk and/or inferior deep cervical (scalene) node.

Left lung: Superior lobe drains to pulmonary and bronchopulmonary (hilar) nodes, inferior tracheobronchial (carinal) nodes, left superior tracheobronchial nodes, left paratracheal nodes and/or (aortic arch) node of ligamentum arteriosum, then to brachiocephalic vein via left bronchomediastinal trunk and thoracic duct. Left inferior lobe also drains to pulmonary and bronchopulmonary (hilar) nodes and to inferior tracheobronchial (carinal) nodes, but then mostly to right superior tracheobronchial nodes, where it follows the same route as lymph from right lung.

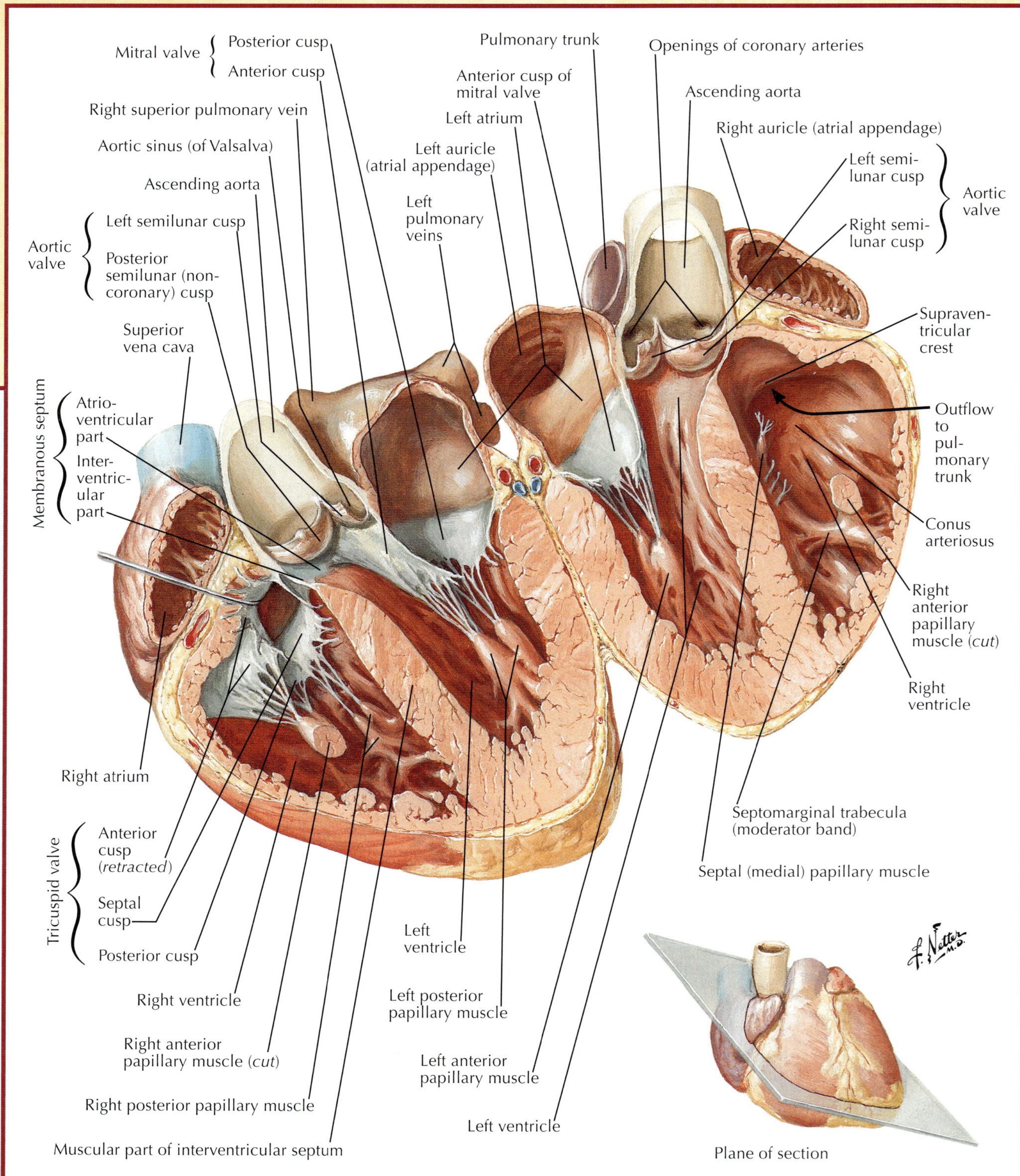
Mitral valve
Posterior cusp
Anterior cusp
Right superior pulmonary vein
Aortic sinus (of Valsalva)
Ascending aorta
Aortic valve
Left semilunar cusp
Posterior semilunar (non-coronary) cusp
Superior vena cava
Membranous septum
Atrio-ventricular part
Inter-ventric-ular part
Right atrium
Tricuspid valve
Anterior cusp (*retracted*)
Septal cusp
Posterior cusp
Right ventricle
Right anterior papillary muscle (*cut*)
Right posterior papillary muscle
Muscular part of interventricular septum
Pulmonary trunk
Anterior cusp of mitral valve
Left atrium
Left auricle (atrial appendage)
Left pulmonary veins
Left ventricle
Left posterior papillary muscle
Left anterior papillary muscle
Left ventricle
Openings of coronary arteries
Ascending aorta
Right auricle (atrial appendage)
Left semi-lunar cusp
Right semi-lunar cusp
Aortic valve
Supraven-tricular crest
Outflow to pul-monary trunk
Conus arteriosus
Right anterior papillary muscle (*cut*)
Right ventricle
Septomarginal trabecula (moderator band)
Septal (medial) papillary muscle
Plane of section

◈ CHAPTER 4 ◈

Cardiovascular System

The cardiovascular system is the body's primary transportation route. Its most important function is the delivery of oxygen to the cells from the lungs and the return of carbon dioxide from the body's cells to the lungs. The cardiovascular system carries other substances, including nutrients, **antibodies**, and waste products, as well. The system is composed of the heart, arteries, arterioles, veins, venules, and capillaries.

The heart powers the flow of blood through the body. The heart is divided into four chambers: right and left **atria** and right and left **ventricles**. In a healthy heart, the right and left sides do not communicate directly. Blood moves through the heart as follows:

1. Deoxygenated blood enters the right atrium through the superior and inferior vena cava.
2. The **tricuspid valve** opens, and blood drops into the right ventricle.
3. The **pulmonary valve** opens, and deoxygenated blood moves into the pulmonary artery.
4. Blood flows through the lungs, depositing carbon dioxide and picking up oxygen from the capillary beds.
5. The pulmonary vein brings oxygenated blood back to the left atrium.
6. The **mitral valve** opens and blood drops into the left ventricle
7. The **aortic valve** opens, and the strong ventricular muscle pumps blood up and out into the body.

With the exception of the pulmonary arteries, arteries carry oxygenated blood. With the exception of the pulmonary veins, veins carry deoxygenated blood.

Because the left ventricle is tasked with propelling blood from the heart into distant regions of the body, it is the chamber of the heart with the biggest and strongest muscles.

Heartbeats are the result of electrical stimulation of heart muscles that cause the heart to contract, or squeeze, to push blood throughout the body. The heart's electrical conduction system can be damaged by age or disease and may require procedures to slow down the contractions or to supplement natural electrical stimulation with artificial electrical pacing.

The heart is encased in the **pericardium** and lubricating fluid to ensure that while it beats, it does not rub against other structures in the **thorax**. The pericardium has two layers: **parietal**, or outer layer, and **visceral**, the inner layer. Pericardial fluid lies between the two layers.

Arteries carry oxygenated blood from the heart to the distant parts of the body. Arteries have thick, elastic muscle layers that can handle high pressure. Clinical blood pressure is a measurement of arterial blood pressure. **Systolic** pressure occurs when the heart is contracting, and **diastolic** pressure occurs when the heart is relaxed.

Blood from an artery flows into **arterioles** and then into **capillaries**. Oxygen exchange occurs in capillaries. **Venules** pick up capillary blood and carried it to veins, which return deoxygenated blood to the heart. Veins have thinner muscles and contain **valves** that prevent **backflow** of blood.

Problems can occur in the circulatory system when blood flow is blocked within a blood vessel or when the heart is defective and cannot pump blood efficiently. These problems can be **congenital** or **acquired**, and their onset may be **chronic** or **acute**.

FIGURE 4-1. The Pericardium and the Heart

The pericardium surrounds the heart and attaches to the sternum, diaphragm, and **anterior** mediastinum. The pericardium also encloses the roots of the great vessels and venae cavae, anchoring the heart in the thorax. **Cardiac tamponade** occurs when fluid (effusion) accumulates in the **inelastic** pericardial sac to the point where it exerts pressure against the exterior of the heart, limiting cardiac filling.

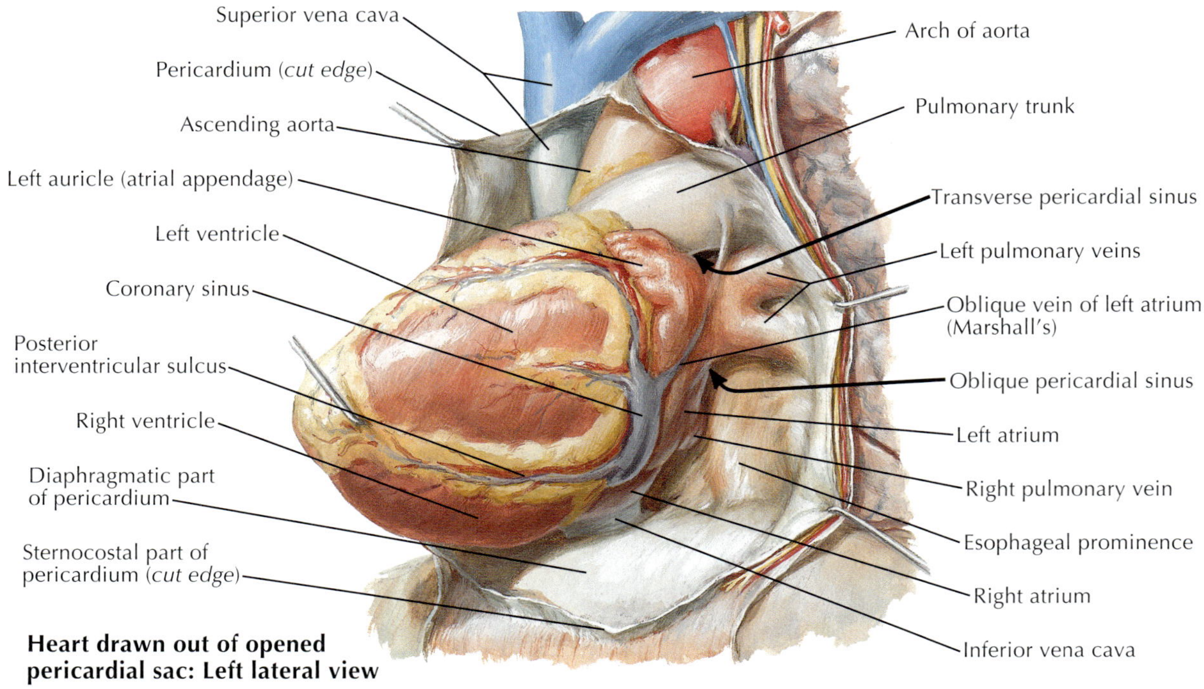

Heart drawn out of opened pericardial sac: Left lateral view

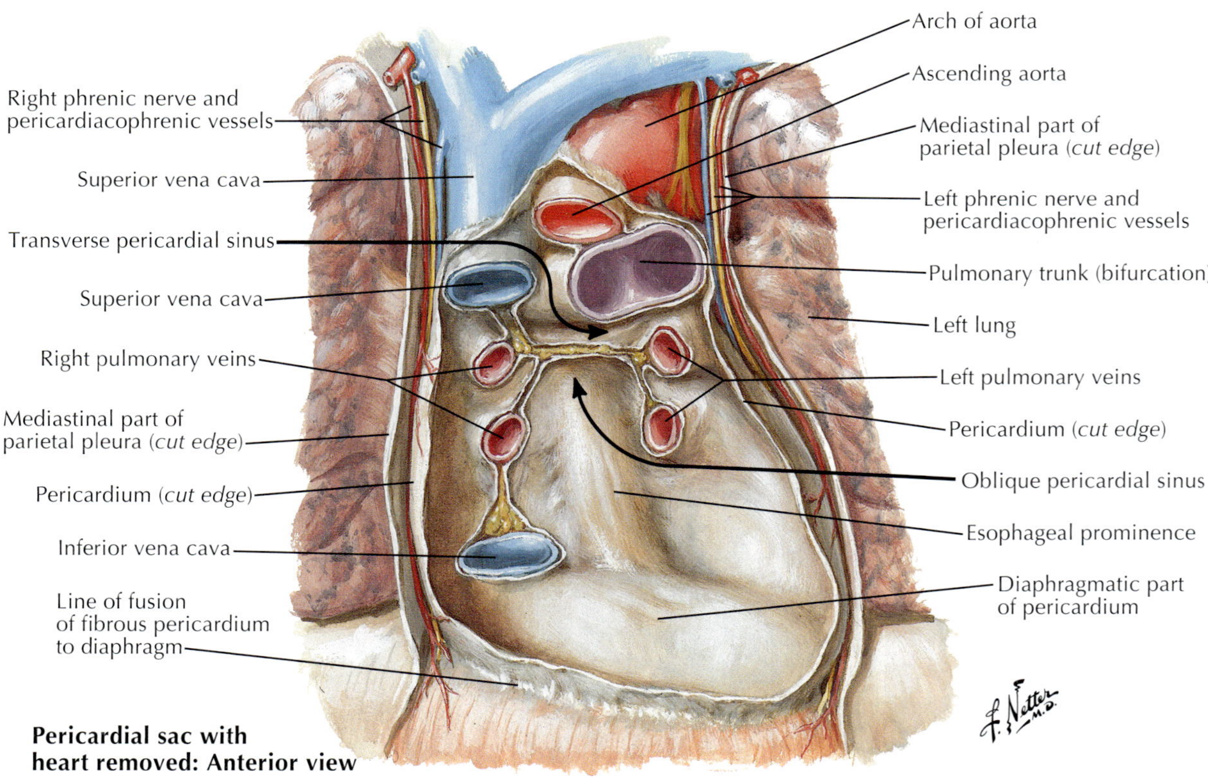

Pericardial sac with heart removed: Anterior view

Heart and Pericardium

Pericardium

Coding Atlas

Pericardial **effusion** is abnormal fluid build-up in the pericardium. It may be caused by inflammation, infection, **malignancy**, injury, kidney failure, or **myocardial infarction**. If fluid builds up in the pericardium, the increased pressure may impede heart function. **Pericardiocentesis** may be performed or a **pericardial window** may be created in the pericardial wall to reduce the pressure. If a pericardial window is created using video-assisted thoracoscopic thoracic system (VATS), code 32659 is reported.

⊙ 33010 Pericardiocentesis; initial

⊙ 33011 subsequent

33015 Tube pericardiostomy

33020 Pericardiotomy for removal of clot or foreign body (primary procedure)

33025 Creation of pericardial window or partial resection for drainage

33030 Pericardiectomy, subtotal or complete; without cardiopulmonary bypass

33031 with cardiopulmonary bypass

33050 Resection of pericardial cyst or tumor

Cardiac Tumor

Coding Atlas

The CPT codes used to report cardiac **tumors** excision do not differentiate between **benign** and **malignant** tumors. Instead, code choice is based on the location of the tumor; a tumor can be located on the exterior surface of the heart (code 33130) or within heart tissues or chambers, requiring **cardiopulmonary bypass** for excision (code 33120).

33120 Excision of intracardiac tumor, resection with cardiopulmonary bypass

33130 Resection of external cardiac tumor

Transmyocardial Revascularization

Coding Atlas

Transmyocardial laser revascularization (TMR) creates channels in the arterioluminal sinusoids, connecting directly with the left ventricular cavity. This increases blood supply to the muscle of the left ventricle. In a typical TMR, 30 to 40 channels that are about 1 cm apart are created using a laser.

33140 Transmyocardial laser revascularization, by thoracotomy; (separate procedure)

✚ 33141 performed at the time of other open cardiac procedure(s) (List separately in addition to code for primary procedure)

Pacemaker or Implantable Defibrillator

Coding Atlas

Pacemakers and implantable defibrillators are systems for regulating the heart's electrical **conduction**. These systems have two main components: **pulse generators** and **leads**. A pacemaker system supplements the electrical activity of the heart by emitting electrical pulses that keep the heart beat and heart rate regular. Implantable defibrillators sense and treat **ventricular tachycardia** or **ventricular fibrillation** by administering shocks to correct the erratic beats (**cardioversion**) through a **defibrillator** lead. There are two types of implantable defibrillators: transvenous pacing implantable cardioverter defibrillators (ICDs), which also supply pacing to control heart rate and beat, and subcutaneous implantable cardioverter-defibrillators (S-ICD). S-ICDs differ from ICDs in that S-ICDs do not provide chronic pacing.

33202 Insertion of epicardial electrode(s); open incision (eg, thoracotomy, median sternotomy, subxiphoid approach)

33203 endoscopic approach (eg, thoracoscopy, pericardioscopy)

⊙ 33206 Insertion of new or replacement of permanent pacemaker with transvenous electrode(s); atrial

⊙ 33207 ventricular

⊙ 33208 atrial and ventricular

⊙ 33210 Insertion or replacement of temporary transvenous single chamber cardiac electrode or pacemaker catheter (separate procedure)

⊙ 33211 Insertion or replacement of temporary transvenous dual chamber pacing electrodes (separate procedure)

FIGURE 4-2. Implantable Pacing Transvenous Cardioverter-Defibrillator

A transvenous implantable cardioverter-defibrillator (ICD) uses a combination of anti-**tachycardia** pacing, low-energy **cardioversion**, or defibrillating electrical shocks to treat **ventricular tachycardia** or **ventricular fibrillation**. The ICD **pulse generator** may be implanted in the abdomen or chest and attached to leads with electrodes in the heart. These devices help control events that can lead to sudden cardiac arrest (SCA). Note: Tools, implants, and/or equipment depicted in the illustration may be outdated but the procedural approach is valid.

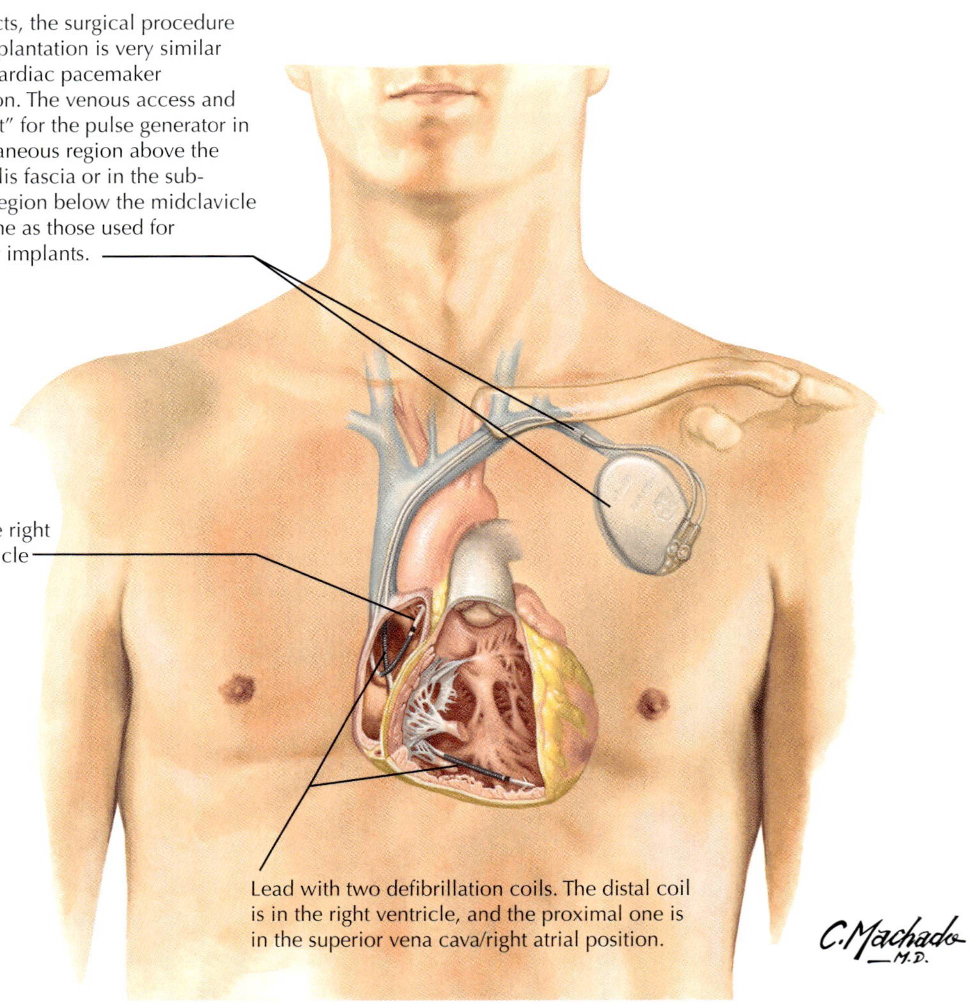

The defibrillation coils that are part of the ICD leads are not found on standard pacemaker leads. At least one coil (in the right ventricle) is necessary for defibrillation. Some models have a second defibrillation coil, which is positioned in the superior vena cava/right atrium.

⊙ **33212** Insertion of pacemaker pulse generator only; with existing single lead

⊙ **33213** with existing dual leads

#⊙ **33221** with existing multiple leads

⊙ **33214** Upgrade of implanted pacemaker system, conversion of single chamber system to dual chamber system (includes removal of previously placed pulse generator, testing of existing lead, insertion of new lead, insertion of new pulse generator)

33215 Repositioning of previously implanted transvenous pacemaker or implantable defibrillator (right atrial or right ventricular) electrode

⊙ **33216** Insertion of a single transvenous electrode, permanent pacemaker or implantable defibrillator

⊙ **33217** Insertion of 2 transvenous electrodes, permanent pacemaker or implantable defibrillator

⊙ **33218** Repair of single transvenous electrode, permanent pacemaker or implantable defibrillator

⊙ 33220 Repair of 2 transvenous electrodes for permanent pacemaker or implantable defibrillator

33221 Code is out of numerical sequence. See 33202-33249

⊙ 33222 Relocation of skin pocket for pacemaker

⊙ 33223 Relocation of skin pocket for implantable defibrillator

33224 Insertion of pacing electrode, cardiac venous system, for left ventricular pacing, with attachment to previously placed pacemaker or implantable defibrillator pulse generator (including revision of pocket, removal, insertion, and/or replacement of existing generator)

✚ 33225 Insertion of pacing electrode, cardiac venous system, for left ventricular pacing, at time of insertion of implantable defibrillator or pacemaker pulse generator (eg, for upgrade to dual chamber system) (List separately in addition to code for primary procedure)

33226 Repositioning of previously implanted cardiac venous system (left ventricular) electrode (including removal, insertion and/or replacement of existing generator)

33227 Code is out of numerical sequence. See 33202-33249

33228 Code is out of numerical sequence. See 33202-33249

33229 Code is out of numerical sequence. See 33202-33249

33230 Code is out of numerical sequence. See 33202-33249

33231 Code is out of numerical sequence. See 33202-33249

⊙ 33233 Removal of permanent pacemaker pulse generator only

#⊙ 33227 Removal of permanent pacemaker pulse generator with replacement of pacemaker pulse generator; single lead system

#⊙ 33228 dual lead system

#⊙ 33229 multiple lead system

⊙ 33234 Removal of transvenous pacemaker electrode(s); single lead system, atrial or ventricular

⊙ 33235 dual lead system

33236 Removal of permanent epicardial pacemaker and electrodes by thoracotomy; single lead system, atrial or ventricular

33237 dual lead system

33238 Removal of permanent transvenous electrode(s) by thoracotomy

⊙ 33240 Insertion of implantable defibrillator pulse generator only; with existing single lead

#⊙ 33230 with existing dual leads

#⊙ 33231 with existing multiple leads

⊙ 33241 Removal of implantable defibrillator pulse generator only

#⊙ 33262 Removal of implantable defibrillator pulse generator with replacement of implantable defibrillator pulse generator; single lead system

#⊙ 33263 dual lead system

#⊙ 33264 multiple lead system

33243 Removal of single or dual chamber implantable defibrillator electrode(s); by thoracotomy

⊙ 33244 by transvenous extraction

⊙ 33249 Insertion or replacement of permanent implantable defibrillator system, with transvenous lead(s), single or dual chamber

33270 Insertion or replacement of permanent subcutaneous implantable defibrillator system, with subcutaneous electrode, including defibrillation threshold evaluation, induction of arrhythmia, evaluation of sensing for arrhythmia termination, and programming or reprogramming of sensing or therapeutic parameters, when performed

33271 Insertion of subcutaneous implantable defibrillator electrode

33272 Removal of subcutaneous implantable defibrillator electrode

33273 Repositioning of previously implanted subcutaneous implantable defibrillator electrode

Electrophysiologic Operative Procedures

Coding Atlas

Ablation along the heart's electrical pathway is performed to reduce rhythm disorders caused by **aberrant** electrical transmissions. The **destruction** of heart tissue creates erratic heart beats that may eliminate the problem. **Ablation** can be performed using an **open** approach, with or without **cardiopulmonary bypass**, or an **endoscopic** approach. Code 33265 is used to report an endoscopic ablation for **paroxysmal** or short-duration **atrial fibrillation** or **flutter**; atrial incision(s) and the ablation technique are limited to use in the left atrium. Work does not extend to the atrioventricular (AV) **annulus**. Code 33266 is used to report endoscopic ablation for **chronic** atrial fibrillation or flutter using a maze technique, with treatment of AV annular lesions.

Incision

33250 Operative ablation of supraventricular arrhythmogenic focus or pathway (eg, Wolff-Parkinson-White, atrioventricular node re-entry), tract(s) and/or focus (foci); without cardiopulmonary bypass

33251 with cardiopulmonary bypass

FIGURE 4-3. Conduction System of the Heart

The sinoatrial (SA) node in the right atrium initiates electrical waves that create heart beats. The SA node's impulse is carried to the atrioventricular (AV) node at the **septum**, near the **tricuspid valve**. The AV checks the impulse and sends it along a track called the AV bundles or bundle of His, which is divided into a right bundle branch and left bundle branch, to the **Purkinje fibers**. When electricity stimulates the heart muscles, they contract: first atria, then ventricles. While contracting, the left ventricle pumps blood into the body, and the right ventricle pumps blood into the lungs.

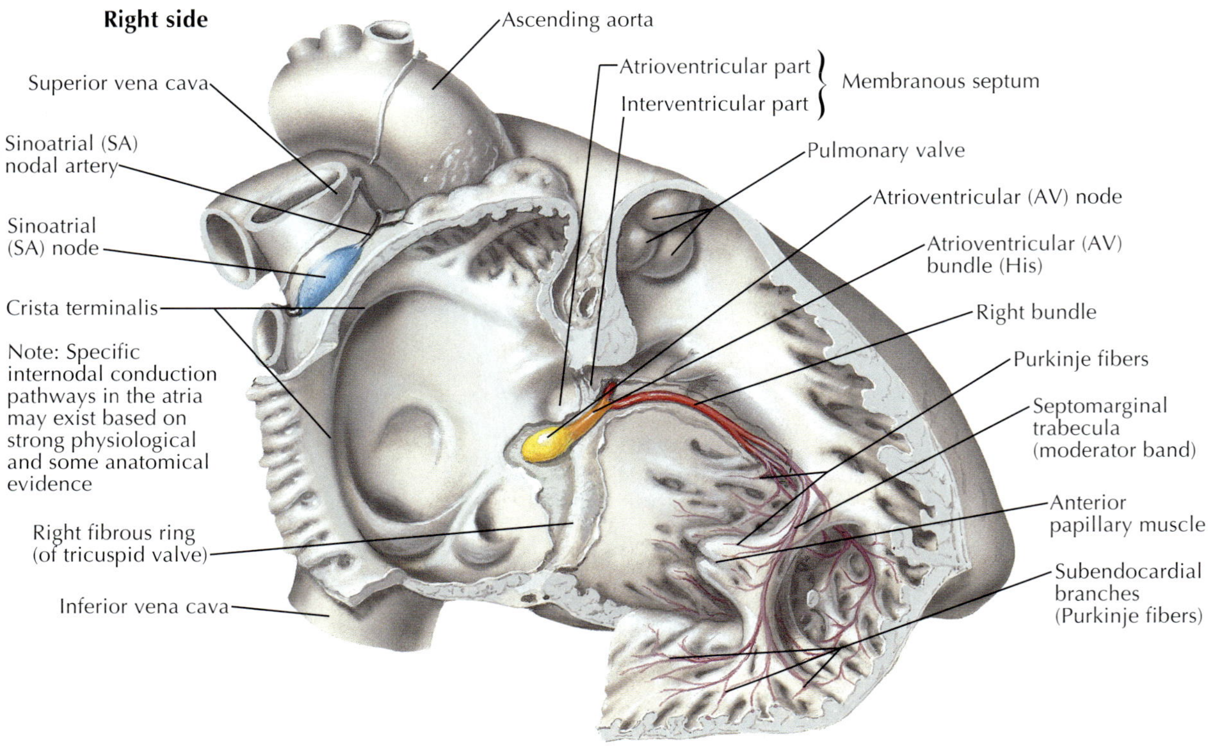

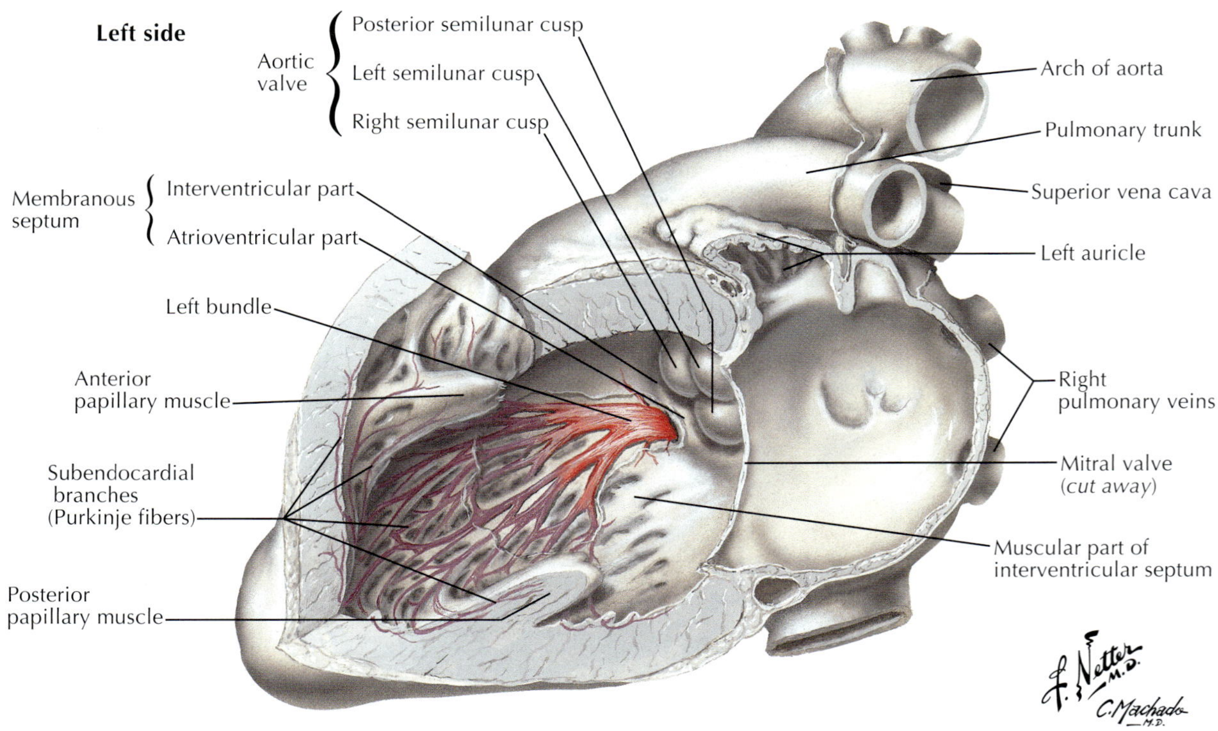

33254 Operative tissue ablation and reconstruction of atria, limited (eg, modified maze procedure)

33255 Operative tissue ablation and reconstruction of atria, extensive (eg, maze procedure); without cardiopulmonary bypass

33256 with cardiopulmonary bypass

✚ **33257** Operative tissue ablation and reconstruction of atria, performed at the time of other cardiac procedure(s), limited (eg, modified maze procedure) (List separately in addition to code for primary procedure)

✚ **33258** Operative tissue ablation and reconstruction of atria, performed at the time of other cardiac procedure(s), extensive (eg, maze procedure), without cardiopulmonary bypass (List separately in addition to code for primary procedure)

✚ **33259** Operative tissue ablation and reconstruction of atria, performed at the time of other cardiac procedure(s), extensive (eg, maze procedure), with cardiopulmonary bypass (List separately in addition to code for primary procedure)

33261 Operative ablation of ventricular arrhythmogenic focus with cardiopulmonary bypass

33262 Code is out of numerical sequence. See 33202-33264

33263 Code is out of numerical sequence. See 33202-33264

33264 Code is out of numerical sequence. See 33202-33264

Endoscopy

33265 Endoscopy, surgical; operative tissue ablation and reconstruction of atria, limited (eg, modified maze procedure), without cardiopulmonary bypass

33266 operative tissue ablation and reconstruction of atria, extensive (eg, maze procedure), without cardiopulmonary bypass

33270 Code is out of numerical sequence. See 33202-33270

33271 Code is out of numerical sequence. See 33202-33271

33272 Code is out of numerical sequence. See 33202-33272

33273 Code is out of numerical sequence. See 33202-33273

Patient-Activated Event Recorder

Coding Atlas

Codes 33282 and 33284 are used to report the surgical implantation and removal of a device that records electrical impulses from the heart. The initial programming is included in the implantation of the device, which is activated by the patient using a remote control device. Analysis and subsequent reprogramming are reported using codes 93285, 93291, 93298, and 93299.

⊙ **33282** Implantation of patient-activated cardiac event recorder

⊙ **33284** Removal of an implantable, patient-activated cardiac event recorder

Heart (Including Valves) and Great Vessels

Coding Atlas

When the heart chambers are incised during open surgery, the patient may require cardiopulmonary bypass to ensure delivery of oxygen to the distal areas of the body. Cannulae are inserted into the venous and arterial vasculatures, and circulation is supported by a heart–lung machine.

33300 Repair of cardiac wound; without bypass

33305 with cardiopulmonary bypass

33310 Cardiotomy, exploratory (includes removal of foreign body, atrial or ventricular thrombus); without bypass

33315 with cardiopulmonary bypass

33320 Suture repair of aorta or great vessels; without shunt or cardiopulmonary bypass

33321 with shunt bypass

33322 with cardiopulmonary bypass

33330 Insertion of graft, aorta or great vessels; without shunt, or cardiopulmonary bypass

33335 with cardiopulmonary bypass

Cardiac Valves

Coding Atlas

The heart valves open and close during contractions of the heart in a sequential fashion. Valve problems usually involve stenosis or insufficiency. In stenosis, the valve narrows and fails to open fully. Insufficiency occurs when the valve fails to close completely, allowing regurgitation, or backflow, of blood. Both of these conditions can be corrected, either in an open procedure exposing the heart or in a transcatheter endoscopic procedure.

Aortic Valve

33361 Transcatheter aortic valve replacement (TAVR/TAVI) with prosthetic valve; percutaneous femoral artery approach

33362 open femoral artery approach

33363 open axillary artery approach

FIGURE 4-4. Path of Blood Through the Heart

In Figure 4-4, oxygenated blood is red and deoxygenated blood is blue. The right atrium accepts deoxygenated blood from the body, and the blood moves through the **tricuspid valve** to the right ventricle, which pumps the blood through the **pulmonary valve** to the lungs. There, the blood is oxygenated. Oxygenated blood enters the left atrium, travels through the **mitral valve** into the left ventricle, and is pumped out the **aortic valve** into the body.

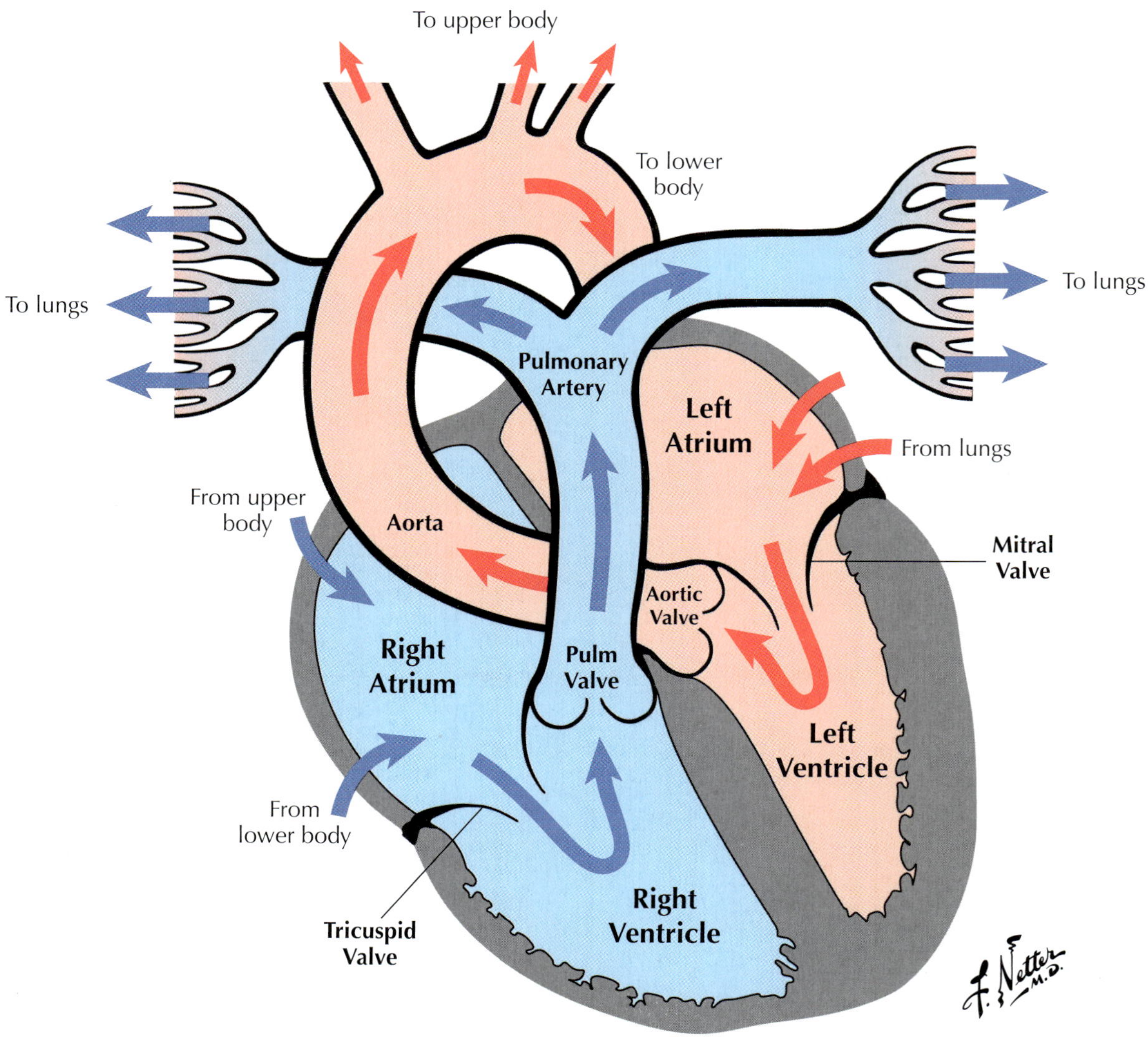

33364 open iliac artery approach

33365 transaortic approach (eg, median sternotomy, mediastinotomy)

33366 transapical exposure (eg, left thoracotomy)

+ 33367 cardiopulmonary bypass support with percutaneous peripheral arterial and venous cannulation (eg, femoral vessels) (List separately in addition to code for primary procedure)

+ 33368 cardiopulmonary bypass support with open peripheral arterial and venous cannulation (eg, femoral, iliac, axillary vessels) (List separately in addition to code for primary procedure)

+ 33369 cardiopulmonary bypass support with central arterial and venous cannulation (eg, aorta, right atrium, pulmonary artery) (List separately in addition to code for primary procedure)

33400 Valvuloplasty, aortic valve; open, with cardiopulmonary bypass

33401 open, with inflow occlusion

⊙=Moderate sedation ✚=Add-on code ⊘=Modifier 51 exempt #=Resequenced code

FIGURE 4-5. The Great Vessels

The **great vessels** refer to the group of large arteries and veins that transport oxygenated and deoxygenated blood to and from the heart. Great vessels include the **superior** and **inferior** vena cava, pulmonary arteries and pulmonary veins, and the aorta. The aorta begins at the left ventricle and curves toward the left, forming the **aortic arch**.

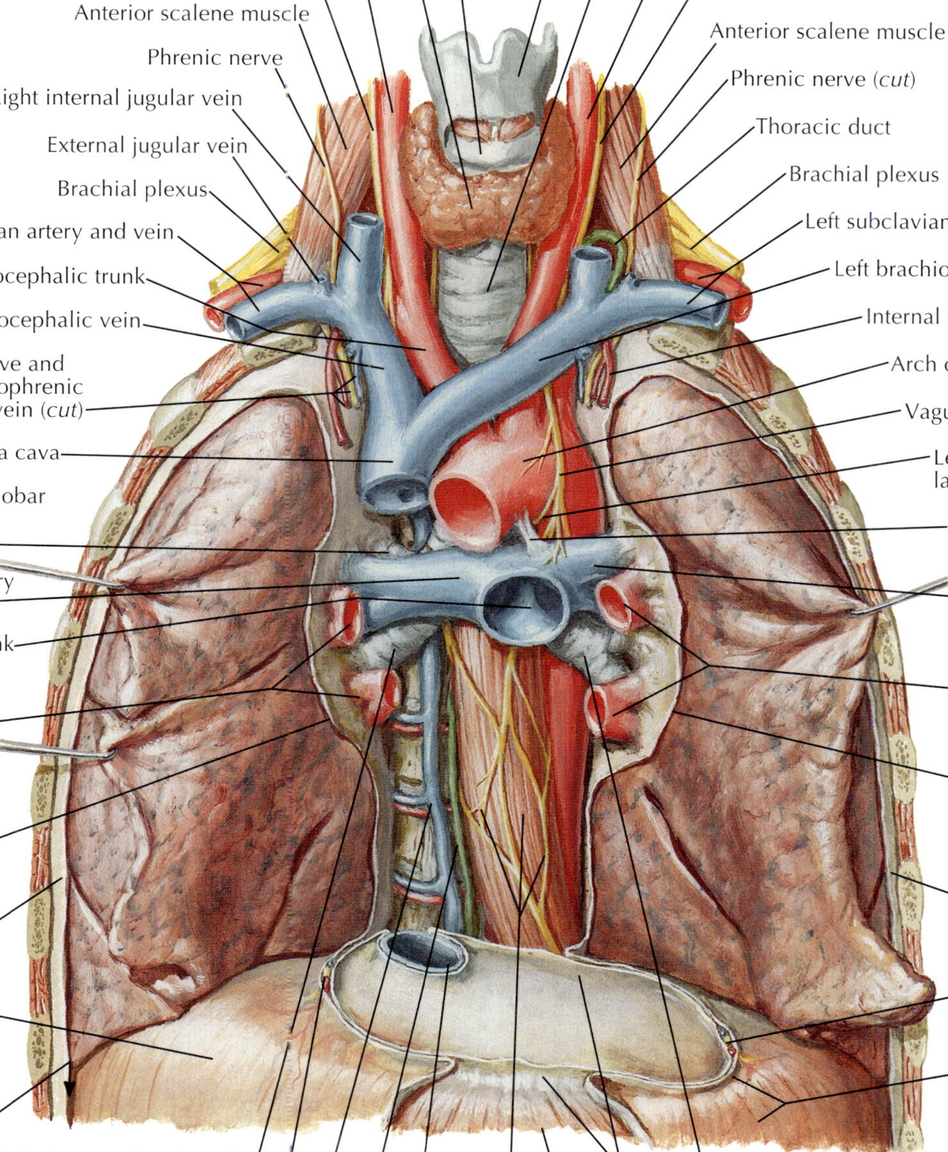

33403 using transventricular dilation, with cardiopulmonary bypass

33404 Construction of apical-aortic conduit

33405 Replacement, aortic valve, with cardiopulmonary bypass; with prosthetic valve other than homograft or stentless valve

33406 with allograft valve (freehand)

33410 with stentless tissue valve

33411 Replacement, aortic valve; with aortic annulus enlargement, noncoronary sinus

33412 with transventricular aortic annulus enlargement (Konno procedure)

33413 by translocation of autologous pulmonary valve with allograft replacement of pulmonary valve (Ross procedure)

33414 Repair of left ventricular outflow tract obstruction by patch enlargement of the outflow tract

33415 Resection or incision of subvalvular tissue for discrete subvalvular aortic stenosis

33416 Ventriculomyotomy (-myectomy) for idiopathic hypertrophic subaortic stenosis (eg, asymmetric septal hypertrophy)

33417 Aortoplasty (gusset) for supravalvular stenosis

Mitral Valve

33418 Transcatheter mitral valve repair, percutaneous approach, including transseptal puncture when performed; initial prosthesis

✚ **33419** additional prosthesis(es) during same session (List separately in addition to code for primary procedure)

33420 Valvotomy, mitral valve; closed heart

33422 open heart, with cardiopulmonary bypass

33425 Valvuloplasty, mitral valve, with cardiopulmonary bypass;

33426 with prosthetic ring

33427 radical reconstruction, with or without ring

33430 Replacement, mitral valve, with cardiopulmonary bypass

Tricuspid Valve

33460 Valvectomy, tricuspid valve, with cardiopulmonary bypass

33463 Valvuloplasty, tricuspid valve; without ring insertion

33464 with ring insertion

33465 Replacement, tricuspid valve, with cardiopulmonary bypass

33468 Tricuspid valve repositioning and plication for Ebstein anomaly

Pulmonary Valve

33470 Valvotomy, pulmonary valve, closed heart; transventricular

33471 via pulmonary artery

33474 Valvotomy, pulmonary valve, open heart, with cardiopulmonary bypass

33475 Replacement, pulmonary valve

33476 Right ventricular resection for infundibular stenosis, with or without commissurotomy

33478 Outflow tract augmentation (gusset), with or without commissurotomy or infundibular resection

Other Valvular Procedures

33496 Repair of non-structural prosthetic valve dysfunction with cardiopulmonary bypass (separate procedure)

Coronary Artery Anomalies

Coding Atlas

Congenital heart anomalies (CHAs) may be associated with coronary artery anomalies (CAAs). Code 33502 is used to report the open repair of a coronary artery with a congenital pulmonary artery origin. This is seen in young patients who present with tachypnea, poor feeding, and cardiomegaly. Because the pulmonary artery contains deoxygenated blood, its contents will fail to oxygenate the heart. Code 33507 is used to report a repair of a coronary artery from an anomalous origin on the aorta.

33500 Repair of coronary arteriovenous or arteriocardiac chamber fistula; with cardiopulmonary bypass

33501 without cardiopulmonary bypass

33502 Repair of anomalous coronary artery from pulmonary artery origin; by ligation

33503 by graft, without cardiopulmonary bypass

33504 by graft, with cardiopulmonary bypass

33505 with construction of intrapulmonary artery tunnel (Takeuchi procedure)

33506 by translocation from pulmonary artery to aorta

33507 Repair of anomalous (eg, intramural) aortic origin of coronary artery by unroofing or translocation

FIGURE 4-6. Valves of the Heart

The **mitral valve** has only two leaflets, while the pulmonary, aortic, and **tricuspid valves** each have three leaflets. The leaflets open and close in response to the heart's contractions. During **diastole**, the tricuspid and mitral valves open, while the pulmonary and aortic valves close. During **systole**, the opposite occurs. In **transcatheter** aortic valve replacement (TAVR), an artificial valve is secured over the open leaflets of the existing aortic valve.

Heart in diastole: Viewed from base with atria removed

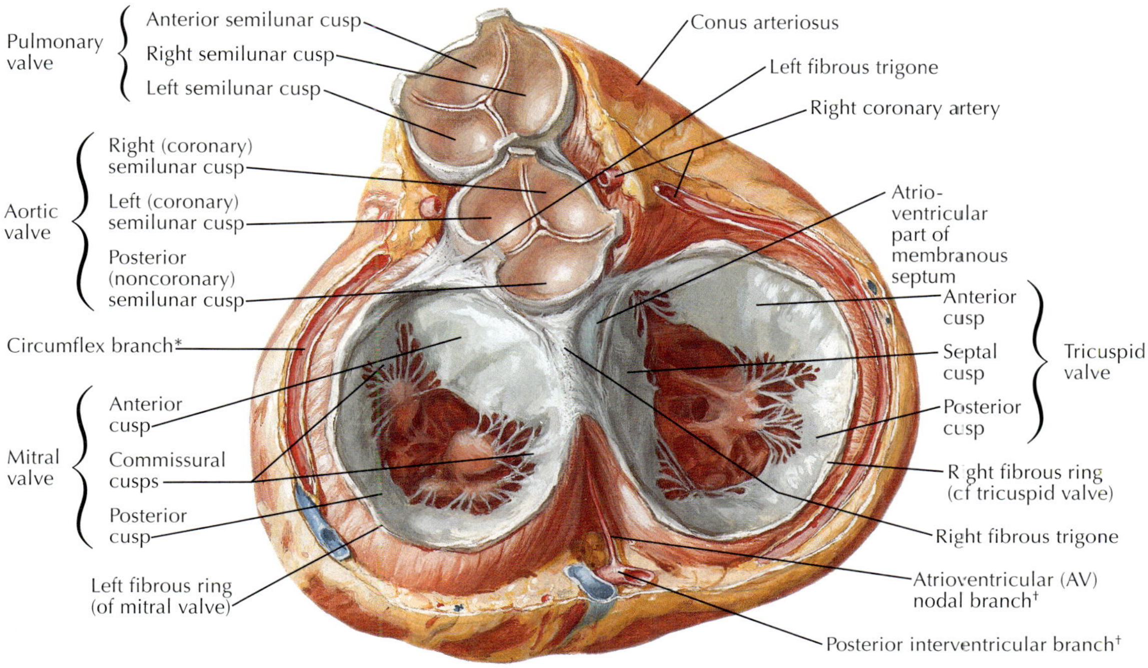

Heart in systole: Viewed from base with atria removed

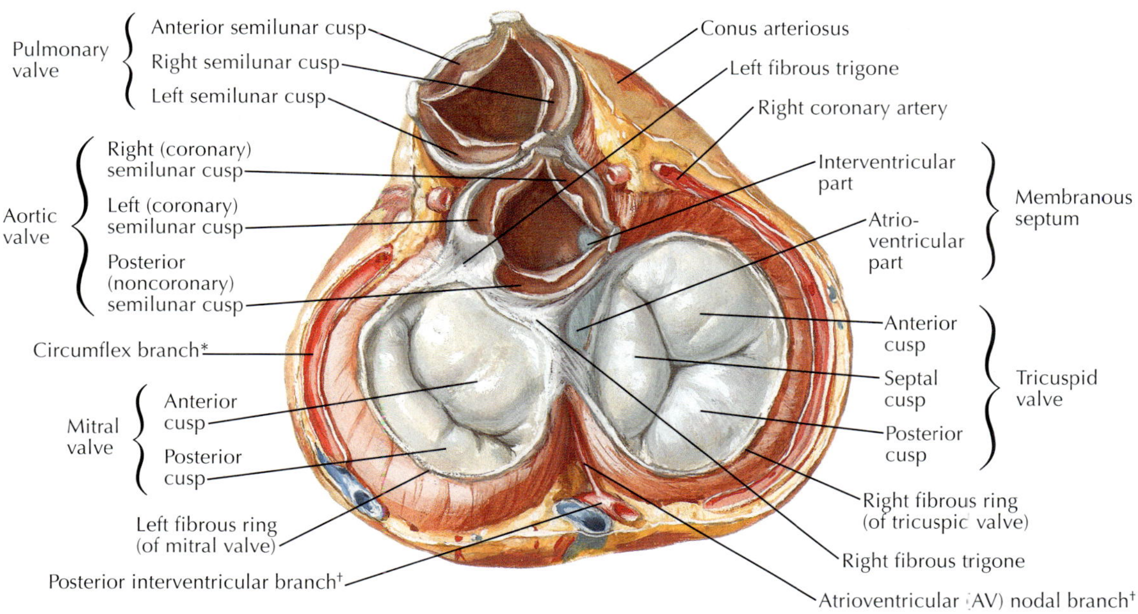

*Of left coronary artery
†Of right coronary artery

Endoscopy

+ 33508 Endoscopy, surgical, including video-assisted harvest of vein(s) for coronary artery bypass procedure (List separately in addition to code for primary procedure)

Venous Grafting Only for Coronary Artery Bypass

Coding Atlas

Codes for bypass grafts of the coronary artery are chosen based on the number of grafts created and the type of material used for the graft (artery, vein, or combination artery and vein). Codes 33510-33516 are used to describe procedures that involve the use of venous grafts. Harvest of the saphenous vein graft is included in the descriptions of work for these codes; however, harvest of an upper extremity vein would be reported in addition to the primary procedure.

33510 Coronary artery bypass, vein only; single coronary venous graft

33511 2 coronary venous grafts

33512 3 coronary venous grafts

33513 4 coronary venous grafts

33514 5 coronary venous grafts

33516 6 or more coronary venous grafts

Combined Arterial-Venous Grafting for Coronary Bypass

Coding Atlas

Codes 33517-33523 are add-on codes that are used to report combined arterial-venous coronary artery bypass grafting (CABG). These codes are reported in addition to the appropriate arterial graft code (codes 33533-33548). Procurement of the saphenous vein graft is included in the descriptions of work for these codes; however, harvest of an upper extremity vein would be reported in addition to the primary procedure.

+ 33517 Coronary artery bypass, using venous graft(s) and arterial graft(s); single vein graft (List separately in addition to code for primary procedure)

+ 33518 2 venous grafts (List separately in addition to code for primary procedure)

+ 33519 3 venous grafts (List separately in addition to code for primary procedure)

+ 33521 4 venous grafts (List separately in addition to code for primary procedure)

+ 33522 5 venous grafts (List separately in addition to code for primary procedure)

+ 33523 6 or more venous grafts (List separately in addition to code for primary procedure)

+ 33530 Reoperation, coronary artery bypass procedure or valve procedure, more than 1 month after original operation (List separately in addition to code for primary procedure)

Arterial Grafting for Coronary Artery Bypass

Coding Atlas

Codes for bypass grafts of the coronary artery are chosen based on the number of grafts created and the type of material used for the graft (artery, vein, or combination artery and vein). These codes describe procedures that involve the use of arterial grafts. Harvest of an upper extremity artery (eg, radial artery) would be reported in addition to the primary procedure.

33533 Coronary artery bypass, using arterial graft(s); single arterial graft

33534 2 coronary arterial grafts

33535 3 coronary arterial grafts

33536 4 or more coronary arterial grafts

33542 Myocardial resection (eg, ventricular aneurysmectomy)

33545 Repair of postinfarction ventricular septal defect, with or without myocardial resection

33548 Surgical ventricular restoration procedure, includes prosthetic patch, when performed (eg, ventricular remodeling, SVR, SAVER, Dor procedures)

Coronary Endarterectomy

Coding Atlas

Coronary endarterectomy is the removal of plaque or other occluding material from a coronary artery.

+ 33572 Coronary endarterectomy, open, any method, of left anterior descending, circumflex, or right coronary artery performed in conjunction with coronary artery bypass graft procedure, each vessel (List separately in addition to primary procedure)

FIGURE 4-7. Coronary Arteries and Veins

Coronary arteries extend from the aorta to supply oxygen to heart muscle. There are two main coronary arteries: right coronary artery (RCA) and left coronary artery (LCA). There are two LCA branches: left **anterior** descending (LAD) and left circumflex (LCX). The great cardiac vein drains blood from anterior ventricles. The small cardiac vein drains blood from the **lateral** and **posterior** right ventricle and atrium. The great and small cardiac veins merge with the coronary **sinus**, which empties into the right **atrium**.

Sternocostal surface

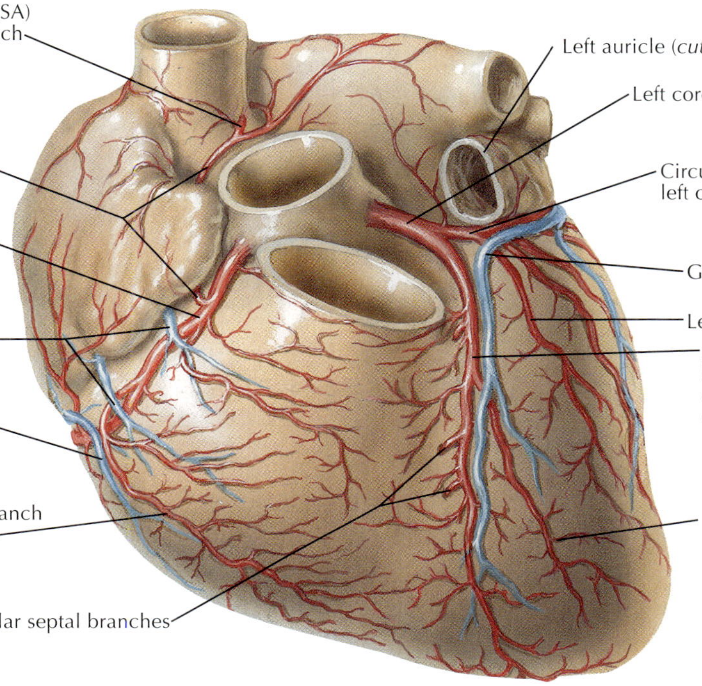

Diaphragmatic surface

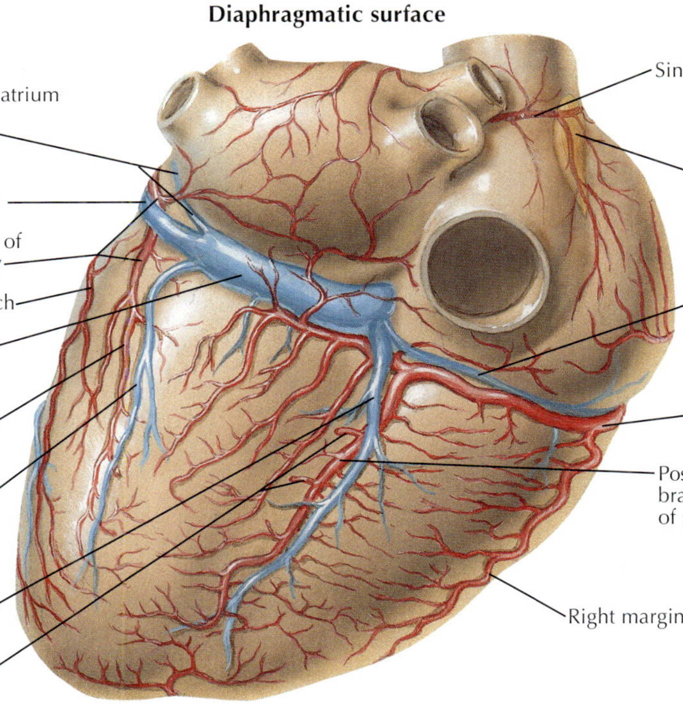

FIGURE 4-8. Coronary Artery Bypass Graft

A coronary artery bypass graft (CABG) is used to treat **coronary artery disease** (CAD) by providing a patent route around a **stenosed** segment of coronary artery. One end of a harvested artery or vein is grafted to the coronary artery **distal** to the blockage, and the other end is grafted to the aorta. In this way, oxygenated blood is delivered from the aorta to the coronary artery below the blockage. In CABG, one **graft** or multiple grafts may be performed. Code selection is based on the number and type of grafts. Note: Tools, implants, and/or equipment depicted in the illustration may be outdated but the procedural approach is valid.

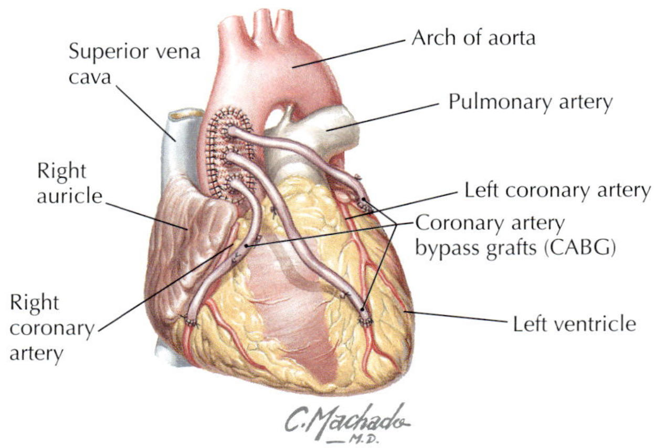

Single Ventricle and Other Complex Cardiac Anomalies

Coding Atlas

Single ventricle heart **anomaly** describes a category of serious **congenital** heart defects in which the right or left ventricle is underdeveloped and **septal** defects allow for mixture of oxygenated and deoxygenated blood within the heart. Repair of a single ventricle defect requires multiple surgeries over time.

33600 Closure of atrioventricular valve (mitral or tricuspid) by suture or patch

33602 Closure of semilunar valve (aortic or pulmonary) by suture or patch

33606 **Anastomosis** of pulmonary artery to aorta (Damus-Kaye-Stansel procedure)

33608 Repair of complex cardiac **anomaly** other than pulmonary **atresia** with ventricular **septal** defect by construction or replacement of conduit from right or left ventricle to pulmonary artery

33610 Repair of complex cardiac anomalies (eg, single ventricle with subaortic obstruction) by surgical enlargement of ventricular septal defect

33611 Repair of double outlet right ventricle with intraventricular tunnel repair;

33612 with repair of right ventricular outflow tract obstruction

33615 Repair of complex cardiac anomalies (eg, tricuspid atresia) by closure of atrial septal defect and anastomosis of atria or vena cava to pulmonary artery (simple Fontan procedure)

33617 Repair of complex cardiac anomalies (eg, single ventricle) by modified Fontan procedure

33619 Repair of single ventricle with aortic outflow obstruction and aortic arch **hypoplasia** (hypoplastic left heart syndrome) (eg, Norwood procedure)

33620 Application of right and left pulmonary artery bands (eg, hybrid approach stage 1)

33621 **Transthoracic** insertion of catheter for **stent** placement with **catheter** removal and closure (eg, hybrid approach stage 1)

33622 Reconstruction of complex cardiac anomaly (eg, single ventricle or hypoplastic left heart) with **palliation** of single ventricle with aortic outflow obstruction and aortic arch hypoplasia, creation of cavopulmonary anastomosis, and removal of right and left pulmonary bands (eg, hybrid approach stage 2, Norwood, bidirectional Glenn, pulmonary artery debanding)

Septal Defect

Coding Atlas

An atrial septal defect (ASD) is a communication between the right and left atria, and a ventricular septal defect (VSD) is a communication between the right and left ventricles. If, in an open procedure, a previously placed ASD device is removed and the ASD is surgically closed, code 33315 is used to report the removal of the device and code 33641 is used to report the ASD repair. The pulmonary artery is banded in order to reduce blood flow to the lungs. Excessive blood flow into the lungs through the pulmonary artery is associated with anomalies such as multiple VSDs or single ventricles in infants and children.

33641 Repair atrial **septal** defect, secundum, with **cardiopulmonary bypass**, with or without patch

33645 Direct or patch closure, sinus venosus, with or without anomalous pulmonary venous drainage

33647 Repair of atrial septal defect and ventricular septal defect, with direct or patch closure

33660 Repair of incomplete or partial atrioventricular canal (ostium primum atrial septal defect), with or without atrioventricular valve repair

33665 Repair of intermediate or transitional atrioventricular canal, with or without atrioventricular valve repair

33670 Repair of complete atrioventricular canal, with or without **prosthetic** valve

33675 Closure of multiple ventricular septal defects;

33676 with pulmonary **valvotomy** or infundibular resection (acyanotic)

33677 with removal of pulmonary artery band, with or without **gusset**

33681 Closure of single ventricular septal defect, with or without patch;

33684 with pulmonary valvotomy or infundibular resection (acyanotic)

33688 with removal of pulmonary artery band, with or without gusset

33690 Banding of pulmonary artery

33692 Complete repair tetralogy of Fallot without pulmonary **atresia**;

33694 with **transannular** patch

33697 Complete repair tetralogy of Fallot with pulmonary atresia including construction of conduit frcm right ventricle to pulmonary artery and closure of ventricular septal defect

Sinus of Valsalva

Coding Atlas

The ascending aorta adjacent to the aortic valve contains three anatomic **dilations** known as the aortic sinuses, or **sinus** of Valsalva. The right and left coronary arteries originate from the right and left sinus of Valsalva. The **ostium** of the right coronary artery is in the right sinus of Valsalva, and the ostium of the left coronary artery is in the left sinus of Valsalva. The third sinus is called the noncoronary sinus.

33702 Repair sinus of Valsalva **fistula**, with **cardiopulmonary bypass**;

33710 with repair of ventricular **septal** defect

33720 Repair sinus of Valsalva **aneurysm**, with cardiopulmonary bypass

33722 Closure of aortico-left ventricular tunnel

Venous Anomalies

Coding Atlas

Scimitar Syndrome, also referred to as hypogenetic lung syndrome or pulmonary venolobar syndrome, presents with a **congenital** and **anomalous** vein that carries oxygenated blood from the lung into the venous system rather than to the left atrium. It is called Scimitar Syndrome because, on X ray, the pulmonary vein has the shape of a curved sword.

33724 Repair of isolated partial **anomalous** pulmonary venous return (eg, Scimitar Syndrome)

33726 Repair of pulmonary venous **stenosis**

33730 Complete repair of anomalous pulmonary venous return (**supracardiac**, **intracardiac**, or **infracardiac** types)

33732 Repair of **cor triatriatum** or **supravalvular** mitral ring by resection of left atrial membrane

FIGURE 4-9. Ventricular Septal Defects

Ventricular **septal defects** (VSDs) are one of the most common **congenital** birth defects. A patient with a VSD may be asymptomatic or have severe symptoms similar to heart failure. Often, a large VSD allows deoxygenated blood to flow into the left ventricle and from there out into the body. A large defect can be corrected with insertion of a **prosthesis** that seals the hole or by surgery.

Muscular interventricular septal defect

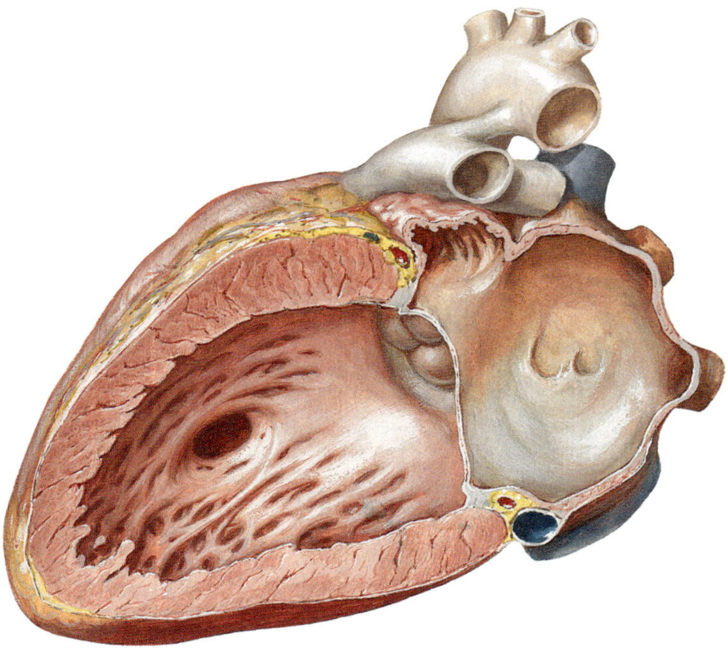

Subpulmonic defect

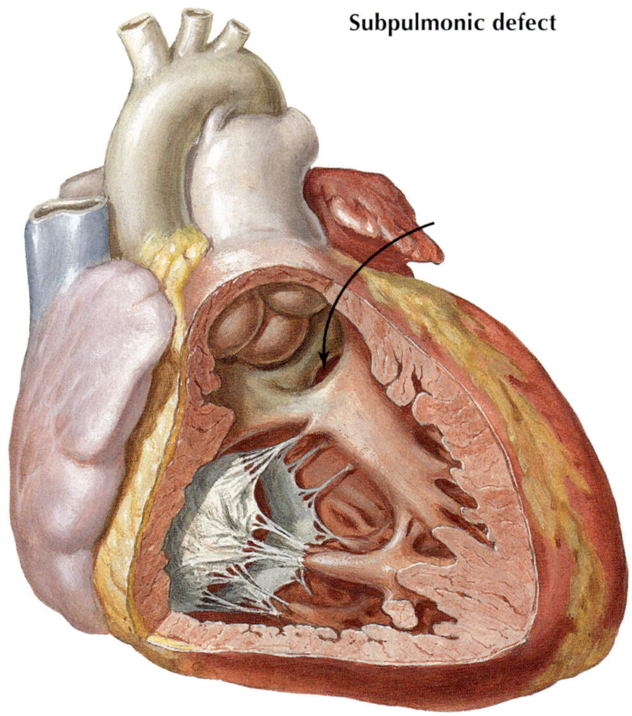

Ventricular septal defect

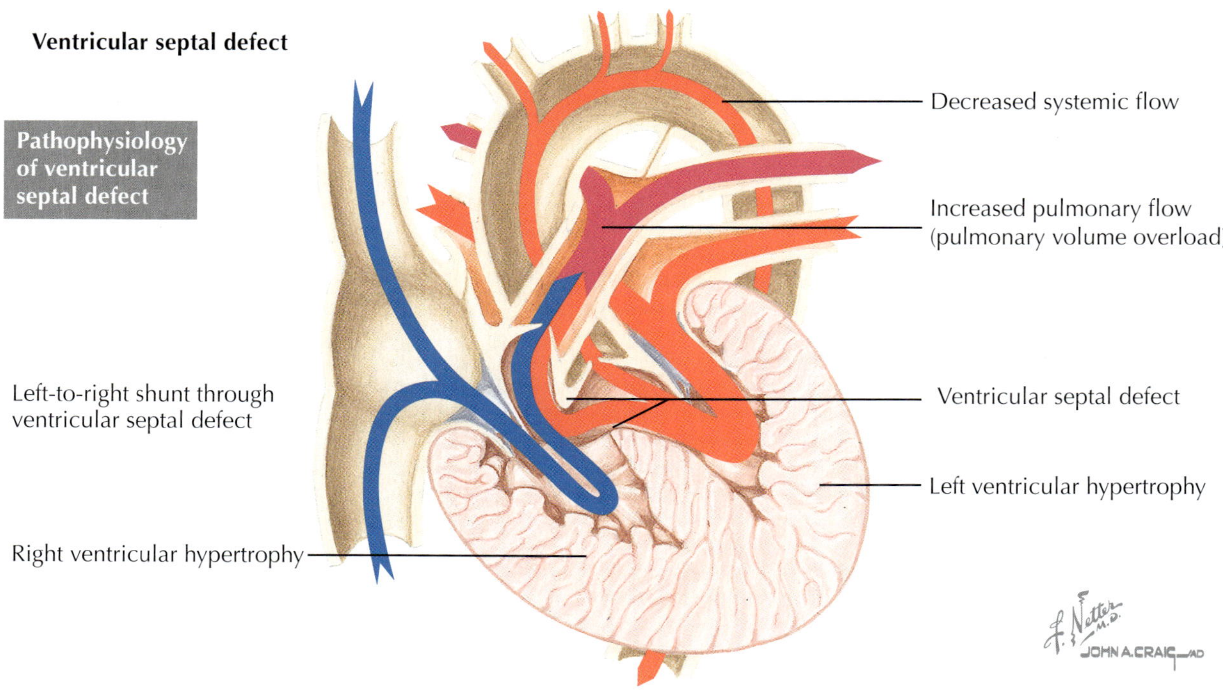

FIGURE 4-10. Tetralogy of Fallot

Tetralogy of Fallot (TOF) is a **congenital** heart defect that includes four elements: a large ventricular **septal defect** (VSD); **stenosis** of the **pulmonary valve**, right ventricular **hypertrophy**, and an aorta that is incorrectly attached between the right and left ventricles, directly over the VSD. Usually, the aorta is attached to the left ventricle. TOF may be corrected surgically. Note: Tools, implants, and/or equipment depicted in the illustration may be outdated but the procedural approach is valid.

Pathophysiology

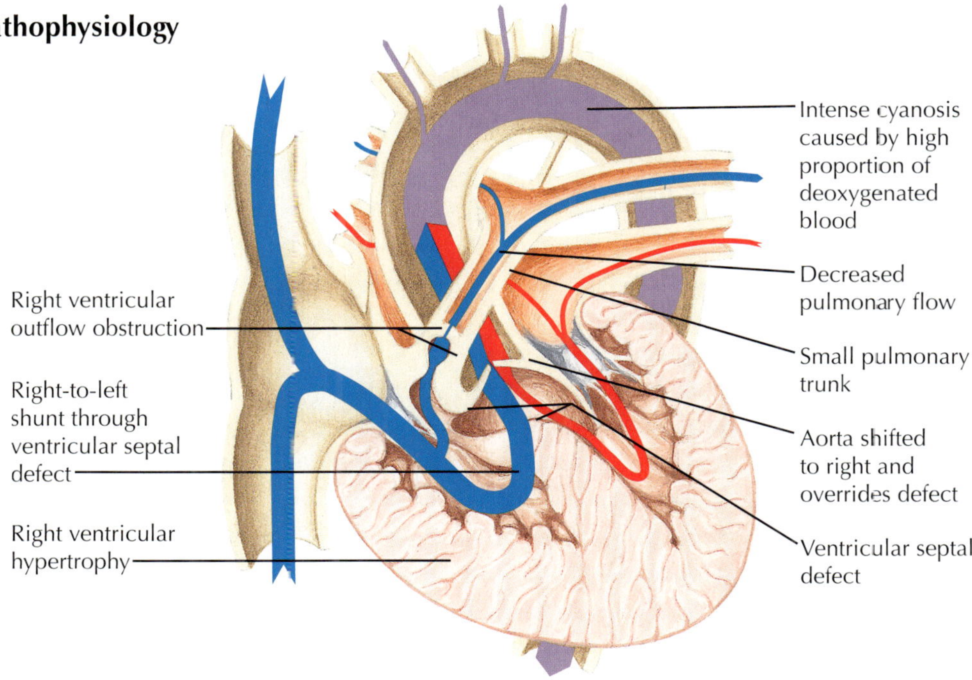

Blalock-Taussig Operation (Palliative)

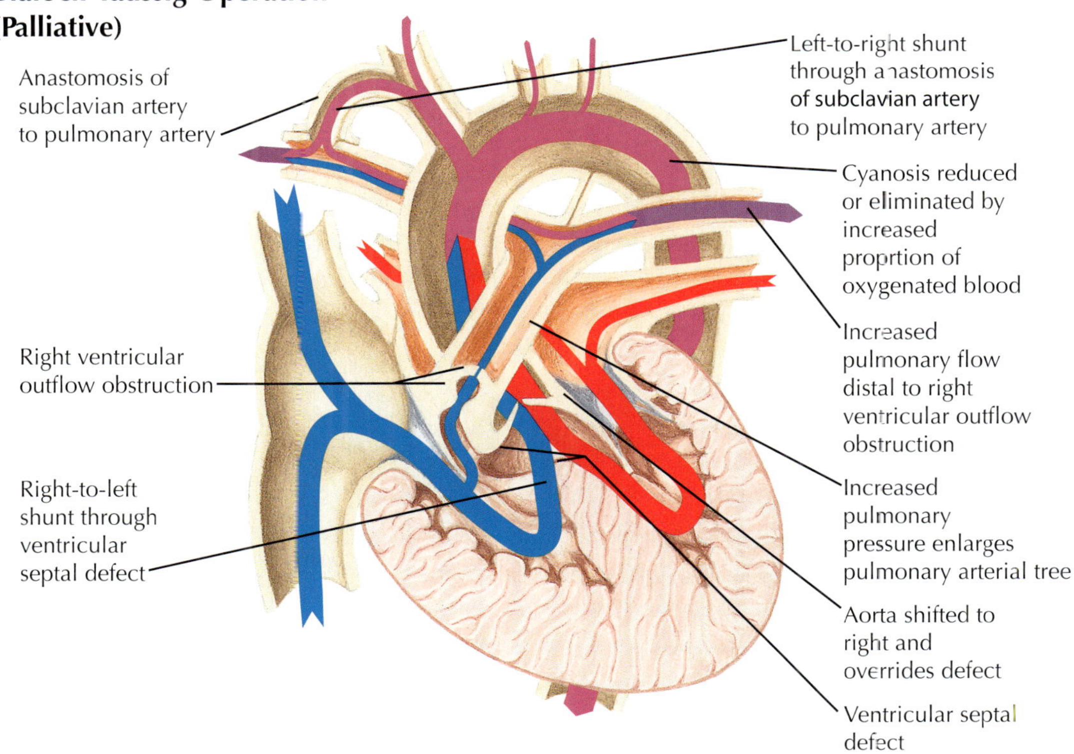

Shunting Procedures

Coding Atlas

A **shunt** is an unnatural passage for diversion of blood that is created surgically within cardiothoracic circulation.

33735 Atrial septectomy or septostomy; closed heart (Blalock-Hanlon type operation)

33736 open heart with cardiopulmonary bypass

33737 open heart, with inflow occlusion

33750 Shunt; subclavian to pulmonary artery (Blalock-Taussig type operation)

33755 ascending aorta to pulmonary artery (Waterston type operation)

33762 descending aorta to pulmonary artery (Potts-Smith type operation)

33764 central, with prosthetic graft

33766 superior vena cava to pulmonary artery for flow to 1 lung (classical Glenn procedure)

33767 superior vena cava to pulmonary artery for flow to both lungs (bidirectional Glenn procedure)

+ 33768 Anastomosis, cavopulmonary, second superior vena cava (List separately in addition to primary procedure)

Transposition of the Great Vessels

Coding Atlas

Transposition of the great vessels (TGV) is a **congenital** anomaly in which oxygenated blood is routed to the lungs and deoxygenated blood is pumped to **distal** portions of the circulatory system causing **cyanosis**. An arterial switch is required to permanently correct the problem. This condition may require multiple surgeries; the first surgery is usually performed during a **neonate**'s first week of life. TGV may occur with other cardiac **anomalies** that may be corrected during the same open-heart surgical session.

33770 Repair of transposition of the great arteries with ventricular septal defect and subpulmonary stenosis; without surgical enlargement of ventricular septal defect

33771 with surgical enlargement of ventricular septal defect

33774 Repair of transposition of the great arteries, atrial baffle procedure (eg, Mustard or Senning type) with cardiopulmonary bypass;

33775 with removal of pulmonary band

33776 with closure of ventricular septal defect

33777 with repair of subpulmonic obstruction

33778 Repair of transposition of the great arteries, aortic pulmonary artery reconstruction (eg, Jatene type);

33779 with removal of pulmonary band

33780 with closure of ventricular septal defect

33781 with repair of subpulmonic obstruction

33782 Aortic root translocation with ventricular septal defect and pulmonary stenosis repair (ie, Nikaidoh procedure); without coronary ostium reimplantation

33783 with reimplantation of 1 or both coronary ostia

Truncus Arteriosus

Coding Atlas

In a **truncus arteriosus** defect, a single blood vessel replaces the pulmonary artery and aorta coming off the right and left ventricles. In this **congenital** condition, there is usually a large ventricular **septal** defect. Surgical intervention is required. Usually, the existing vessel becomes the aorta, and a pulmonary artery is fashioned from graft tissue. The septal defect is repaired.

33786 Total repair, truncus arteriosus (Rastelli type operation)

33788 Reimplantation of an anomalous pulmonary artery

Aortic Anomalies

Coding Atlas

Not all **congenital** anomalies of the heart cause dysfunction sufficient to be diagnosed at birth. Some defects are not detected until later in life, usually due to symptoms of shortness of breath, exercise intolerance, or heart murmur. The defect may become symptomatic as other heart stressors occur, eg, a child's growth spurt or a comorbidity such as coronary artery disease in an older adult.

33800 Aortic suspension (aortopexy) for tracheal decompression (eg, for tracheomalacia) (separate procedure)

33802 Division of aberrant vessel (vascular ring);

33803 with reanastomosis

33813 Obliteration of aortopulmonary septal defect; without cardiopulmonary bypass

33814 with cardiopulmonary bypass

33820 Repair of patent ductus arteriosus; by ligation

33822 by division, younger than 18 years

33824 by division, 18 years and older

FIGURE 4-11. Truncus Arteriosis and Transposition of the Great Vessels

In persistent **truncus arteriosis**, the pulmonary artery and aorta are replaced with a single vessel. This **congenital** defect is usually accompanied by a large ventricular **septal** defect. In transposition of great vessels (TGV), also documented as transposition of great arteries (TGA), oxygenated blood travels a **blind loop** within the heart and lung. Deoxygenated blood is pumped into the heart and returns to the body without oxygenation. Symptoms of TGV vary, depending upon coexisting cardiac anomalies.

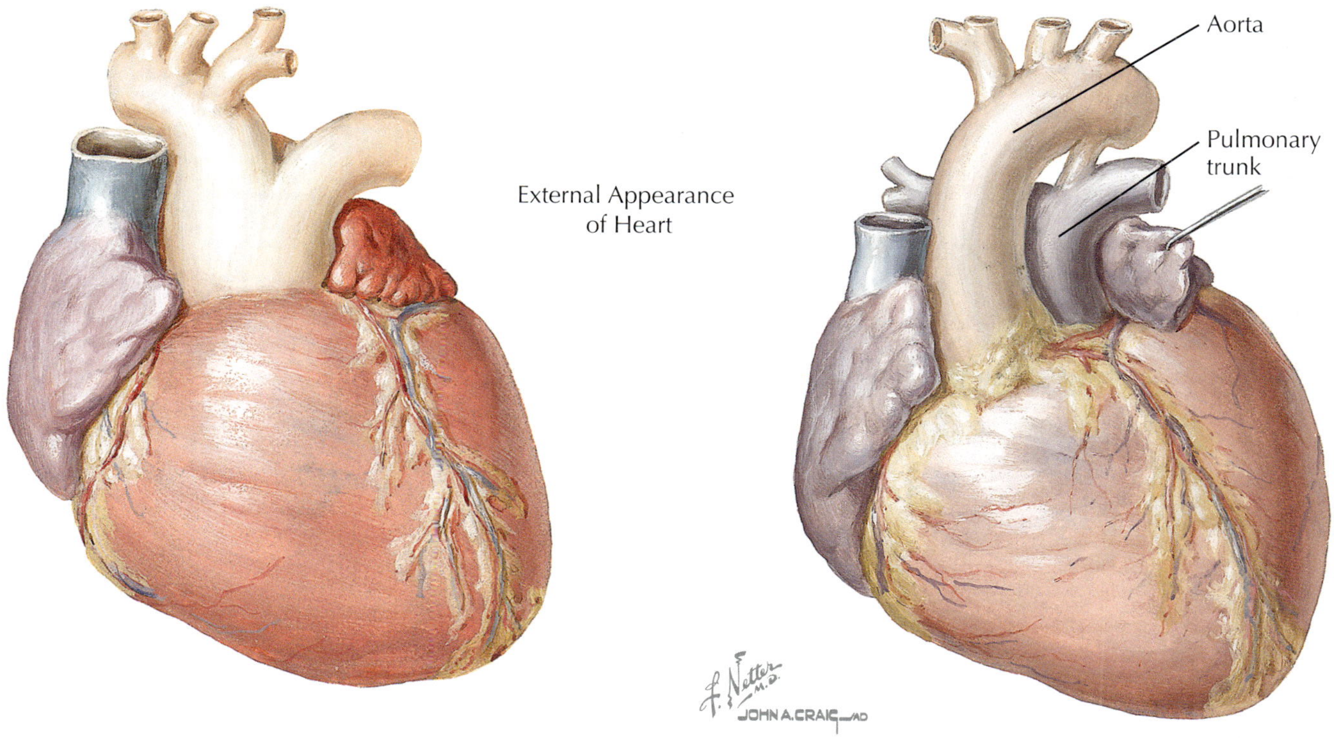

33840 Excision of **coarctation** of aorta, with or without associated patent ductus arteriosus; with direct anastomosis

33845 with **graft**

33851 repair using either left subclavian artery or **prosthetic** material as gusset for enlargement

33852 Repair of **hypoplastic** or interrupted aortic arch using **autogenous** or prosthetic material; without cardiopulmonary bypass

33853 with cardiopulmonary bypass

Thoracic Aortic Aneurysm

Coding Atlas

A thoracic aortic **aneurysm** (TAA) is a ballooning out of the aortic artery wall in the chest cavity. The risk of TAA is rupture and **hemorrhage** at the site of the weakened wall, leading to shock or death. TAAs are often treated surgically because of their high mortality rate.

33860 Ascending aorta **graft**, with **cardiopulmonary bypass**, includes valve suspension, when performed

33863 Ascending aorta graft, with cardiopulmonary bypass, with aortic root replacement using valved conduit and coronary reconstruction (eg, Bentall)

33864 Ascending aorta graft, with cardiopulmonary bypass with valve suspension, with coronary reconstruction and valve-sparing aortic root remodeling (eg, David Procedure, Yacoub Procedure)

FIGURE 4-12. Fetal and Newborn Circulation

Before birth, the aorta and pulmonary artery are connected by a blood vessel called the **ductus arteriosus. Patent** ductus arteriosus (PDA) occurs when this connection, which normally closes soon after birth, remains open. PDA allows oxygenated blood from the aorta to mix with deoxygenated blood from the pulmonary artery, increasing blood pressure in the lungs, overworking the muscles of the heart, and reducing the concentration of oxygen in the oxygenated blood being pumped from the heart to the body.

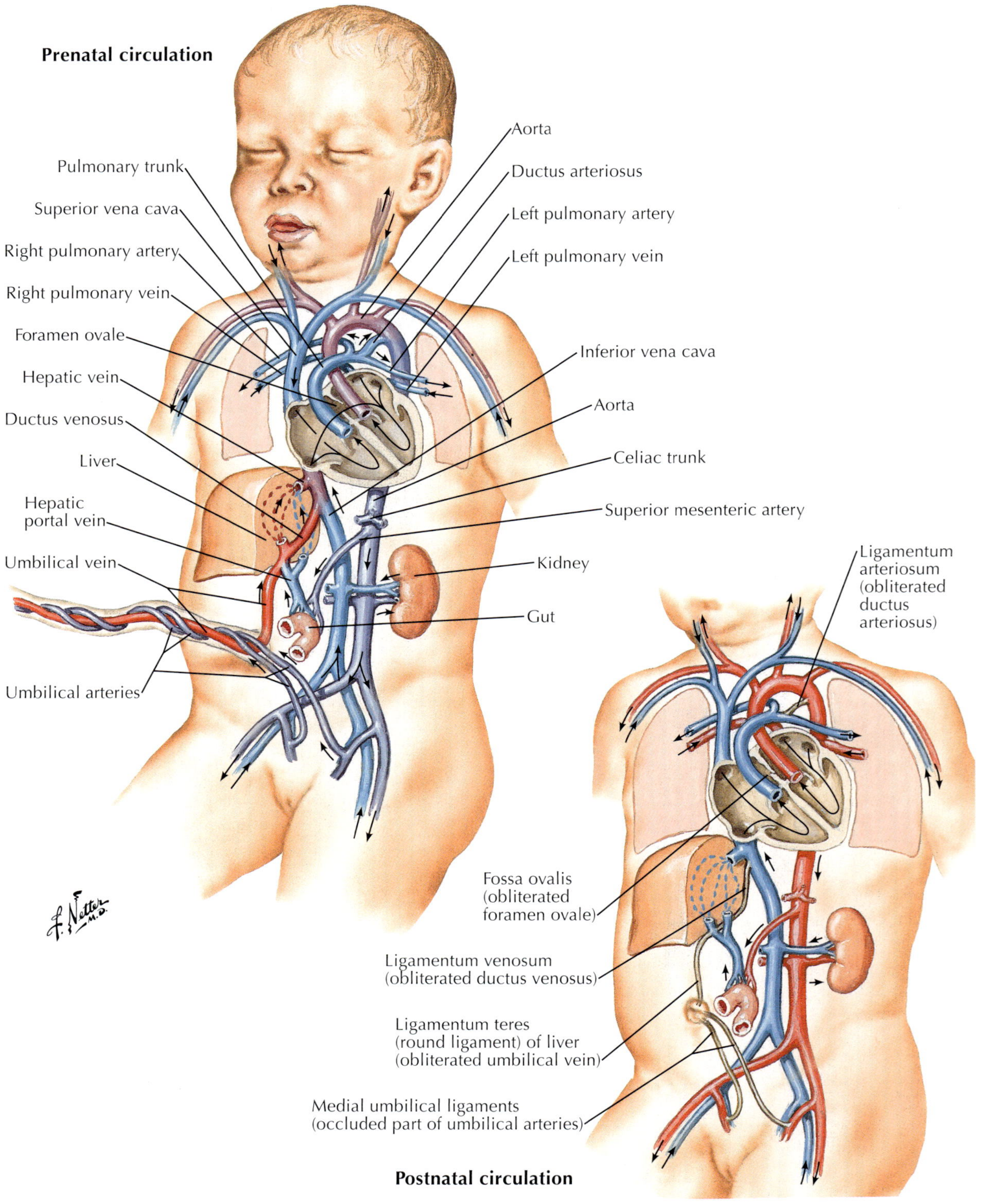

33870 Transverse arch graft, with cardiopulmonary bypass

33875 Descending thoracic aorta graft, with or without bypass

33877 Repair of thoracoabdominal aortic aneurysm with graft, with or without cardiopulmonary bypass

Endovascular Repair of Descending Thoracic Aorta

Coding Atlas

In **endovascular** repair of the descending thoracic aorta, an **endoprosthesis** is carried through a scope to the site of an **aneurysm**, **ulcer**, or other abnormality and secured over the defect endoscopically. The thoracic aorta is the origin of several paired arteries: bronchial, mediastinal, esophageal, and pericardial. The **superior** phrenic artery also branches from the thoracic aorta, as do the **posterior** intercostal arteries. In some cases, an aneurysm bridges an area with an arterial branch, and prosthetic extension(s) are placed in the artery forking from the aorta to complete the repair.

33880 Endovascular repair of descending thoracic aorta (eg, aneurysm, pseudoaneurysm, dissection, penetrating ulcer, intramural hematoma, or traumatic disruption); involving coverage of left subclavian artery origin, initial endoprosthesis plus descending thoracic aortic extension(s), if required, to level of celiac artery origin

33881 not involving coverage of left subclavian artery origin, initial endoprosthesis plus descending thoracic aortic extension(s), if required, to level of celiac artery origin

33883 Placement of proximal extension prosthesis for endovascular repair of descending thoracic aorta (eg, aneurysm, pseudoaneurysm, dissection, penetrating ulcer, intramural hematoma, or traumatic disruption); initial extension

+ 33884 each additional proximal extension (List separately in addition to code for primary procedure)

33886 Placement of distal extension prosthesis(s) delayed after endovascular repair of descending thoracic aorta

33889 Open subclavian to carotid artery transposition performed in conjunction with endovascular repair of descending thoracic aorta, by neck incision, unilateral

33891 Bypass graft, with other than vein, transcervical retropharyngeal carotid-carotid, performed in conjunction with endovascular repair of descending thoracic aorta, by neck incision

Pulmonary Artery

Coding Atlas

The main pulmonary artery (MPA), also referred to as pulmonary trunk, begins at the **pulmonary valve**, splitting into the left pulmonary artery (LPA) and right pulmonary artery (RPA) after it emerges from the **pericardium**. The RPA is longer than the LPA, as the RPA must cross the mediastinum. The LPA's arc is effectively a continuation of the MPA's arc.

33910 Pulmonary artery embolectomy; with cardiopulmonary bypass

33915 without cardiopulmonary bypass

33916 Pulmonary endarterectomy, with or without embolectomy, with cardiopulmonary bypass

33917 Repair of pulmonary artery stenosis by reconstruction with patch or graft

33920 Repair of pulmonary atresia with ventricular septal defect, by construction or replacement of conduit from right or left ventricle to pulmonary artery

33922 Transection of pulmonary artery with cardiopulmonary bypass

+ 33924 Ligation and takedown of a systemic-to-pulmonary artery shunt, performed in conjunction with a congenital heart procedure (List separately in addition to code for primary procedure)

33925 Repair of pulmonary artery arborization anomalies by unifocalization; without cardiopulmonary bypass

33926 with cardiopulmonary bypass

Heart/Lung Transplantation

Coding Atlas

A **transplant** has three components: acquiring the donor organ, in the case of a heart or heart-lung transplant, from a **cadaver**; trimming and preparing the donor organ for transplant; and transplanting the donor organ into the patient, with or without removal of the patient's **native** organ.

33930 Donor cardiectomy-pneumonectomy (including cold preservation)

33933 Backbench standard preparation of cadaver donor heart/lung allograft prior to transplantation, including dissection of allograft from surrounding soft tissues to prepare aorta, superior vena cava, inferior vena cava, and trachea for implantation

FIGURE 4-13. Thoracic Aorta

The aorta in the **thorax** is divided into three segments: the ascending aorta (not shown), which begins at the aortic valve and continues to the arch; the aortic arch; and the descending aorta, which begins at the **aortic arch** and continues distally to the **diaphragm**. At the diaphragm, the abdominal aorta begins. The descending aorta is situated on the left of the **esophagus** and continues to the diaphragm where it is nearly centered over the vertebral column.

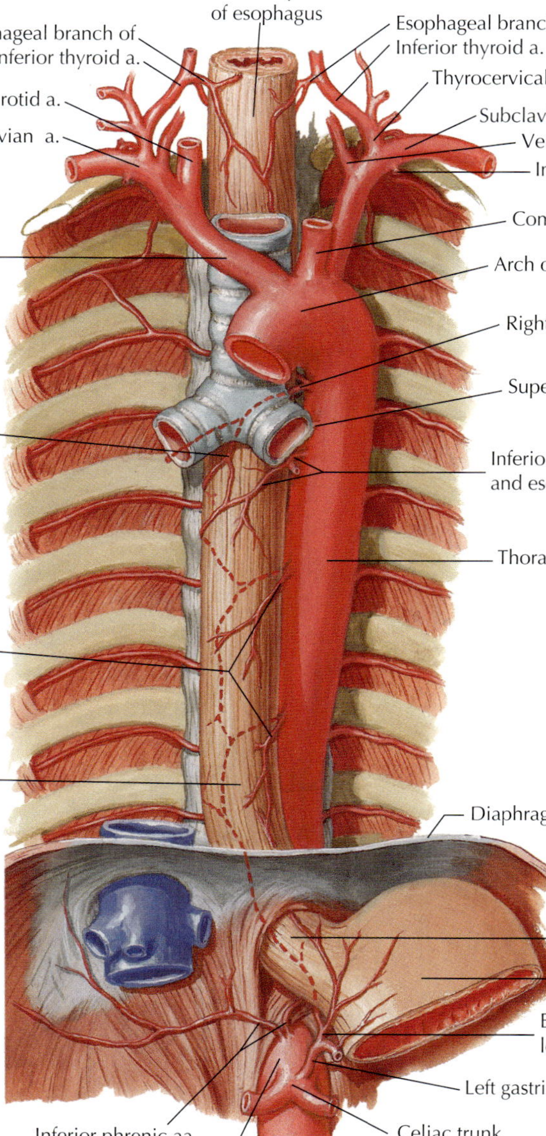

FIGURE 4-14. Pulmonary Arteries and Veins

After birth, the pulmonary arteries are the only arteries that carry deoxygenated blood and the pulmonary veins are the only veins that carry oxygenated blood. In most illustrations in this book, red signifies arteries and blue signifies veins. In Figure 4-14, the colors of pulmonary vessels are reversed to signify their reversed functions. Each lobe of the lung has its own independent vascularization.

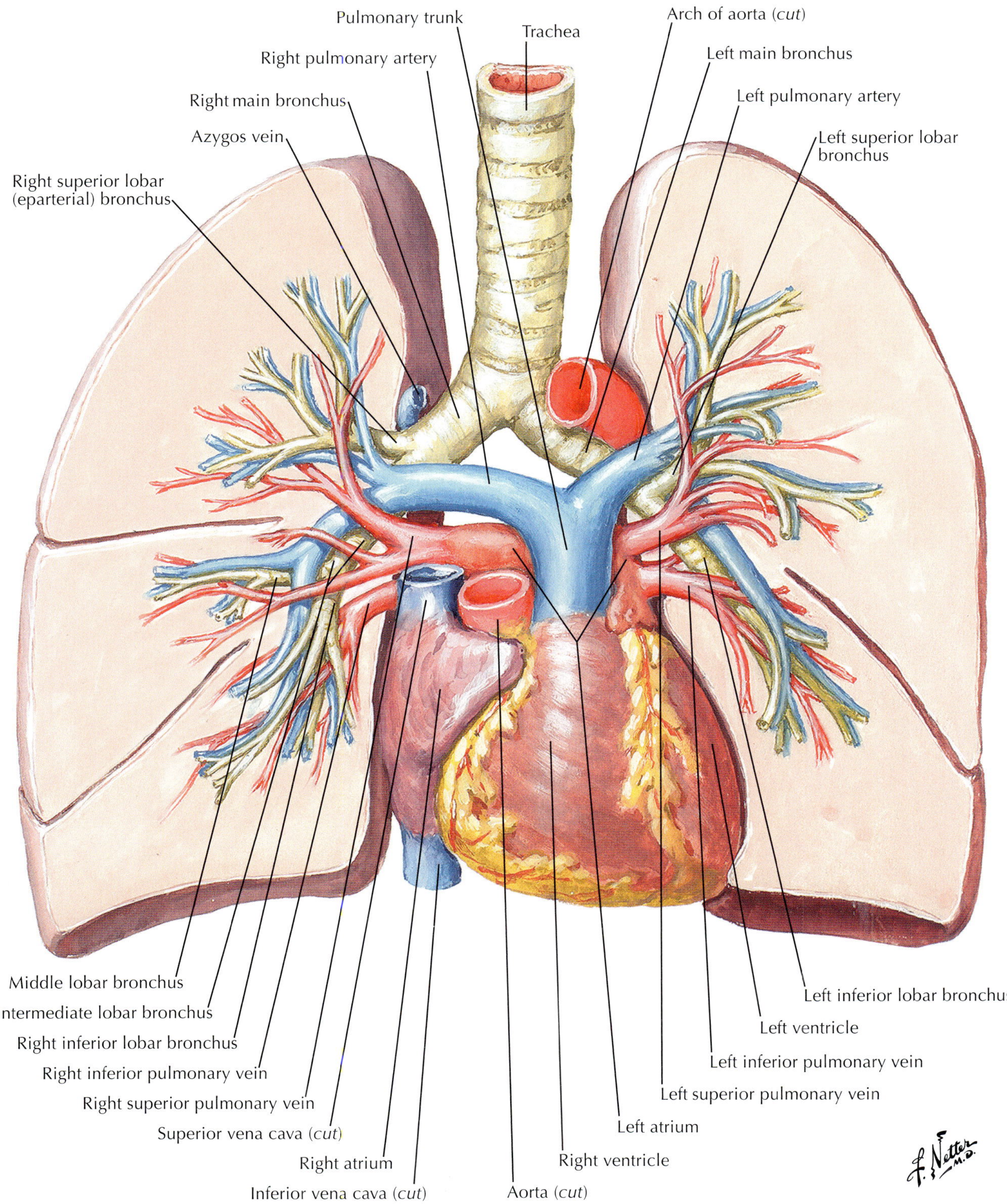

33935 Heart-lung transplant with recipient cardiectomy-pneumonectomy

33940 Donor cardiectomy (including cold preservation)

33944 Backbench standard preparation of cadaver donor heart allograft prior to transplantation, including dissection of allograft from surrounding soft tissues to prepare aorta, superior vena cava, inferior vena cava, pulmonary artery, and left atrium for implantation

33945 Heart transplant, with or without recipient cardiectomy

Extracorporeal Membrane Oxygenation or Extracorporeal Life Support Services

Coding Atlas

Extracorporeal membrane oxygenation (ECMO) and extracorporeal life support (ECLS) are performed to provide prolonged cardiac and/or respiratory support. Blood is pumped out of the body. The blood is infused with oxygen and carbon dioxide is removed. The blood is then warmed and returned to the body. If a cannula is inserted into an artery and another cannula is inserted into a vein during the procedure, it is called veno-arterial ECMO/ECLS. If two cannulas are inserted into a vein, it is called veno-venous ECMO/ECLS.

33946 Extracorporeal membrane oxygenation (ECMO)/ extracorporeal life support (ECLS) provided by physician; initiation, veno-venous

33947 initiation, veno-arterial

33948 daily management, each day, veno-venous

33949 daily management, each day, veno-arterial

33951 insertion of peripheral (arterial and/or venous) cannula(e), percutaneous, birth through 5 years of age (includes fluoroscopic guidance, when performed)

33952 insertion of peripheral (arterial and/or venous) cannula(e), percutaneous, 6 years and older (includes fluoroscopic guidance, when performed)

33953 insertion of peripheral (arterial and/or venous) cannula(e), open, birth through 5 years of age

33954 insertion of peripheral (arterial and/or venous) cannula(e), open, 6 years and older

33955 insertion of central cannula(e) by sternotomy or thoracotomy, birth through 5 years of age

33956 insertion of central cannula(e) by sternotomy or thoracotomy, 6 years and older

33957 reposition peripheral (arterial and/or venous) cannula(e), percutaneous, birth through 5 years of age (includes fluoroscopic guidance, when performed)

33958 reposition peripheral (arterial and/or venous) cannula(e), percutaneous, 6 years and older (includes fluoroscopic guidance, when performed)

33959 reposition peripheral (arterial and/or venous) cannula(e), open, birth through 5 years of age (includes fluoroscopic guidance, when performed)

\# **33962** reposition peripheral (arterial and/or venous) cannula(e), open, 6 years and older (includes fluoroscopic guidance, when performed)

\# **33963** reposition of central cannula(e) by sternotomy or thoracotomy, birth through 5 years of age (includes fluoroscopic guidance, when performed)

\# **33964** reposition central cannula(e) by sternotomy or thoracotomy, 6 years and older (includes fluoroscopic guidance, when performed)

\# **33965** removal of peripheral (arterial and/or venous) cannula(e), percutaneous, birth through 5 years of age

\# **33966** removal of peripheral (arterial and/or venous) cannula(e), percutaneous, 6 years and older

\# **33969** removal of peripheral (arterial and/or venous) cannula(e), open, birth through 5 years of age

\# **33984** removal of peripheral (arterial and/or venous) cannula(e), open, 6 years and older

\# **33985** removal of central cannula(e) by sternotomy or thoracotomy, birth through 5 years of age

\# **33986** removal of central cannula(e) by sternotomy or thoracotomy, 6 years and older

\#✚ **33987** Arterial exposure with creation of graft conduit (eg, chimney graft) to facilitate arterial perfusion for ECMO/ ECLS (List separately in addition to code for primary procedure)

\# **33988** Insertion of left heart vent by thoracic incision (eg, sternotomy, thoracotomy) for ECMO/ECLS

\# **33989** Removal of left heart vent by thoracic incision (eg, sternotomy, thoracotomy) for ECMO/ECLS

Cardiac Assist

Coding Atlas

A ventricular assist device (VAD) supports the heart's weakened ventricle to pump blood throughout the body, usually in patients who are in **end stage heart failure** or who are awaiting transplant. CPT codes 33975 and 33977 are used to report the insertion and removal of VADs by open surgical techniques. Percutaneous VAD (pVAD) devices are used to assist patients who have impaired ventricular function and are undergoing high-risk procedures or those with severe ventricular dysfunction who require medical stabilization. Codes 33990-33993 describe the insertion, removal, and repositioning of a pVAD.

33962 Code is out of numerical sequence. See 33946-33993

33963 Code is out of numerical sequence. See 33946-33993

33964 Code is out of numerical sequence. See 33946-33993

33965 Code is out of numerical sequence. See 33946-33993

33966 Code is out of numerical sequence. See 33946-33993

33967 Insertion of intra-aortic balloon assist device, percutaneous

33968 Removal of intra-aortic balloon assist device, percutaneous

33969 Code is out of numerical sequence. See 33946-33993

33970 Insertion of intra-aortic balloon assist device through the femoral artery, open approach

33971 Removal of intra-aortic balloon assist device including repair of femoral artery, with or without graft

33973 Insertion of intra-aortic balloon assist device through the ascending aorta

33974 Removal of intra-aortic balloon assist device from the ascending aorta, including repair of the ascending aorta, with or without graft

33975 Insertion of ventricular assist device; extracorporeal, single ventricle

33976 extracorporeal, biventricular

33977 Removal of ventricular assist device; extracorporeal, single ventricle

33978 extracorporeal, biventricular

33979 Insertion of ventricular assist device, implantable intracorporeal, single ventricle

33980 Removal of ventricular assist device, implantable intracorporeal, single ventricle

33981 Replacement of extracorporeal ventricular assist device, single or biventricular, pump(s), single or each pump

33982 Replacement of ventricular assist device pump(s); implantable intracorporeal, single ventricle, without cardiopulmonary bypass

33983 implantable intracorporeal, single ventricle, with cardiopulmonary bypass

33984 Code is out of numerical sequence. See 33946-33993

33985 Code is out of numerical sequence. See 33946-33993

33986 Code is out of numerical sequence. See 33946-33993

33987 Code is out of numerical sequence. See 33946-33993

33988 Code is out of numerical sequence. See 33946-33993

33989 Code is out of numerical sequence. See 33946-33993

⊙ **33990** Insertion of ventricular assist device, percutaneous including radiological supervision and interpretation; arterial access only

⊙ **33991** both arterial and venous access, with transseptal puncture

⊙ **33992** Removal of percutaneous ventricular assist device at separate and distinct session from insertion

⊙ **33993** Repositioning of percutaneous ventricular assist device with imaging guidance at separate and distinct session from insertion

Arteries and Veins

Embolectomy/Thrombectomy

Coding Atlas

A **thrombus** is a blood clot that has formed **in situ**. A thrombus becomes an **embolus** if it breaks free and is carried downstream of the site at which it formed. An embolus may consist of matter other than blood, eg, a fat globule or air bubble. When the traveling embolus becomes lodged in the bloodstream, it is called an embolism. Both thrombi and emboli narrow or totally occlude the vessels in which they become lodged. Codes 34001-34490 are used to report the open treatment of a thrombus or embolus, indicating that the physician made an incision into the skin overlying the vessel to locate the defect and then incised the vessel to remove the defect. A catheter may be used in the procedure. The procedure is reported once even if multiple vessels are accessed through the single incision. In **thromboendarterectomy**, the thrombus is removed along with a portion of the inner lining of the artery. Thromboendarterectomy is reported using CPT codes 35301-35372.

FIGURE 4-15. Major Arteries and Pulse Points

Arteries, which deliver oxygenated blood throughout the body, contain three layers: the tunica intima, a smooth, inner layer lined with **endothelium**; the tunica media, a muscular middle layer; and the tunica adventitia, a strong outer layer formed from a connective structure that anchors the arteries to adjacent tissues. A pulse point is the site on the surface of the body in which arterial pulsations can be easily palpated, ie, where a finger pressing the skin wedges the artery against bone so that the finger can feel the rhythm of the heart beat in the blood flowing through the artery.

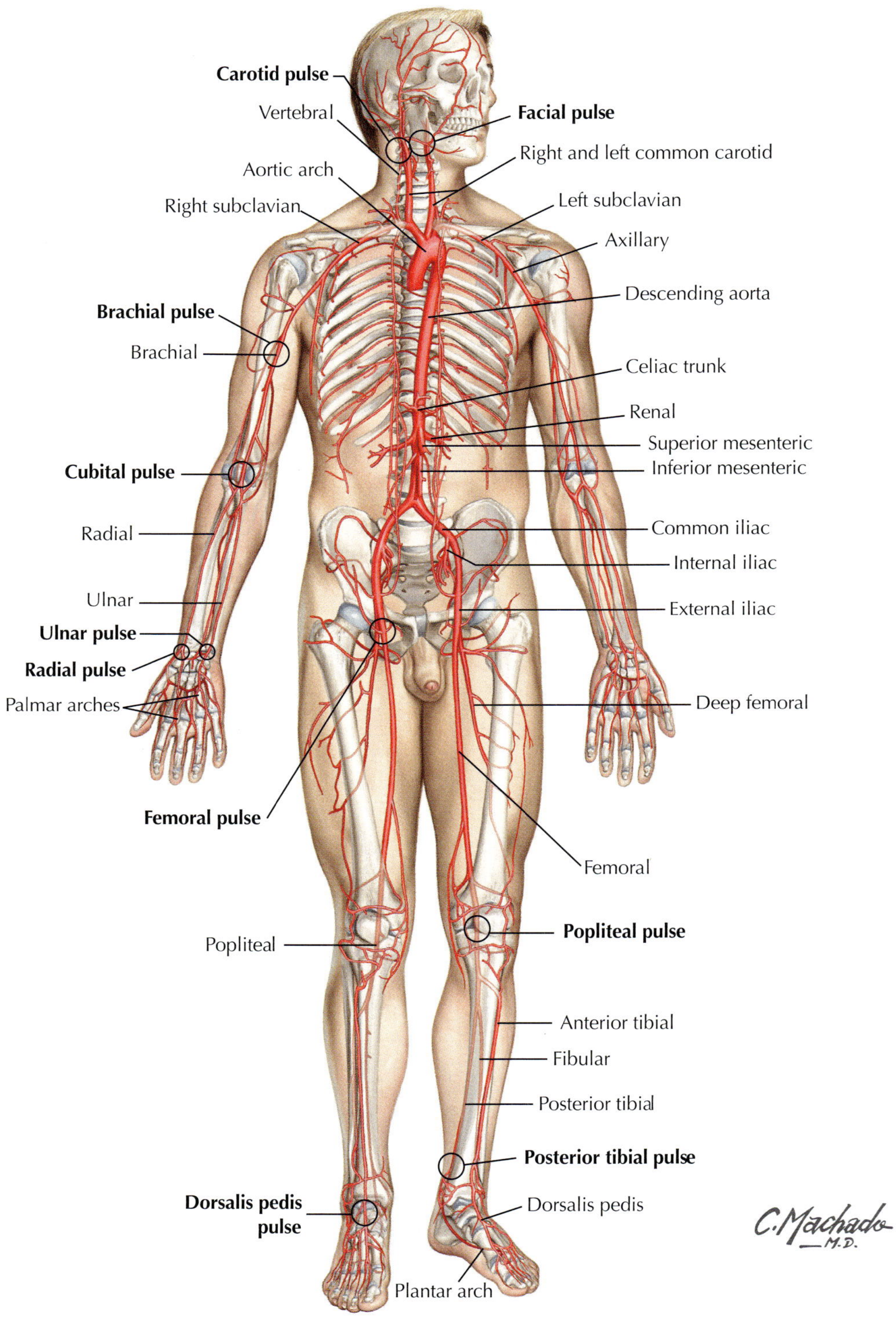

FIGURE 4-16. Major Veins

Veins return blood from the periphery back to the heart and lungs. Most veins have only one layer, although some larger veins have a thin muscular layer. The action of muscles in the lower extremities during exertion works in conjunction with **valves** in the veins to return blood against the pull of gravity to the heart. Venous dysfunction is usually attributed to obstructions or to venous valve **incompetence**.

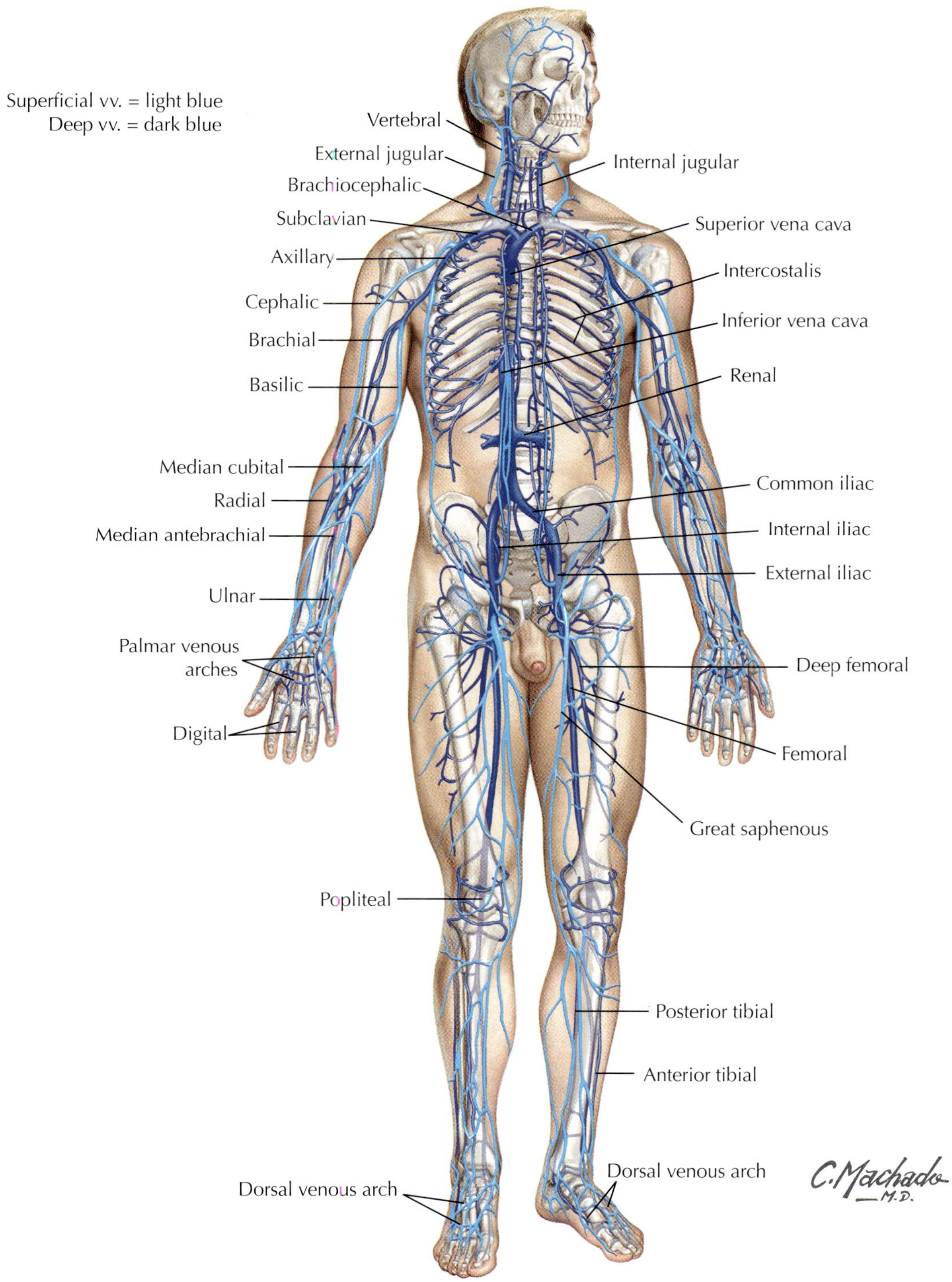

Arterial, With or Without Catheter

34001 Embolectomy or thrombectomy, with or without catheter; carotid, subclavian or innominate artery, by neck incision

34051 innominate, subclavian artery, by thoracic incision

34101 axillary, brachial, innominate, subclavian artery, by arm incision

34111 radial or ulnar artery, by arm incision

34151 renal, celiac, mesentery, aortoiliac artery, by abdominal incision

34201 femoropopliteal, aortoiliac artery, by leg incision

34203 popliteal-tibio-peroneal artery, by leg incision

Venous, Direct or With Catheter

34401 Thrombectomy, direct or with catheter; vena cava, iliac vein, by abdominal incision

34421 vena cava, iliac, femoropopliteal vein, by leg incision

34451 vena cava, iliac, femoropopliteal vein, by abdominal and leg incision

34471 subclavian vein, by neck incision

34490 axillary and subclavian vein, by arm incision

Venous Reconstruction

Coding Atlas

When the venous valves are **incompetent**, blood flows **retrograde** into the lower leg, causing chronic venous insufficiency (CVI) and venous congestion. Veins commonly affected by CVI include the great saphenous vein (GSV); small saphenous vein (SSV); and anterior tibial, posterior tibial, peroneal, popliteal, deep femoral, superficial femoral, and iliac veins.

34501 Valvuloplasty, femoral vein

34502 Reconstruction of vena cava, any method

34510 Venous valve transposition, any vein donor

34520 Cross-over vein graft to venous system

34530 Saphenopopliteal vein anastomosis

Endovascular Repair of Abdominal Aortic Aneurysm

Coding Atlas

An **aneurysm** is a weakened wall, or bulge, in an artery. Abdominal aortic aneurysms (AAAs) may be described as **fusiform**, meaning the defect extends around the circumference of the vessel completely, or **saccular**, meaning the defect is localized. In **endovascular** aortic aneurysm repair (EVAR), a **prosthesis**, which is usually constructed of cloth and a stent exoskeleton, is placed within the aorta at the site of the aneurysm. The **stent** may have branches that extend into local arteries.

34800 Endovascular repair of infrarenal abdominal aortic aneurysm or dissection; using aorto-aortic tube prosthesis

34802 using modular bifurcated prosthesis (1 docking limb)

34803 using modular bifurcated prosthesis (2 docking limbs)

34804 using unibody bifurcated prosthesis

34805 using aorto-uniiliac or aorto-unifemoral prosthesis

+ 34806 Transcatheter placement of wireless physiologic sensor in aneurysmal sac during endovascular repair, including radiological supervision and interpretation, instrument calibration, and collection of pressure data (List separately in addition to code for primary procedure)

+ 34808 Endovascular placement of iliac artery occlusion device (List separately in addition to code for primary procedure)

34812 Open femoral artery exposure for delivery of endovascular prosthesis, by groin incision, unilateral

+ 34813 Placement of femoral-femoral prosthetic graft during endovascular aortic aneurysm repair (List separately in addition to code for primary procedure)

34820 Open iliac artery exposure for delivery of endovascular prosthesis or iliac occlusion during endovascular therapy, by abdominal or retroperitoneal incision, unilateral

34825 Placement of proximal or distal extension prosthesis for endovascular repair of infrarenal abdominal aortic or iliac aneurysm, false aneurysm, or dissection; initial vessel

+ 34826 each additional vessel (List separately in addition to code for primary procedure)

34830 Open repair of infrarenal aortic aneurysm or dissection, plus repair of associated arterial trauma, following unsuccessful endovascular repair; tube prosthesis

34831 aorto-bi-iliac prosthesis

34832 aorto-bifemoral prosthesis

FIGURE 4-17. Aortic Aneurysm

Aortic aneurysms may be treated with **endoscopic** or **open** repair. Regardless of approach, the goal of surgery is to provide support to the existing aorta wall, which is stretched thin and bulging. The aorta wall may dissect into layers, and blood may course between the layers, increasing the risk of rupture. Aortic aneurysms are most commonly caused by **artherosclerosis** but may also be caused by infection or injury. Pictured here is a dissecting aortic aneurysm. Note: Tools, implants, and/or equipment depicted in the illustration may be outdated but the procedural approach is valid.

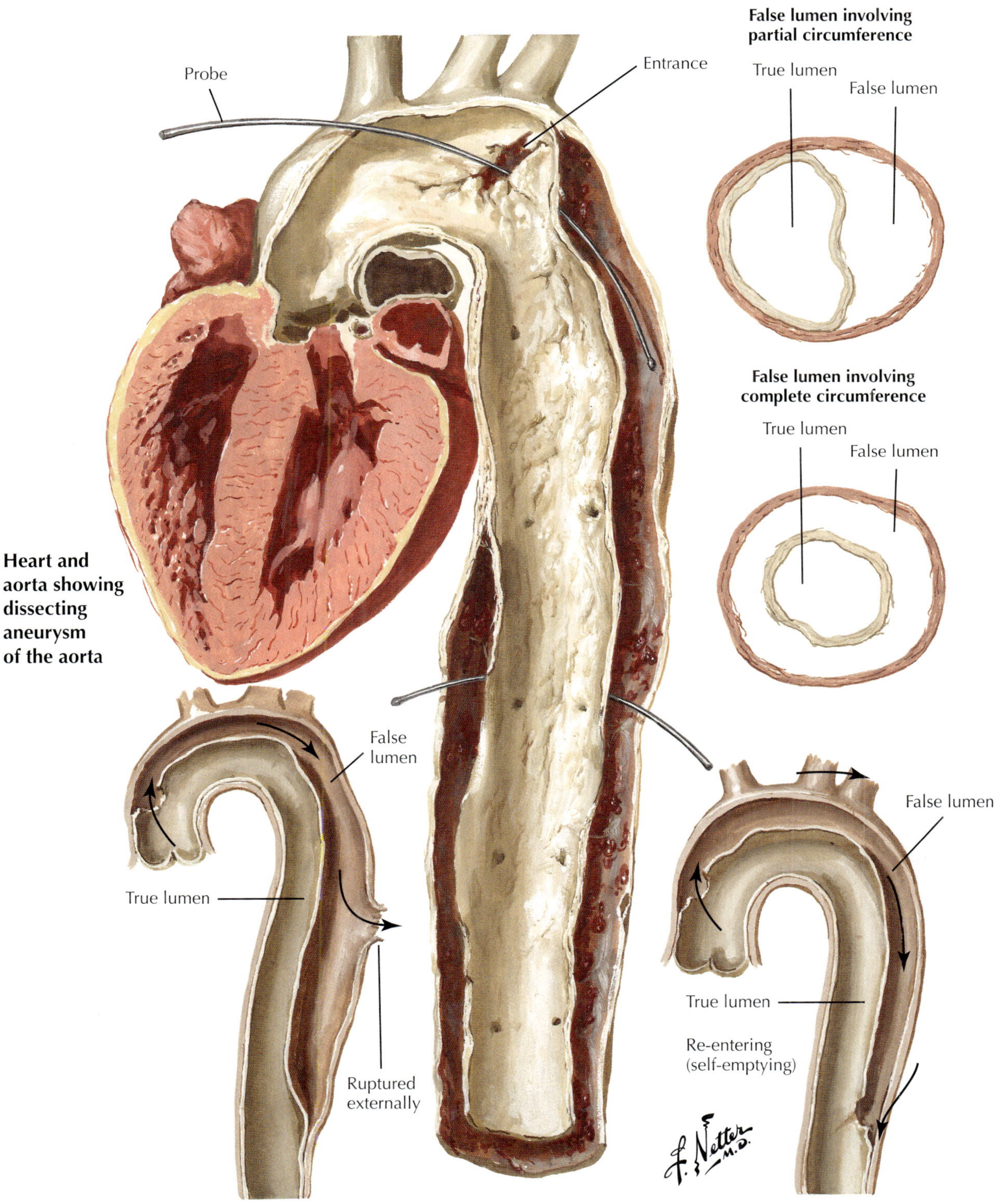

34833 Open iliac artery exposure with creation of conduit for delivery of aortic or iliac endovascular prosthesis, by abdominal or retroperitoneal incision, unilateral

34834 Open brachial artery exposure to assist in the deployment of aortic or iliac endovascular prosthesis by arm incision, unilateral

Fenestrated Endovascular Repair of the Visceral and Infrarenal Aorta

Coding Atlas

An aneurysm is a weakened wall, or bulge, in an artery. Abdominal aortic aneurysms (AAAs) may be described as fusiform, meaning the defect extends around the circumference of the vessel, or saccular, meaning the defect is localized. In fenestrated endovascular repair (FEVR), a computer is used to map arterial branches from the aorta to create a blueprint for an endoprosthesis customized to the patient's aorta. The prosthesis contains windows (fenestrations) that match up with the arterial branches off the visceral and/or infrarenal aorta, as well as one or more prosthetic extensions.

34839 Physician planning of a patient-specific fenestrated visceral aortic endograft requiring a minimum of 90 minutes of physician time

34841 Endovascular repair of visceral aorta (eg, aneurysm, pseudoaneurysm, dissection, penetrating ulcer, intramural hematoma, or traumatic disruption) by deployment of a fenestrated visceral aortic endograft and all associated radiological supervision and interpretation, including target zone angioplasty, when performed; including one visceral artery endoprosthesis (superior mesenteric, celiac or renal artery)

34842 including two visceral artery endoprostheses (superior mesenteric, celiac and/or renal artery[s])

34843 including three visceral artery endoprostheses (superior mesenteric, celiac and/or renal artery[s])

34844 including four or more visceral artery endoprostheses (superior mesenteric, celiac and/or renal artery[s])

34845 Endovascular repair of visceral aorta and infrarenal abdominal aorta (eg, aneurysm, pseudoaneurysm, dissection, penetrating ulcer, intramural hematoma, or traumatic disruption) with a fenestrated visceral aortic endograft and concomitant unibody or modular infrarenal aortic endograft and all associated radiological supervision and interpretation, including target zone angioplasty, when performed; including one visceral artery endoprosthesis (superior mesenteric, celiac or renal artery)

34846 including two visceral artery endoprostheses (superior mesenteric, celiac and/or renal artery[s])

34847 including three visceral artery endoprostheses (superior mesenteric, celiac and/or renal artery[s])

34848 including four or more visceral artery endoprostheses (superior mesenteric, celiac and/or renal artery[s])

Endovascular Repair of Iliac Aneurysm

Coding Atlas

In endovascular repair of an iliac aneurysm, a graft is deployed to treat an arteriovenous malformation (AVM), aneurysm, pseudoaneurysm, or traumatic injury of the common, hypogastric, or external iliac artery. Balloon angioplasty and stent placement may be included in the procedure.

34900 Endovascular repair of iliac artery (eg, aneurysm, pseudoaneurysm, arteriovenous malformation, trauma) using ilio-iliac tube endoprosthesis

Direct Repair of Aneurysm or Excision (Partial or Total) and Graft Insertion for Aneurysm, Pseudoaneurysm, Ruptured Aneurysm, and Associated Occlusive Disease

Coding Atlas

An aneurysm is a weakened wall, or bulge, in an artery. Endovascular repair has replaced open repair of aneurysms in many cases, as it is less invasive and has a lower mortality rate. However, open repair is still performed when direct visualization of the aneurysm is desired, eg, in the case of a ruptured AAA and also some cases in which the vessels are close to the skin.

35001 Direct repair of aneurysm, pseudoaneurysm, or excision (partial or total) and graft insertion, with or without patch graft; for aneurysm and associated occlusive disease, carotid, subclavian artery, by neck incision

35002 for ruptured aneurysm, carotid, subclavian artery, by neck incision

35005 for aneurysm, pseudoaneurysm, and associated occlusive disease, vertebral artery

35011 for aneurysm and associated occlusive disease, axillary-brachial artery, by arm incision

35013 for ruptured aneurysm, axillary-brachial artery, by arm incision

35021 for aneurysm, pseudoaneurysm, and associated occlusive disease, innominate, subclavian artery, by thoracic incision

35022	for ruptured aneurysm, innominate, subclavian artery, by thoracic incision
35045	for aneurysm, pseudoaneurysm, and associated occlusive disease, radial or ulnar artery
35081	for aneurysm, pseudoaneurysm, and associated occlusive disease, abdominal aorta
35082	for ruptured aneurysm, abdominal aorta
35091	for aneurysm, pseudoaneurysm, and associated occlusive disease, abdominal aorta involving visceral vessels (mesenteric, celiac, renal)
35092	for ruptured aneurysm, abdominal aorta involving visceral vessels (mesenteric, celiac, renal)
35102	for aneurysm, pseudoaneurysm, and associated occlusive disease, abdominal aorta involving iliac vessels (common, hypogastric, external)
35103	for ruptured aneurysm, abdominal aorta involving iliac vessels (common, hypogastric, external)
35111	for aneurysm, pseudoaneurysm, and associated occlusive disease, splenic artery
35112	for ruptured aneurysm, splenic artery
35121	for aneurysm, pseudoaneurysm, and associated occlusive disease, hepatic, celiac, renal, or mesenteric artery
35122	for ruptured aneurysm, hepatic, celiac, renal, or mesenteric artery
35131	for aneurysm, pseudoaneurysm, and associated occlusive disease, iliac artery (common, hypogastric, external)
35132	for ruptured aneurysm, iliac artery (common, hypogastric, external)
35141	for aneurysm, pseudoaneurysm, and associated occlusive disease, common femoral artery (profunda femoris, superficial femoral)
35142	for ruptured aneurysm, common femoral artery (profunda femoris, superficial femoral)
35151	for aneurysm, pseudoaneurysm, and associated occlusive disease, popliteal artery
35152	for ruptured aneurysm, popliteal artery

Repair Arteriovenous Fistula

Coding Atlas

Congenital arteriovenous **fistulas** may also be called **arteriovenous malformations** (AVMs). Arteriovenous fistulas (AVFs) may form when two vessels are injured; they heal with an **anomalous** connection. An AVF may be created surgically, usually to provide a stable **port** for **hemodialysis**. Repair of hemodialysis fistulas are reported using codes 36831-36833 and 36870.

35180	Repair, **congenital** arteriovenous **fistula**; head and neck
35182	thorax and abdomen
35184	extremities
35188	Repair, **acquired** or traumatic arteriovenous fistula; head and neck
35189	thorax and abdomen
35190	extremities

Repair Blood Vessel Other Than for Fistula, With or Without Patch Angioplasty

Coding Atlas

Codes 35201-35286 are used to report the repair of a vein or artery through an open incision with **direct visualization**. For some cases, a **donor** piece of vein is used as a **graft** patch; in other cases, the graft is made of material other than vein.

35201	Repair blood vessel, direct; neck
35206	upper extremity
35207	hand, finger
35211	intrathoracic, with **bypass**
35216	intrathoracic, without bypass
35221	intra-abdominal
35226	lower extremity
35231	Repair blood vessel with vein **graft**; neck
35236	upper extremity
35241	intrathoracic, with bypass
35246	intrathoracic, without bypass
35251	intra-abdominal
35256	lower extremity
35261	Repair blood vessel with graft other than vein; neck
35266	upper extremity
35271	intrathoracic, with bypass
35276	intrathoracic, without bypass
35281	intra-abdominal
35286	lower extremity

Thromboendarterectomy

Coding Atlas

All blood vessels contain a thin layer of **endothelium** cells on their interior surface. Defects in the endothelial layer, commonly called **plaque**, can lead to the formation of **blood clots** (**thrombi**) on the endothelium. At times, a layer of vessel lining and plaque are removed with the thrombus. This is called **thromboendarterectomy**.

35301 Thromboendarterectomy, including patch graft, if performed; carotid, vertebral, subclavian, by neck incision

35302 superficial femoral artery

35303 popliteal artery

35304 tibioperoneal trunk artery

35305 tibial or peroneal artery, initial vessel

✚ **35306** each additional tibial or peroneal artery (List separately in addition to code for primary procedure)

35311 subclavian, innominate, by thoracic incision

35321 axillary-brachial

35331 abdominal aorta

35341 mesenteric, celiac, or renal

35351 iliac

35355 iliofemoral

35361 combined aortoiliac

35363 combined aortoiliofemoral

35371 common femoral

35372 deep (profunda) femoral

✚ **35390** Reoperation, carotid, thromboendarterectomy, more than 1 month after original operation (List separately in addition to code for primary procedure)

Angioscopy

Coding Atlas

Intraoperative angioscopy involves the use of a **fiberoptic** catheter to provide **endovascular** visualization for assessment of vessel walls.

✚ **35400** Angioscopy (non-coronary vessels or grafts) during therapeutic intervention (List separately in addition to code for primary procedure)

Transluminal Angioplasty

Coding Atlas

In **transluminal angioplasty**, the **lumen** of a partly occluded blood vessel is enlarged, usually by inserting a deflated balloon into it, and the balloon is inflated to mechanically widen the lumen. In both the **open** approach and **percutaneous** approach, a catheter is fed to the site to be treated. In the open approach, an incision is made to expose and enter the vessel. In the percutaneous approach, a needle is inserted into the vessel, and a guidewire and catheter are then inserted.

Open

35450 Transluminal balloon angioplasty, open; renal or other visceral artery

35452 aortic

35458 brachiocephalic trunk or branches, each vessel

35460 venous

Percutaneous

⊙ **35471** Transluminal balloon angioplasty, percutaneous; renal or visceral artery

⊙ **35472** aortic

⊙ **35475** brachiocephalic trunk or branches, each vessel

⊙ **35476** venous

Bypass Graft

Coding Atlas

Bypass grafting is a surgical technique used to treat **peripheral vascular disease** (PVD). In a bypass **graft**, blood is redirected around a blocked or damaged artery and through an alternative route that may be made of a segment of vein, artery, or synthetic graft. In the CPT code descriptions, the listed arteries are separated by a hyphen. The first vessel listed identifies the upstream attachment point, and the second vessel listed is the downstream attachment point for the graft. In some cases, one combined word without a hypen identifies both vessels, eg, aortobifemoral describes a graft from the aorta that branches to the right and left femoral arteries.

FIGURE 4-18. Bypass Grafts

Balloon angioplasty increases the size of a **lumen** by stretching it using an intravascular balloon. Peripheral artery **bypass** grafting allows for blood to flow around a damaged or **atherosclerotic** artery, which may be recorded or noted with **peripheral artery disease** (PAD). Pain is caused by the demand for oxygen by the leg's muscles during walking and the decrease in oxygen flow to the muscle tissue. The graft may be **synthetic** (as shown here) or a **harvested** vein or artery. Note: Tools, implants, and/or equipment depicted in the illustration may be outdated but the procedural approach is valid.

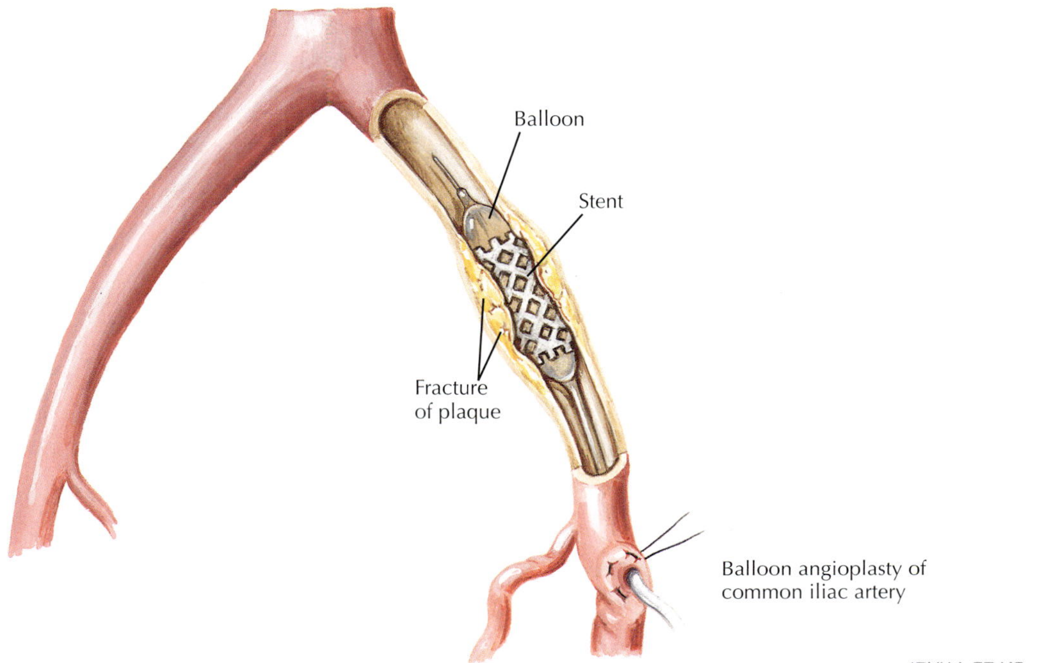

Surgical Bypass Procedures

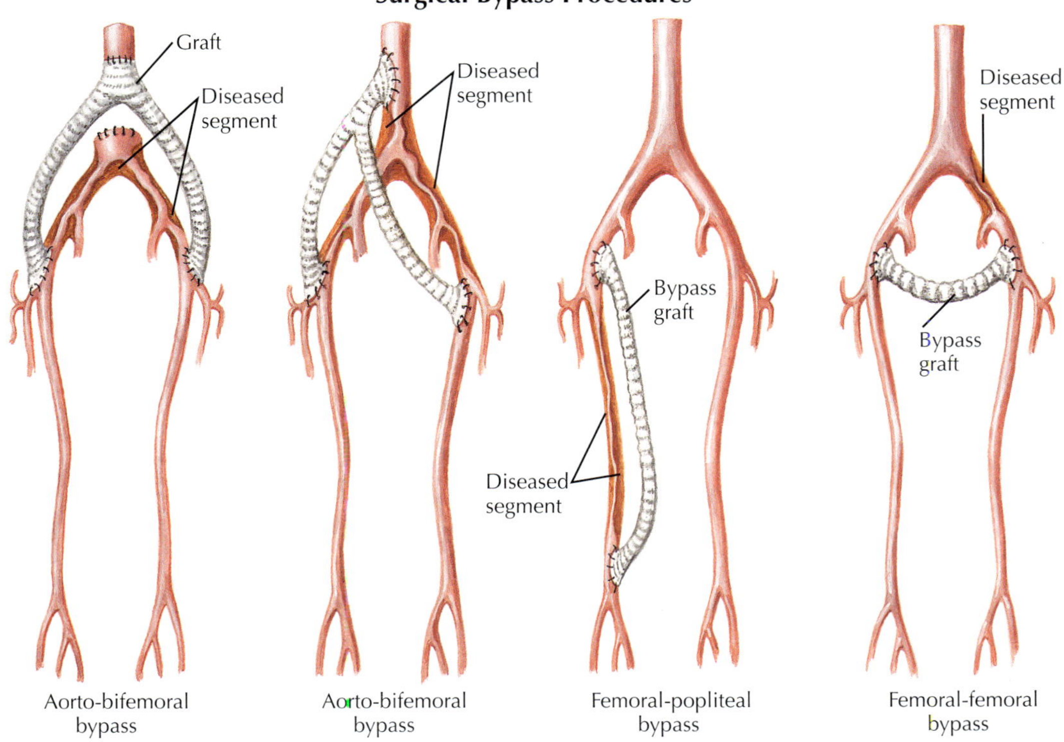

Vein

+ 35500 **Harvest** of upper extremity vein, 1 segment, for lower extremity or coronary artery **bypass** procedure (List separately in addition to code for primary procedure)

35501 Bypass **graft**, with vein; common carotid-**ipsilateral** internal carotid

35506 carotid-subclavian or subclavian-carotid

35508 carotid-vertebral

35509 carotid-**contralateral** carotid

35510 carotid-brachial

35511 subclavian-subclavian

35512 subclavian-brachial

35515 subclavian-vertebral

35516 subclavian-axillary

35518 axillary-axillary

35521 axillary-femoral

35522 axillary-brachial

35523 brachial-ulnar or -radial

35525 brachial-brachial

35526 aortosubclavian, aortoinnominate, or aortocarotid

35531 aortoceliac or aortomesenteric

35533 axillary-femoral-femoral

35535 hepatorenal

35536 splenorenal

35537 aortoiliac

35538 aortobi-iliac

35539 aortofemoral

35540 aortobifemoral

35556 femoral-popliteal

35558 femoral-femoral

35560 aortorenal

35563 ilioiliac

35565 iliofemoral

35566 femoral-anterior tibial, posterior tibial, peroneal artery or other **distal** vessels

35570 tibial-tibial, peroneal-tibial, or tibial/peroneal trunk-tibial

35571 popliteal-tibial, -peroneal artery or other distal vessels

+ 35572 **Harvest** of femoropopliteal vein, 1 segment, for vascular reconstruction procedure (eg, aortic, vena caval, coronary, peripheral artery) (List separately in addition to code for primary procedure)

In-Situ Vein

35583 **In-situ** vein bypass; femoral-popliteal

35585 femoral-anterior tibial, posterior tibial, or peroneal artery

35587 popliteal-tibial, peroneal

Other Than Vein

+ 35600 **Harvest** of upper extremity artery, 1 segment, for coronary artery **bypass** procedure (List separately in addition to code for primary procedure)

35601 Bypass graft, with other than vein; common carotid-ipsilateral internal carotid

35606 carotid-subclavian

35612 subclavian-subclavian

35616 subclavian-axillary

35621 axillary-femoral

35623 axillary-popliteal or -tibial

35626 aortosubclavian, aortoinnominate, or aortocarotid

35631 aortoceliac, aortomesenteric, aortorenal

35632 ilio-celiac

35633 ilio-mesenteric

35634 iliorenal

35636 splenorenal (splenic to renal arterial anastomosis)

35637 aortoiliac

35638 aortobi-iliac

35642 carotid-vertebral

35645 subclavian-vertebral

35646 aortobifemoral

35647 aortofemoral

35650 axillary-axillary

35654 axillary-femoral-femoral

35656 femoral-popliteal

35661 femoral-femoral

35663 ilioiliac

35665 iliofemoral

35666 femoral-anterior tibial, posterior tibial, or peroneal artery

35671 popliteal-tibial or -peroneal artery

FIGURE 4-19. Venous Valves

Venous valves prevent the backflow (reflux) of blood in veins of the leg when the valves are functioning properly. When the valves are malfunctioning, chronic venous insufficiency (CVI) may result. In CVI, blood may pool in the affected veins, resulting in a condition called venous stasis. CVI is also associated with varicose veins and stasis ulcers.

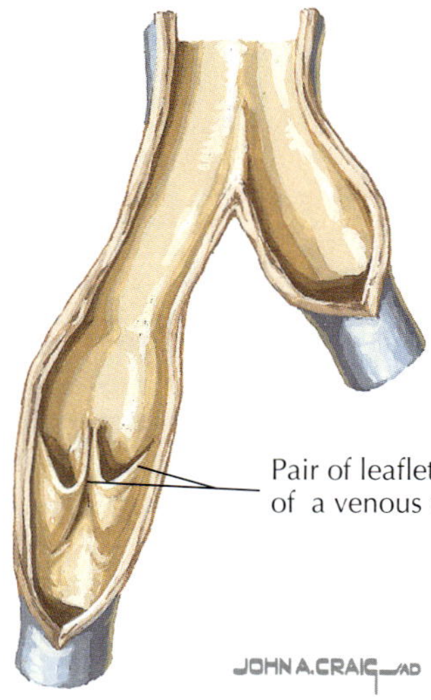

Composite Grafts

Coding Atlas

Composite grafts are made of more than one unique segment. Multiple segments are anastamosed to form the composite graft.

✚ 35681 Bypass graft; composite, prosthetic and vein (List separately in addition to code for primary procedure)

✚ 35682 autogenous composite, 2 segments of veins from 2 locations (List separately in addition to code for primary procedure)

✚ 35683 autogenous composite, 3 or more segments of vein from 2 or more locations (List separately in addition to code for primary procedure)

Adjuvant Techniques

Coding Atlas

An adjuvant technique is one that enhances another procedure. For example, a vein patch or cuff applied during the primary synthetic graft procedure is an adjuvant technique for femoral-popliteal, femoral-tibial, or popliteal-tibial bypass grafts. In some cases, an autogenous vein is used to create an arteriovenous fistula (AVF) between the tibial or peroneal artery and vein at or beyond the distal primary bypass anastomosis site; this would also be considered adjuvant.

✚ 35685 Placement of vein patch or cuff at distal anastomosis of bypass graft, synthetic conduit (List separately in addition to code for primary procedure)

✚ 35686 Creation of distal arteriovenous fistula during lower extremity bypass surgery (non-hemodialysis) (List separately in addition to code for primary procedure)

Arterial Transposition

Coding Atlas

Transposition of an artery is usually performed to provide an oxygenated blood supply to an area affected by a stenotic or damaged artery.

35691 Transposition and/or reimplantation; vertebral to carotid artery

35693 vertebral to subclavian artery

35694 subclavian to carotid artery

35695 carotid to subclavian artery

✚ **35697** Reimplantation, visceral artery to infrarenal aortic prosthesis, each artery (List separately in addition to code for primary procedure)

Excision, Exploration, Repair, Revision

Coding Atlas

Open procedures on the circulatory system are typically performed because direct visualization or direct access is required for the operative goal, eg, exploration for postoperative hemorrhage or excision of an infected graft.

✚ **35700** Reoperation, femoral-popliteal or femoral (popliteal)-anterior tibial, posterior tibial, peroneal artery, or other distal vessels, more than 1 month after original operation (List separately in addition to code for primary procedure)

35701 Exploration (not followed by surgical repair), with or without lysis of artery; carotid artery

35721 femoral artery

35741 popliteal artery

35761 other vessels

35800 Exploration for postoperative hemorrhage, thrombosis or infection; neck

35820 chest

35840 abdomen

35860 extremity

35870 Repair of graft-enteric fistula

35875 Thrombectomy of arterial or venous graft (other than hemodialysis graft or fistula);

35876 with revision of arterial or venous graft

35879 Revision, lower extremity arterial bypass, without thrombectomy, open; with vein patch angioplasty

35881 with segmental vein interposition

35883 Revision, femoral anastomosis of synthetic arterial bypass graft in groin, open; with nonautogenous patch graft (eg, Dacron, ePTFE, bovine pericardium)

35884 with autogenous vein patch graft

35901 Excision of infected graft; neck

35903 extremity

35905 thorax

35907 abdomen

Vascular Injection Procedures

Coding Atlas

For selective catheter placement, documented vascular access refers to the location at which the vascular system is entered. The common femoral artery (CFA) in the groin is the most commonly used. Non-selective catheter placement indicates that the catheter remains in the accessed vessel or is advanced to the aorta. Selective catheter placement refers to a branching off from the aorta or access vessel. The first branch off of the aorta or access vessel is considered first order. Each branch represents smaller vessels and further distance. Branches after the first order are second order. For code selection purposes, the highest level of branching, which represents the most work and smallest vessels, is third order.

Intravenous

36000 Introduction of needle or intracatheter, vein

36002 Injection procedures (eg, thrombin) for percutaneous treatment of extremity pseudoaneurysm

36005 Injection procedure for extremity venography (including introduction of needle or intracatheter)

⊙ **36010** Introduction of catheter, superior or inferior vena cava

36011 Selective catheter placement, venous system; first order branch (eg, renal vein, jugular vein)

36012 second order, or more selective, branch (eg, left adrenal vein, petrosal sinus)

36013 Introduction of catheter, right heart or main pulmonary artery

36014 Selective catheter placement, left or right pulmonary artery

36015 Selective catheter placement, segmental or subsegmental pulmonary artery

FIGURE 4-20. Vascular Access

From the common femoral artery, a **percutaneous** vascular access can be threaded through the vascular system to the site needing treatment or diagnostic evaluation. Depending on the procedure and the patient's physiology, other vascular-access sites may be selected. Vascular-access codes are used to report the vessel order required for the procedure, and the procedure is often reported separately using codes from the Cardiovascular or Medicine code sets. Codes for **percutaneous** transluminal coronary **angioplasty** are found in the Medicine code set. Note: Tools, implants, and/or equipment depicted in the illustration may be outdated but the procedural approach is valid.

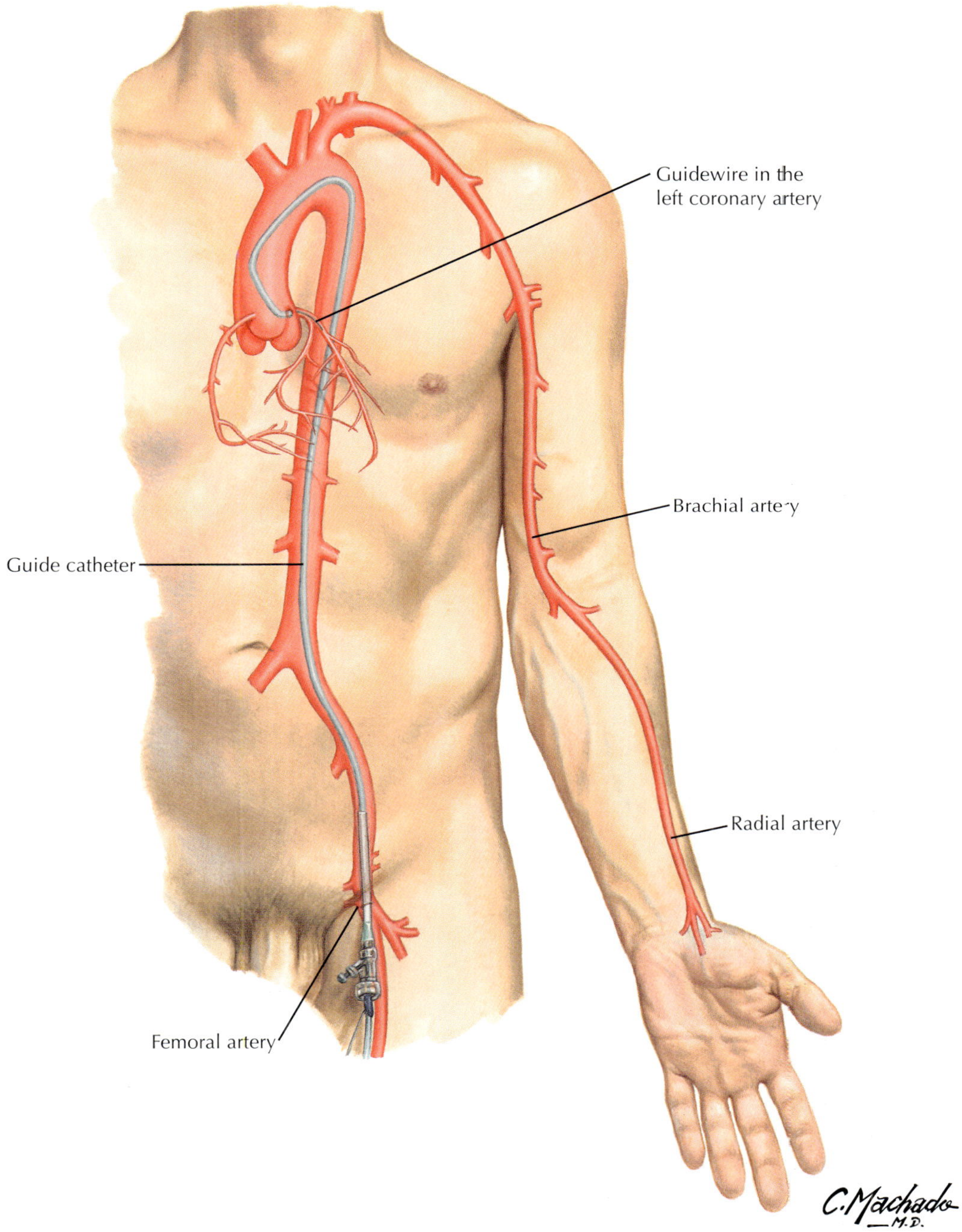

Intra-Arterial—Intra-Aortic

36100 Introduction of needle or intracatheter, carotid or vertebral artery

36120 Introduction of needle or intracatheter; retrograde brachial artery

⊙ **36140** extremity artery

⊙ **36147** Introduction of needle and/or catheter, **arteriovenous** shunt created for **dialysis** (**graft/fistula**); initial access with complete radiological evaluation of dialysis access, including fluoroscopy, image documentation and report (includes access of **shunt**, injection[s] of contrast, and all necessary imaging from the arterial **anastomosis** and adjacent artery through entire venous outflow including the **inferior** or **superior** vena cava)

⊙✚ **36148** additional access for **therapeutic** intervention (List separately in addition to code for primary procedure)

36160 Introduction of needle or intracatheter, aortic, **translumbar**

⊙ **36200** Introduction of catheter, aorta

36215 Selective catheter placement, arterial system; each first order thoracic or brachiocephalic branch, within a vascular family

36216 initial **second order** thoracic or brachiocephalic branch, within a vascular family

36217 initial **third order** or more selective thoracic or brachiocephalic branch, within a vascular family

✚ **36218** additional second order, third order, and beyond, thoracic or brachiocephalic branch, within a vascular family (List in addition to code for initial second or third order vessel as appropriate)

⊙ **36221** **Non-selective catheter placement**, thoracic aorta, with angiography of the **extracranial** carotid, vertebral, and/or **intracranial** vessels, **unilateral** or **bilateral**, and all associated radiological supervision and interpretation, includes angiography of the cervicocerebral arch, when performed

⊙ **36222** Selective catheter placement, common carotid or innominate artery, unilateral, any approach, with angiography of the **ipsilateral** extracranial carotid circulation and all associated radiological supervision and interpretation, includes angiography of the cervicocerebral arch, when performed

⊙ **36223** Selective catheter placement, common carotid or innominate artery, unilateral, any approach, with angiography of the ipsilateral intracranial carotid circulation and all associated radiological supervision and interpretation, includes angiography of the extracranial carotid and cervicocerebral arch, when performed

⊙ **36224** Selective catheter placement, internal carotid artery, unilateral, with angiography of the ipsilateral intracranial carotid circulation and all associated radiological supervision and interpretation, includes angiography of the extracranial carotid and cervicocerebral arch, when performed

⊙ **36225** Selective catheter placement, subclavian or innominate artery, unilateral, with angiography of the ipsilateral vertebral circulation and all associated radiological supervision and interpretation, includes angiography of the cervicocerebral arch, when performed

⊙ **36226** Selective catheter placement, vertebral artery, unilateral, with angiography of the ipsilateral vertebral circulation and all associated radiological supervision and interpretation, includes angiography of the cervicocerebral arch, when performed

⊙✚ **36227** Selective catheter placement, external carotid artery, unilateral, with angiography of the ipsilateral external carotid circulation and all associated radiological supervision and interpretation (List separately in addition to code for primary procedure)

⊙✚ **36228** Selective catheter placement, each intracranial branch of the internal carotid or vertebral arteries, unilateral, with angiography of the selected vessel circulation and all associated radiological supervision and interpretation (eg, middle cerebral artery, posterior inferior cerebellar artery) (List separately in addition to code for primary procedure)

⊙ **36245** Selective catheter placement, arterial system; each first order abdominal, pelvic, or lower extremity artery branch, within a vascular family

⊙ **36246** initial second order abdominal, pelvic, or lower extremity artery branch, within a vascular family

⊙ **36247** initial third order or more selective abdominal, pelvic, or lower extremity artery branch, within a vascular family

⊙✚ **36248** additional second order, third order, and beyond, abdominal, pelvic, or lower extremity artery branch, within a vascular family (List in addition to code for initial second or third order vessel as appropriate)

⊙ **36251** Selective catheter placement (first-order), main renal artery and any accessory renal artery(s) for renal angiography, including arterial puncture and catheter placement(s), fluoroscopy, contrast injection(s), image postprocessing, permanent recording of images, and radiological supervision and interpretation, including pressure gradient measurements when performed, and flush aortogram when performed; unilateral

⊙ **36252** bilateral

⊙ **36253** Superselective catheter placement (one or more second order or higher renal artery branches) renal artery and any accessory renal artery(s) for renal angiography, including arterial puncture, catheterization, fluoroscopy, contrast injection(s), image postprocessing, permanent recording of images, and radiological supervision and interpretation, including pressure gradient measurements when performed, and flush **aortogram** when performed; unilateral

⊙ **36254** bilateral

36260 Insertion of implantable intra-arterial infusion pump (eg, for **chemotherapy** of liver)

36261 Revision of implanted intra-arterial infusion pump

36262 Removal of implanted intra-arterial infusion pump

Venous

36400 **Venipuncture**, younger than age 3 years, necessitating the skill of a physician or other qualified health care professional, not to be used for routine venipuncture; femoral or jugular vein

36405 scalp vein

36406 other vein

36410 Venipuncture, age 3 years or older, necessitating the skill of a physician or other qualified health care professional (separate procedure), for diagnostic or therapeutic purposes (not to be used for routine venipuncture)

36415 Collection of venous blood by venipuncture

36416 Collection of capillary blood specimen (eg, finger, heel, ear stick)

36420 Venipuncture, **cutdown**; younger than age 1 year

36425 age 1 or over

36430 **Transfusion**, blood or blood components

36440 **Push transfusion**, blood, 2 years or younger

36450 **Exchange transfusion**, blood; **newborn**

36455 other than newborn

36460 Transfusion, **intrauterine**, fetal

36468 Single or multiple injections of **sclerosing** solutions, spider veins (**telangiectasia**), limb or trunk

36470 Injection of sclerosing solution; single vein

36471 multiple veins, same leg

36475 Endovenous **ablation** therapy of incompetent vein, extremity, inclusive of all imaging guidance and monitoring, percutaneous, radiofrequency; first vein treated

✚ **36476** second and subsequent veins treated in a single extremity, each through separate access sites (List separately in addition to code for primary procedure)

36478 **Endovenous** ablation therapy of incompetent vein, extremity, inclusive of all imaging guidance and monitoring, percutaneous, laser; first vein treated

✚ **36479** second and subsequent veins treated in a single extremity, each through separate access sites (List separately in addition to code for primary procedure)

⊙ **36481** **Percutaneous** portal vein **catheterization** by any method

36500 Venous catheterization for selective organ blood sampling

36510 Catheterization of umbilical vein for diagnosis or therapy, newborn

36511 Therapeutic **apheresis**; for white blood cells

36512 for red blood cells

36513 for platelets

36514 for plasma pheresis

36515 with extracorporeal immunoadsorption and plasma reinfusion

36516 with **extracorporeal** selective adsorption or selective filtration and plasma reinfusion

36522 **Photopheresis**, extracorporeal

Central Venous Access Procedures

Insertion of Central Venous Access Device

⊙ **36555** Insertion of non-tunneled centrally inserted **central venous catheter**; younger than 5 years of age

36556 age 5 years or older

⊙ **36557** Insertion of tunneled centrally inserted central venous catheter, without **subcutaneous** port or pump; younger than 5 years of age

⊙ **36558** age 5 years or older

⊙ **36560** Insertion of tunneled centrally inserted central venous access device, with subcutaneous port; younger than 5 years of age

⊙ **36561** age 5 years or older

⊙ **36563** Insertion of tunneled centrally inserted central venous access device with subcutaneous pump

⊙ **36565** Insertion of **tunneled** centrally inserted central venous access device, requiring 2 catheters via 2 separate venous access sites; without subcutaneous port or pump (eg, Tesio type catheter)

⊙ **36566** with subcutaneous port(s)

⊙ **36568** Insertion of **peripherally inserted central venous catheter** (PICC), without subcutaneous port or pump; younger than 5 years of age

36569 age 5 years or older

FIGURE 4-21. Catheter Placement

A **central venous catheter**, sometimes referred to as a central line, can be left in place for a longer period of time than an intravenous (IV) catheter. The central venous catheter tip is threaded through the vein until it reaches a vein near the heart. The central venous catheter can be inserted into a large vein in the chest, or in a peripheral vein. A **peripherally inserted central catheter** (PICC or PICC line) is frequently used to obtain central venous access for patients in acute care. Note: Tools, implants, and/or equipment depicted in the illustration may be outdated but the procedural approach is valid.

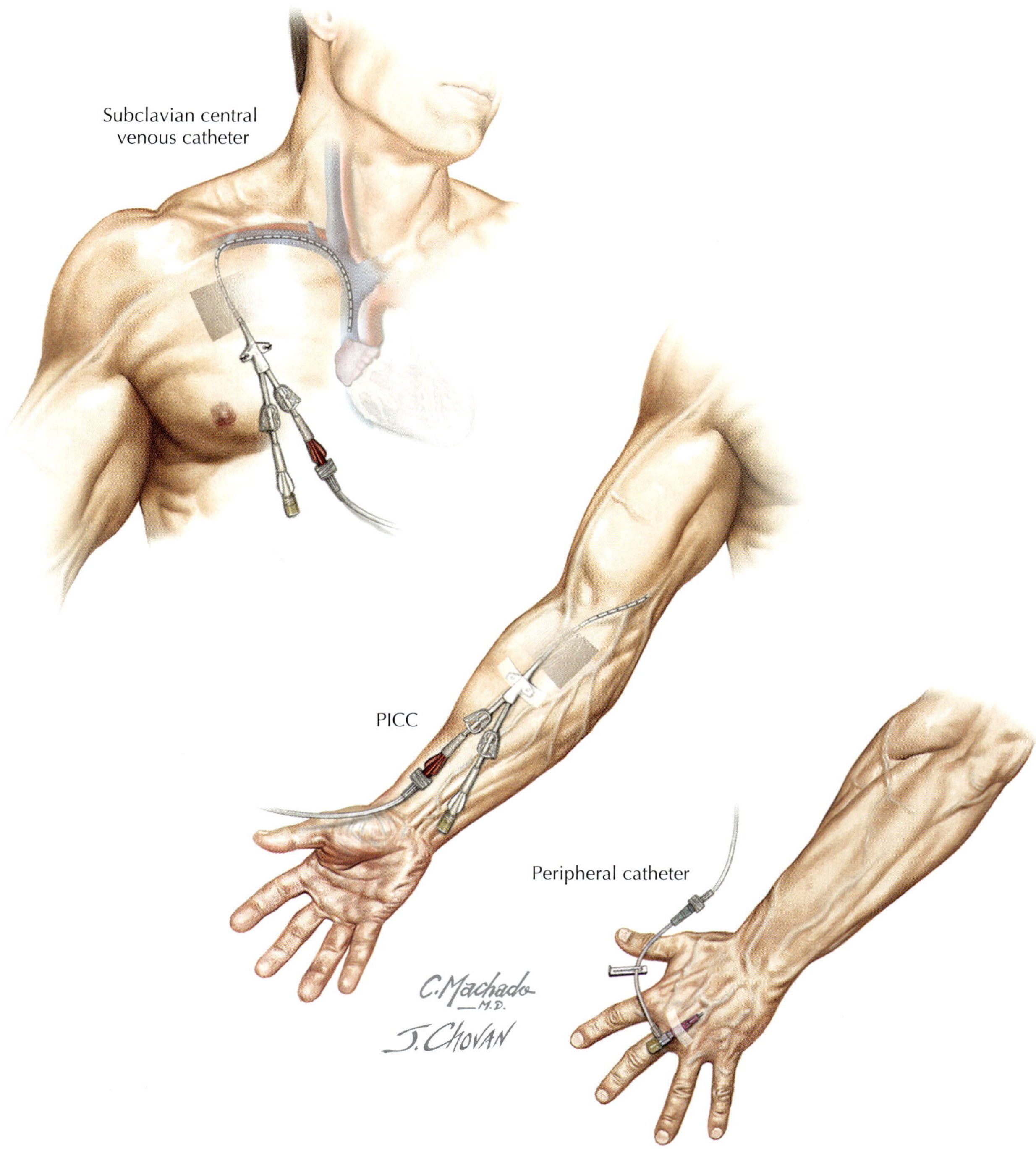

⊙ **36570** Insertion of peripherally inserted central venous access device, with subcutaneous port; younger than 5 years of age

⊙ **36571** age 5 years or older

Repair of Central Venous Access Device

36575 Repair of tunneled or non-tunneled central venous access catheter, without subcutaneous port or pump, central or peripheral insertion site

⊙ **36576** Repair of central venous access device, with subcutaneous port or pump, central or peripheral insertion site

Partial Replacement of Central Venous Access Device (Catheter Only)

⊙ **36578** Replacement, catheter only, of central venous access device, with subcutaneous port or pump, central or peripheral insertion site

Complete Replacement of Central Venous Access Device Through Same Venous Access Site

36580 Replacement, complete, of a non-tunneled centrally inserted central venous catheter, without subcutaneous port or pump, through same venous access

⊙ **36581** Replacement, complete, of a tunneled centrally inserted central venous catheter, without subcutaneous port or pump, through same venous access

⊙ **36582** Replacement, complete, of a tunneled centrally inserted central venous access device, with subcutaneous port, through same venous access

⊙ **36583** Replacement, complete, of a tunneled centrally inserted central venous access device, with subcutaneous pump, through same venous access

36584 Replacement, complete, of a peripherally inserted central venous catheter (PICC), without subcutaneous port or pump, through same venous access

⊙ **36585** Replacement, complete, of a peripherally inserted central venous access device, with subcutaneous port, through same venous access

Removal of Central Venous Access Device

36589 Removal of tunneled central venous catheter, without subcutaneous port or pump

⊙ **36590** Removal of tunneled central venous access device, with subcutaneous port or pump, central or peripheral insertion

Other Central Venous Access Procedures

36591 Collection of blood specimen from a completely implantable venous access device

36592 Collection of blood specimen using established central or peripheral catheter, venous, not otherwise specified

36593 Declotting by thrombolytic agent of implanted vascular access device or catheter

36595 Mechanical removal of pericatheter obstructive material (eg, fibrin sheath) from central venous device via separate venous access

36596 Mechanical removal of intraluminal (intracatheter) obstructive material from central venous device through device lumen

36597 Repositioning of previously placed central venous catheter under fluoroscopic guidance

36598 Contrast injection(s) for radiologic evaluation of existing central venous access device, including fluoroscopy, image documentation and report

Arterial

Coding Atlas

Because arterial blood is oxygenated, arterial blood can be analyzed to identify factors that are not seen when deoxygenated venous blood is analyzed. In some cases, infusion of therapeutic agents is more effective when it occurs arterially.

36600 Arterial puncture, withdrawal of blood for diagnosis

⊘ **36620** Arterial catheterization or cannulation for sampling, monitoring or transfusion (separate procedure); percutaneous

36625 cutdown

36640 Arterial catheterization for prolonged infusion therapy (chemotherapy), cutdown

36660 Catheterization, umbilical artery, newborn, for diagnosis or therapy

Intraosseous

36680 Placement of needle for intraosseous infusion

Hemodialysis Access, Intervascular Cannulation for Extracorporeal Circulation, or Shunt Insertion

Coding Atlas

A high volume of blood is extracted from, and returned to, a patient during **hemodialysis**, making robust vascular access crucial to success. There are three types of vascular access for hemodialysis: venous catheter, **AV graft**, and **AV fistula**. A venous catheter is a tube placed into the neck, chest, or groin. A catheter is used on a temporary basis because complications related to catheters are common. An AV graft surgically connects the artery to the vein using synthetic vein. An AV fistula is created by surgically connecting an artery directly to a vein, usually in the forearm.

36800 Insertion of cannula for hemodialysis, other purpose (separate procedure); vein to vein

36810 arteriovenous, external (Scribner type)

36815 arteriovenous, external revision, or closure

36818 Arteriovenous anastomosis, open; by upper arm cephalic vein transposition

36819 by upper arm basilic vein transposition

36820 by forearm vein transposition

36821 direct, any site (eg, Cimino type) (separate procedure)

36823 Insertion of arterial and venous cannula(s) for isolated extracorporeal circulation including regional chemotherapy perfusion to an extremity, with or without hyperthermia, with removal of cannula(s) and repair of arteriotomy and venotomy sites

36825 Creation of arteriovenous fistula by other than direct arteriovenous anastomosis (separate procedure); autogenous graft

36830 nonautogenous graft (eg, biological collagen, thermoplastic graft)

36831 Thrombectomy, open, arteriovenous fistula without revision, autogenous or nonautogenous dialysis graft (separate procedure)

36832 Revision, open, arteriovenous fistula; without thrombectomy, autogenous or nonautogenous dialysis graft (separate procedure)

36833 with thrombectomy, autogenous or nonautogenous dialysis graft (separate procedure)

36835 Insertion of Thomas shunt (separate procedure)

36838 Distal revascularization and interval ligation (DRIL), upper extremity hemodialysis access (steal syndrome)

36860 External cannula declotting (separate procedure); without balloon catheter

36861 with balloon catheter

⊙ **36870** Thrombectomy, percutaneous, arteriovenous fistula, autogenous or nonautogenous graft (includes mechanical thrombus extraction and intra-graft thrombolysis)

Portal Decompression Procedures

Coding Atlas

Portal hypertension refers to increased blood pressure in the hepatic vein, a common complication of **cirrhosis**. A **transvenous** intrahepatic portosystemic **shunt** (TIPS), or **stent**, is inserted **endoscopically** into the liver to create an artificial channel between the (inflow) portal vein and (outflow) hepatic vein in order to reduce portal hypertension.

37140 Venous anastomosis, open; portocaval

37145 renoportal

37160 caval-mesenteric

37180 splenorenal, proximal

37181 splenorenal, distal (selective decompression of esophagogastric varices, any technique)

37182 Insertion of transvenous intrahepatic portosystemic shunt(s) (TIPS) (includes venous access, hepatic and portal vein catheterization, portography with hemodynamic evaluation, intrahepatic tract formation/dilatation, stent placement and all associated imaging guidance and documentation)

⊙ **37183** Revision of transvenous intrahepatic portosystemic shunt(s) (TIPS) (includes venous access, hepatic and portal vein catheterization, portography with hemodynamic evaluation, intrahepatic tract recanulization/dilatation, stent placement and all associated imaging guidance and documentation)

Transcatheter Procedures

Coding Atlas

A **transcatheter** procedure code describes a treatment or diagnostic procedure on a vessel after an endoscopic tool has been advanced to the targeted site.

FIGURE 4-22. Hepatic Portal Vein and Tributaries

The hepatic portal vein, or simply portal vein (PV), drains blood from the gastrointestinal system and spleen into the liver. Nutrients extracted from food are present in the blood as it enters the liver, where they are processed and advanced into the circulatory system. The liver also acts as a filter for toxins that may be ingested.

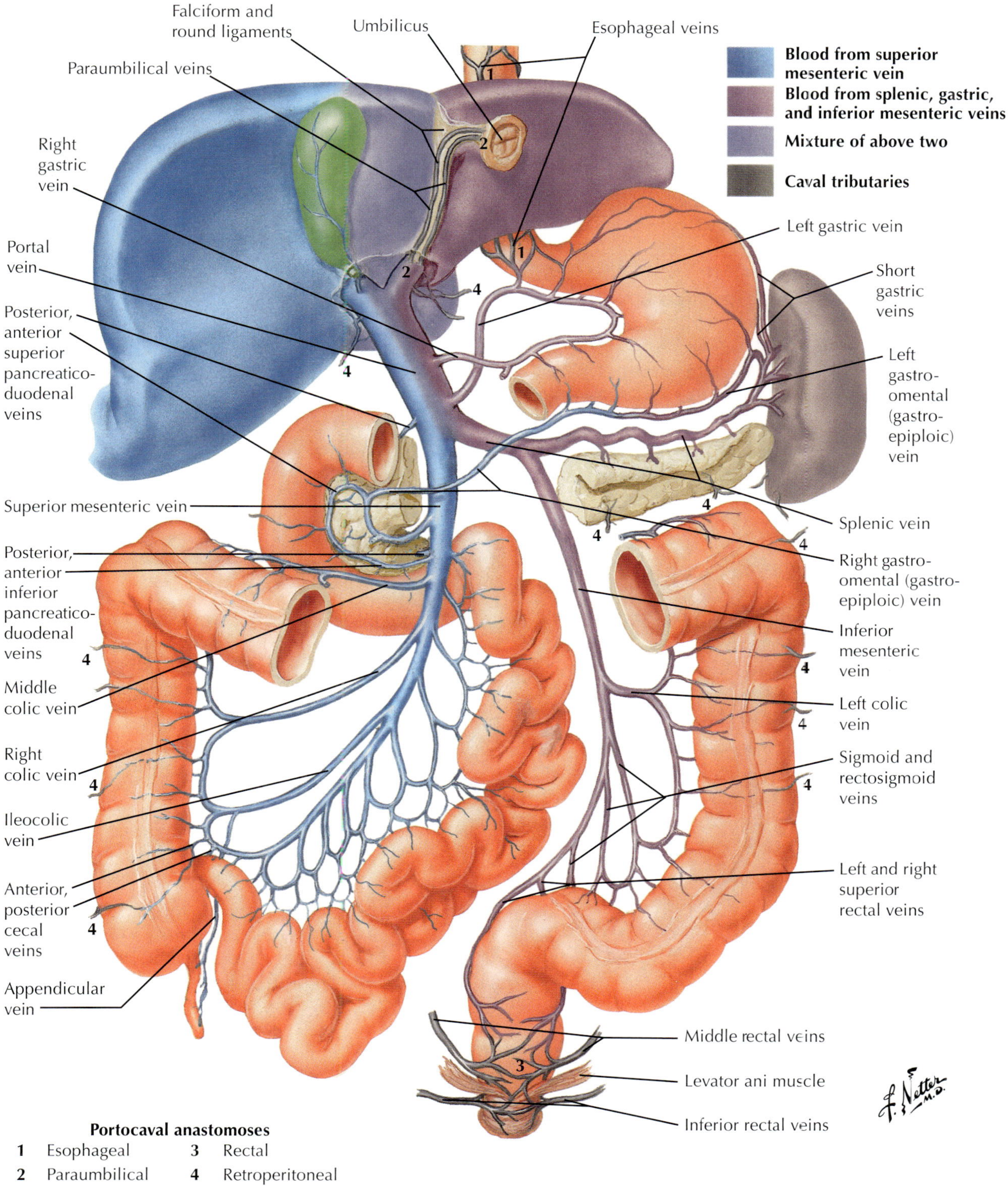

Arterial Mechanical Thrombectomy

⊙ **37184** Primary percutaneous transluminal mechanical thrombectomy, noncoronary, arterial or arterial bypass graft, including fluoroscopic guidance and intraprocedural pharmacological thrombolytic injection(s); initial vessel

⊙✚ **37185** second and all subsequent vessel(s) within the same vascular family (List separately in addition to code for primary mechanical thrombectomy procedure)

⊙✚ **37186** Secondary percutaneous transluminal thrombectomy (eg, nonprimary mechanical, snare basket, suction technique), noncoronary, arterial or arterial bypass graft, including fluoroscopic guidance and intraprocedural pharmacological thrombolytic injections, provided in conjunction with another percutaneous intervention other than primary mechanical thrombectomy (List separately in addition to code for primary procedure)

Venous Mechanical Thrombectomy

⊙ **37187** Percutaneous transluminal mechanical thrombectomy, vein(s), including intraprocedural pharmacological thrombolytic injections and fluoroscopic guidance

⊙ **37188** Percutaneous transluminal mechanical thrombectomy, vein(s), including intraprocedural pharmacological thrombolytic injections and fluoroscopic guidance, repeat treatment on subsequent day during course of thrombolytic therapy

Other Procedures

⊙ **37191** Insertion of intravascular vena cava filter, endovascular approach including vascular access, vessel selection, and radiological supervision and interpretation, intraprocedural roadmapping, and imaging guidance (ultrasound and fluoroscopy), when performed

⊙ **37192** Repositioning of intravascular vena cava filter, endovascular approach including vascular access, vessel selection, and radiological supervision and interpretation, intraprocedural roadmapping, and imaging guidance (ultrasound and fluoroscopy), when performed

⊙ **37193** Retrieval (removal) of intravascular vena cava filter, endovascular approach including vascular access, vessel selection, and radiological supervision and interpretation, intraprocedural roadmapping, and imaging guidance (ultrasound and fluoroscopy), when performed

37195 Thrombolysis, cerebral, by intravenous infusion

⊙ **37197** Transcatheter retrieval, percutaneous, of intravascular foreign body (eg, fractured venous or arterial catheter), includes radiological supervision and interpretation, and imaging guidance (ultrasound or fluoroscopy), when performed

37200 Transcatheter biopsy

#⊙ **37211** Transcatheter therapy, arterial infusion for thrombolysis other than coronary, any method, including radiological supervision and interpretation, initial treatment day

#⊙ **37212** Transcatheter therapy, venous infusion for thrombolysis, any method, including radiological supervision and interpretation, initial treatment day

#⊙ **37213** Transcatheter therapy, arterial or venous infusion for thrombolysis other than coronary, any method, including radiological supervision and interpretation, continued treatment on subsequent day during course of thrombolytic therapy, including follow-up catheter contrast injection, position change, or exchange, when performed;

#⊙ **37214** cessation of thrombolysis including removal of catheter and vessel closure by any method

37202 Transcatheter therapy, infusion other than for thrombolysis, any type (eg, spasmolytic, vasoconstrictive)

37211 Code is out of numerical sequence. See 37191-37216

37212 Code is out of numerical sequence. See 37191-37216

37213 Code is out of numerical sequence. See 37191-37216

37214 Code is out of numerical sequence. See 37191-37216

⊙ **37215** Transcatheter placement of intravascular stent(s), cervical carotid artery, open or percutaneous, including angioplasty, when performed, and radiological supervision and interpretation; with distal embolic protection

⊙ **37216** without distal embolic protection

37217 Transcatheter placement of intravascular stent(s), intrathoracic common carotid artery or innominate artery by retrograde treatment, open ipsilateral cervical carotid artery exposure, including angioplasty, when performed, and radiological supervision and interpretation

⊙ **37218** Transcatheter placement of intravascular stent(s), intrathoracic common carotid artery or innominate artery, open or percutaneous antegrade approach, including angioplasty, when performed, and radiological supervision and interpretation

Endovascular Revascularization (Open or Percutaneous, Transcatheter)

Coding Atlas

Codes 37220-37239 are used to report procedures performed to treat **occlusive** disease of peripheral arteries and veins. The site of the occlusion is accessed **endoscopically** and treated with **angioplasty**, **atherectomy**, and/or **stent** placement.

⊙ **37220** Revascularization, endovascular, open or percutaneous, iliac artery, unilateral, initial vessel; with transluminal angioplasty

⊙ **37221** with transluminal stent placement(s), includes angioplasty within the same vessel, when performed

⊙✚ **37222** Revascularization, endovascular, open or percutaneous, iliac artery, each additional ipsilateral iliac vessel; with transluminal angioplasty (List separately in addition to code for primary procedure)

⊙✚ **37223** with transluminal stent placement(s), includes angioplasty within the same vessel, when performed (List separately in addition to code for primary procedure)

⊙ **37224** Revascularization, endovascular, open or percutaneous, femoral, popliteal artery(s), unilateral; with transluminal angioplasty

⊙ **37225** with atherectomy, includes angioplasty within the same vessel, when performed

⊙ **37226** with transluminal stent placement(s), includes angioplasty within the same vessel, when performed

⊙ **37227** with transluminal stent placement(s) and atherectomy, includes angioplasty within the same vessel, when performed

⊙ **37228** Revascularization, endovascular, open or percutaneous, tibial, peroneal artery, unilateral, initial vessel; with transluminal angioplasty

⊙ **37229** with atherectomy, includes angioplasty within the same vessel, when performed

⊙ **37230** with transluminal stent placement(s), includes angioplasty within the same vessel, when performed

⊙ **37231** with transluminal stent placement(s) and atherectomy, includes angioplasty within the same vessel, when performed

⊙✚ **37232** Revascularization, endovascular, open or percutaneous, tibial/peroneal artery, unilateral, each additional vessel; with transluminal angioplasty (List separately in addition to code for primary procedure)

⊙✚ **37233** with atherectomy, includes angioplasty within the same vessel, when performed (List separately in addition to code for primary procedure)

⊙✚ **37234** with transluminal stent placement(s), includes angioplasty within the same vessel, when performed (List separately in addition to code for primary procedure)

⊙✚ **37235** with transluminal stent placement(s) and atherectomy, includes angioplasty within the same vessel, when performed (List separately in addition to code for primary procedure)

⊙ **37236** Transcatheter placement of an intravascular stent(s) (except lower extremity artery(s) for occlusive disease, cervical carotid, extracranial vertebral or intrathoracic carotid, intracranial, or coronary), open or percutaneous, including radiological supervision and interpretation and including all angioplasty within the same vessel, when performed; initial artery

⊙✚ **37237** each additional artery (List separately in addition to code for primary procedure)

⊙ **37238** Transcatheter placement of an intravascular stent(s), open or percutaneous, including radiological supervision and interpretation and including angioplasty within the same vessel, when performed; initial vein

⊙✚ **37239** each additional vein (List separately in addition to code for primary procedure)

Vascular Embolization and Occlusion

Coding Atlas

In vascular embolization, a **transcatheter** approach is used to reach the site in which a vessel is targeted for **occlusion**. A vessel may be occluded to cause **ischemia** in aberrant tissue, eg, a **tumor**, or to mitigate an **arteriovenous malformation** (AVM) or **hemorrhage**. Codes 37241-37244 are not used to report embolization procedures of the head and neck, which are reported using codes 61624, 61626, and 61710.

⊙ **37241** Vascular embolization or occlusion, inclusive of all radiological supervision and interpretation, intraprocedural roadmapping, and imaging guidance necessary to complete the intervention; venous, other than hemorrhage (eg, congenital or acquired venous malformations, venous and capillary hemangiomas, varices, varicoceles)

⊙ **37242** arterial, other than hemorrhage or tumor (eg, congenital or acquired arterial malformations, arteriovenous malformations, arteriovenous fistulas, aneurysms, pseudoaneurysms)

⊙ **37243** for tumors, organ ischemia, or infarction

⊙ **37244** for arterial or venous hemorrhage or lymphatic extravasation

Intravascular Ultrasound Services

Coding Atlas

Intravascular **ultrasound** is a diagnostic procedure in which a tiny ultrasound wand is carried within a **catheter** through a vessel to the vessel site targeted for examination. This procedure is very different from a more typical ultrasound in which a wand is place on the skin overlying the vessel.

+ 37250 Intravascular ultrasound (non-coronary vessel) during diagnostic evaluation and/or therapeutic intervention; initial vessel (List separately in addition to code for primary procedure)

+ 37251 each additional vessel (List separately in addition to code for primary procedure)

Endoscopy

Coding Atlas

Subfascial endoscopic perforator surgery (SEPS) is performed to treat advanced chronic venous insufficiency (CVI). Using a small endoscopic camera and trocar inserted through a small incision into the vein, blood flow to the vein is severed. This decreases venous **reflux**.

37500 Vascular endoscopy, surgical, with ligation of perforator veins, subfascial (SEPS)

Ligation

Coding Atlas

Ligation is the tying off of a lumen so that nothing travels through it. Codes 37565-37660 are used to report the ligation of vessels using an open technique in which an incision is made in the skin overlying the vessel being accessed. In **vein stripping**, a length of vein is removed through a small incision. In **stab phlebectomy**, a small piece, or small pieces, of vein is excised through a stab incision to treat varicosities.

37565 Ligation, internal jugular vein

37600 Ligation; external carotid artery

37605 internal or common carotid artery

37606 internal or common carotid artery, with gradual occlusion, as with Selverstone or Crutchfield clamp

37607 Ligation or banding of angioaccess arteriovenous fistula

37609 Ligation or biopsy, temporal artery

37615 Ligation, major artery (eg, post-traumatic, rupture); neck

37616 chest

37617 abdomen

37618 extremity

37619 Ligation of inferior vena cava

37650 Ligation of femoral vein

37660 Ligation of common iliac vein

37700 Ligation and division of long saphenous vein at saphenofemoral junction, or distal interruptions

37718 Ligation, division, and stripping, short saphenous vein

37722 Ligation, division, and stripping, long (greater) saphenous veins from saphenofemoral junction to knee or below

37735 Ligation and division and complete stripping of long or short saphenous veins with radical excision of ulcer and skin graft and/or interruption of communicating veins of lower leg, with excision of deep fascia

37760 Ligation of perforator veins, subfascial, radical (Linton type), including skin graft, when performed, open,1 leg

37761 Ligation of perforator vein(s), subfascial, open, including ultrasound guidance, when performed, 1 leg

37765 Stab phlebectomy of varicose veins, 1 extremity; 10-20 stab incisions

37766 more than 20 incisions

37780 Ligation and division of short saphenous vein at saphenopopliteal junction (separate procedure)

37785 Ligation, division, and/or excision of varicose vein cluster(s), 1 leg

Other Procedures

37788 Penile revascularization, artery, with or without vein graft

37790 Penile venous occlusive procedure

FIGURE 4-23. Arteries to the Brain

Optimal brain function is dependent on adequate supply of oxygen and nutrients, which are delivered by the paired common carotid arteries and paired vertebral arteries. The common carotids divide into the external and internal carotids. The external carotids supply the face and scalp, while the internal carotids supply the anterior cerebrum. Any reduction in flow through the internal carotids impairs function of the frontal lobe. The vertebrobasilar arteries supply the posterior cerebrum, part of the cerebellum, and the brain stem.

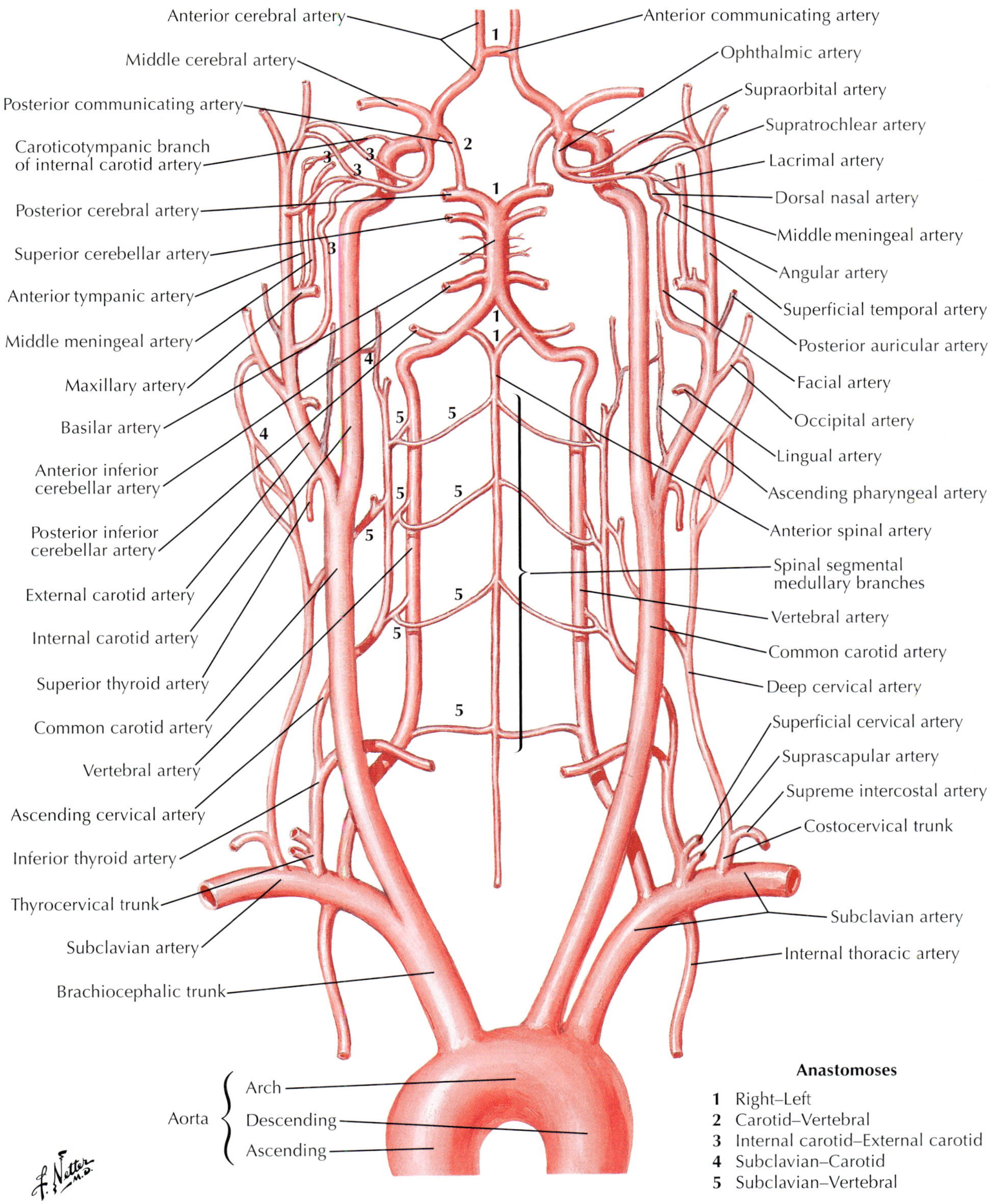

Anastomoses

1 Right–Left
2 Carotid–Vertebral
3 Internal carotid–External carotid
4 Subclavian–Carotid
5 Subclavian–Vertebral

FIGURE 4-24. Superficial Veins of the Lower Extremity

Superficial veins help to cool the body by transferring heat to the skin surface; they are not as critical to **circulation** as deep veins. Superficial veins, especially those of the lower extremities, may develop **varicosities** or valve disorders. These **aberrant** vessels may be removed or **ligated** and left **in situ** to reduce **venous congestion**.

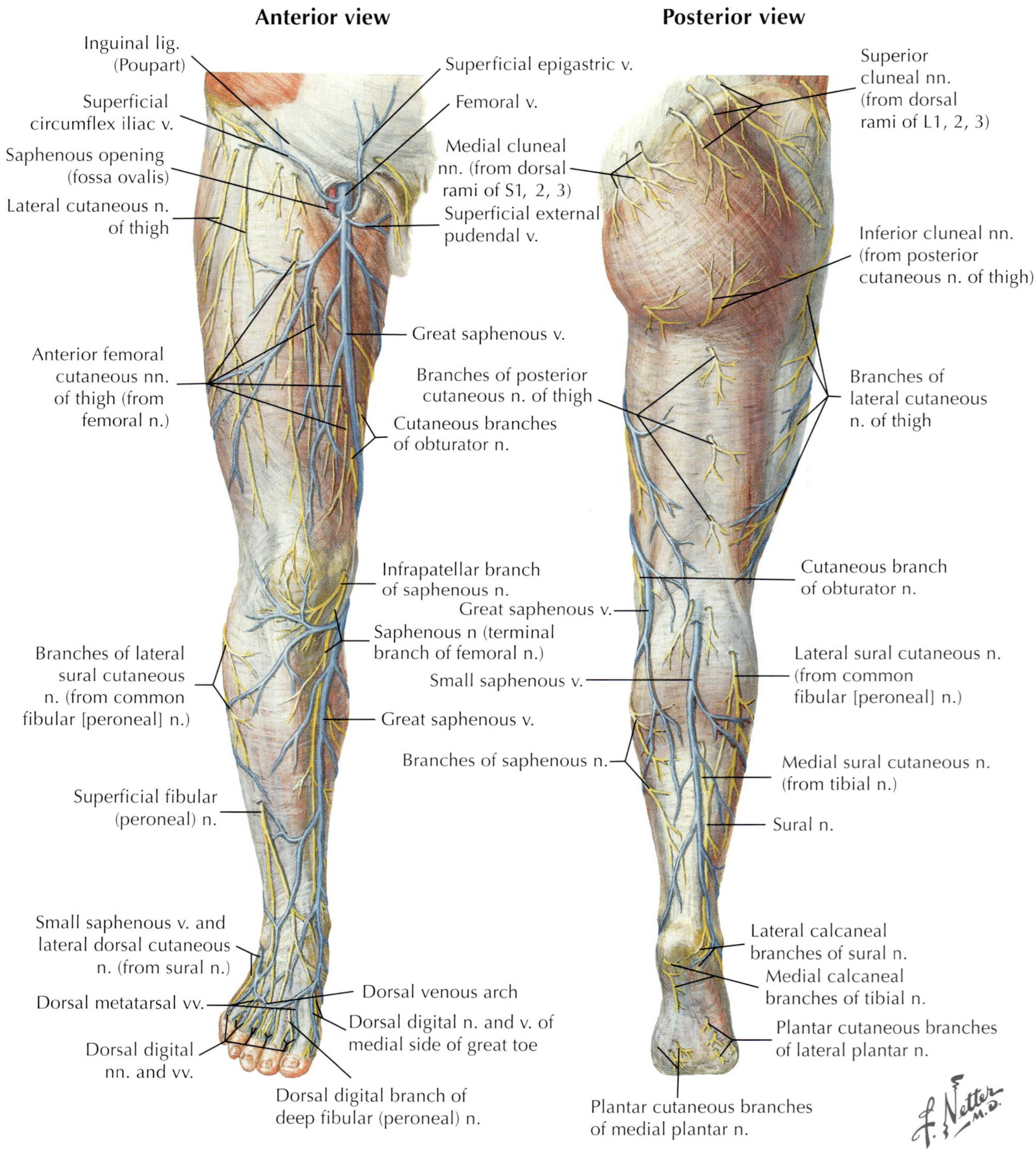

Hemic and Lymphatic Systems

Spleen

Excision

Coding Atlas

The normal **spleen** is about the size of a fist and highly vascularized. A **splenectomy** may be complete (total) or partial. Typically an open splenectomy (codes 38100-38102) is performed in emergent situations or when **direct visualization** and **exploration** is desired, eg, following traumatic injury.

38100 Splenectomy; total (separate procedure)

38101 partial (separate procedure)

+ **38102** total, en bloc for extensive disease, in conjunction with other procedure (List in addition to code for primary procedure)

Repair

Coding Atlas

The **spleen** is protected by its tough exterior capsule. When this capsule ruptures, the highly vascularized tissue within **hemorrhages** into the abdomen. A ruptured spleen usually is the result of **blunt trauma** and may be treated with a suture repair (**splenorrhaphy**) or complete or partial **splenectomy**.

38115 Repair of ruptured spleen (splenorrhaphy) with or without partial splenectomy

Laparoscopy

38120 Laparoscopy, surgical, splenectomy

Introduction

Coding Atlas

Splenoportography is the introduction of **radiopaque** material into the spleen to enhance visualization of the splenic and main portal veins of the portal circulation in a radiograph.

38200 Injection procedure for splenoportography

General

Bone Marrow or Stem Cell Services/Procedures

Coding Atlas

Bone marrow transplant procedures are used to treat leukemia, lymphoma, breast cancer, multiple myeloma, renal cell cancer, neuroblastoma, ovarian cancer, aplastic anemia, inherited inborn errors of metabolism, and **immunodeficiencies**. The **harvest** and modification procedures vary depending on the type of cell being sought.

38204 Management of recipient hematopoietic progenitor cell donor search and cell acquisition

38205 Blood-derived hematopoietic progenitor cell harvesting for transplantation, per collection; allogeneic

38206 autologous

38207 Transplant preparation of hematopoietic progenitor cells; cryopreservation and storage

38208 thawing of previously frozen harvest, without washing, per donor

38209 thawing of previously frozen harvest, with washing, per donor

38210 specific cell depletion within harvest, T-cell depletion

38211 tumor cell depletion

38212 red blood cell removal

38213 platelet depletion

38214 plasma (volume) depletion

38215 cell concentration in plasma, mononuclear, or buffy coat layer

38220 Bone marrow; aspiration only

38221 biopsy, needle or trocar

38230 Bone marrow harvesting for transplantation; allogeneic

38232 autologous

FIGURE 4-25. The Spleen

The **spleen** is a large, vascular lymphatic organ located in the upper part of the abdominal cavity on the left side between the stomach and **diaphragm**. The spleen filters old or damaged red blood cells out of the bloodstream, destroys worn out and damaged **platelets**, and produces infection-fighting agents. It is composed of **lymph** tissue that produces **antibodies** (proteins that destroy certain microorganisms), **phagocytes** (cells that ingest certain microorganisms), and **lymphocytes** (a type of white blood cell).

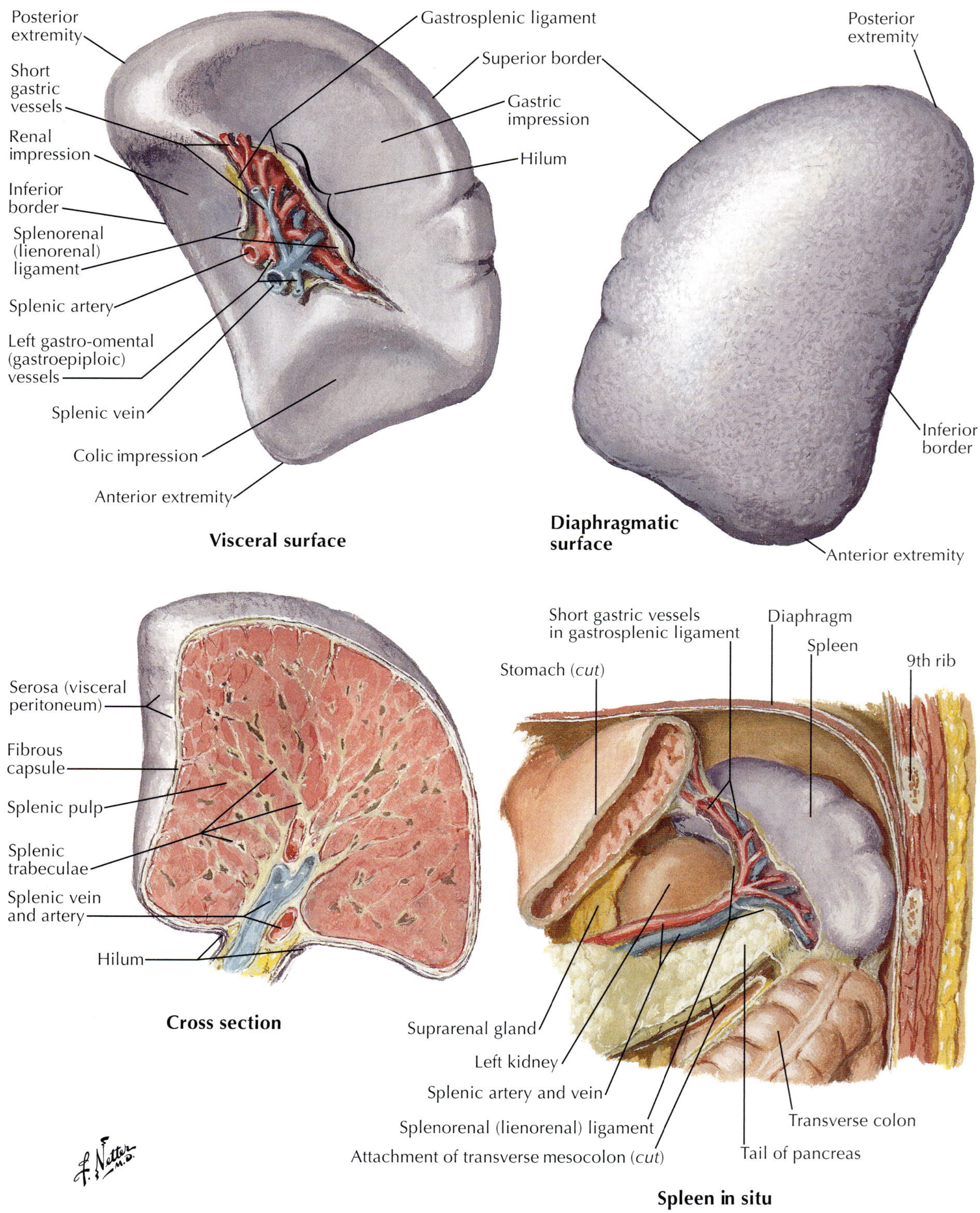

Transplantation and Post-Transplantation Cellular Infusions

Coding Atlas

Hematopoietic progenitor cells (HPCs) are also referred to as stem cells. Code 38240 is used to report each allogeneic stem cell transplant, whether derived from **bone marrow**, blood-derived peripheral stem cells, or cord blood stem cell sources. Code 38241 is used to report infusion of cells that were earlier extracted from the same patient. Code 38243 is used to report an HPC boost given due to complications from administration of marrow suppressive medications used to restore normal blood counts in patients with infection post-transplant. Code 38242 is used to report donor lymphocyte infusions (DLIs) to treat relapse or viral infections in **allogeneic** transplant recipients.

38240 Hematopoietic progenitor cell (HPC); allogeneic transplantation per donor

38241 autologous transplantation

38243 HPC boost

38242 Allogeneic lymphocyte infusions

38243 Code is out of numerical sequence. See 38240-38242

Lymph Nodes and Lymphatic Channels

Incision

Coding Atlas

The **thoracic duct** is the largest **lymphatic** vessel and is also referred to as the **left lymphatic duct**, **alimentary duct**, **chyliferous** duct, or **Van Hoorne's canal**. The thoracic duct parallels the spinal column from the abdomen to the neck. Lymph within the duct is pushed forward by the action of breathing.

38300 Drainage of lymph node abscess or lymphadenitis; simple

38305 extensive

38308 Lymphangiotomy or other operations on lymphatic channels

38380 Suture and/or ligation of thoracic duct; cervical approach

38381 thoracic approach

38382 abdominal approach

Excision

Coding Atlas

The first lymph node draining away from the site of a malignancy is called the **sentinel node**. **Metastatic** cancer normally is established at the sentinel node before moving on to other parts of the body. The sentinel node is often targeted for examination in the staging of a malignancy. Open **biopsy** of a sentinel node usually requires two codes: code 38792 to report the injection procedure that identifies the sentinel node and a code from the code range 38500-38542 to report the excision.

38500 Biopsy or excision of lymph node(s); open, superficial

38505 by needle, superficial (eg, cervical, inguinal, axillary)

38510 open, deep cervical node(s)

38520 open, deep cervical node(s) with excision scalene fat pad

38525 open, deep axillary node(s)

38530 open, internal mammary node(s)

38542 Dissection, deep jugular node(s)

38550 Excision of cystic hygroma, axillary or cervical; without deep neurovascular dissection

38555 with deep neurovascular dissection

Limited Lymphadenectomy for Staging

Coding Atlas

Staging describes the evaluation of a **malignancy** to determine the severity and extent of **metastasis**. Cancer cells may break away from the main **tumor** and enter the bloodstream or lymphatic system. Sampling of regional lymph nodes for metastatic disease may be a component of staging to inform the treatment plan for the **primary** cancer.

38562 Limited lymphadenectomy for staging (separate procedure); pelvic and para-aortic

38564 retroperitoneal (aortic and/or splenic)

FIGURE 4-26. The Lymphatic System

The **lymphatic system** is a network of **ducts**, **valves**, vessels, nodes, and organs that creates and circulate clear lymph fluid throughout the body. The lymphatic system plays a major role in **immunity**. Lymph nodes filter circulating lymphatic fluid to remove bacteria and other foreign matter including **cancer** cells. During digestion, **emulsified** fat combines with lymph to form **chyle**, which is then carried into the **circulation**. The tonsils, adenoids, **spleen**, and **thymus gland** are included in the lymphatic system.

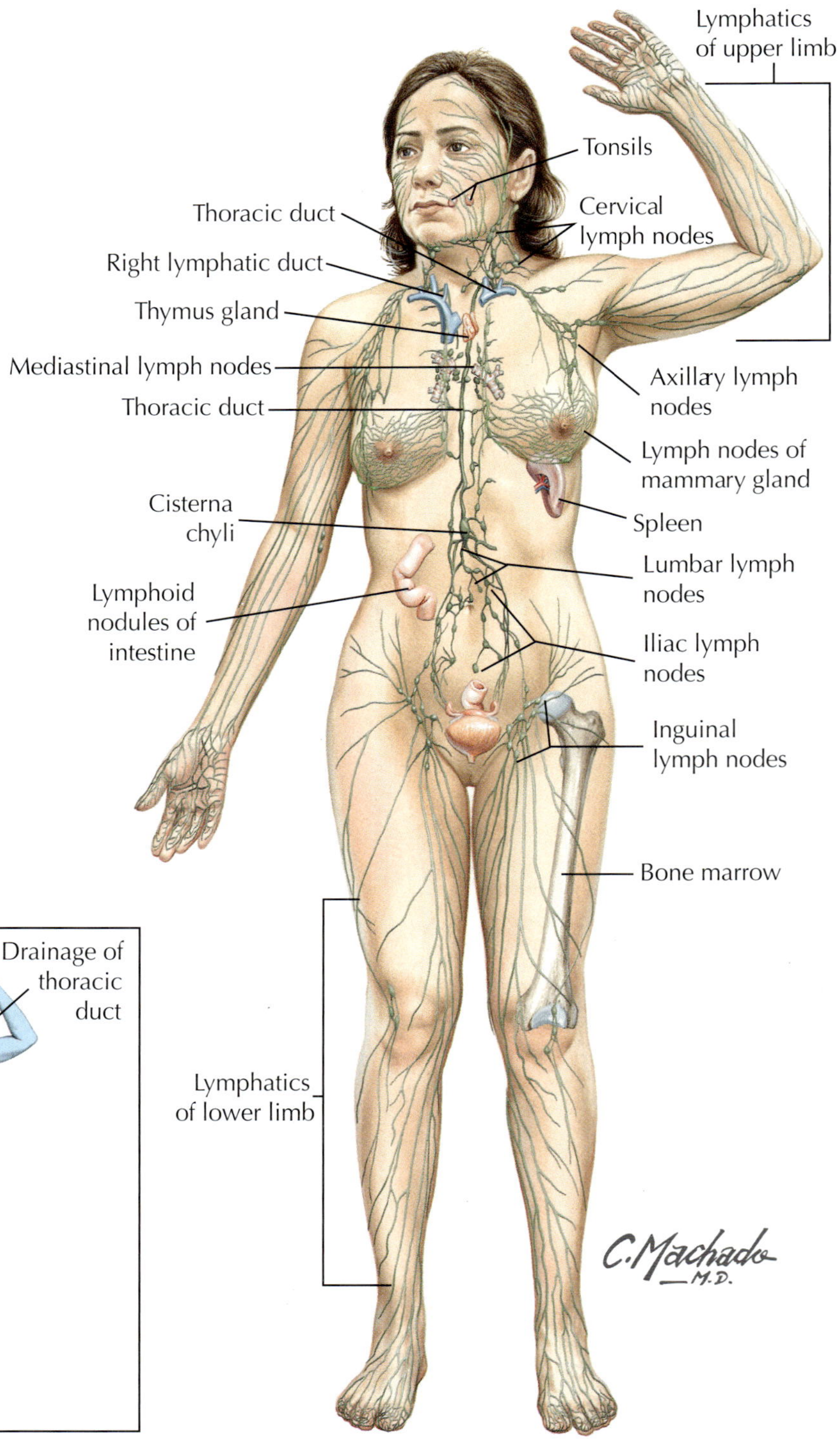

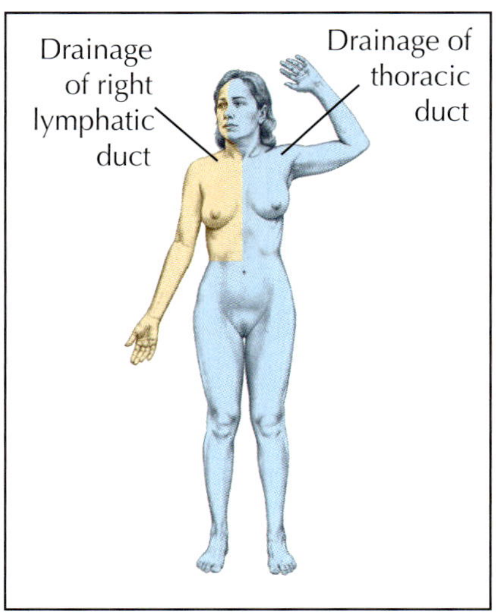

Laparoscopy

Coding Atlas

Laparoscopy is an approach that involves use of multiple small portals to enter the body and perform surgery, with tools, optics, and lighting placed through these portals. It is less invasive than **open** surgical techniques but lacks **direct visualization**. Sampling of regional lymph nodes for **metastatic** disease may be a component of **staging** to inform the treatment plan for the **primary** cancer.

38570 Laparoscopy, surgical; with retroperitoneal lymph node sampling (biopsy), single or multiple

38571 with bilateral total pelvic lymphadenectomy

38572 with bilateral total pelvic lymphadenectomy and peri-aortic lymph node sampling (biopsy), single or multiple

38589 Unlisted laparoscopy procedure, lymphatic system

Radical Lymphadenectomy (Radical Resection of Lymph Nodes)

Coding Atlas

The **lymphatic system** is one of the main routes through which cancer can spread. Nearly a third of all lymph nodes are located in the head and neck. In the treatment of head and neck cancer, a radical (complete) neck dissection (RND) or a modified radical neck dissection (MRND) may be indicated. Since the goal of the neck dissection is to prevent spread of the disease, some nonlymphatic structures (eg, muscles, glands, arteries, and/or veins) may be excised depending on the extent to which the cancer has spread. Suprahyoid lymphadenectomy and supraomohyoid lymphadenectomy are sometimes documented as suprahyoid/supraomohyoid neck dissection. Lymphadenectomy is a unilateral procedure. Because there is no single code to use for resection of a primary tumor with a modified radical neck dissection, one code is used to report the tumor resection (eg, 42420) and one code is used to report the modified radical neck dissection (eg, code 38724).

38700 Suprahyoid lymphadenectomy

38720 Cervical lymphadenectomy (complete)

38724 Cervical lymphadenectomy (modified radical neck dissection)

38740 Axillary lymphadenectomy; superficial

38745 complete

✚ 38746 Thoracic lymphadenectomy by thoracotomy, mediastinal and regional lymphadenectomy (List separately in addition to code for primary procedure)

✚ 38747 Abdominal lymphadenectomy, regional, including celiac, gastric, portal, peripancreatic, with or without para-aortic and vena caval nodes (List separately in addition to code for primary procedure)

38760 Inguinofemoral lymphadenectomy, superficial, including Cloquets node (separate procedure)

38765 Inguinofemoral lymphadenectomy, superficial, in continuity with pelvic lymphadenectomy, including external iliac, hypogastric, and obturator nodes (separate procedure)

38770 Pelvic lymphadenectomy, including external iliac, hypogastric, and obturator nodes (separate procedure)

38780 Retroperitoneal transabdominal lymphadenectomy, extensive, including pelvic, aortic, and renal nodes (separate procedure)

Introduction

Coding Atlas

The first lymph node draining away from the site of a malignancy is called the **sentinel node**. **Metastatic** cancer normally is established there before moving on to other parts of the body. The sentinel node is often targeted for examination in the **staging** of a malignancy. Open biopsy of a sentinel node is reported with two codes: code 38792 to report the injection procedure that identifies the sentinel node and a code from code range 38500-38542 to report the **excision**.

38790 Injection procedure; lymphangiography

38792 radioactive tracer for identification of sentinel node

38794 Cannulation, thoracic duct

Other Procedures

✚ 38900 Intraoperative identification (eg, mapping) of sentinel lymph node(s) includes injection of non-radioactive dye, when performed (List separately in addition to code for primary procedure)

FIGURE 4-27. The Mediastinum

The **mediastinum** is not an organ but rather a location in the chest. The mediastinum describes the area bound by the right and left lung, the **sternum**, and the vertebral column. The mediastinum contains the heart, **thymus gland**, portions of the esophagus and trachea, and other structures. Most often the term is used to describe the space and tissues between these organs.

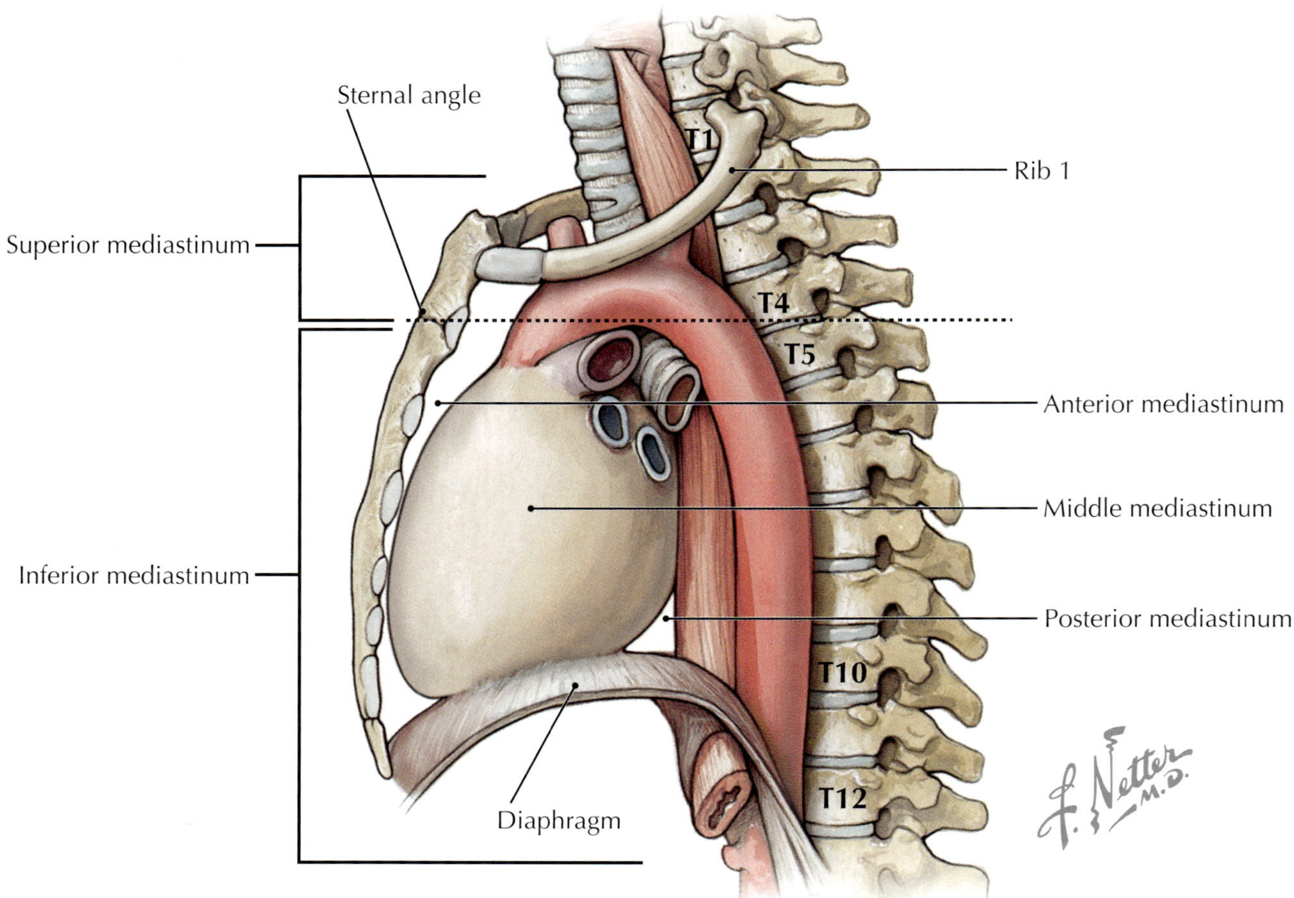

Mediastinum and Diaphragm

Mediastinum

Incision

Coding Atlas

Codes 39000 and 39010 are used to report **open** approaches to the **thoracic cavity**, with code selection based on the site of the incision, ie, cervical or median **sternotomy**. For video-assisted thoracic surgery (VATS) pericardial biopsy, see code 32604.

39000 Mediastinotomy with exploration, drainage, removal of foreign body, or biopsy; cervical approach

39010 transthoracic approach, including either transthoracic or median sternotomy

Excision/Resection

Coding Atlas

Mediastinal **tumors** are somewhat rare. Those found in children are most commonly **benign** neoplasms of neurological origin. Those found in adults are commonly **malignant** lymphomas.

39200 Resection of mediastinal cyst

39220 Resection of mediastinal tumor

Endoscopy

Coding Atlas

In **mediastinoscopy**, a scope is inserted into a small incision in the neck and passed into the chest cavity to examine the **mediastinum**. Tissue samples may be removed.

39400 Mediastinoscopy, includes biopsy(ies), when performed

Diaphragm

Repair

Coding Atlas

A diaphragmatic **hernia** is an abnormal opening in the diaphragm that causes abdominal organs to protrude into the thoracic cavity.

39501 Repair, laceration of diaphragm, any approach

39503 Repair, neonatal diaphragmatic hernia, with or without chest tube insertion and with or without creation of ventral hernia

39540 Repair, diaphragmatic hernia (other than neonatal), traumatic; acute

39541 chronic

39545 Imbrication of diaphragm for eventration, transthoracic or transabdominal, paralytic or nonparalytic

39560 Resection, diaphragm; with simple repair (eg, primary suture)

39561 with complex repair (eg, prosthetic material, local muscle flap)

FIGURE 4-28. Abdominal Surface of the Diaphragm

The **diaphragm** is a thin sheet of muscle that separates the **thoracic cavity** from the **abdominal cavity**. Shaped like a dome, the diaphragm contracts during inhalation, thereby enlarging the thoracic cavity, and expands during exhalation to the opposite result. The diaphragm is also involved in the prevention of **acid reflux** when pressure is applied on the **esophagus**. In Figure 4-28, the **inferior** dome of the diaphragm is viewed from the abdomen.

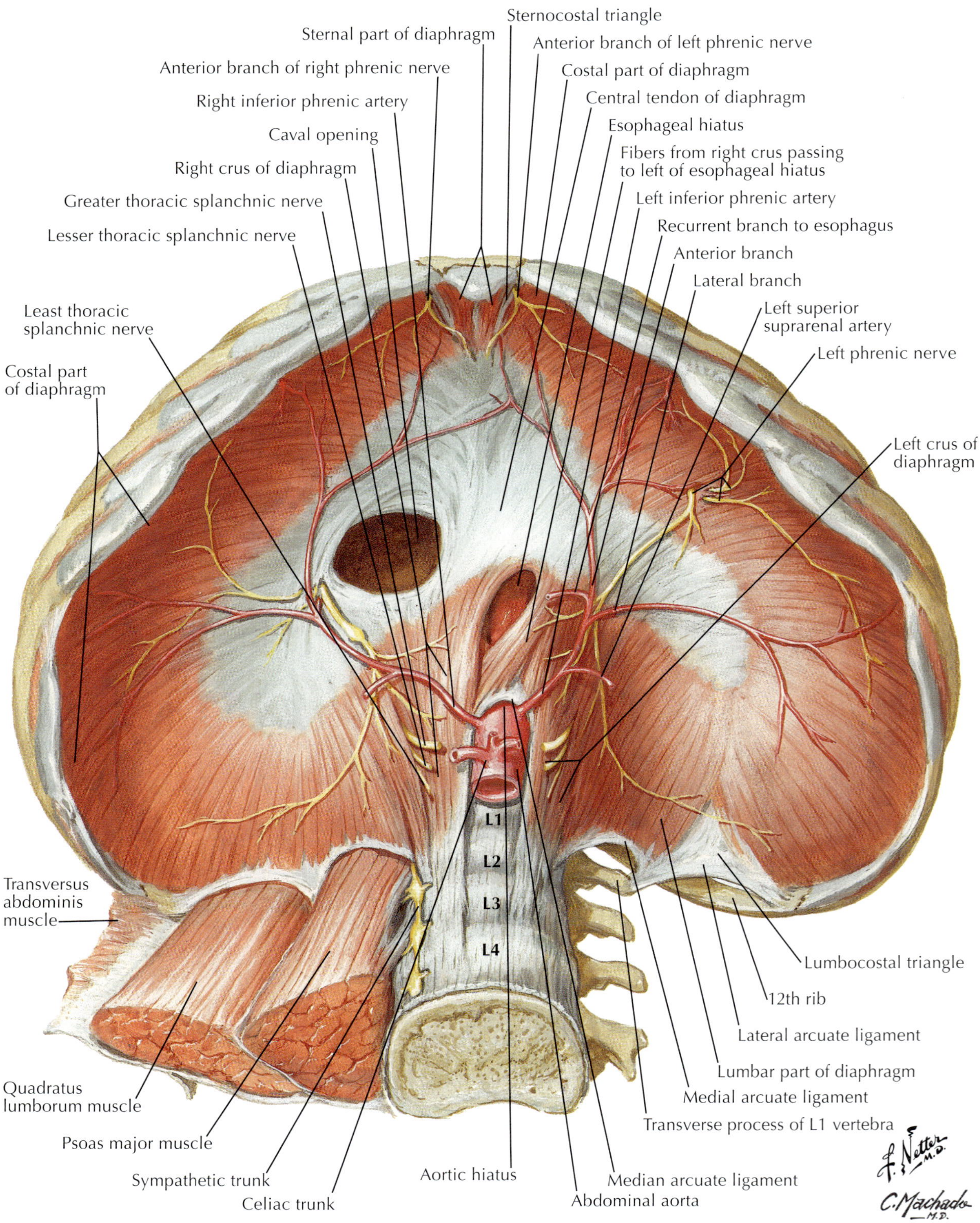

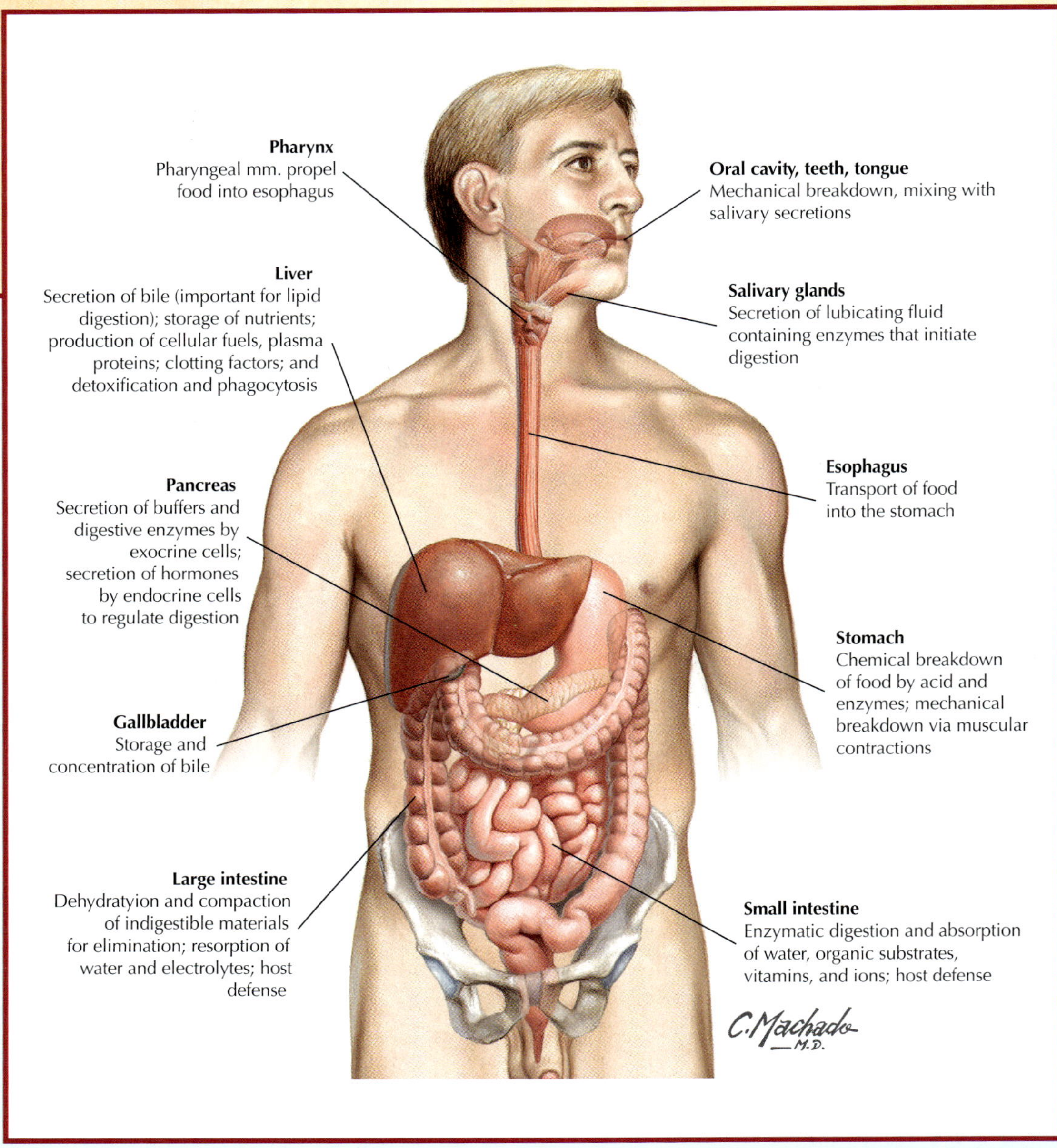

Pharynx
Pharyngeal mm. propel food into esophagus
Oral cavity, teeth, tongue
Mechanical breakdown, mixing with salivary secretions
Liver
Secretion of bile (important for lipid digestion); storage of nutrients; production of cellular fuels, plasma proteins; clotting factors; and detoxification and phagocytosis
Salivary glands
Secretion of lubicating fluid containing enzymes that initiate digestion
Esophagus
Transport of food into the stomach
Pancreas
Secretion of buffers and digestive enzymes by exocrine cells; secretion of hormones by endocrine cells to regulate digestion
Stomach
Chemical breakdown of food by acid and enzymes; mechanical breakdown via muscular contractions
Gallbladder
Storage and concentration of bile
Large intestine
Dehydratyion and compaction of indigestible materials for elimination; resorption of water and electrolytes; host defense
Small intestine
Enzymatic digestion and absorption of water, organic substrates, vitamins, and ions; host defense
C.Machado M.D.

CHAPTER 5

Digestive System

The digestive system is responsible for the ingestion, digestion, and assimilation of food, as well as the elimination of residual digestive waste products. The food that enters the mouth follows the **alimentary tract** in an uninterrupted pathway that travels from one compartment to the next: mouth to esophagus to stomach to small intestine to large intestine to rectum to anus. By the time food reaches the large intestine, nutrients have been transferred into the circulatory system, leaving behind only waste in the form of **feces**. In addition, the large intestine also plays an important role in water balance in that it absorbs a considerable quantity of water and electrolytes (particularly sodium). In the process of breaking down materials in the large intestine, these bacteria also produce a lot of gas. Other digestive organs (liver, pancreas, gallbladder) communicate through **ducts** along the alimentary tract to provide digestive **enzymes** and **bile**.

Smell and taste are important and intermingled components of eating. We consider eating a social and pleasurable experience, but smell and taste are also components of survival. The lips and tongue screen food entering the alimentary tract. If the food tastes odd or is too prickly or hot, it is rejected, protecting the rest of the body. Smell serves as a checkpoint for food safety as well.

Digestion begins with **mastication**. Saliva produced in the salivary glands contains enzymes that help to break down the starch in food through salivary amylase. The saliva helps to moisten food and create a **bolus** so it can be swallowed easily. Once swallowed, the bolus travels to the pharynx and esophagus, then through the esophageal **sphincter** into the stomach.

The stomach controls the rate at which food enters the small intestines. It also provides a temporary storage area for food and it is the first part of the gastrointestinal (GI) tract that breaks down proteins into peptides. Food then passes through the pyloric **valve** into the duodenum of the small intestine.

The small intestine has three segments: duodenum, jejunum, and ileum. Further aiding the breakdown of food in the duodenum are pancreatic enzymes and bile that originates in the liver and is stored and released by the gallbladder. Once the food reaches the jejunum and ileum, its nutrients are further broken down for uptake into the bloodstream. What remains is waste and water.

The small intestine empties into the large intestine through the ileocecal valve, which empties into the cecum of the ascending colon. Water is removed from waste as it travels up the ascending colon, across the transverse colon, and into the descending colon, which is attached to the rectum. The rectum contains nerves that alert the brain to the need to defecate. The anal sphincter controls this urge.

Food, nutrients, and feces move through the gastrointestinal system via a series of smooth muscle contractions called **peristalsis**. Valves and sphincters between organ structures prevent **backflow**.

The walls of the alimentary tract have the same basic structure throughout their length: **mucosa** with epithelial lining, submucosa, and **smooth muscle**.

When a person eats, the gallbladder contracts, releasing bile into ducts that lead into the common bile duct. The sphincter at the ampulla of Vater opens, and the bile flows into the duodenum. If the gallbladder is removed, bile flows directly from the liver with little change in functional result. The pancreas, in addition to producing digestive enzymes, is an **endocrine** gland that produces **insulin**, **glucagon**, **somatostatin**, and pancreatic polypeptide.

Because the gastrointestinal system is essentially a continuous **lumen** with a few connecting ducts, **endoscopy** is a common surgical approach for both diagnostic and therapeutic procedures.

FIGURE 5-1. Mouth Features

The lips rim the entrance to the oral cavity and function as a type of "valve" to keep the mouth closed during **mastication**. Lips also perform a significant role in speech. Procedures on the lips are significant in that the lips play a vital role in aesthetics and in facial expression, making **cosmesis** an important component of lip surgery.

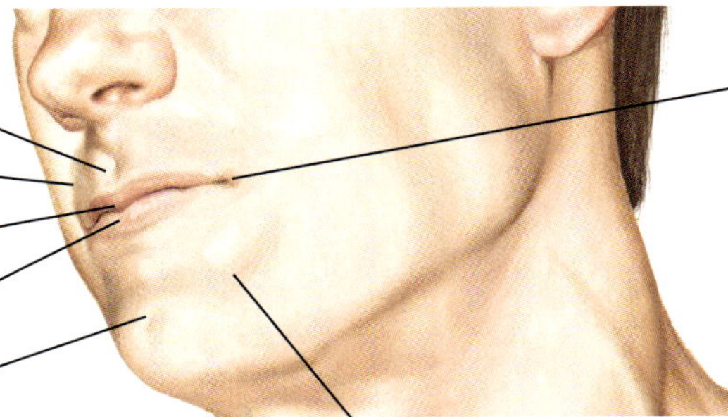

Lips

Excision

Coding Atlas

The **vermilion** is the darker skin, or "lipstick region," that rims the mouth. It is the only oral **mucosa** that is always exposed. When a procedure involves only the skin of the lip, codes from the Integumentary System code set should be consulted rather than those from the Digestive System code set.

40490 Biopsy of lip

40500 Vermilionectomy (lip shave), with mucosal advancement

40510 Excision of lip; transverse wedge excision with primary closure

40520 V-excision with primary direct linear closure

40525 full thickness, reconstruction with local flap (eg, Estlander or fan)

40527 full thickness, reconstruction with cross lip flap (Abbe-Estlander)

40530 Resection of lip, more than one-fourth, without reconstruction

Repair (Cheiloplasty)

Coding Atlas

A cleft lip (**cheiloschisis**) develops during the embryonic stage and is usually repaired in infancy or childhood. The cleft lip defect may range from a small groove on the border of the upper lip to a large deformity extending into the floor of the nostril, and it may be **unilateral** or **bilateral**. A cleft lip may occur with a cleft palate (**palatoschisis**).

40650 Repair lip, full thickness; vermilion only

40652 up to half vertical height

40654 over one-half vertical height, or complex

40700 Plastic repair of cleft lip/nasal deformity; primary, partial or complete, unilateral

40701 primary bilateral, 1-stage procedure

40702 primary bilateral, 1 of 2 stages

40720 secondary, by recreation of defect and reclosure

40761 with cross lip pedicle flap (Abbe-Estlander type), including sectioning and inserting of pedicle

FIGURE 5-2. The Oral Cavity

The oral cavity includes the **dentoalveolar** structures, palate, tonsils, uvula, tongue, floor of mouth, and vestibule of mouth. The vestibule of mouth is the area inside the oral cavity that is beyond the dental arch. It includes the interior cheek **mucosa** and submucosa that continues in a U-shape to meet the **gingiva** at the teeth. Note: Tools, implants, and/or equipment depicted in the illustration may be outdated but the procedural approach is valid.

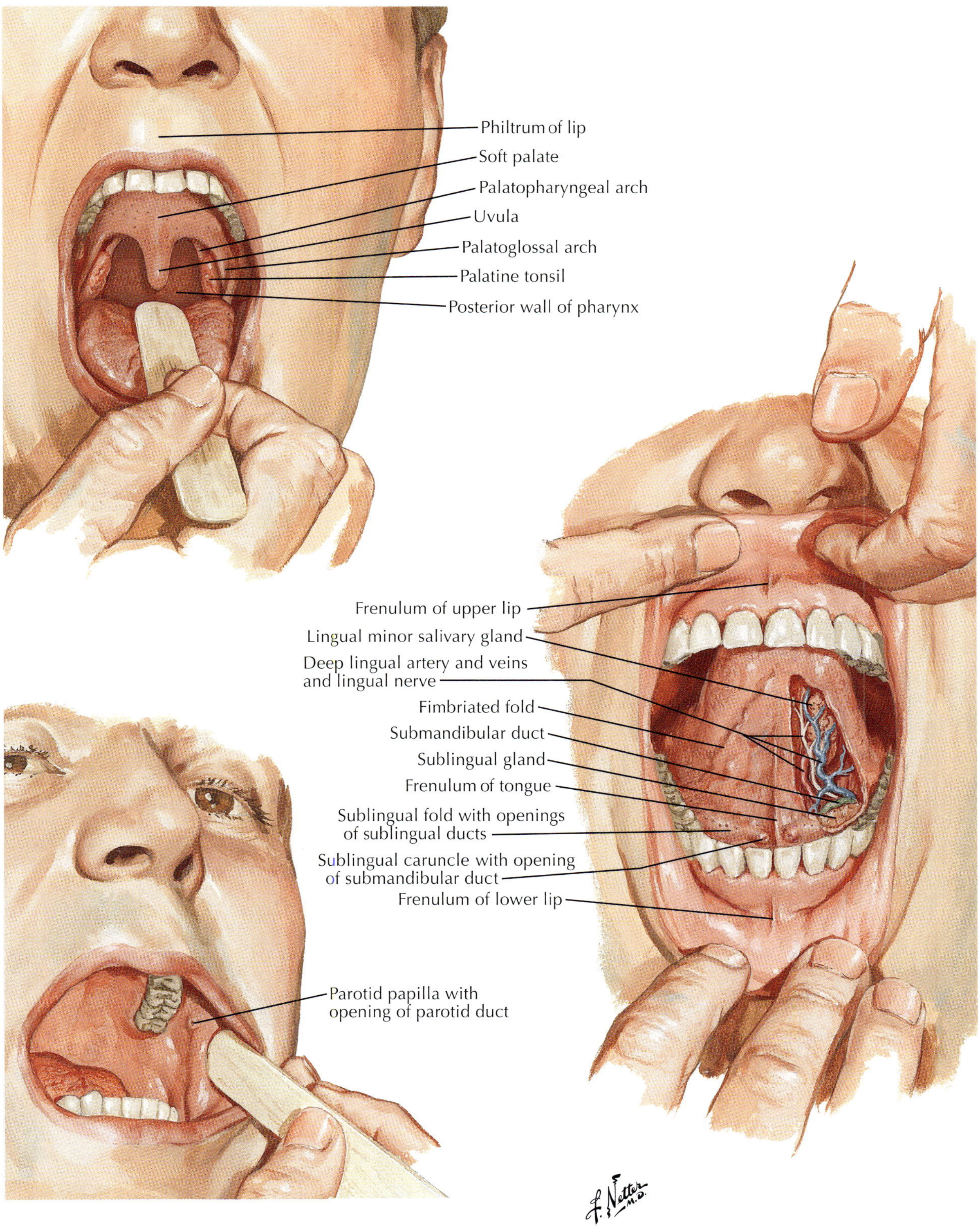

Vestibule of Mouth

Incision

Coding Atlas

The labial **frenum**, or frenulum, is a thin band of oral **mucosa** that attaches each lip at its base midline to alveolar mucosal tissue of the vestibule of the mouth. In most people, this attachment is insignificant; however, in cases in which the frenum is too bulky or too restrictive, it may be severed surgically.

40800 Drainage of abscess, cyst, hematoma, vestibule of mouth; simple

40801 complicated

40804 Removal of embedded foreign body, vestibule of mouth; simple

40805 complicated

40806 Incision of labial frenum (frenotomy)

Excision, Destruction

Coding Atlas

The mucosal lining of the cheek is called **buccal** mucosa and is a common source of **graft** material for procedures involving sites with mucosal linings. In some cases, the CPT codes for these procedures include **harvest** of buccal **mucosa** in their descriptions. In other cases, the harvest of buccal mucosa is reported separately with code 40818.

40808 Biopsy, vestibule of mouth

40810 Excision of lesion of mucosa and submucosa, vestibule of mouth; without repair

40812 with simple repair

40814 with complex repair

40816 complex, with excision of underlying muscle

40818 Excision of mucosa of vestibule of mouth as donor graft

40819 Excision of frenum, labial or buccal (frenumectomy, frenulectomy, frenectomy)

40820 Destruction of lesion or scar of vestibule of mouth by physical methods (eg, laser, thermal, cryo, chemical)

Repair

Coding Atlas

In **vestibuloplasty**, the gingival-mucosal membranes of the vestibule of the mouth are incised and rearranged. Vestibuloplasty is also called vestibulo-sulcoplasty or vestibular extension. This procedure is typically performed to prepare the mouth for or improve the fit and function of, dentures.

40830 Closure of laceration, vestibule of mouth; 2.5 cm or less

40831 over 2.5 cm or complex

40840 Vestibuloplasty; anterior

40842 posterior, unilateral

40843 posterior, bilateral

40844 entire arch

40845 complex (including ridge extension, muscle repositioning)

Tongue and Floor of Mouth

Incision

Coding Atlas

An **intraoral** incision is performed by accessing the site through an opened mouth. An **extraoral** excision is performed by accessing the site through an incision on the skin, in this case, of the face, typically the cheek or chin. Incision of a **lingual frenum** is performed in patients with tongue tie, a condition in which a tight band of mucosal skin connects the underside of the tongue to the floor of the mouth, restricting tongue movement. In **frenotomy**, the frenum is cut, but no tissue is removed.

41000 Intraoral incision and drainage of abscess, cyst, or hematoma of tongue or floor of mouth; lingual

41005 sublingual, superficial

41006 sublingual, deep, supramylohyoid

41007 submental space

41008 submandibular space

41009 masticator space

41010 Incision of lingual frenum (frenotomy)

41015 Extraoral incision and drainage of abscess, cyst, or hematoma of floor of mouth; sublingual

41016 submental

FIGURE 5-3. The Tongue

The tongue is covered with papillae and mucosa. It is attached at its base to the hyoid bone. The tongue moves food around in the mouth to aid in mastication, swallowing, and speech. The tongue is composed of both intrinsic and extrinsic muscles that contribute to its dexterity, strength, and ability to change shape. Taste buds are typically found between papillae. Each taste bud has multiple gustatory receptor cells that transmit information about taste to the brain.

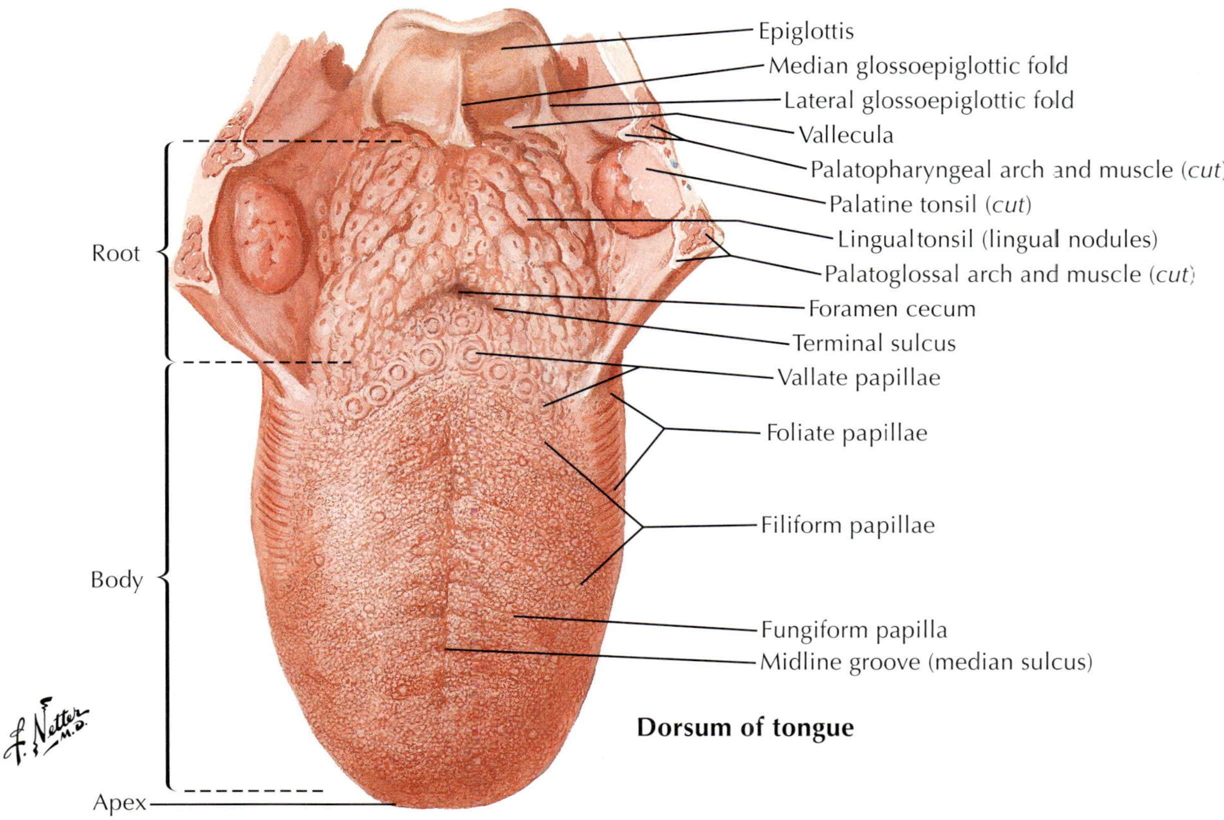

Dorsum of tongue

41017 submandibular

41018 masticator space

41019 Placement of needles, catheters, or other device(s) into the head and/or neck region (percutaneous, transoral, or transnasal) for subsequent interstitial radioelement application

Excision

Coding Atlas

In a tongue biopsy, tissue is excised for examination, without attention to margins. A glossectomy is excision of all or part of the tongue and is usually performed alone or in combination with neck dissection or other wide dissections to treat squamous cell carcinoma (SCC). SCC accounts for more than 95% of tongue malignancies. Any reconstruction may be reported separately.

41100 Biopsy of tongue; anterior two-thirds

41105 posterior one-third

41108 Biopsy of floor of mouth

41110 Excision of lesion of tongue without closure

41112 Excision of lesion of tongue with closure; anterior two-thirds

41113 posterior one-third

41114 with local tongue flap

41115 Excision of lingual frenum (frenectomy)

41116 Excision, lesion of floor of mouth

41120 Glossectomy; less than one-half tongue

41130 hemiglossectomy

41135 partial, with unilateral radical neck dissection

41140 complete or total, with or without tracheostomy, without radical neck dissection

41145 complete or total, with or without tracheostomy, with unilateral radical neck dissection

41150 composite procedure with resection floor of mouth and mandibular resection, without radical neck dissection

41153 composite procedure with resection floor of mouth, with suprahyoid neck dissection

41155 composite procedure with resection floor of mouth, mandibular resection, and radical neck dissection (Commando type)

Repair

Coding Atlas

The most common cause of a tongue laceration is a fall in which the tongue is between the teeth, injuring the muscle of the tongue. A laceration may also be the result of seizure or from penetrating injury. Repair of a laceration of the tongue must take into consideration the tongue's layered muscle anatomy.

41250 Repair of laceration 2.5 cm or less; floor of mouth and/or anterior two-thirds of tongue

41251 posterior one-third of tongue

41252 Repair of laceration of tongue, floor of mouth, over 2.6 cm or complex

Other Procedures

Coding Atlas

Code 41500 is used to report the use of K-wire in a nonsuture technique to attach and position the tongue. Code 41512 is used to report a suture technique that treats snoring and obstructive sleep apnea (OSA).

41500 Fixation of tongue, mechanical, other than suture (eg, K-wire)

41510 Suture of tongue to lip for micrognathia (Douglas type procedure)

41512 Tongue base suspension, permanent suture technique

41520 Frenoplasty (surgical revision of frenum, eg, with Z-plasty)

41530 Submucosal ablation of the tongue base, radiofrequency, 1 or more sites, per session

Dentoalveolar Structures

Incision

Coding Atlas

A dentoalveolar structure is any anatomical structure in the oral cavity that consists of teeth or the sockets in the jaw that hold the roots of teeth (alveoli). Included in the CPT code range for dentoalveolar structures are procedures relating to dental bone, gingiva, pericoronal tissues, and alveolar mucosa.

41800 Drainage of abscess, cyst, hematoma from dentoalveolar structures

41805 Removal of embedded foreign body from dentoalveolar structures; soft tissues

41806 bone

Excision, Destruction

Coding Atlas

In gingivectomy, gum tissue is excised to eliminate pockets of periodontal disease or for cosmesis in cases of overgrowth. In alveolectomy, bone that forms the socket for a tooth root is excised. Operculectomy is the excision of a flap of mucosal tissue at the site of an erupting molar.

41820 Gingivectomy, excision gingiva, each quadrant

41821 Operculectomy, excision pericoronal tissues

41822 Excision of fibrous tuberosities, dentoalveolar structures

41823 Excision of osseous tuberosities, dentoalveolar structures

41825 Excision of lesion or tumor (except listed above), dentoalveolar structures; without repair

41826 with simple repair

41827 with complex repair

41828 Excision of hyperplastic alveolar mucosa, each quadrant (specify)

41830 Alveolectomy, including curettage of osteitis or sequestrectomy

41850 Destruction of lesion (except excision), dentoalveolar structures

FIGURE 5-4. Roof of the Mouth

The roof of the mouth separates the oral and nasal cavities. It consists of an anterior **hard palate** that is lined in maxillary bone and a posterior and boneless **soft palate** (**velum**) that terminates at the **uvula**. The soft palate closes off the nasal cavity from the oral cavity during speech, swallowing, and sucking.

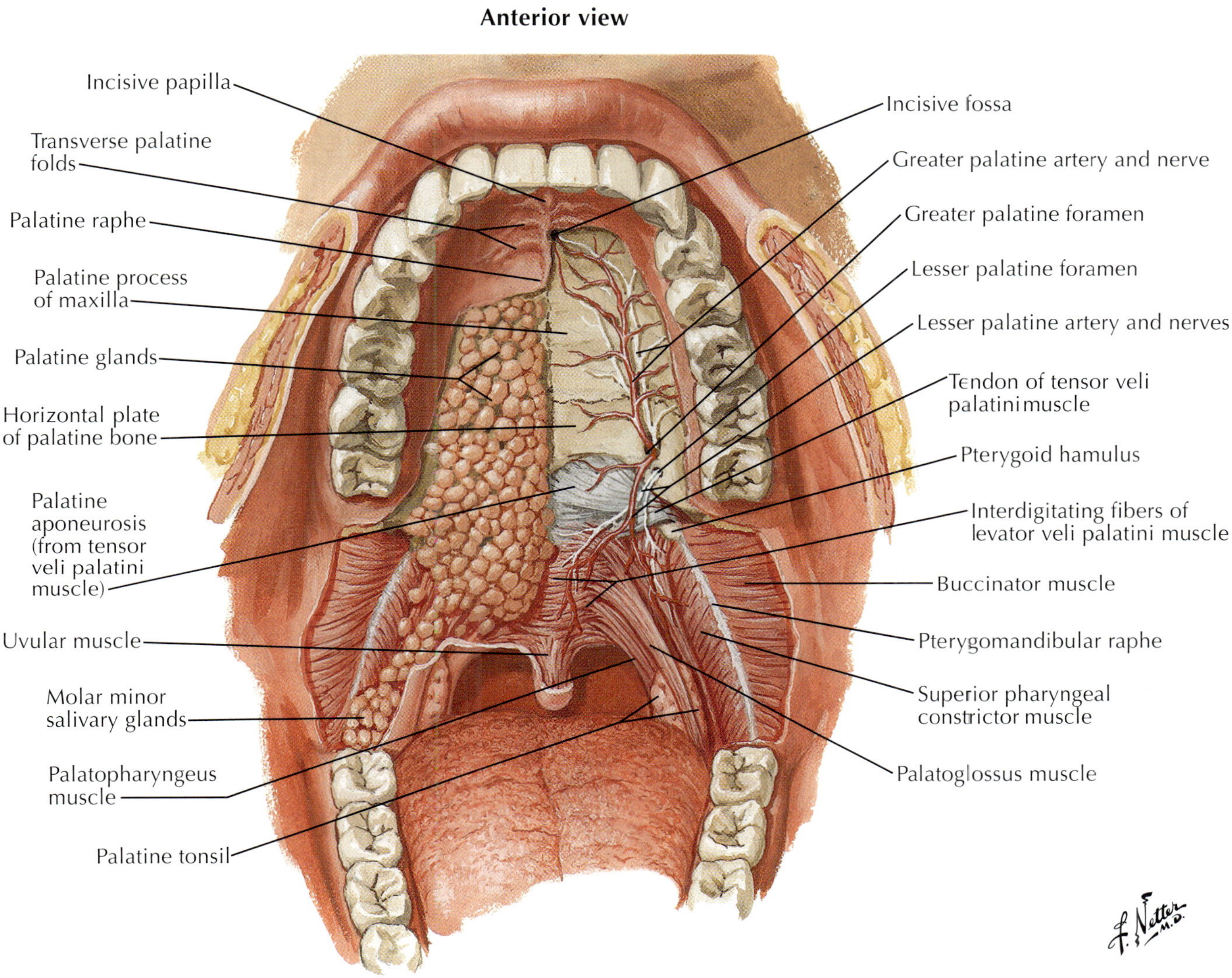

Other Procedures

Coding Atlas

In **gingivoplasty**, diseased gum tissue is removed and reshaped to remove pockets between the gums and teeth. In **alveoloplasty**, alveolar bone is removed to aid in the fitting of a dental **prosthesis**, to gain better access to a tooth, or to smooth the jaw bone.

41870 Periodontal mucosal grafting

41872 Gingivoplasty, each quadrant (specify)

41874 Alveoloplasty, each quadrant (specify)

Palate and Uvula

Incision

42000 Drainage of abscess of palate, uvula

Excision, Destruction

Coding Atlas

In **palatopharyngoplasty**, excess tissue of the **palate** and **oropharynx** is resected to open the airway in an effort to reduce snoring. This is often often called a **uvulopalatopharyngoplasty** (UPPP or UP3).

42100 Biopsy of palate, uvula

42104 Excision, lesion of palate, uvula; without closure

42106 with simple primary closure

42107 with local flap closure

42120 Resection of palate or extensive resection of lesion

42140 Uvulectomy, excision of uvula

42145 Palatopharyngoplasty (eg, uvulopalatopharyngoplasty, uvulopharyngoplasty)

42160 Destruction of lesion, palate or uvula (thermal, cryo or chemical)

Repair

Coding Atlas

A cleft palate (**palatoschisis**) is a **congenital** deformity in which the right and left plates of the **hard palate** do not fuse. Usually, the **soft palate** has a cleft as well. The resulting hole in the roof of the mouth communicates directly with the nasal cavity in what is often referred to as a **velopharyngeal inadequacy** (VPI). The VPI causes difficulties in feeding, speech, and socialization. A cleft palate may occur with a cleft lip (**cheiloschisis**). Both conditions may be repaired surgically.

42180 Repair, laceration of palate; up to 2 cm

42182 over 2 cm or complex

42200 Palatoplasty for cleft palate, soft and/or hard palate only

42205 Palatoplasty for cleft palate, with closure of alveolar ridge; soft tissue only

42210 with bone graft to alveolar ridge (includes obtaining graft)

42215 Palatoplasty for cleft palate; major revision

42220 secondary lengthening procedure

42225 attachment pharyngeal flap

42226 Lengthening of palate, and pharyngeal flap

42227 Lengthening of palate, with island flap

42235 Repair of anterior palate, including vomer flap

42260 Repair of nasolabial fistula

42280 Maxillary impression for palatal prosthesis

42281 Insertion of pin-retained palatal prosthesis

FIGURE 5-5. The Salivary Glands

Salivary glands produce saliva that lubricates and dissolves food. Three sets of major salivary glands occur in **bilateral** pairs: parotid, submandibular, and sublingual. Parotid glands are the largest salivary glands; they release saliva into the mouth through Stensen's ducts in each cheek. Submandibular glands lie beneath the jaw and release saliva through Wharton's ducts on either side of the lingual **frenum** and are sometimes referred to as submaxillary glands. Sublingual glands are in the floor of the mouth and on the sides of the tongue.

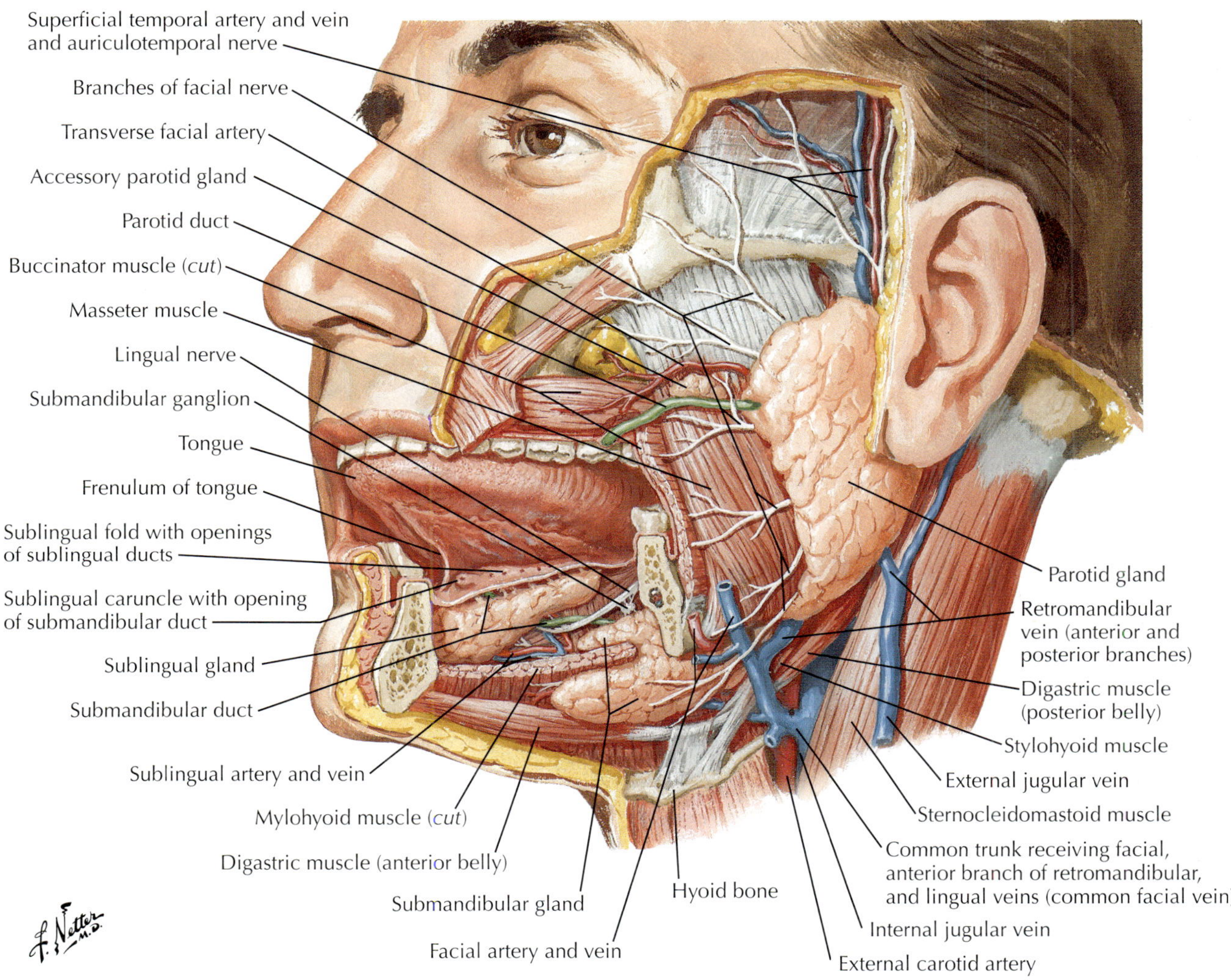

Salivary Gland and Ducts

Incision

Coding Atlas

Sialolithiasis is a condition in which a calculus forms from calcium and other deposits within a salivary gland or salivary duct. Removal that requires incision is called sialolithotomy. The submandibular glands beneath the jaw are the most common site for sialolithiasis, but calculi can form in any of the salivary glands or ducts.

42300 Drainage of abscess; parotid, simple

42305 parotid, complicated

42310 Drainage of abscess; submaxillary or sublingual, intraoral

42320 submaxillary, external

42330 Sialolithotomy; submandibular (submaxillary), sublingual or parotid, uncomplicated, intraoral

42335 submandibular (submaxillary), complicated, intraoral

42340 parotid, extraoral or complicated intraoral

Excision

Coding Atlas

There is no single combined code for the resection of a primary tumor and a modified radical neck dissection (MRND). Therefore, one code is used to report the tumor resection and one code is used to report the MRND (code 38724). Radical neck dissection includes excision of the tumor and is reported using CPT code 38700.

42400 Biopsy of salivary gland; needle

42405 incisional

42408 Excision of sublingual salivary cyst (ranula)

42409 Marsupialization of sublingual salivary cyst (ranula)

42410 Excision of parotid tumor or parotid gland; lateral lobe, without nerve dissection

42415 lateral lobe, with dissection and preservation of facial nerve

42420 total, with dissection and preservation of facial nerve

42425 total, en bloc removal with sacrifice of facial nerve

42426 total, with unilateral radical neck dissection

42440 Excision of submandibular (submaxillary) gland

42450 Excision of sublingual gland

Repair

Coding Atlas

Parotid duct diversion is a treatment for sialorrhea (drooling, ptyalism) that occurs due to neurological damage, for example, in patients with cerebral palsy. In some cases, submandibular glands or ducts may be treated during the parotid duct diversion.

42500 Plastic repair of salivary duct, sialodochoplasty; primary or simple

42505 secondary or complicated

42507 Parotid duct diversion, bilateral (Wilke type procedure);

42509 with excision of both submandibular glands

42510 with ligation of both submandibular (Wharton's) ducts

Other Procedures

Coding Atlas

Ducts of the parotid gland are called Stensen's ducts, while ducts of the submaxillary glands are called Wharton's ducts. The sublingual gland has ducts called the duct of Rivinus, the largest of which is Bartholin's duct.

42550 Injection procedure for sialography

42600 Closure salivary fistula

42650 Dilation salivary duct

42660 Dilation and catheterization of salivary duct, with or without injection

42665 Ligation salivary duct, intraoral

FIGURE 5-6. Opened Posterior View of the Pharynx

The pharynx is divided into three segments: nasopharynx, oropharynx, and laryngopharynx. The oropharynx begins at the back of the mouth and continues down to the epiglottis, which is the flap of tissue at the top of the larynx. The oropharynx is shared by the respiratory and digestive systems. Another view of the pharynx can be seen in Figure 3-7.

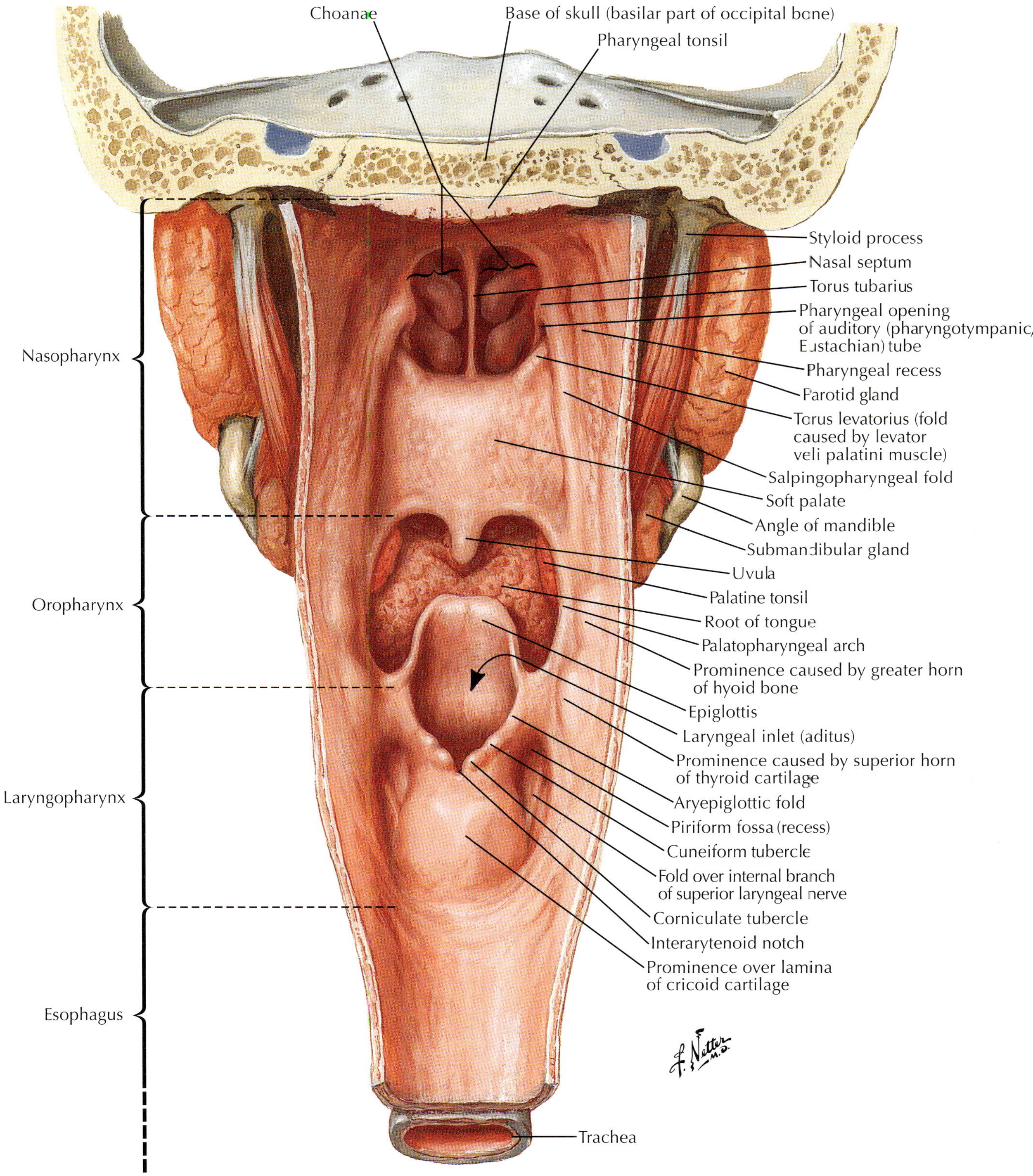

Pharynx, Adenoids, and Tonsils

Incision

Coding Atlas

A peritonsillar abscess is sometimes called a PTA or quinsy. Occurring in patients with tonsillitis, PTA can lead to serious complications including a blocked airway or aspiration of a ruptured abscess. Pharyngeal abscesses may be approached through the mouth (intraoral) or through a cut in the skin of the neck (extraoral).

42700 Incision and drainage abscess; peritonsillar

42720 retropharyngeal or parapharyngeal, intraoral approach

42725 retropharyngeal or parapharyngeal, external approach

Excision, Destruction

Coding Atlas

A branchial cleft cyst is a congenital malformation that arises in the embryo stage. It presents as an epithelium-lined cyst in the neck, usually along the angle of the sternocleidomastoid muscle, and may be limited to subcutaneous tissue or may have deeper structures. Adenoids, also documented as pharyngeal tonsils, are located at the pharyngeal apex. Like all tonsils, adenoids are made of lymphatic tissue.

42800 Biopsy; oropharynx

42804 nasopharynx, visible lesion, simple

42806 nasopharynx, survey for unknown primary lesion

42808 Excision or destruction of lesion of pharynx, any method

42809 Removal of foreign body from pharynx

42810 Excision branchial cleft cyst or vestige, confined to skin and subcutaneous tissues

42815 Excision branchial cleft cyst, vestige, or fistula, extending beneath subcutaneous tissues and/or into pharynx

42820 Tonsillectomy and adenoidectomy; younger than age 12

42821 age 12 or over

42825 Tonsillectomy, primary or secondary; younger than age 12

42826 age 12 or over

42830 Adenoidectomy, primary; younger than age 12

42831 age 12 or over

42835 Adenoidectomy, secondary; younger than age 12

42836 age 12 or over

42842 Radical resection of tonsil, tonsillar pillars, and/or retromolar trigone; without closure

42844 closure with local flap (eg, tongue, buccal)

42845 closure with other flap

42860 Excision of tonsil tags

42870 Excision or destruction lingual tonsil, any method (separate procedure)

42890 Limited pharyngectomy

42892 Resection of lateral pharyngeal wall or pyriform sinus, direct closure by advancement of lateral and posterior pharyngeal walls

42894 Resection of pharyngeal wall requiring closure with myocutaneous or fasciocutaneous flap or free muscle, skin, or fascial flap with microvascular anastomosis

Repair

Coding Atlas

Pharyngoplasty may be performed if cleft palate repair does not provide satisfactory results for speech. A pharyngoplasty improves the function of the soft palate in order to limit the escape of air through the nose during speech.

42900 Suture pharynx for wound or injury

42950 Pharyngoplasty (plastic or reconstructive operation on pharynx)

42953 Pharyngoesophageal repair

Other Procedures

Coding Atlas

Hemorrhage occurs in 1% to 2% of post-tonsillectomy or post-adenoidectomy patients; bleeding may occur in the first 24 hours (primary) or later (secondary). Bleeding may be simple and treatable in the office setting with a technique such as cautery. Persistent or copious bleeding that requires emergency services that may include fluid replacement, pain control, and/or hematologic study may be considered more complex.

42955 Pharyngostomy (fistulization of pharynx, external for feeding)

42960 Control oropharyngeal hemorrhage, primary or secondary (eg, post-tonsillectomy); simple

42961 complicated, requiring hospitalization

42962 with secondary surgical intervention

42970 Control of nasopharyngeal hemorrhage, primary or secondary (eg, postadenoidectomy); simple, with posterior nasal packs, with or without anterior packs and/or cautery

42971 complicated, requiring hospitalization

42972 with secondary surgical intervention

Esophagus

Incision

Coding Atlas

The cricopharyngeous muscle is also known as the upper esophageal sphincter (UES). **Myotomy** describes use of an open approach to incise this muscle in order to treat persistent spasm and symptoms of **dysphagia** and **achalasia**.

43020 Esophagotomy, cervical approach, with removal of foreign body

43030 Cricopharyngeal myotomy

43045 Esophagotomy, thoracic approach, with removal of foreign body

Excision

Coding Atlas

An **esophagectomy** is the excision of all or part of the esophagus. Because the entire **alimentary tract** is composed of similar tissue, a graft from a segment of the intestine or a portion of the stomach may be used to replace the excised portion of esophagus. An open esophagectomy may be performed using a transhiatal (with incisions in the neck and upper abdomen) or transthoracic (with incisions in the chest and upper abdomen) approach.

43100 Excision of lesion, esophagus, with primary repair; cervical approach

43101 thoracic or abdominal approach

43107 Total or near total esophagectomy, without thoracotomy; with pharyngogastrostomy or cervical esophagogastrostomy, with or without pyloroplasty (transhiatal)

43108 with colon interposition or small intestine reconstruction, including intestine mobilization, preparation and anastomosis(es)

43112 Total or near total esophagectomy, with thoracotomy; with pharyngogastrostomy or cervical esophagogastrostomy, with or without pyloroplasty

43113 with colon interposition or small intestine reconstruction, including intestine mobilization, preparation, and anastomosis(es)

43116 Partial esophagectomy, cervical, with free intestinal graft, including microvascular anastomosis, obtaining the graft and intestinal reconstruction

43117 Partial esophagectomy, distal two-thirds, with thoracotomy and separate abdominal incision, with or without proximal gastrectomy; with thoracic esophagogastrostomy, with or without pyloroplasty (Ivor Lewis)

43118 with colon interposition or small intestine reconstruction, including intestine mobilization, preparation, and anastomosis(es)

43121 Partial esophagectomy, distal two-thirds, with thoracotomy only, with or without proximal gastrectomy, with thoracic esophagogastrostomy, with or without pyloroplasty

43122 Partial esophagectomy, thoracoabdominal or abdominal approach, with or without proximal gastrectomy; with esophagogastrostomy, with or without pyloroplasty

43123 with colon interposition or small intestine reconstruction, including intestine mobilization, preparation, and anastomosis(es)

43124 Total or partial esophagectomy, without reconstruction (any approach), with cervical esophagostomy

43130 Diverticulectomy of hypopharynx or esophagus, with or without myotomy; cervical approach

43135 thoracic approach

FIGURE 5-7. Esophagus In Situ

The esophagus is a muscular **lumen** that extends from the pharynx to the stomach. It is divided into three sections: the cervical portion that extends from the pharyngoesophageal junction to the **suprasternal notch**, the thoracic portion that extends from the suprasternal notch to the **diaphragm**, and the abdominal portion that extends from the diaphragm to the cardiac portion of the stomach.

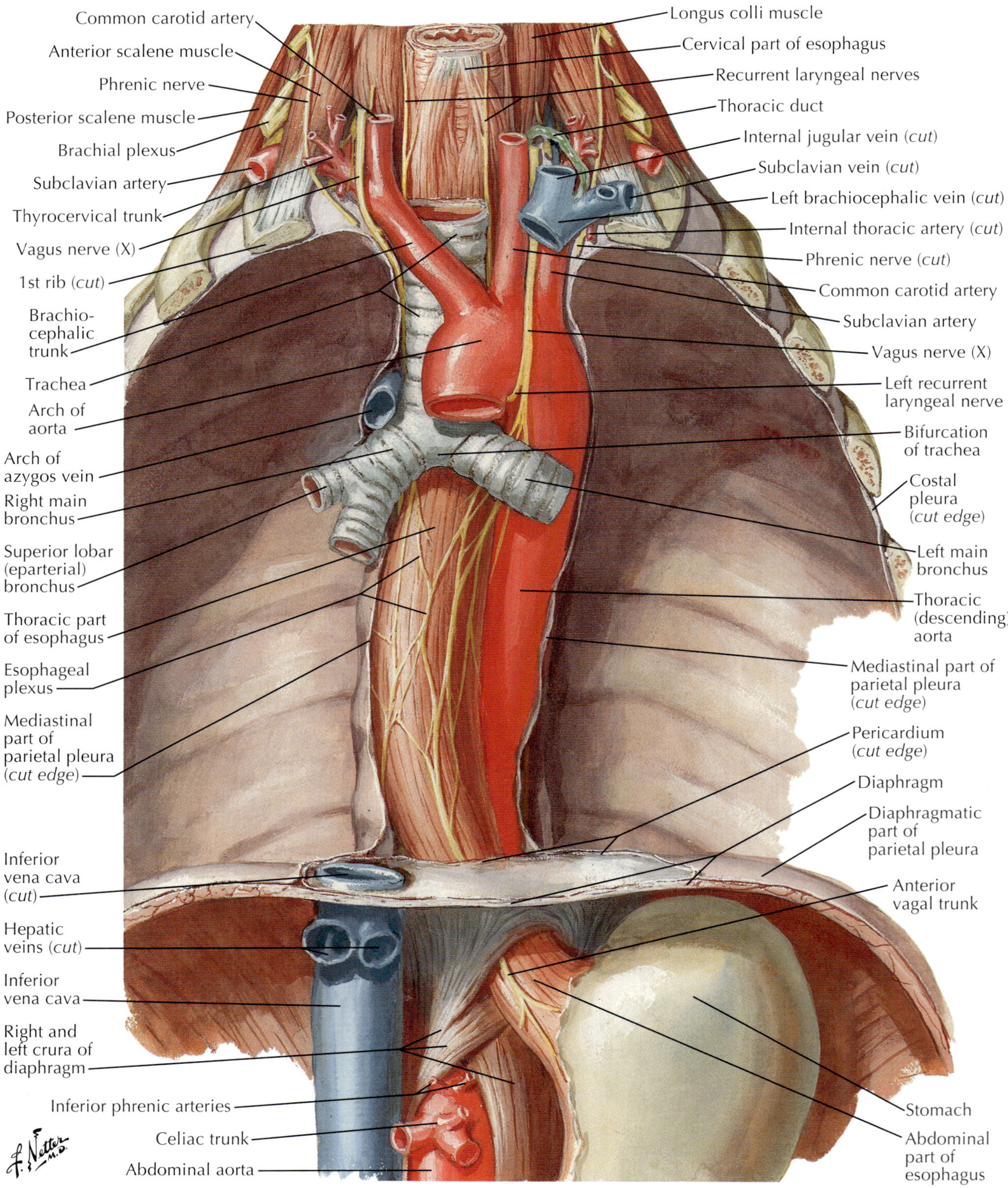

Endoscopy

Coding Atlas

Endoscopy codes within the CPT code set of the Esophagus subsection describe **esophagoscopy** (esophagus only), **esophagogastroduodenoscopy** (EGD; esophagus, stomach, and duodenum), and **endoscopic retrograde cholangiopancreatography** (ERCP; esophagus, stomach, duodenum, and gallbladder [if present] and one or more of the following: pancreatic duct, hepatic duct, common bile duct, or ampulla of Vater). In each case, a camera, light, and tool are threaded along the **alimentary tract** to the site of examination or the site of a known defect. The physician performs the procedure through the lining of the **lumen** without making an external incision. The physician views the camera image on a video display or through an eyepiece. A **percutaneous** endoscopic gastrostomy (PEG) tube is reported using code 43246.

Esophagoscopy

43180 Esophagoscopy, rigid, transoral with diverticulectomy of hypopharynx or cervical esophagus (eg, Zenker's diverticulum), with cricopharyngeal myotomy, includes use of telescope or operating microscope and repair, when performed

43191 Esophagoscopy, rigid, transoral; diagnostic, including collection of specimen(s) by brushing or washing when performed (separate procedure)

43192 with directed submucosal injection(s), any substance

43193 with biopsy, single or multiple

43194 with removal of foreign body(s)

43195 with balloon dilation (less than 30 mm diameter)

43196 with insertion of guide wire followed by dilation over guide wire

43197 Esophagoscopy, flexible, transnasal; diagnostic, including collection of specimen(s) by brushing or washing, when performed (separate procedure)

43198 with biopsy, single or multiple

⊙ **43200** Esophagoscopy, flexible, transoral; diagnostic, including collection of specimen(s) by brushing or washing, when performed (separate procedure)

⊙ **43201** with directed submucosal injection(s), any substance

⊙ **43202** with biopsy, single or multiple

⊙ **43204** with injection sclerosis of esophageal varices

⊙ **43205** with band ligation of esophageal varices

⊙ **43206** with optical endomicroscopy

43211 Code is out of numerical sequence. See 43191-43232

43212 Code is out of numerical sequence. See 43191-43232

43213 Code is out of numerical sequence. See 43191-43232

43214 Code is out of numerical sequence. See 43191-43232

⊙ **43215** with removal of foreign body(s)

⊙ **43216** with removal of tumor(s), polyp(s), or other lesion(s) by hot biopsy forceps

⊙ **43217** with removal of tumor(s), polyp(s), or other lesion(s) by snare technique

#⊙ **43211** with endoscopic mucosal resection

#⊙ **43212** with placement of endoscopic stent (includes pre- and post-dilation and guide wire passage, when performed)

⊙ **43220** with transendoscopic balloon dilation (less than 30 mm diameter)

#⊙ **43213** with dilation of esophagus, by balloon or dilator, retrograde (includes fluoroscopic guidance, when performed)

#⊙ **43214** with dilation of esophagus with balloon (30 mm diameter or larger) (includes fluoroscopic guidance, when performed)

⊙ **43226** with insertion of guide wire followed by passage of dilator(s) over guide wire

⊙ **43227** with control of bleeding, any method

⊙ **43229** with ablation of tumor(s), polyp(s), or other lesion(s) (includes pre- and post-dilation and guide wire passage, when performed)

⊙ **43231** with endoscopic ultrasound examination

⊙ **43232** with transendoscopic ultrasound-guided intramural or transmural fine needle aspiration/biopsy(s)

43233 Code is out of numerical sequence. See 43180-43232

FIGURE 5-8. Esophagograpy and Esophagoscopy

Esophagoscopy can be rigid or flexible, and flexible is preferred in most situations. In esophagoscopy, the scope is advanced to examine the upper esophageal sphincter (cricopharyngeus muscle), esophagus, and gastroesophageal junction. In some cases, tools are carried through the scope to the site of a defect. A camera in the scope transmits images onto a video display. Note: Tools, implants, and/or equipment depicted in the illustration may be outdated but the procedural approach is valid.

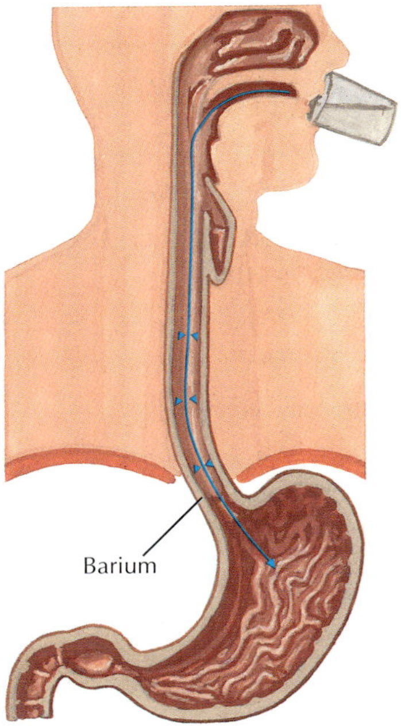

Barium esophagography demonstrates hernia, stricture, ulcer, or other complications in patients with symptomatic reflux

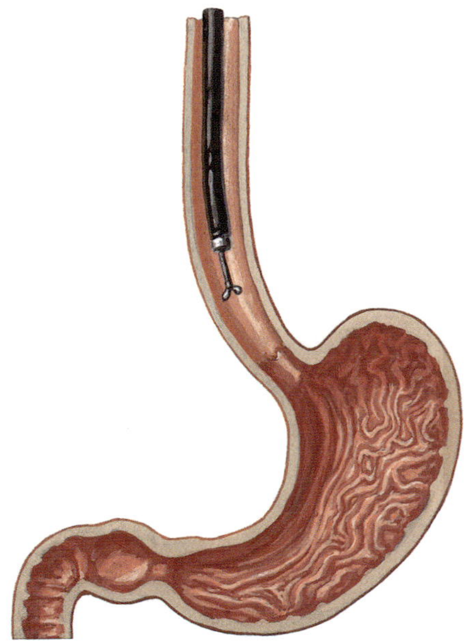

Endoscopy demonstrates esophagitis

Normal esophagoscopic views

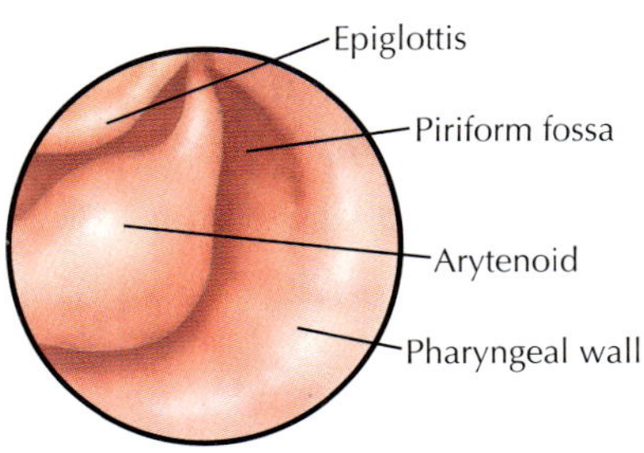

Exposure of piriform fossa

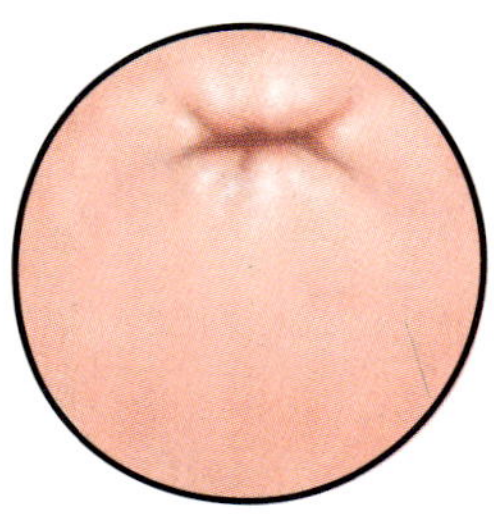

Mouth of esophagus (cricopharyngeus)

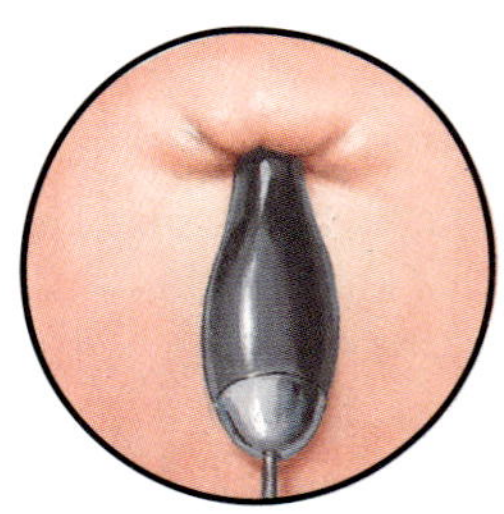

Introduction of lumen-finding bougie to relax cricopharyngeus

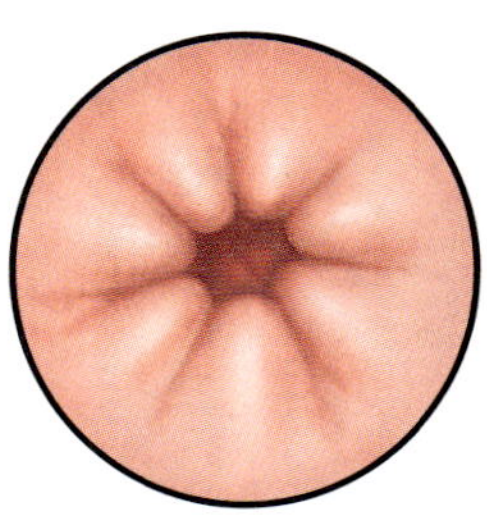

Thoracic esophagus (expiration)

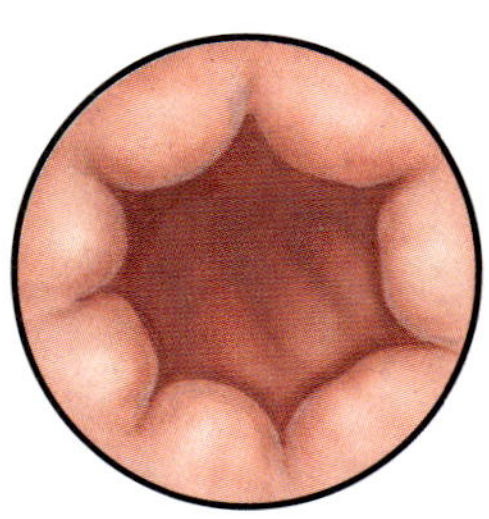

Thoracic esophagus (inspiration)

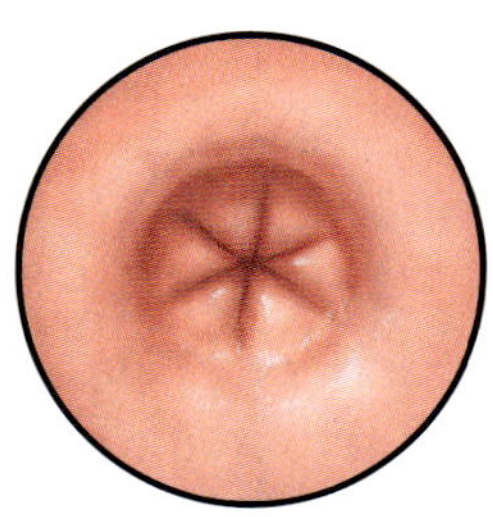

Inferior esophageal sphincter

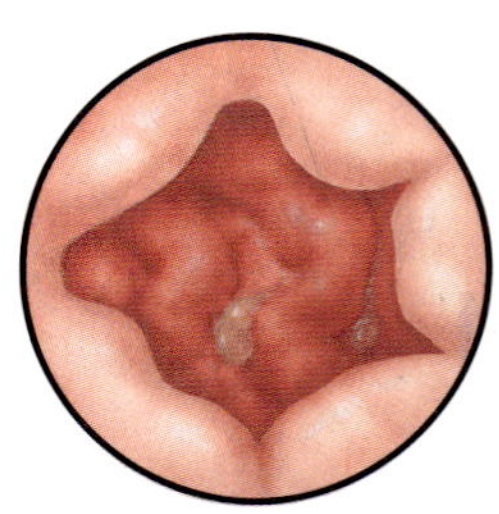

Gastro-esophageal juncture

Esophagogastroduodenoscopy

⊙ **43235** Esophagogastroduodenoscopy, flexible, transoral; diagnostic, including collection of specimen(s) by brushing or washing, when performed (separate procedure)

⊙ **43236** with directed submucosal injection(s), any substance

⊙ **43237** with endoscopic ultrasound examination limited to the esophagus, stomach or duodenum, and adjacent structures

⊙ **43238** with transendoscopic ultrasound-guided intramural or transmural fine needle aspiration/biopsy(s), (includes endoscopic ultrasound examination limited to the esophagus, stomach or duodenum, and adjacent structures)

⊙ **43239** with biopsy, single or multiple

⊙ **43240** with transmural drainage of pseudocyst (includes placement of transmural drainage catheter[s]/stent[s], when performed, and endoscopic ultrasound, when performed)

⊙ **43241** with insertion of intraluminal tube or catheter

⊙ **43242** with transendoscopic ultrasound-guided intramural or transmural fine needle aspiration/biopsy(s) (includes endoscopic ultrasound examination of the esophagus, stomach, and either the duodenum or a surgically altered stomach where the jejunum is examined distal to the anastomosis)

⊙ **43243** with injection sclerosis of esophageal/gastric varices

⊙ **43244** with band ligation of esophageal/gastric varices

⊙ **43245** with dilation of gastric/duodenal stricture(s) (eg, balloon, bougie)

⊙ **43246** with directed placement of percutaneous gastrostomy tube

⊙ **43247** with removal of foreign body(s)

⊙ **43248** with insertion of guide wire followed by passage of dilator(s) through esophagus over guide wire

⊙ **43249** with transendoscopic balloon dilation of esophagus (less than 30 mm diameter)

#⊙ **43233** with dilation of esophagus with balloon (30 mm diameter or larger) (includes fluoroscopic guidance, when performed)

⊙ **43250** with removal of tumor(s), polyp(s), or other lesion(s) by hot biopsy forceps

⊙ **43251** with removal of tumor(s), polyp(s), or other lesion(s) by snare technique

⊙ **43252** with optical endomicroscopy

⊙ **43253** with transendoscopic ultrasound-guided transmural injection of diagnostic or therapeutic substance(s) (eg, anesthetic, neurolytic agent) or fiducial marker(s) (includes endoscopic ultrasound examination of the esophagus, stomach, and either the duodenum or a surgically altered stomach where the jejunum is examined distal to the anastomosis)

⊙ **43254** with endoscopic mucosal resection

⊙ **43255** with control of bleeding, any method

#⊙ **43266** with placement of endoscopic stent (includes pre- and post-dilation and guide wire passage, when performed)

⊙ **43257** with delivery of thermal energy to the muscle of lower esophageal sphincter and/or gastric cardia, for treatment of gastroesophageal reflux disease

#⊙ **43270** with ablation of tumor(s), polyp(s), or other lesion(s) (includes pre- and post-dilation and guide wire passage, when performed)

⊙ **43259** with endoscopic ultrasound examination, including the esophagus, stomach, and either the duodenum or a surgically altered stomach where the jejunum is examined distal to the anastomosis

Endoscopic Retrograde Cholangiopancreatography (ERCP)

⊙ **43260** Endoscopic retrograde cholangiopancreatography (ERCP); diagnostic, including collection of specimen(s) by brushing or washing, when performed (separate procedure)

⊙ **43261** with biopsy, single or multiple

⊙ **43262** with sphincterotomy/papillotomy

⊙ **43263** with pressure measurement of sphincter of Oddi

⊙ **43264** with removal of calculi/debris from biliary/pancreatic duct(s)

⊙ **43265** with destruction of calculi, any method (eg, mechanical, electrohydraulic, lithotripsy)

43266 Code is out of numerical sequence. See 43235-43273

43270 Code is out of numerical sequence. See 43235-43273

#⊙ **43274** with placement of endoscopic stent into biliary or pancreatic duct, including pre- and post-dilation and guide wire passage, when performed, including sphincterotomy, when performed, each stent

#⊙ **43275** with removal of foreign body(s) or stent(s) from biliary/pancreatic duct(s)

#⊙ **43276** with removal and exchange of stent(s), biliary or pancreatic duct, including pre- and post-dilation and guide wire passage, when performed, including sphincterotomy, when performed, each stent exchanged

FIGURE 5-9. Stomach Anatomy and Esophagogastroduodenoscopy

Esophagogastroduodenoscopy (EGD) includes examination of the lining of the esophagus, stomach, and duodenum; the scope must advance beyond the pylorus in an EGD. Strong acids that digest food in the stomach can also contribute to erosion of the stomach's lining (ulcer). The visualization provided by an EGD may aid in the identification of the source of upper gastrointestinal bleeding from a gastric ulcer. Also, an EGD may be used to deliver tools for therapeutic interventions, eg, control of bleeding.

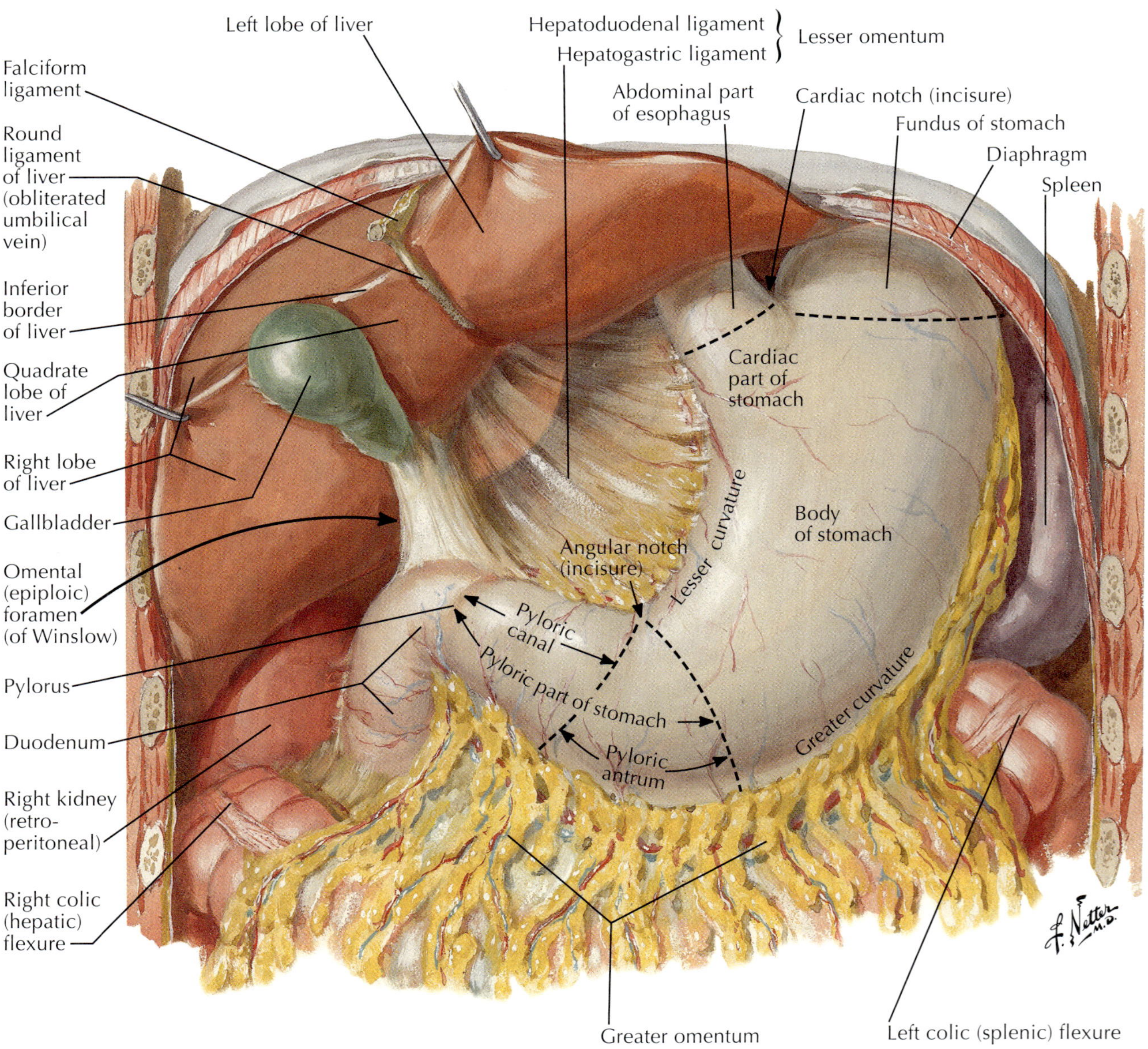

FIGURE 5-10. Duodenum In Situ

The duodenum lies immediately **distal** to the pylorus and is the connection site for ducts carrying enzymes, bicarbonate, and **bile** from the liver, pancreas, and gallbladder. The **superior** segment of the duodenum is the segment of the intestine that is exposed to the highest level of acidic gastric secretions and consequently is a common site for ulcers.

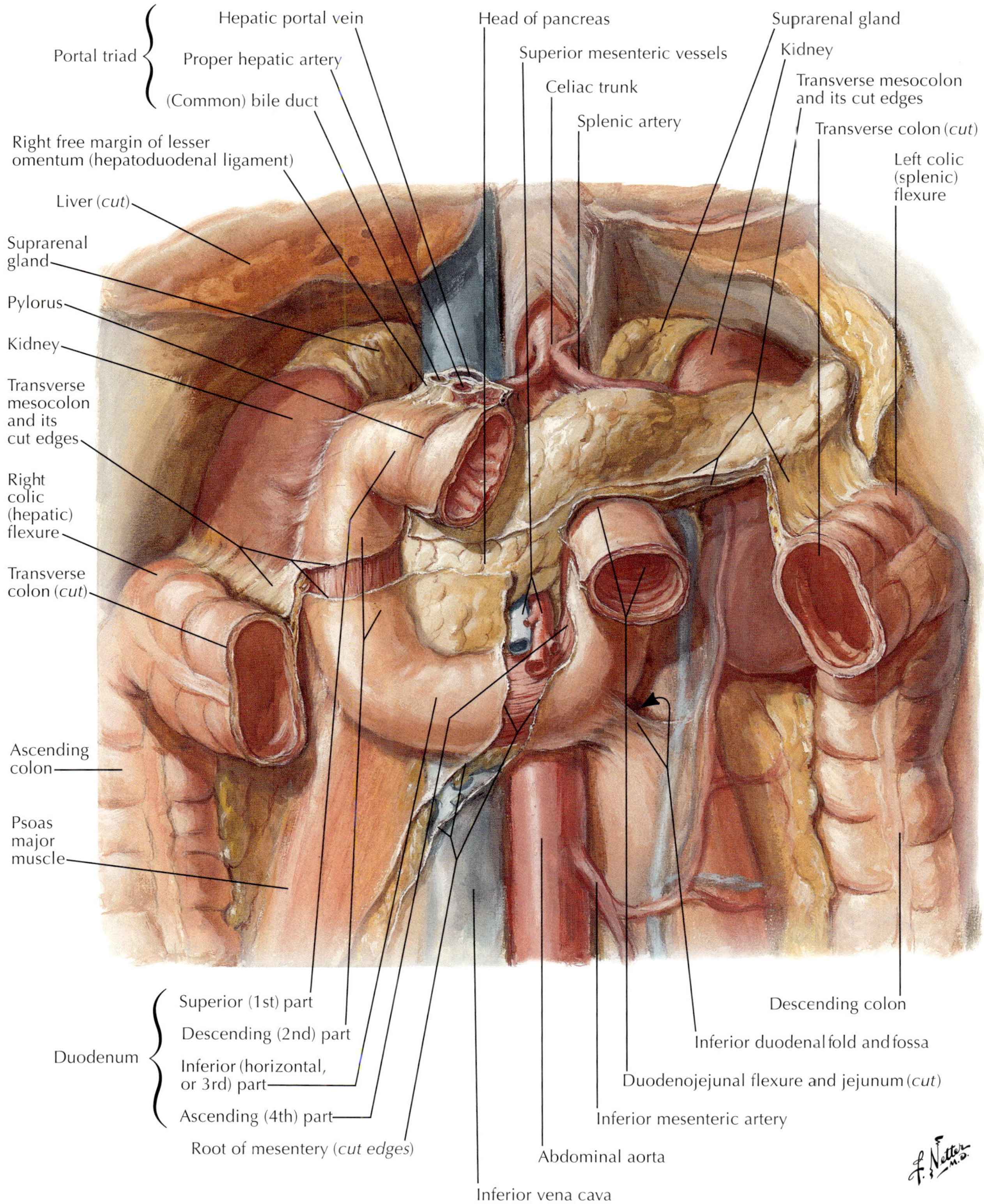

FIGURE 5-11. Endoscopic Retrograde Cholangiopancreatography Imaging Studies

Endoscopic retrograde cholangiopancreatography (ERCP) includes an upper gastrointestinal endoscopic evaluation. In addition, a catheter attached to the endoscope is guided into the papillary opening in the duodenum, and contrast medium is injected into the ducts. This contrast is visible on X ray and reveals any stenosis or blockage in the ducts. Procedures to treat the blockage or stenosis may be performed during ERCP. Note: Tools, implants, and/or equipment depicted in the illustration may be outdated but the procedural approach is valid.

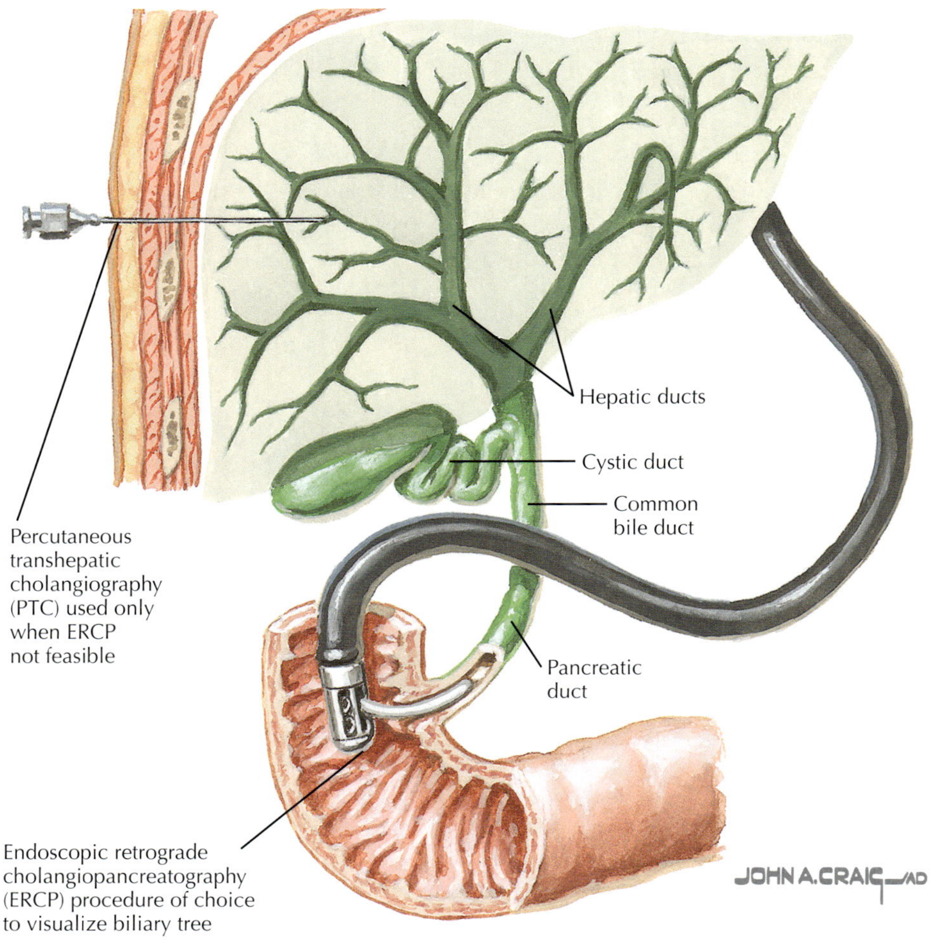

#⊙ **43277** with trans-endoscopic balloon dilation of biliary/pancreatic duct(s) or of ampulla (sphincteroplasty), including sphincterotomy, when performed, each duct

#⊙ **43278** with ablation of tumor(s), polyp(s), or other lesion(s), including pre- and post-dilation and guide wire passage, when performed

⊙✚ **43273** Endoscopic cannulation of papilla with direct visualization of pancreatic/common bile duct(s) (List separately in addition to code(s) for primary procedure)

43274 Code is out of numerical sequence. See 43260-43273

43275 Code is out of numerical sequence. See 43260-43273

43276 Code is out of numerical sequence. See 43260-43273

43277 Code is out of numerical sequence. See 43260-43273

43278 Code is out of numerical sequence. See 43260-43273

Laparoscopy

Coding Atlas

An esophagogastric **fundoplasty** (Nissen, Belsey, Toupet, or Dor fundoplication) creates a new valve between the esophagus and the stomach. This is achieved by wrapping a portion of the fundus of the stomach around the lower end of the esophagus; it is usually a treatment for **gastric reflux**. Esophagogastric fundoplasty can be performed laparoscopically, ie, through multiple small incisions in the abdomen and using a camera for visualization of the operation site. CPT codes 43327 and 43328 are used to report an open approach for esophagogastric fundoplasty.

43279 Laparoscopy, surgical, esophagomyotomy (Heller type), with fundoplasty, when performed

43280 Laparoscopy, surgical, esophagogastric fundoplasty (eg, Nissen, Toupet procedures)

43281 Laparoscopy, surgical, repair of paraesophageal hernia, includes fundoplasty, when performed; without implantation of mesh

43282 with implantation of mesh

✚ **43283** Laparoscopy, surgical, esophageal lengthening procedure (eg, Collis gastroplasty or wedge gastroplasty) (List separately in addition to code for primary procedure)

Repair

Coding Atlas

An esophagogastric **fundoplasty** (Nissen, Belsey, Toupet, or Dor **fundoplication**) creates a new valve between the esophagus and the stomach. This is done by wrapping a portion of the fundus of the stomach around the lower end of the esophagus; it is often used to treat **gastric reflux**. Esophagogastric fundoplasty can be performed by **laparotomy** (code 43327) or **thoracotomy** (code 43328), ie, through a single incision in the abdomen or chest with **direct visualization** of the operation site. CPT code 43280 is used to report a **laparoscopic** approach for esophagogastric fundoplasty.

43300 Esophagoplasty (plastic repair or reconstruction), cervical approach; without repair of tracheoesophageal fistula

43305 with repair of tracheoesophageal fistula

43310 Esophagoplasty (plastic repair or reconstruction), thoracic approach; without repair of tracheoesophageal fistula

43312 with repair of tracheoesophageal fistula

43313 Esophagoplasty for congenital defect (plastic repair or reconstruction), thoracic approach; without repair of congenital tracheoesophageal fistula

43314 with repair of congenital tracheoesophageal fistula

43320 Esophagogastrostomy (cardioplasty), with or without vagotomy and pyloroplasty, transabdominal or transthoracic approach

43325 Esophagogastric fundoplasty; with fundic patch (Thal-Nissen procedure)

43327 Esophagogastric fundoplasty partial or complete; laparotomy

43328 thoracotomy

43330 Esophagomyotomy (Heller type); abdominal approach

43331 thoracic approach

43332 Repair, paraesophageal hiatal hernia (including fundoplication), via laparotomy, except neonatal; without implantation of mesh or other prosthesis

43333 with implantation of mesh or other prosthesis

43334 Repair, paraesophageal hiatal hernia (including fundoplication), via thoracotomy, except neonatal; without implantation of mesh or other prosthesis

43335 with implantation of mesh or other prosthesis

43336 Repair, paraesophageal hiatal hernia, (including fundoplication), via thoracoabdominal incision, except neonatal; without implantation of mesh or other prosthesis

43337 with implantation of mesh or other prosthesis

✚ **43338** Esophageal lengthening procedure (eg, Collis gastroplasty or wedge gastroplasty) (List separately in addition to code for primary procedure)

43340 Esophagojejunostomy (without total gastrectomy); abdominal approach

43341 thoracic approach

43351 Esophagostomy, fistulization of esophagus, external; thoracic approach

43352 cervical approach

43360 Gastrointestinal reconstruction for previous esophagectomy, for obstructing esophageal lesion or fistula, or for previous esophageal exclusion; with stomach, with or without pyloroplasty

43361 with colon interposition or small intestine reconstruction, including intestine mobilization, preparation, and anastomosis(es)

43400 Ligation, direct, esophageal varices

43401 Transection of esophagus with repair, for esophageal varices

43405 Ligation or stapling at gastroesophageal junction for pre-existing esophageal perforation

FIGURE 5-12. Nissen Fundoplication

In a Nissen **fundoplication**, the upper curve of the stomach (**fundus**) is wrapped around the esophagus to strengthen the esophageal valve; it is used to treat gastric **reflux** that, in some cases, is caused by a hiatal **hernia**. The procedure can be performed as an **open** surgery through the abdomen or chest, as shown in Figure 5-12; however, the laparoscopic approach is more common. Note: Tools, implants, and/or equipment depicted in the illustration may be outdated but the procedural approach is valid.

A. Crural closure. Thick bites of crural pillars are taken with nonabsorbable suture, ensuring traversal of endoabdominal fascia to help prevent recurrence.

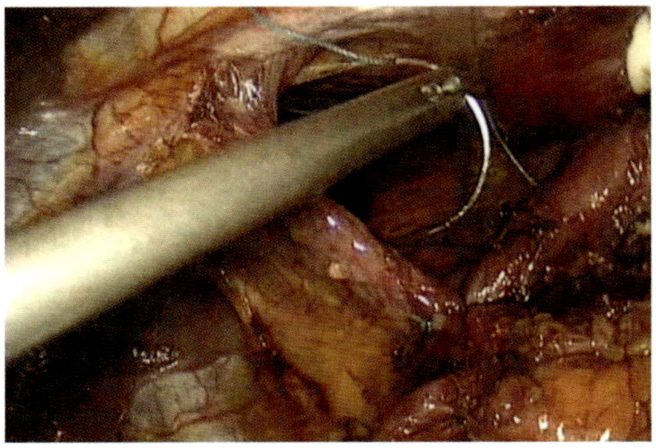

B. Posterior gastric fundus

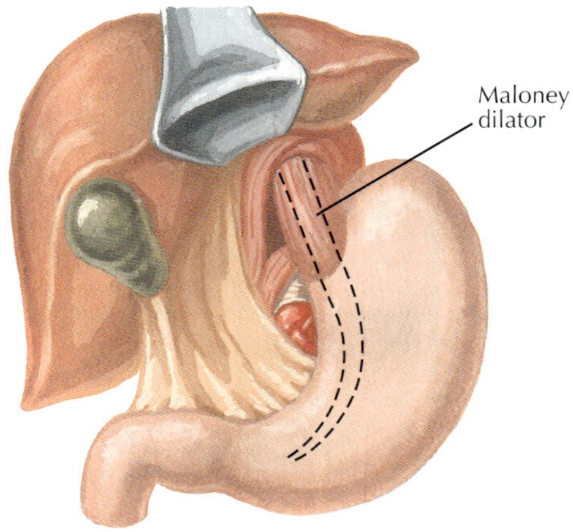

1. Esophagogastric junction exposed through upper abdominal incision. Hernia reduced and Maloney dilator passed into stomach.

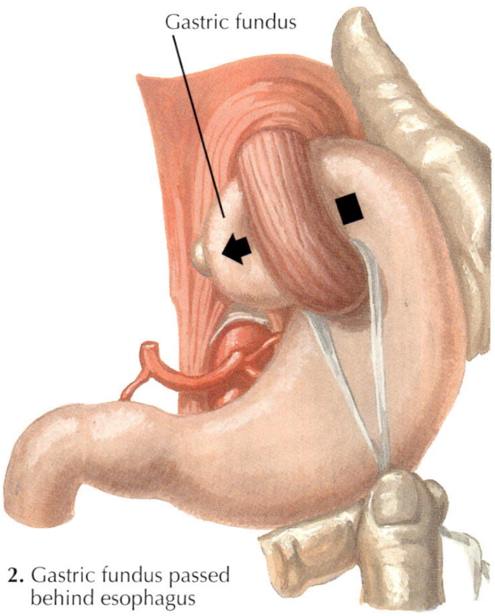

2. Gastric fundus passed behind esophagus

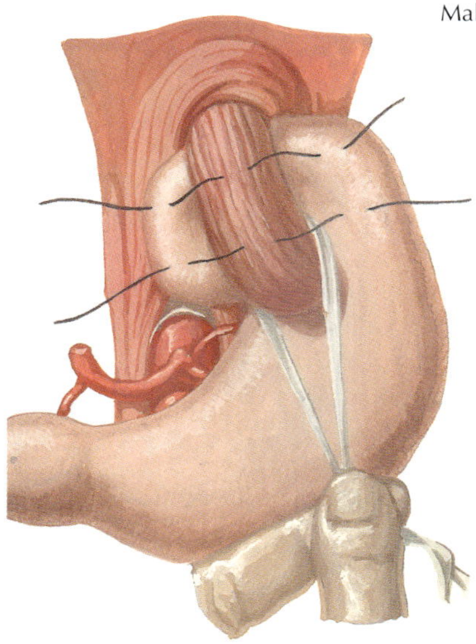

3. Heavy interrupted silk sutures passed through seromuscular layers of fundus, lightly incorporating anterior esophageal wall.

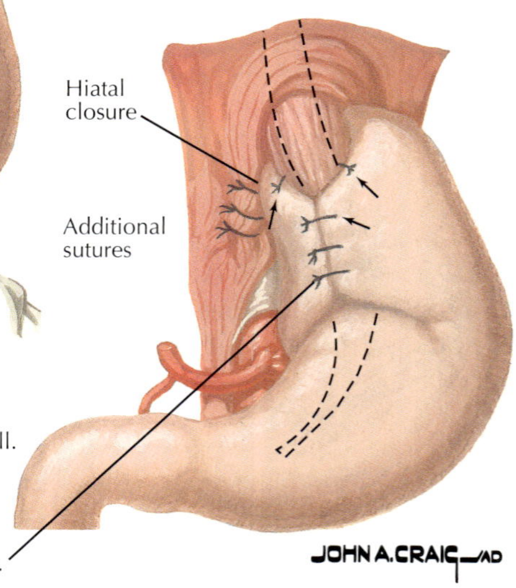

4. Sutures tied, creating 360° fundoplication around distal esophagus.

43410 Suture of esophageal wound or injury; cervical approach

43415 transthoracic or transabdominal approach

43420 Closure of esophagostomy or fistula; cervical approach

43425 transthoracic or transabdominal approach

Manipulation

Coding Atlas

Stenosis of the esophagus can be treated by **dilation** to stretch the esophageal **lumen**. Codes in this section are used to is used to report a direct, **intraoral** approach. The esophagus can be dilated with a sound or bougie (code 43450) or dilated following the insertion of a guidewire, which is generally placed using **fluoroscopic guidance** and without the use of an endoscope (code 43453). An esophageal **tamponade** with balloon is used to treat **hemorrhage** of esophageal **varices**.

43450 Dilation of esophagus, by unguided sound or bougie, single or multiple passes

⊙ 43453 Dilation of esophagus, over guide wire

43460 Esophagogastric tamponade, with balloon (Sengstaken type)

Other Procedures

43496 Free jejunum transfer with microvascular anastomosis

Stomach

Incision

Coding Atlas

Pyloromyotomy is used to treat pyloric **stenosis**; the pyloric muscle is incised along its length to increase the size of the **lumen**. Code 43520 is used to report an open procedure to access the pylorus. This procedure is usually performed on infants with **hypertrophic** pyloric stenosis.

43500 Gastrotomy; with exploration or foreign body removal

43501 with suture repair of bleeding ulcer

43502 with suture repair of pre-existing esophagogastric laceration (eg, Mallory-Weiss)

43510 with esophageal dilation and insertion of permanent intraluminal tube (eg, Celestin or Mousseaux-Barbin)

43520 Pyloromyotomy, cutting of pyloric muscle (Fredet-Ramstedt type operation)

Excision

Coding Atlas

CPT codes 43605-43641 are used to report an **open** approach through an incision in the skin, subcutaneous tissue, and omentum. This approach provides **direct visualization** of the surgical site within the stomach.

43605 Biopsy of stomach, by laparotomy

43610 Excision, local; ulcer or benign tumor of stomach

43611 malignant tumor of stomach

43620 Gastrectomy, total; with esophagoenterostomy

43621 with Roux-en-Y reconstruction

43622 with formation of intestinal pouch, any type

43631 Gastrectomy, partial, distal; with gastroduodenostomy

43632 with gastrojejunostomy

43633 with Roux-en-Y reconstruction

43634 with formation of intestinal pouch

✚ 43635 Vagotomy when performed with partial distal gastrectomy (List separately in addition to code[s] for primary procedure)

43640 Vagotomy including pyloroplasty, with or without gastrostomy; truncal or selective

43641 parietal cell (highly selective)

Laparoscopy

Coding Atlas

Bariatrics refers to medical prevention and treatment of obesity, and bariatric surgery is performed to limit the assimilation of calories by **obese** patients. This may be accomplished by surgically reducing the size of the stomach or by surgically altering the small intestine, where nutritional uptake to the bloodstream occurs. In the CPT code set, bariatric procedures are reported using codes 43644-43645, 43770-43775, and 43886-43888.

43644 Laparoscopy, surgical, gastric restrictive procedure; with gastric bypass and Roux-en-Y gastroenterostomy (roux limb 150 cm or less)

43645 with gastric bypass and small intestine reconstruction to limit absorption

43647 Laparoscopy, surgical; implantation or replacement of gastric neurostimulator electrodes, antrum

43648 revision or removal of gastric neurostimulator electrodes, antrum

FIGURE 5-13. The Stomach

The lining of the stomach contains **rugae**, or folds, that relax to increase capacity during gustation. The pyloric valve is at the stomach base and empties into the duodenum. The main function of the pyloric valve is to prevent **backflow** of food from the small intestine. Gastric ulcers occur in the lining of the stomach or in the first part of the small intestine (duodenum). The condition is often called peptic ulcer disease (PUD).

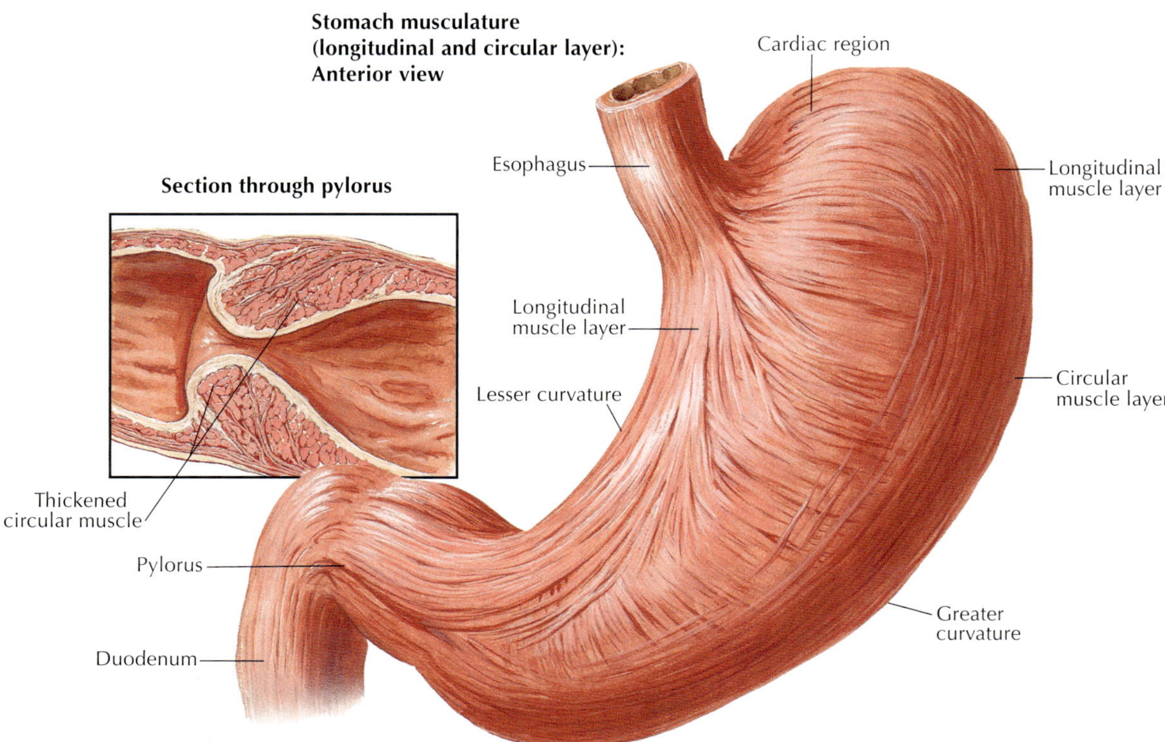

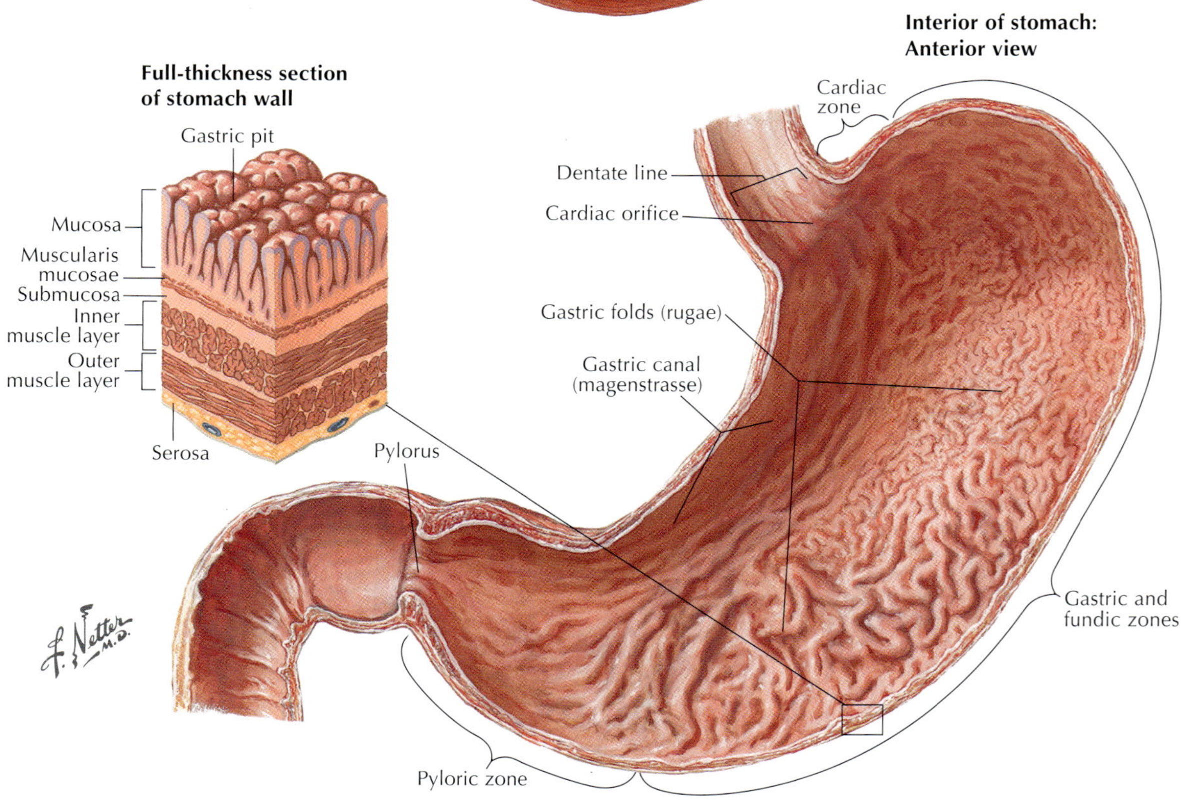

FIGURE 5-14. Abdominal Regions and Planes

For **diagnostic** purposes, the abdomen is divided into imaginary regions and **planes** using skeletal and soft tissue landmarks. These regions and planes are often noted in documentation, as symptoms associated with specific regions or planes may align with specific differential diagnoses being explored. For example, pain in the right lower quadrant may be associated with appendicitis, while pain in the epigastric region may point to biliary disease or hiatal hernia.

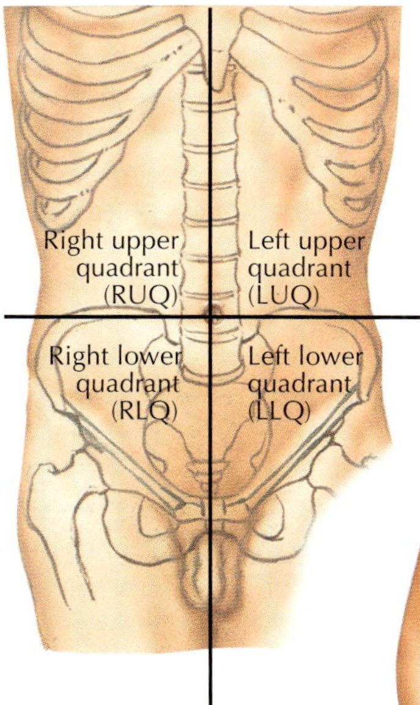

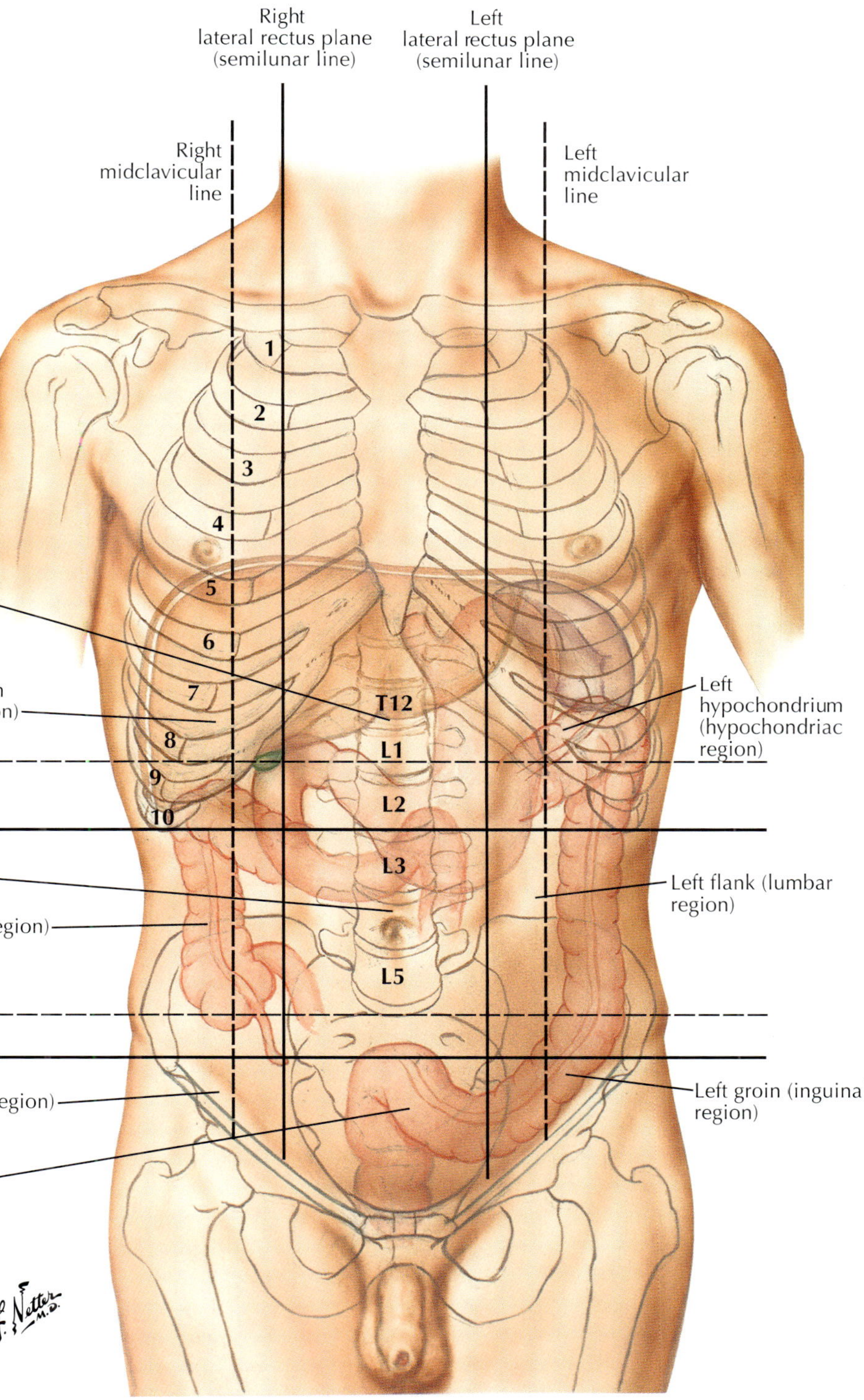

43651 Laparoscopy, surgical; transection of vagus nerves, truncal

43652 transection of vagus nerves, selective or highly selective

43653 gastrostomy, without construction of gastric tube (eg, Stamm procedure) (separate procedure)

Introduction

Coding Atlas

Nasogastric (NG) and orogastric (OG) tubes are advanced into the stomach for therapeutic **aspiration** or **lavage**, eg, for poisoning or gastrointestinal hemorrhage; for feeding or administration of **contrast**; or for diagnostic testing, eg, stomach content analysis. In some cases, the NG/OG tube is advanced past the pyloric valve into the duodenum.

43752 Naso- or oro-gastric tube placement, requiring physician's skill and fluoroscopic guidance (includes fluoroscopy, image documentation and report)

43753 Gastric intubation and aspiration(s) therapeutic, necessitating physician's skill (eg, for gastrointestinal hemorrhage), including lavage if performed

43754 Gastric intubation and aspiration, diagnostic; single specimen (eg, acid analysis)

43755 collection of multiple fractional specimens with gastric stimulation, single or double lumen tube (gastric secretory study) (eg, histamine, insulin, pentagastrin, calcium, secretin), includes drug administration

43756 Duodenal intubation and aspiration, diagnostic, includes image guidance; single specimen (eg, bile study for crystals or afferent loop culture)

43757 collection of multiple fractional specimens with pancreatic or gallbladder stimulation, single or double lumen tube, includes drug administration

43760 Change of gastrostomy tube, percutaneous, without imaging or endoscopic guidance

43761 Repositioning of a naso- or oro-gastric feeding tube, through the duodenum for enteric nutrition

Bariatric Surgery

Coding Atlas

Bariatrics refers to medical prevention and treatment of obesity, and bariatric surgery is performed to limit the assimilation of calories by **obese** patients. This may be accomplished by surgically reducing the size of the stomach or by surgically altering the small intestine, where nutritional uptake to the bloodstream occurs. In the CPT code set, bariatric procedures are reported using codes 43644-43645, 43770-43775, and 43886-43888.

Laparoscopy

43770 Laparoscopy, surgical, gastric restrictive procedure; placement of adjustable gastric restrictive device (eg, gastric band and subcutaneous port components)

43771 revision of adjustable gastric restrictive device component only

43772 removal of adjustable gastric restrictive device component only

43773 removal and replacement of adjustable gastric restrictive device component only

43774 removal of adjustable gastric restrictive device and subcutaneous port components

43775 longitudinal gastrectomy (ie, sleeve gastrectomy)

Other Procedures

Coding Atlas

The vagus nerve may be resected in a patient with duodenal or gastric peptic ulcer disease (PUD) if medications are unsuccessful in controlling stomach acid secretions. In highly selective **vagotomy** (HSV), only the **fundus** and body of the stomach are **denervated**. This is sometimes called a parietal cell vagotomy (PCV) or proximal gastric vagotomy (PGV). A Janeway **gastrostomy** differs from a Stamm gastrostomy in that in the Janeway procedure, a full-thickness stomach flap is taken from the greater curvature of the stomach to create an ostomy tunnel that is sutured to the skin. The mucosa-lined stomach tissue is secured as a tube around a catheter and heals to become a permanent tunnel and ostomy site not requiring a catheter. In the Stamm procedure, the ostomy site is fitted with a catheter but is not lined in mucosa and is considered a temporary communication.

FIGURE 5-15. Bariatric Options

Options for **bariatric** surgery include **gastric bypass** with **Roux-en-Y**, gastric **stapling**, and gastric banding. While bypass and stapling both result in permanent changes to the patient's anatomy, a banding procedure can be reversed. In gastric banding, an adjustable band encircles the stomach, creating a small pouch that limits the amount of food intake. A laparoscopic adjustable gastric band (lap-band, LAGB) is inflatable and can be adjusted through a subcutaneous portal as the patient loses weight. Note: Tools, implants, and/or equipment depicted in the illustration may be outdated but the procedural approach is valid.

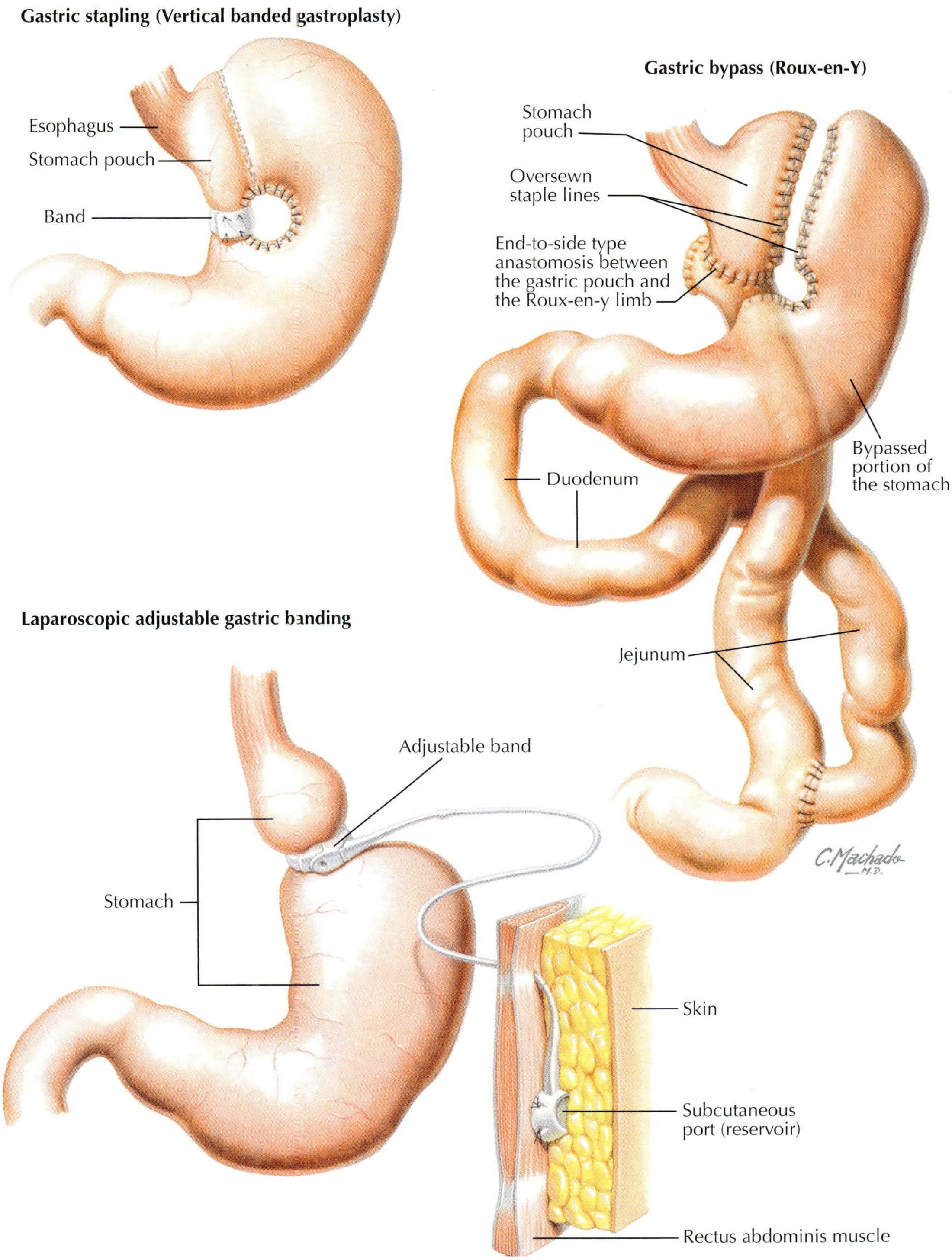

43800 Pyloroplasty

43810 Gastroduodenostomy

43820 Gastrojejunostomy; without vagotomy

43825 with vagotomy, any type

43830 Gastrostomy, open; without construction of gastric tube (eg, Stamm procedure) (separate procedure)

43831 neonatal, for feeding

43832 with construction of gastric tube (eg, Janeway procedure)

43840 Gastrorrhaphy, suture of perforated duodenal or gastric ulcer, wound, or injury

43842 Gastric restrictive procedure, without gastric bypass, for morbid obesity; vertical-banded gastroplasty

43843 other than vertical-banded gastroplasty

43845 Gastric restrictive procedure with partial gastrectomy, pylorus-preserving duodenoileostomy and ileoileostomy (50 to 100 cm common channel) to limit absorption (biliopancreatic diversion with duodenal switch)

43846 Gastric restrictive procedure, with gastric bypass for morbid obesity; with short limb (150 cm or less) Roux-en-Y gastroenterostomy

43847 with small intestine reconstruction to limit absorption

43848 Revision, open, of gastric restrictive procedure for morbid obesity, other than adjustable gastric restrictive device (separate procedure)

43850 Revision of gastroduodenal anastomosis (gastroduodenostomy) with reconstruction; without vagotomy

43855 with vagotomy

43860 Revision of gastrojejunal anastomosis (gastrojejunostomy) with reconstruction, with or without partial gastrectomy or intestine resection; without vagotomy

43865 with vagotomy

43870 Closure of gastrostomy, surgical

43880 Closure of gastrocolic fistula

43881 Implantation or replacement of gastric neurostimulator electrodes, antrum, open

43882 Revision or removal of gastric neurostimulator electrodes, antrum, open

43886 Gastric restrictive procedure, open; revision of subcutaneous port component only

43887 removal of subcutaneous port component only

43888 removal and replacement of subcutaneous port component only

Intestines (Except Rectum)

Incision

Coding Atlas

Adult small and large intestines are more than 20 feet in combined length, and any kink or disruption in the **lumen** can result in blockage of the flow of nutrients, gas, and **feces** through the **alimentary tract**. In **enterolysis**, intestinal tissue is freed from fibrous scars. **Malrotation** is an anomalous twisting of the intestine, while **volvulus** is the complete twisting of a loop of intestine around its mesenteric attachment. **Intussusception** is a condition in which the intestine collapses into itself, causing a blockage.

44005 Enterolysis (freeing of intestinal adhesion) (separate procedure)

44010 Duodenotomy, for exploration, biopsy(s), or foreign body removal

✚ 44015 Tube or needle catheter jejunostomy for enteral alimentation, intraoperative, any method (List separately in addition to primary procedure)

44020 Enterotomy, small intestine, other than duodenum; for exploration, biopsy(s), or foreign body removal

44021 for decompression (eg, Baker tube)

44025 Colotomy, for exploration, biopsy(s), or foreign body removal

44050 Reduction of volvulus, intussusception, internal hernia, by laparotomy

44055 Correction of malrotation by lysis of duodenal bands and/or reduction of midgut volvulus (eg, Ladd procedure)

FIGURE 5-16. The Large Intestine

The large intestine begins at the cecum and continues with ascending, transverse, and descending segments before connecting to the rectum. Intestinal contents are liquid when they enter the large intestine, where most of the water is absorbed before defecation. The word "colon" is a synonym for large intestine; thus, a colonoscopy is an endoscopy of the entire large intestine.

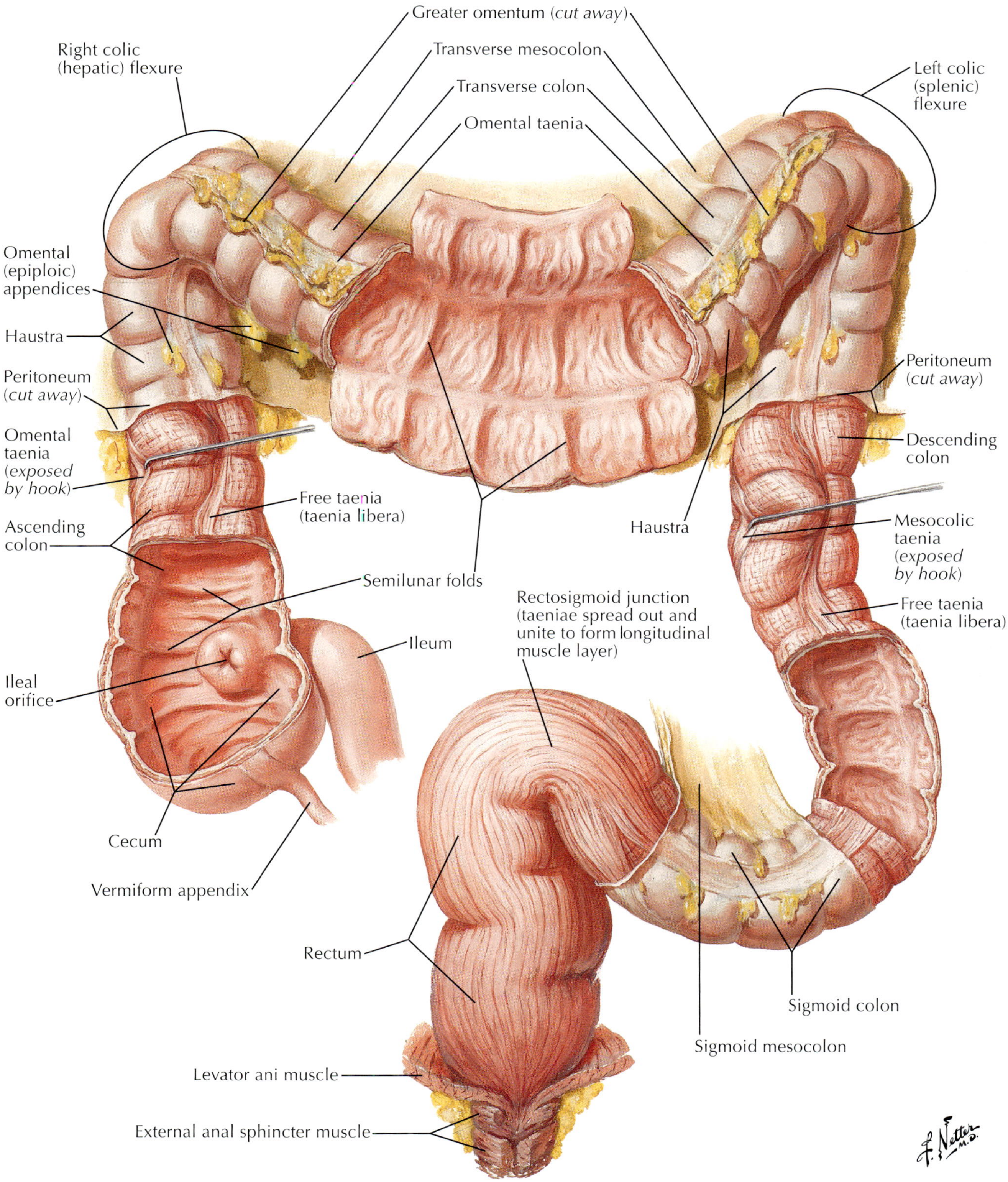

Excision

Coding Atlas

Enterectomy is the excision of a segment of small intestine, while **colectomy** is the excision of a segment of large intestine. When a segment of intestine is excised, the remaining **proximal** and **distal** ends are sutured so that the **lumen**'s continuity is restored. This suturing is called **anastamosis**. If the ends being sutured are not the same dimension, one end may be surgically tapered so that the anastomosis provides a smooth transition.

44100 Biopsy of intestine by capsule, tube, peroral (1 or more specimens)

44110 Excision of 1 or more lesions of small or large intestine not requiring anastomosis, exteriorization, or fistulization; single enterotomy

44111 multiple enterotomies

44120 Enterectomy, resection of small intestine; single resection and anastomosis

+ 44121 each additional resection and anastomosis (List separately in addition to code for primary procedure)

44125 with enterostomy

44126 Enterectomy, resection of small intestine for congenital atresia, single resection and anastomosis of proximal segment of intestine; without tapering

44127 with tapering

+ 44128 each additional resection and anastomosis (List separately in addition to code for primary procedure)

44130 Enteroenterostomy, anastomosis of intestine, with or without cutaneous enterostomy (separate procedure)

44132 Donor enterectomy (including cold preservation), open; from cadaver donor

44133 partial, from living donor

44135 Intestinal allotransplantation; from cadaver donor

44136 from living donor

44137 Removal of transplanted intestinal allograft, complete

+ 44139 Mobilization (take-down) of splenic flexure performed in conjunction with partial colectomy (List separately in addition to primary procedure)

44140 Colectomy, partial; with anastomosis

44141 with skin level cecostomy or colostomy

44143 with end colostomy and closure of distal segment (Hartmann type procedure)

44144 with resection, with colostomy or ileostomy and creation of mucofistula

44145 with coloproctostomy (low pelvic anastomosis)

44146 with coloproctostomy (low pelvic anastomosis), with colostomy

44147 abdominal and transanal approach

44150 Colectomy, total, abdominal, without proctectomy; with ileostomy or ileoproctostomy

44151 with continent ileostomy

44155 Colectomy, total, abdominal, with proctectomy; with ileostomy

44156 with continent ileostomy

44157 with ileoanal anastomosis, includes loop ileostomy, and rectal mucosectomy, when performed

44158 with ileoanal anastomosis, creation of ileal reservoir (S or J), includes loop ileostomy, and rectal mucosectomy, when performed

44160 Colectomy, partial, with removal of terminal ileum with ileocolostomy

Laparoscopy

Coding Atlas

Laparotomy, or **open** incision into the abdomen, provides the physician **direct visualization** of the operative site; however, it also requires significant recuperation time for the patient. **Laparoscopy** is a technique developed to reduce risk and recovery time during abdominal surgery. In a laparoscopy, several small abdominal incisions act as portals for a tiny video camera (laparoscope), light source, and surgical tools. The physician manipulates the surgical tools while viewing the surgical site on a video display screen or through an eyepiece. To enhance visibility, the abdomen may be filled with gas (**pneumoperitoneum**) during the procedure.

Incision

44180 Laparoscopy, surgical, enterolysis (freeing of intestinal adhesion) (separate procedure)

Enterostomy—External Fistulization of Intestines

44186 Laparoscopy, surgical; jejunostomy (eg, for decompression or feeding)

44187 ileostomy or jejunostomy, non-tube

44188 Laparoscopy, surgical, colostomy or skin level cecostomy

Excision

44202 Laparoscopy, surgical; enterectomy, resection of small intestine, single resection and anastomosis

✚ 44203 each additional small intestine resection and anastomosis (List separately in addition to code for primary procedure)

44204 colectomy, partial, with anastomosis

44205 colectomy, partial, with removal of terminal ileum with ileocolostomy

44206 colectomy, partial, with end colostomy and closure of distal segment (Hartmann type procedure)

44207 colectomy, partial, with anastomosis, with coloproctostomy (low pelvic anastomosis)

44208 colectomy, partial, with anastomosis, with coloproctostomy (low pelvic anastomosis) with colostomy

44210 colectomy, total, abdominal, without proctectomy, with ileostomy or ileoproctostomy

44211 colectomy, total, abdominal, with proctectomy, with ileoanal anastomosis, creation of ileal reservoir (S or J), with loop ileostomy, includes rectal mucosectomy, when performed

44212 colectomy, total, abdominal, with proctectomy, with ileostomy

✚ 44213 Laparoscopy, surgical, mobilization (take-down) of splenic flexure performed in conjunction with partial colectomy (List separately in addition to primary procedure)

Repair

44227 Laparoscopy, surgical, closure of enterostomy, large or small intestine, with resection and anastomosis

Enterostomy—External Fistulization of Intestines

Coding Atlas

At times during the treatment or recovery of a patient, the continuous lumen that is the alimentary canal becomes temporarily or permanently disrupted. The disruption may be a blockage, eg, esophageal or rectal malignancy, or a more generalized problem, eg, malnutrition in a severely weakened patient. The disruption can be bypassed with the creation of a communication from the lumen to the exterior of the body. An enteral stoma is a communication to the skin from the small or large intestine that allows feces to be excreted, bypassing intestines, rectum, and anus distal to the site. An enterostomy tube or cecostomy tube may be placed in the cecum or small intestine so that nutrients can be injected, bypassing the mouth, esophagus, and stomach proximal to the site. This feeding tube is often documented as a J-tube (jejunostomy tube). J-tube placement in an open procedure is reported using code 44300. Percutaneous J-tube placement is reported using code 49441.

44300 Placement, enterostomy or cecostomy, tube open (eg, for feeding or decompression) (separate procedure)

44310 Ileostomy or jejunostomy, non-tube

44312 Revision of ileostomy; simple (release of superficial scar) (separate procedure)

44314 complicated (reconstruction in-depth) (separate procedure)

44316 Continent ileostomy (Kock procedure) (separate procedure)

44320 Colostomy or skin level cecostomy;

44322 with multiple biopsies (eg, for congenital megacolon) (separate procedure)

44340 Revision of colostomy; simple (release of superficial scar) (separate procedure)

44345 complicated (reconstruction in-depth) (separate procedure)

44346 with repair of paracolostomy hernia (separate procedure)

FIGURE 5-17. Gastroenteric Stomas

A **stoma**, or **ostomy** site, is surgically created on the wall of the abdomen as a permanent solution following bowel surgery or as a temporary solution to allow the bowel to heal. Stoma sites are determined based on the site of the defect that is being treated. In **ileostomy**, the ileum is cut and the proximal end is brought to the surface. In **colostomy**, the colon is cut. A **fecal** collection bag is attached to the skin around the stoma. Note: Tools, implants, and/or equipment depicted in the illustration may be outdated but the procedural approach is valid.

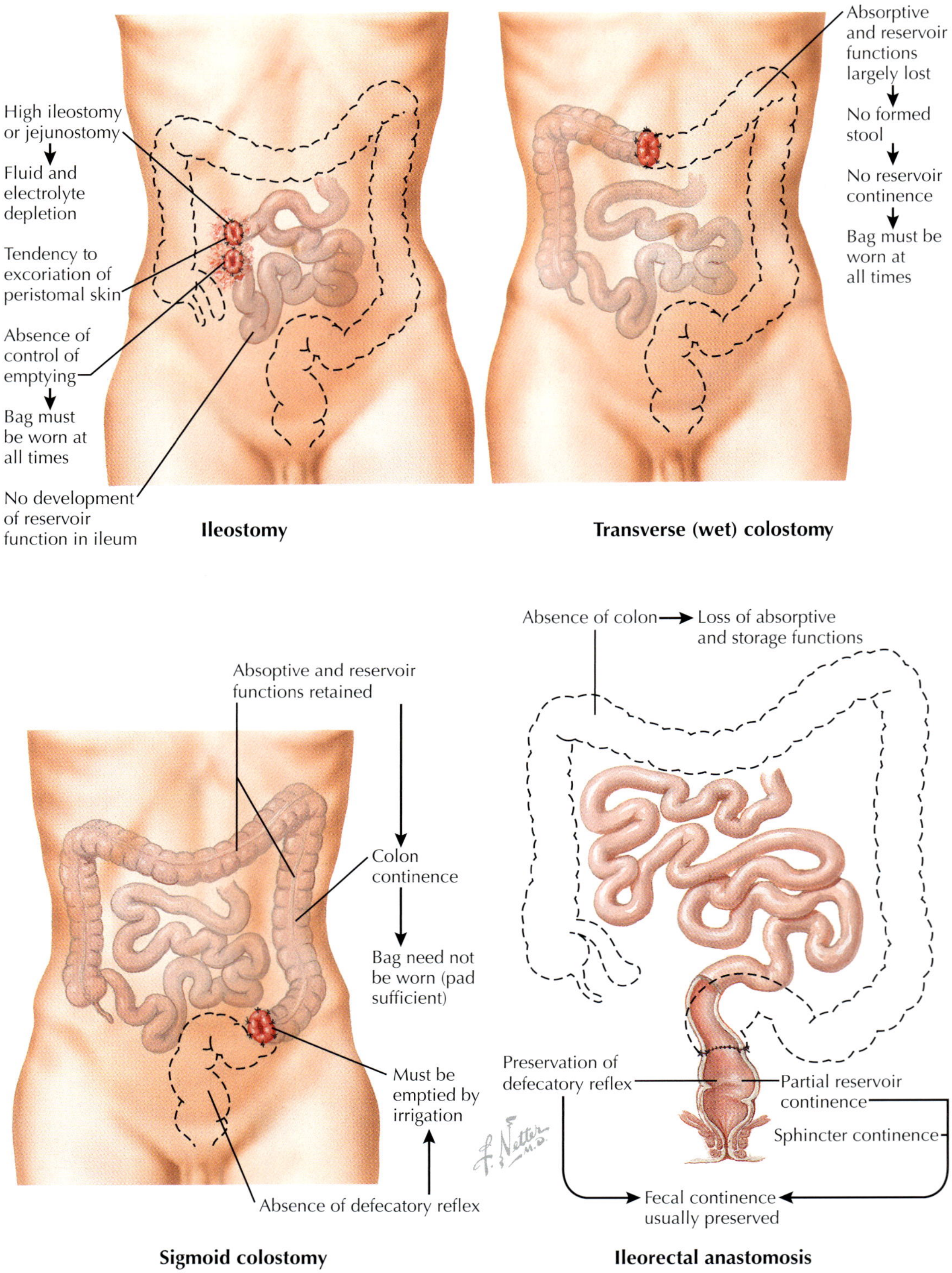

Endoscopy, Small Intestine

Coding Atlas

The small intestine includes the duodenum, jejunum, and ileum. The duodenum begins **distal** to the pyloric valve of the stomach and transitions to jejunum at the duodenojejunal flexture, where it is fixed to the retroperitoneum by the ligament of Treitz. Endoscopic access to the small intestine may be **intraoral** and through the pyloric valve or through a pre-existing **stoma** site.

⊙ **44360** Small intestinal endoscopy, enteroscopy beyond second portion of duodenum, not including ileum; diagnostic, including collection of specimen(s) by brushing or washing, when performed (separate procedure)

⊙ **44361** with biopsy, single or multiple

⊙ **44363** with removal of foreign body(s)

⊙ **44364** with removal of tumor(s), polyp(s), or other lesion(s) by snare technique

⊙ **44365** with removal of tumor(s), polyp(s), or other lesion(s) by hot biopsy forceps or bipolar cautery

⊙ **44366** with control of bleeding (eg, injection, bipolar cautery, unipolar cautery, laser, heater probe, stapler, plasma coagulator)

⊙ **44369** with ablation of tumor(s), polyp(s), or other lesion(s) not amenable to removal by hot biopsy forceps, bipolar cautery or snare technique

⊙ **44370** with transendoscopic stent placement (includes predilation)

⊙ **44372** with placement of percutaneous jejunostomy tube

⊙ **44373** with conversion of percutaneous gastrostomy tube to percutaneous jejunostomy tube

⊙ **44376** Small intestinal endoscopy, enteroscopy beyond second portion of duodenum, including ileum; diagnostic, with or without collection of specimen(s) by brushing or washing (separate procedure)

⊙ **44377** with biopsy, single or multiple

⊙ **44378** with control of bleeding (eg, injection, bipolar cautery, unipolar cautery, laser, heater probe, stapler, plasma coagulator)

⊙ **44379** with transendoscopic stent placement (includes predilation)

Endoscopy, Stomal

Coding Atlas

The small intestine includes the duodenum, jejunum, and ileum. The duodenum begins **distal** to the pyloric valve of the stomach and transitions to jejunum at the duodenojejunal flexture, where it is fixed to the retroperitoneum by the ligament of Treitz. Endoscopic access to the small intestine may be **intraoral** and through the pyloric valve or through a pre-existing **stoma** site.

⊙ **44380** Ileoscopy, through stoma; diagnostic, including collection of specimen(s) by brushing or washing, when performed (separate procedure)

44381 Code is out of numerical sequence. See 44380-44394

⊙ **44382** with biopsy, single or multiple

#⊙ **44381** with transendoscopic balloon dilation

⊙ **44384** with placement of endoscopic stent (includes pre- and post-dilation and guide wire passage, when performed)

⊙ **44385** Endoscopic evaluation of small intestinal pouch (eg, Kock pouch, ileal reservoir [S or J]); diagnostic, including collection of specimen(s) by brushing or washing, when performed (separate procedure)

⊙ **44386** with biopsy, single or multiple

⊙ **44388** Colonoscopy through stoma; diagnostic, including collection of specimen(s) by brushing or washing, when performed (separate procedure)

⊙ **44389** with biopsy, single or multiple

⊙ **44390** with removal of foreign body(s)

⊙ **44391** with control of bleeding, any method

⊙ **44392** with removal of tumor(s), polyp(s), or other lesion(s) by hot biopsy forceps

#⊙ **44401** with ablation of tumor(s), polyp(s), or other lesion(s) (includes pre-and post-dilation and guide wire passage, when performed)

⊙ **44394** with removal of tumor(s), polyp(s), or other lesion(s) by snare technique

44401 Code is out of numerical sequence. See 44380-44408

⊙ **44402** with endoscopic stent placement (including pre- and post-dilation and guide wire passage, when performed)

⊙ **44403** with endoscopic mucosal resection

⊙ **44404** with directed submucosal injection(s), any substance

⊙ **44405** with transendoscopic balloon dilation

⊙ **44406** with endoscopic ultrasound examination, limited to the sigmoid, descending, transverse, or ascending colon and cecum and adjacent structures

FIGURE 5-18. The Small Intestine

The small intestine, or small bowel, is coiled between the ascending and descending colon and below the stomach. The small intestine is connected to mesentery, a fan-shaped double fold of peritoneum attached to the posterior abdominal wall and covering the length of the jejunum and ileum. The ileum is the **distal** end of the small intestine, where it transitions to the colon at the ileocecal junction.

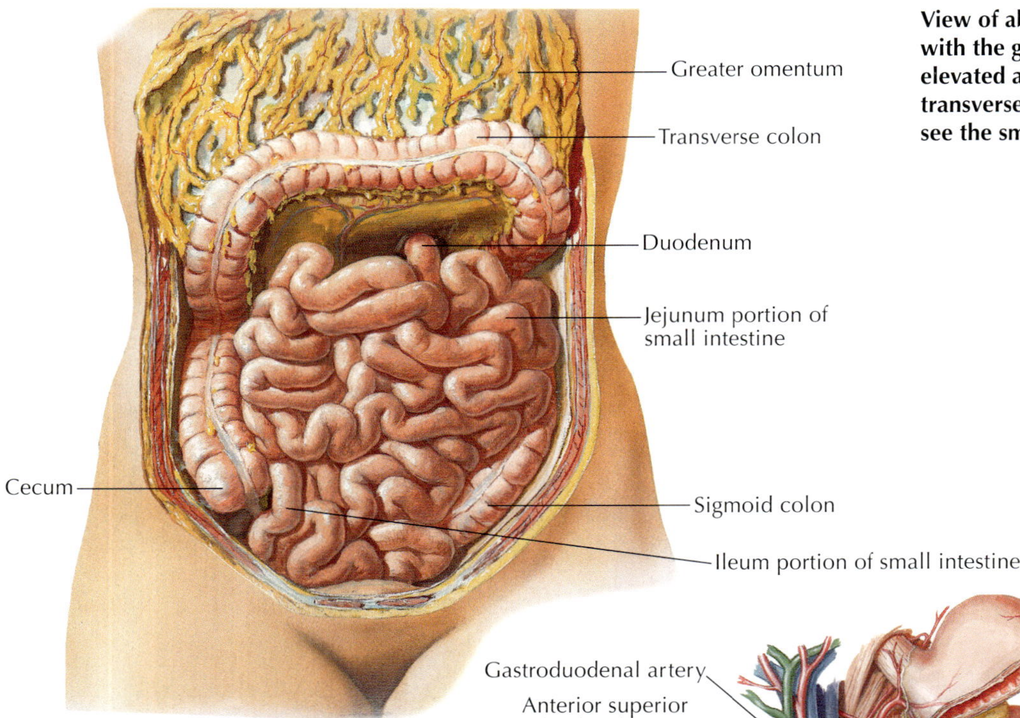

View of abdominal viscera with the greater omentum elevated above the transverse colon to better see the small intestines

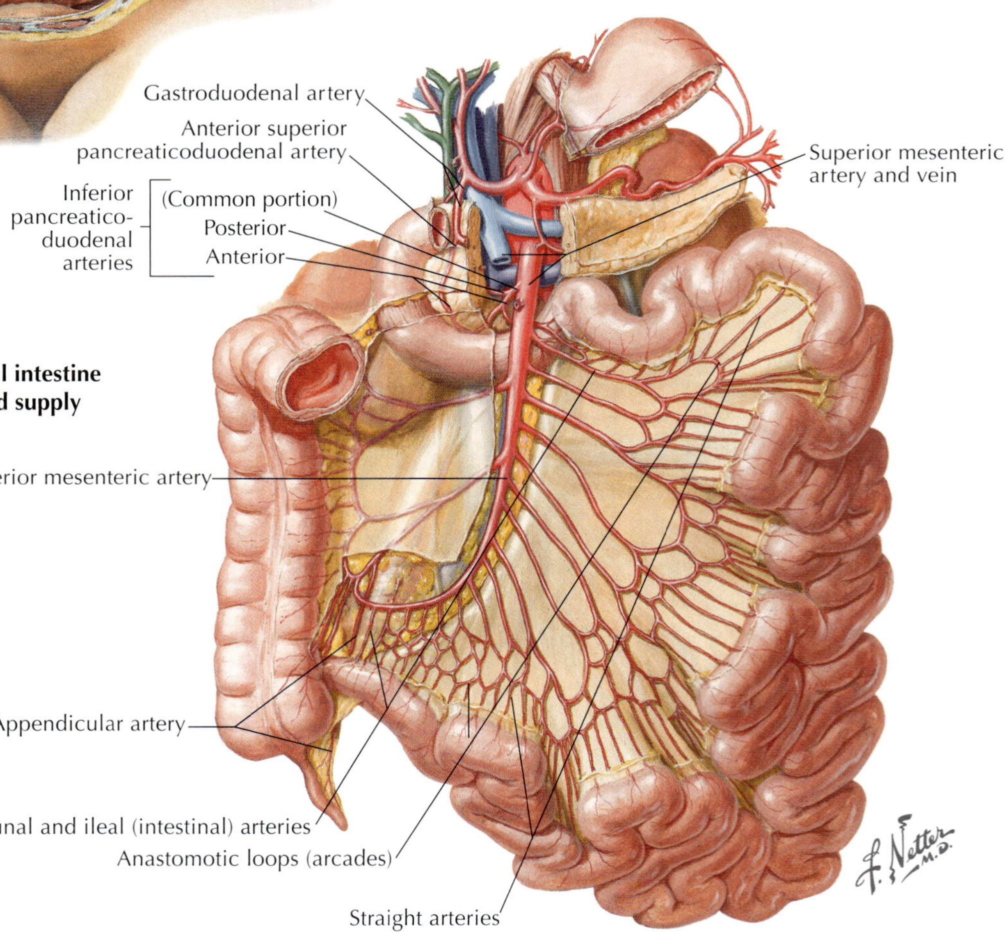

Subdivisions of small intestine and its arterial blood supply

⊙ **44407** with transendoscopic ultrasound guided intramural or transmural fine needle aspiration/biopsy(s), includes endoscopic ultrasound examination limited to the sigmoid, descending, transverse, or ascending colon and cecum and adjacent structures

⊙ **44408** with decompression (for pathologic distention) (eg, volvulus, megacolon), including placement of decompression tube, when performed

Introduction

⊙⊘ **44500** Introduction of long gastrointestinal tube (eg, Miller-Abbott) (separate procedure)

Repair

Coding Atlas

In a Hartmann procedure, the colon is resected and a **colostomy** is formed with the **proximal** bowel, leaving the **distal** bowel and rectum as a stump. At a future time, the colon and rectum may be **reanastomosed** to restore bowel function.

44602 Suture of small intestine (enterorrhaphy) for perforated ulcer, diverticulum, wound, injury or rupture; single perforation

44603 multiple perforations

44604 Suture of large intestine (colorrhaphy) for perforated ulcer, diverticulum, wound, injury or rupture (single or multiple perforations); without colostomy

44605 with colostomy

44615 Intestinal stricturoplasty (enterotomy and enterorrhaphy) with or without dilation, for intestinal obstruction

44620 Closure of enterostomy, large or small intestine;

44625 with resection and anastomosis other than colorectal

44626 with resection and colorectal anastomosis (eg, closure of Hartmann type procedure)

44640 Closure of intestinal cutaneous fistula

44650 Closure of enteroenteric or enterocolic fistula

44660 Closure of enterovesical fistula; without intestinal or bladder resection

44661 with intestine and/or bladder resection

44680 Intestinal plication (separate procedure)

Other Procedures

Coding Atlas

The small intestine may be separated from the true pelvis by prosthesis or native tissue in order to elevate the small intestine out of the targeted pelvic site for radiation therapy. This prevents damage to the intestinal tissue. This open surgical procedure is reported using code 44700.

44700 Exclusion of small intestine from pelvis by mesh or other prosthesis, or native tissue (eg, bladder or omentum)

✚ **44701** Intraoperative colonic lavage (List separately in addition to code for primary procedure)

44705 Preparation of fecal microbiota for instillation, including assessment of donor specimen

44715 Backbench standard preparation of cadaver or living donor intestine allograft prior to transplantation, including mobilization and fashioning of the superior mesenteric artery and vein

44720 Backbench reconstruction of cadaver or living donor intestine allograft prior to transplantation; venous anastomosis, each

44721 arterial anastomosis, each

Meckel's Diverticulum and the Mesentery

Excision

Coding Atlas

Meckel's diverticulum is a **congenital** pouch in the wall of the intestine. The cellular composition of Meckel's diverticulum may be intestinal or **ectopic** pancreatic or stomach tissue. Omphalomesenteric duct is a synonym for **Meckel's diverticulum**, which forms from an embryonic yolk stalk that fails to break down during fetal development.

44800 Excision of Meckel's diverticulum (diverticulectomy) or omphalomesenteric duct

44820 Excision of lesion of mesentery (separate procedure)

Suture

44850 Suture of mesentery (separate procedure)

Appendix

Incision

44900 Incision and drainage of appendiceal abscess, open

Excision

Coding Atlas

The appendix is a finger-sized lumen that extends from the cecum. The end of the appendix is closed, like the fingertip of a glove. An appendicitis is generally caused by an obstruction in the lumen, which in turn leads to swelling, ischemia, and bacterial invasion. Surgical excision of the appendix resolves the condition. An appendectomy may be performed through an abdominal incision (codes 44950-44960) or laparoscopically (code 44970).

44950 Appendectomy;

✚ **44955** when done for indicated purpose at time of other major procedure (not as separate procedure) (List separately in addition to code for primary procedure)

44960 for ruptured appendix with abscess or generalized peritonitis

Laparoscopy

44970 Laparoscopy, surgical, appendectomy

Colon and Rectum

Incision

Coding Atlas

The rectum is the terminal segment of the large intestine that begins at the sigmoid colon and ends at the anus. The rectum acts as a holding area for feces. As the rectal walls stretch to accommodate feces, the nervous system reacts, creating the urge to defecate. Rectal abscesses may be treated by incising the rectal mucosa overlying the abscess (transrectal) or through a skin incision.

45000 Transrectal drainage of pelvic abscess

45005 Incision and drainage of submucosal abscess, rectum

45020 Incision and drainage of deep supralevator, pelvirectal, or retrorectal abscess

Excision

Coding Atlas

A proctectomy is the surgical excision of the rectum, eg, as a treatment for a malignancy or ulcerative colitis. A pull-through is the anastomosis of the proximal stump of the colon to the anus, so called because the distal end of the sigmoid colon is pulled through the sphincter complex and then sutured to the anus.

45100 Biopsy of anorectal wall, anal approach (eg, congenital megacolon)

45108 Anorectal myomectomy

45110 Proctectomy; complete, combined abdominoperineal, with colostomy

45111 partial resection of rectum, transabdominal approach

45112 Proctectomy, combined abdominoperineal, pull-through procedure (eg, colo-anal anastomosis)

45113 Proctectomy, partial, with rectal mucosectomy, ileoanal anastomosis, creation of ileal reservoir (S or J), with or without loop ileostomy

45114 Proctectomy, partial, with anastomosis; abdominal and transsacral approach

45116 transsacral approach only (Kraske type)

45119 Proctectomy, combined abdominoperineal pull-through procedure (eg, colo-anal anastomosis), with creation of colonic reservoir (eg, J-pouch), with diverting enterostomy when performed

45120 Proctectomy, complete (for congenital megacolon), abdominal and perineal approach; with pull-through procedure and anastomosis (eg, Swenson, Duhamel, or Soave type operation)

45121 with subtotal or total colectomy, with multiple biopsies

45123 Proctectomy, partial, without anastomosis, perineal approach

45126 Pelvic exenteration for colorectal malignancy, with proctectomy (with or without colostomy), with removal of bladder and ureteral transplantations, and/or hysterectomy, or cervicectomy, with or without removal of tube(s), with or without removal of ovary(s), or any combination thereof

45130 Excision of rectal procidentia, with anastomosis; perineal approach

45135 abdominal and perineal approach

45136 Excision of ileoanal reservoir with ileostomy

45150 Division of stricture of rectum

45160 Excision of rectal tumor by proctotomy, transsacral or transcoccygeal approach

45171 Excision of rectal tumor, transanal approach; not including muscularis propria (ie, partial thickness)

45172 including muscularis propria (ie, full thickness)

Destruction

45190 Destruction of rectal tumor (eg, electrodesiccation, electrosurgery, laser ablation, laser resection, cryosurgery) transanal approach

Endoscopy

Coding Atlas

Endoscopy of the colon and rectum enables the physician to visually inspect and also treat the large bowel using a camera that projects an image onto a video display or through an eyepiece. Tools can be fed through the scoping device to the site of a defect, and the defect can be treated. Codes for reporting endoscopy of the colon are based on the extent of the examination. In proctosigmoidoscopy, the examination includes the rectum and may include a portion of the sigmoid colon. In sigmoidoscopy, the examination includes the rectum, entire sigmoid colon, and may include a portion of the descending colon. In colonoscopy, a scope is used to examine the colon from the rectum all the way to the cecum; a colonoscopy may include the terminal ileum.

45300 Proctosigmoidoscopy, rigid; diagnostic, with or without collection of specimen(s) by brushing or washing (separate procedure)

⊙ **45303** with dilation (eg, balloon, guide wire, bougie)

⊙ **45305** with biopsy, single or multiple

⊙ **45307** with removal of foreign body

⊙ **45308** with removal of single tumor, polyp, or other lesion by hot biopsy forceps or bipolar cautery

⊙ **45309** with removal of single tumor, polyp, or other lesion by snare technique

⊙ **45315** with removal of multiple tumors, polyps, or other lesions by hot biopsy forceps, bipolar cautery or snare technique

⊙ **45317** with control of bleeding (eg, injection, bipolar cautery, unipolar cautery, laser, heater probe, stapler, plasma coagulator)

⊙ **45320** with ablation of tumor(s), polyp(s), or other lesion(s) not amenable to removal by hot biopsy forceps, bipolar cautery or snare technique (eg, laser)

⊙ **45321** with decompression of volvulus

⊙ **45327** with transendoscopic stent placement (includes predilation)

45330 Sigmoidoscopy, flexible; diagnostic, including collection of specimen(s) by brushing or washing, when performed (separate procedure)

45331 with biopsy, single or multiple

⊙ **45332** with removal of foreign body(s)

⊙ **45333** with removal of tumor(s), polyp(s), or other lesion(s) by hot biopsy forceps

⊙ **45334** with control of bleeding, any method

⊙ **45335** with directed submucosal injection(s), any substance

⊙ **45337** with decompression (for pathologic distention) (eg, volvulus, megacolon), including placement of decompression tube, when performed

⊙ **45338** with removal of tumor(s), polyp(s), or other lesion(s) by snare technique

#⊙ **45346** with ablation of tumor(s), polyp(s), or other lesion(s) (includes pre- and post-dilation and guide wire passage, when performed)

⊙ **45340** with transendoscopic balloon dilation

⊙ **45341** with endoscopic ultrasound examination

⊙ **45342** with transendoscopic ultrasound guided intramural or transmural fine needle aspiration/biopsy(s)

45346 Code is out of numerical sequence. See 45330-45342

⊙ **45347** with placement of endoscopic stent (includes pre- and post-dilation and guide wire passage, when performed)

⊙ **45349** with endoscopic mucosal resection

⊙ **45350** with band ligation(s) (eg, hemorrhoids)

⊙ **45378** Colonoscopy, flexible; diagnostic, including collection of specimen(s) by brushing or washing, when performed (separate procedure)

⊙ **45379** with removal of foreign body(s)

⊙ **45380** with biopsy, single or multiple

⊙ **45381** with directed submucosal injection(s), any substance

⊙ **45382** with control of bleeding, any method

#⊙ **45388** with ablation of tumor(s), polyp(s), or other lesion(s) (includes pre- and post-dilation and guide wire passage, when performed)

⊙ **45384** with removal of tumor(s), polyp(s), or other lesion(s) by hot biopsy forceps

⊙ **45385** with removal of tumor(s), polyp(s), or other lesion(s) by snare technique

FIGURE 5-19. Anoscopy, Sigmoidoscopy, and Colonoscopy

Colonoscopy employs an endoscopic camera, with images displayed on a video screen or through an eyepiece. In colonoscopy, the entire bowel, from the **distal** rectum to the **proximal** cecum, is inspected. Procedures are often performed during screening or diagnostic colonoscopies, when the physician encounters a defect that requires intervention. Note: Tools, implants, and/or equipment depicted in the illustration may be outdated but the procedural approach is valid.

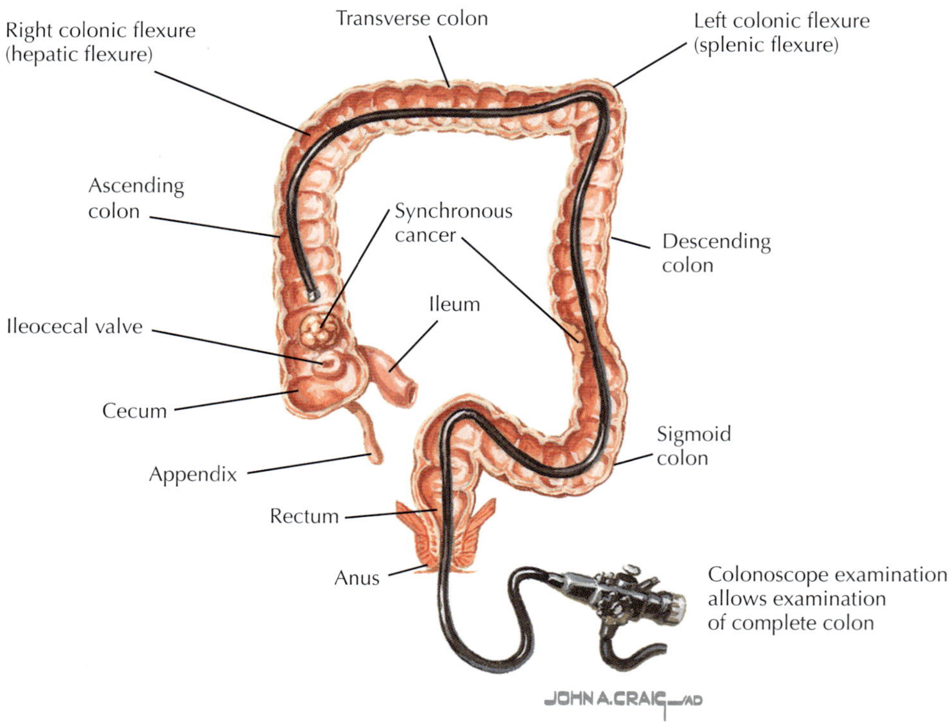

⊙ **45386** with transendoscopic balloon dilation

45388 Code is out of numerical sequence. See 45300-45393

⊙ **45389** with endoscopic stent placement (includes pre- and post-dilation and guide wire passage, when performed)

45390 Code is out of numerical sequence. See 45300-45393

⊙ **45391** with endoscopic ultrasound examination limited to the rectum, sigmoid, descending, transverse, or ascending colon and cecum, and adjacent structures

⊙ **45392** with transendoscopic ultrasound guided intramural or transmural fine needle aspiration/biopsy(s), includes endoscopic ultrasound examination limited to the rectum, sigmoid, descending, transverse, or ascending colon and cecum, and adjacent structures

#⊙ **45390** with endoscopic mucosal resection

⊙ **45393** with decompression (for pathologic distention) (eg, volvulus, megacolon), including placement of decompression tube, when performed

#⊙ **45398** with band ligation(s) (eg, hemorrhoids)

Laparoscopy

Coding Atlas

Laparoscopy is a technique developed to reduce risk and recovery time during abdominal surgery. Several small abdominal incisions act as portals for a tiny video camera (laparoscope), light source, and surgical tools. The physician manipulates the surgical tools while viewing the surgical site on a video display screen or through an eyepiece. To enhance visibility, the abdomen may be filled with gas (**pneumoperitoneum**) during the procedure.

Excision

45395 Laparoscopy, surgical; proctectomy, complete, combined abdominoperineal, with colostomy

45397 proctectomy, combined abdominoperineal pull-through procedure (eg, colo-anal anastomosis), with creation of colonic reservoir (eg, J-pouch), with diverting enterostomy, when performed

45398 Code is out of numerical sequence. See 45395-45399

45399 Code is out of numerical sequence. See 45300-45999

Repair

45400 Laparoscopy, surgical; proctopexy (for prolapse)

45402 proctopexy (for prolapse), with sigmoid resection

45499 Unlisted laparoscopy procedure, rectum

Repair

Coding Atlas

Rectal prolapse is a condition in which the rectal mucosa protrudes from the anus due to weakness of the anal sphincter, overstretching of rectal ligaments, and/or a generally weak pelvic floor. Several surgical alternatives exist for treating prolapse, including **proctopexy** (surgical fixation of the rectum using sutures).

45500 Proctoplasty; for stenosis

45505 for prolapse of mucous membrane

45520 Perirectal injection of sclerosing solution for prolapse

45540 Proctopexy (eg, for prolapse); abdominal approach

45541 perineal approach

45550 with sigmoid resection, abdominal approach

45560 Repair of rectocele (separate procedure)

45562 Exploration, repair, and presacral drainage for rectal injury;

45563 with colostomy

45800 Closure of rectovesical fistula;

45805 with colostomy

45820 Closure of rectourethral fistula;

45825 with colostomy

Manipulation

Coding Atlas

Procidentia is the prolapse of full-thickness rectal tissue through the anus.

45900 Reduction of procidentia (separate procedure) under anesthesia

45905 Dilation of anal sphincter (separate procedure) under anesthesia other than local

45910 Dilation of rectal stricture (separate procedure) under anesthesia other than local

45915 Removal of fecal impaction or foreign body (separate procedure) under anesthesia

Other Procedures

45990 Anorectal exam, surgical, requiring anesthesia (general, spinal, or epidural), diagnostic

Anus

Incision

Coding Atlas

In the transition zone of the anus are anal crypts, or sinuses, lined with anal glands and anal **papillae**. Perianal **abscesses** and **fistulas** are usually caused by infections that begin in the anal glands. An anal fistula is an abnormal **sinus tract** that forms from an anal gland and may lead to the skin surface.

46020 Placement of seton

46030 Removal of anal seton, other marker

46040 Incision and drainage of ischiorectal and/or perirectal abscess (separate procedure)

46045 Incision and drainage of intramural, intramuscular, or submucosal abscess, transanal, under anesthesia

46050 Incision and drainage, perianal abscess, superficial

46060 Incision and drainage of ischiorectal or intramural abscess, with fistulectomy or fistulotomy, submuscular, with or without placement of seton

46070 Incision, anal septum (infant)

46080 Sphincterotomy, anal, division of sphincter (separate procedure)

46083 Incision of thrombosed hemorrhoid, external

FIGURE 5-20. The Rectum and Anal Canal

The anal canal is the terminus for the gastrointestinal tract. There are several anatomical landmarks in the anus. The anorectal ring is about 5 cm from the anus. The pectinate line, also referred to as the dentate line or mucocutaneous line, is at the base of the anal columns. The anal verge is the orifice itself. Although with the same pigmented color as that of the surrounding perianal skin, the verge differs in that it contains no hair, sweat glands, or sebaceous glands.

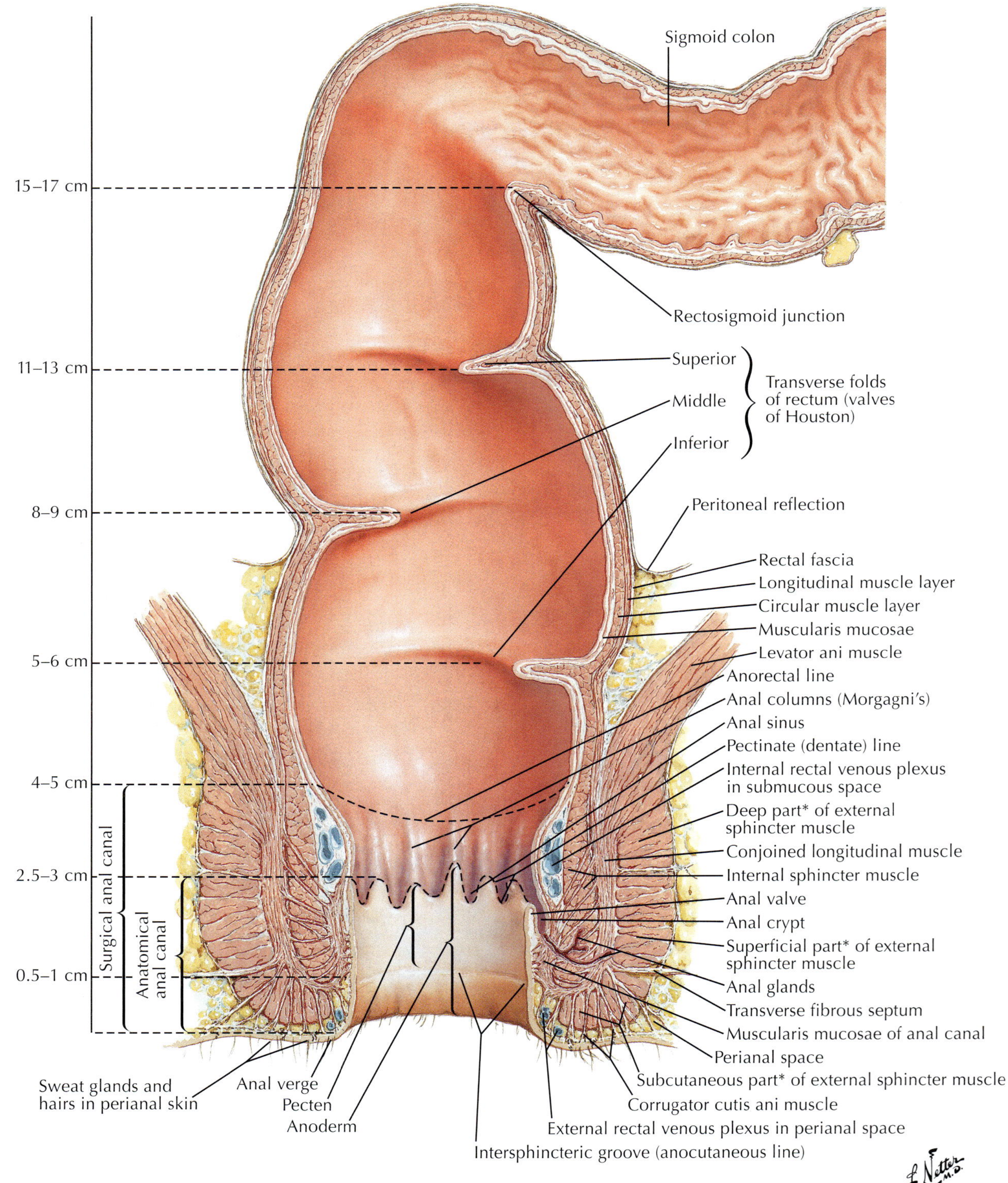

*Parts variable and often indistinct

Excision

Coding Atlas

Hemorrhoidal cushions are normal anatomical structures of the anorectum, with an extensive vascular supply and high sensitivity. Hemorrhoidal cushions commonly **prolapse**, **thrombose**, itch, or cause other symptoms and are then referred to as "hemorrhoids." Hemorrhoids are not varicose veins but rather clusters of venous and arteriolar branches in the anal canal. Hemorrhoids may be excised or treated by banding to induce **ischemia** and death of the hemorrhoidal tissue.

46200 Fissurectomy, including sphincterotomy, when performed

46220 Code is out of numerical sequence. See 46200-46288

46221 Hemorrhoidectomy, internal, by rubber band ligation(s)

46945 Hemorrhoidectomy, internal, by ligation other than rubber band; single hemorrhoid column/group

46946 2 or more hemorrhoid columns/groups

46220 Excision of single external papilla or tag, anus

46230 Excision of multiple external papillae or tags, anus

46320 Excision of thrombosed hemorrhoid, external

46250 Hemorrhoidectomy, external, 2 or more columns/groups

46255 Hemorrhoidectomy, internal and external, single column/group;

46257 with fissurectomy

46258 with fistulectomy, including fissurectomy, when performed

46260 Hemorrhoidectomy, internal and external, 2 or more columns/groups;

46261 with fissurectomy

46262 with fistulectomy, including fissurectomy, when performed

46270 Surgical treatment of anal fistula (fistulectomy/fistulotomy); subcutaneous

46275 intersphincteric

46280 transsphincteric, suprasphincteric, extrasphincteric or multiple, including placement of seton, when performed

46285 second stage

46288 Closure of anal fistula with rectal advancement flap

46320 Code is out of numerical sequence. See 46200-46288

Introduction

Coding Atlas

Injection of a **sclerosing** agent into a hemorrhoid causes an inflammatory response that interrupts the blood flow and creates a **secondary fibrosis**, shrinking the hemorrhoid. **Chemodenervation** of the internal anal sphincter is performed by injecting **botulinum toxin** into the sphincter muscle to loosen the anal opening and promote healing of a **fissure** that has developed there.

46500 Injection of sclerosing solution, hemorrhoids

46505 Chemodenervation of internal anal sphincter

Endoscopy

Coding Atlas

Anoscopy allows for **direct visualization** and treatment of the anus. An **anoscope** may be called an **anal speculum**.

46600 Anoscopy; diagnostic, including collection of specimen(s) by brushing or washing, when performed (separate procedure)

46601 diagnostic, with high-resolution magnification (HRA) (eg, colposcope, operating microscope) and chemical agent enhancement, including collection of specimen(s) by brushing or washing, when performed

46604 with dilation (eg, balloon, guide wire, bougie)

46606 with biopsy, single or multiple

46607 with high-resolution magnification (HRA) (eg, colposcope, operating microscope) and chemical agent enhancement, with biopsy, single or multiple

46608 with removal of foreign body

46610 with removal of single tumor, polyp, or other lesion by hot biopsy forceps or bipolar cautery

46611 with removal of single tumor, polyp, or other lesion by snare technique

46612 with removal of multiple tumors, polyps, or other lesions by hot biopsy forceps, bipolar cautery or snare technique

46614 with control of bleeding (eg, injection, bipolar cautery, unipolar cautery, laser, heater probe, stapler, plasma coagulator)

46615 with ablation of tumor(s), polyp(s), or other lesion(s) not amenable to removal by hot biopsy forceps, bipolar cautery or snare technique

FIGURE 5-21. Injection and Rubber Band Ligation

Rubber band ligation (RBL) is a common treatment for internal hemorrhoids. Using **anoscopy** and under direct visualization, the physician is able to grasp the hemorrhoid with a clamp and place a band around the base of the hemorrhoid. The hemorrhoid then withers from **ischemia** and eventually falls off. A scar forms over the site. Note: Tools, implants, and/or equipment depicted in the illustration may be outdated but the procedural approach is valid.

A. Injection of internal hemorrhoids

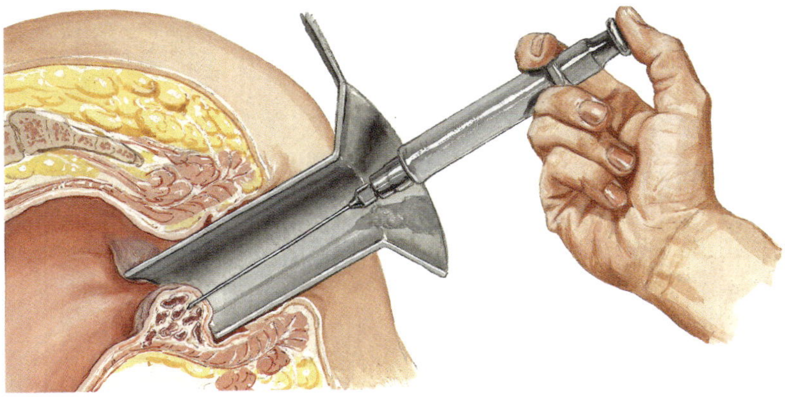

B. Ligature of internal hemorrhoids

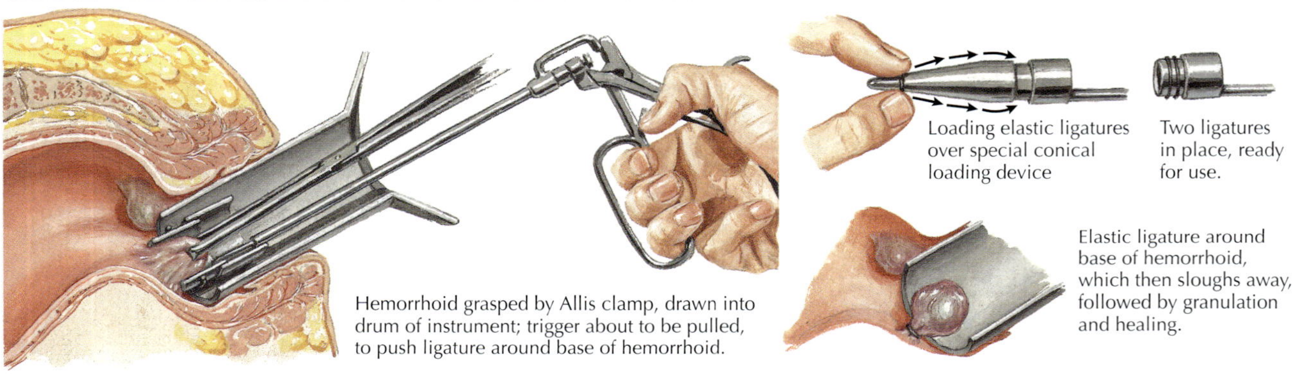

C. Surgical management of internal hemorrhoids: Elastic ligation technique

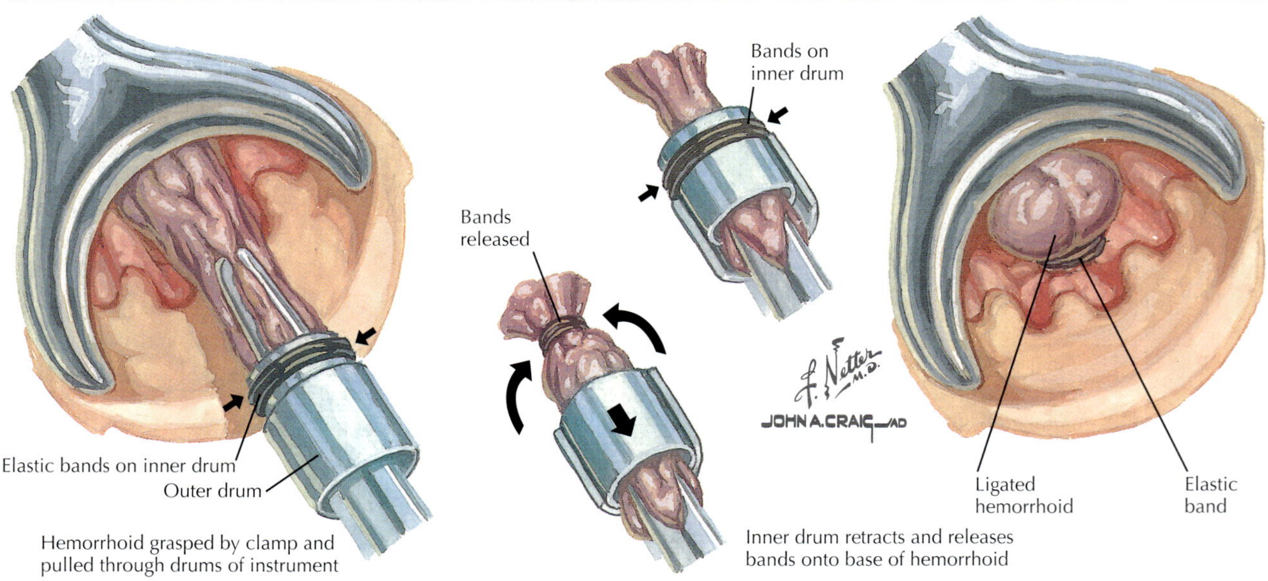

FIGURE 5-22. Hemorrhoids

Hemorrhoids are swollen, symptomatic blood vessels in the rectum and anus. Internal hemorrhoids originate above the dentate line, and external hemorrhoids originate below the dentate line. An internal hemorrhoid may prolapse to extrude through the anus. An engorged hemorrhoid may clot, or **thrombose**, a condition that causes significant pain. Anal **skin tags** or tabs are remnants of hemorrhoids that have resolved.

A. Anatomy of hemorrhoids

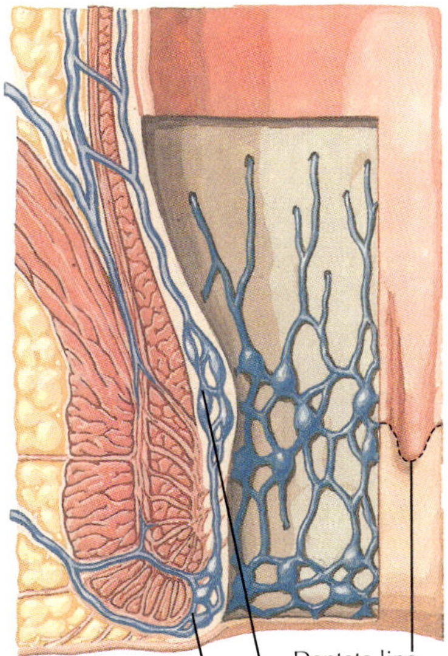

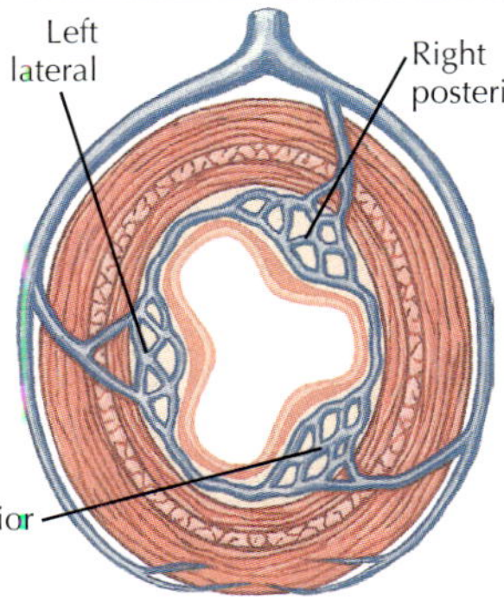

Usual position of internal hemorrhoids, or anal cushions

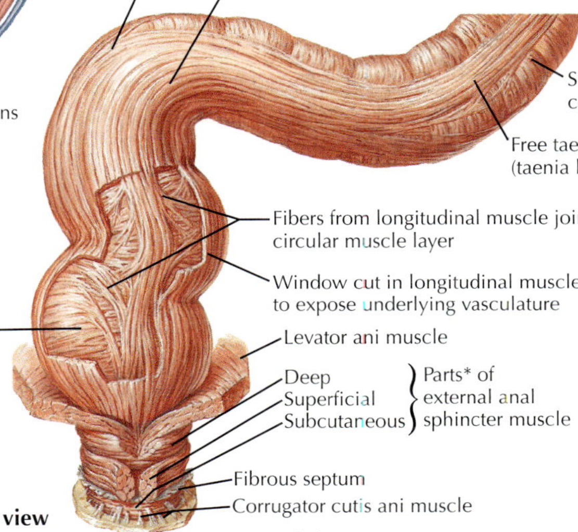

Anterior view

*Parts variable and often indistinct

B. Types of hemorrhoids

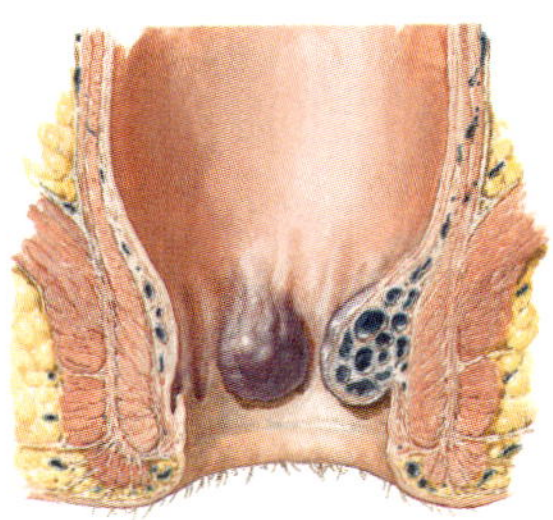

Internal hemorrhoids

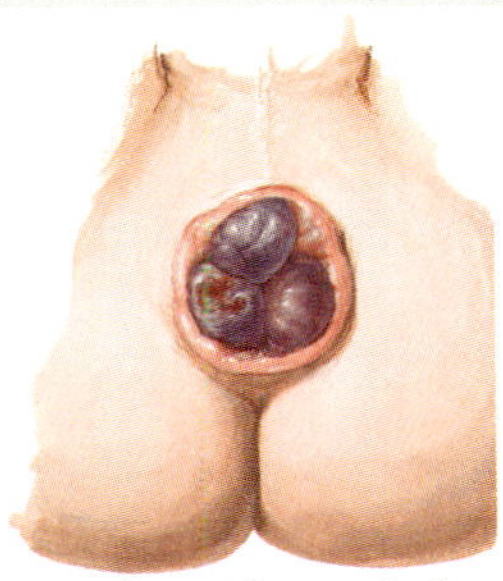

Prolapsed "rosette" of internal hemorrhoids

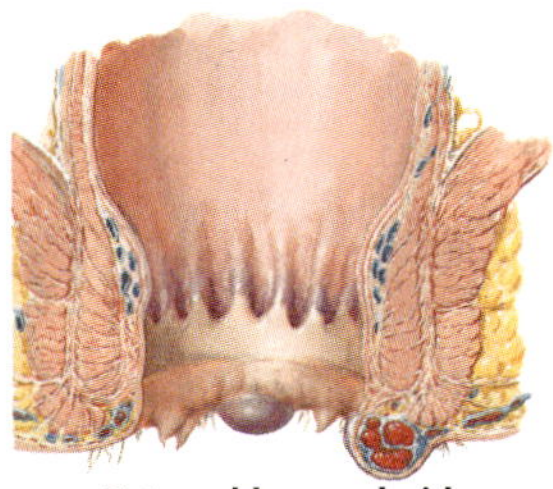

External hemorrhoids and skin tabs

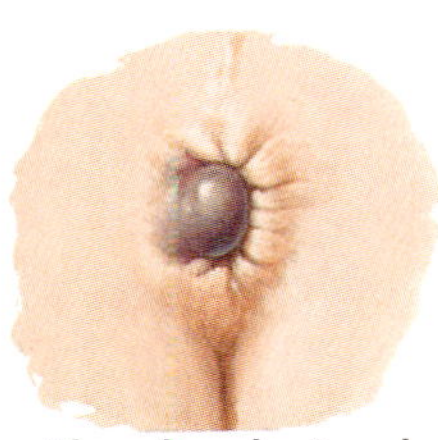

Thrombosed external hemorrhoid

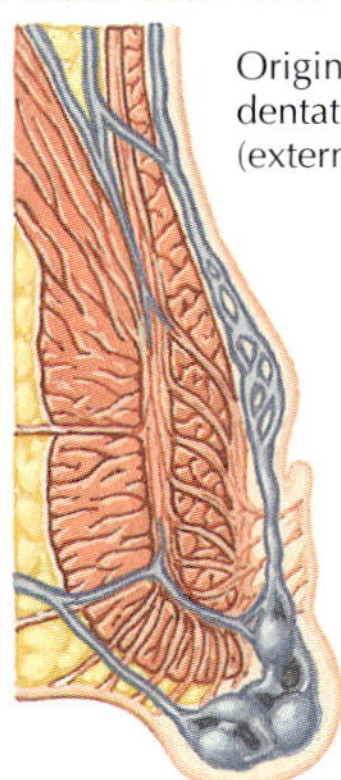

Origin below dentate line (external plexus)

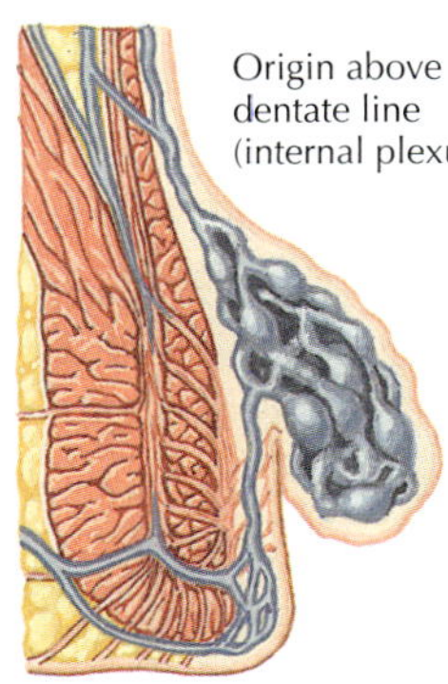

Origin above dentate line (internal plexus)

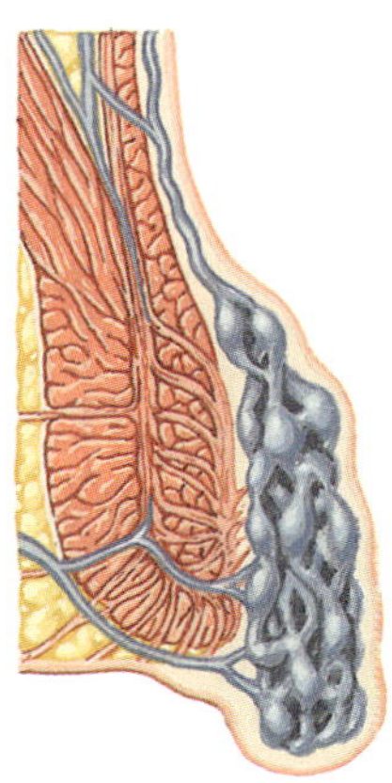

Origin above and below dentate line (internal and external plexus)

Repair

Coding Atlas

Anorectal malformations (ARMs) are congenital defects and include cloacal anomaly and imperforate anus. A low imperforate anus will have a colon close to the skin, with a very stenotic anus or the colon ending in a blind pouch. In high imperforate anus, the colon is higher in the pelvis, with a fistula connecting the rectum to another organ. In a cloacal anomaly, the rectum, vagina, and urinary tract all form a single channel.

46700 Anoplasty, plastic operation for stricture; adult

46705 infant

46706 Repair of anal fistula with fibrin glue

46707 Repair of anorectal fistula with plug (eg, porcine small intestine submucosa [SIS])

46710 Repair of ileoanal pouch fistula/sinus (eg, perineal or vaginal), pouch advancement; transperineal approach

46712 combined transperineal and transabdominal approach

46715 Repair of low imperforate anus; with anoperineal fistula (cut-back procedure)

46716 with transposition of anoperineal or anovestibular fistula

46730 Repair of high imperforate anus without fistula; perineal or sacroperineal approach

46735 combined transabdominal and sacroperineal approaches

46740 Repair of high imperforate anus with rectourethral or rectovaginal fistula; perineal or sacroperineal approach

46742 combined transabdominal and sacroperineal approaches

46744 Repair of cloacal anomaly by anorectovaginoplasty and urethroplasty, sacroperineal approach

46746 Repair of cloacal anomaly by anorectovaginoplasty and urethroplasty, combined abdominal and sacroperineal approach;

46748 with vaginal lengthening by intestinal graft or pedicle flaps

46750 Sphincteroplasty, anal, for incontinence or prolapse; adult

46751 child

46753 Graft (Thiersch operation) for rectal incontinence and/or prolapse

46754 Removal of Thiersch wire or suture, anal canal

46760 Sphincteroplasty, anal, for incontinence, adult; muscle transplant

46761 levator muscle imbrication (Park posterior anal repair)

46762 implantation artificial sphincter

\# **46947** Hemorrhoidopexy (eg, for prolapsing internal hemorrhoids) by stapling

Destruction

Coding Atlas

The codes in this subsection are used to report destruction or excision of lesions in the anus, including anal verge.

46900 Destruction of lesion(s), anus (eg, condyloma, papilloma, molluscum contagiosum, herpetic vesicle), simple; chemical

46910 electrodesiccation

46916 cryosurgery

46917 laser surgery

46922 surgical excision

46924 Destruction of lesion(s), anus (eg, condyloma, papilloma, molluscum contagiosum, herpetic vesicle), extensive (eg, laser surgery, electrosurgery, cryosurgery, chemosurgery)

46930 Destruction of internal hemorrhoid(s) by thermal energy (eg, infrared coagulation, cautery, radiofrequency)

46940 Curettage or cautery of anal fissure, including dilation of anal sphincter (separate procedure); initial

46942 subsequent

46945 Code is out of numerical sequence. See 46200-46288

46946 Code is out of numerical sequence. See 46200-46288

46947 Code is out of numerical sequence. See 46700-46947

FIGURE 5-23. Surfaces and Bed of the Liver

The liver is in the right upper abdominal quadrant, with most of it tucked up under the rib cage. It is covered in a layer of connective tissue called Glisson's capsule. The liver has multiple segments, and each segment has its own independent blood supply and biliary branches. Among the liver's functions are nutrient management; plasma protein synthesis, including **albumin** and clotting factors; vitamin, mineral, and **glycogen** storage; clearance of damaged red blood cells; bile creation; and **biotransformation** of toxins, hormones, and drugs.

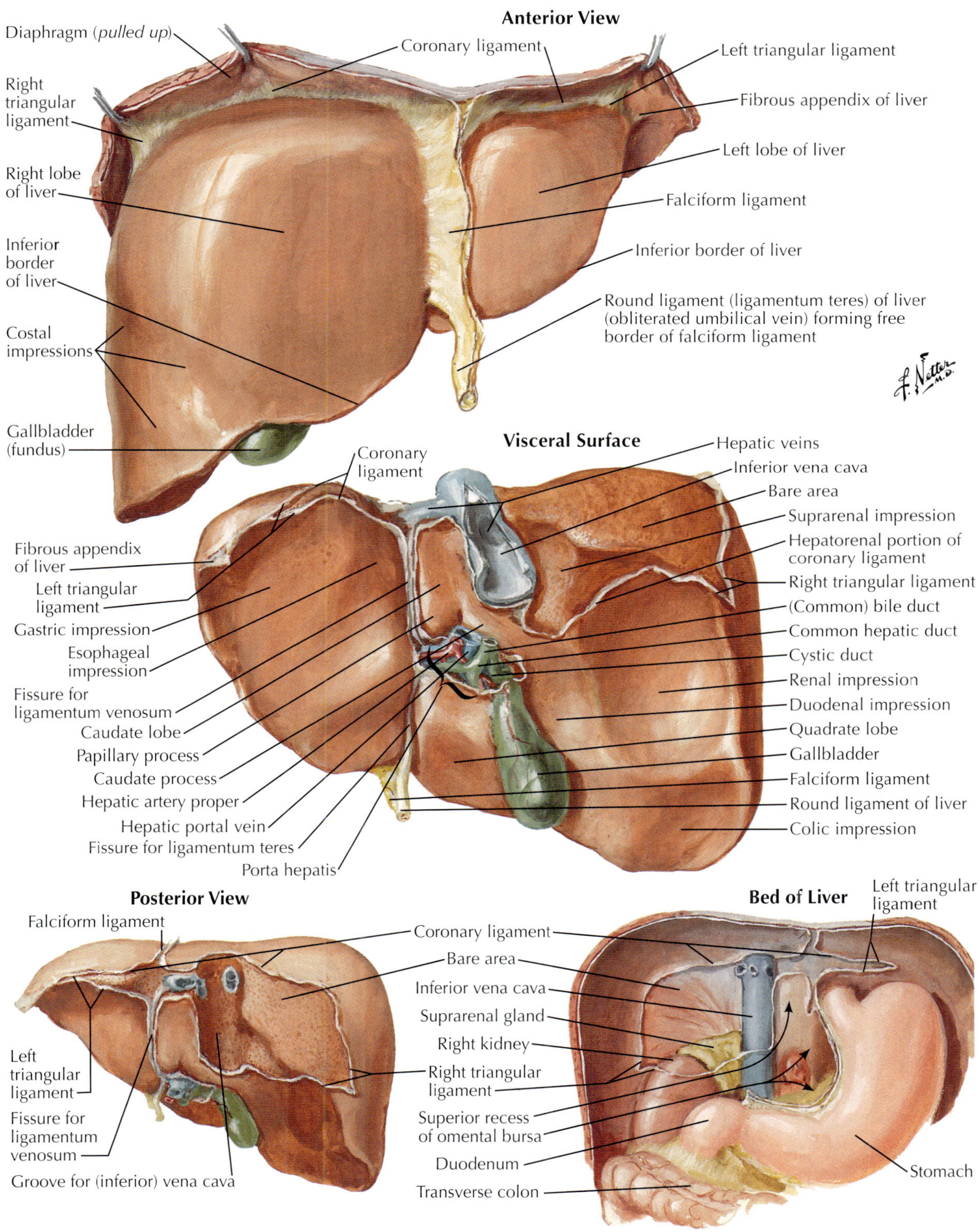

Liver

Incision

Coding Atlas

In percutaneous needle biopsy of the liver, a long needle is introduced through the skin and into the liver to obtain a liver specimen. This may be performed as a follow-up to an abnormal test result, to evaluate a liver mass, or to evaluate the severity of a known disease, eg, alcoholic liver disease, hepatitis, or hemochromatosis. The biopsy may be performed using a cutting needle, a suction needle, or a spring-loaded needle.

⊙ **47000** Biopsy of liver, needle; percutaneous

✚ **47001** when done for indicated purpose at time of other major procedure (List separately in addition to code for primary procedure)

47010 Hepatotomy, for open drainage of abscess or cyst, 1 or 2 stages

47015 Laparotomy, with aspiration and/or injection of hepatic parasitic (eg, amoebic or echinococcal) cyst(s) or abscess(es)

Excision

Coding Atlas

The liver is the body's largest internal organ and is essential for sustaining life. It contains four functional surgical components: the right and left lobes; the medial lobes; the small caudate segment, which extends from the posterior side of the right lobe; and the quadrate lobe, which is inferior to the caudate segment and extends toward the gallbladder. Trisegmentectomy involves excision of the right (or, rarely, left) lobe plus the caudate and quadrate segments (medial segment).

47100 Biopsy of liver, wedge

47120 Hepatectomy, resection of liver; partial lobectomy

47122 trisegmentectomy

47125 total left lobectomy

47130 total right lobectomy

Liver Transplantation

Coding Atlas

Donor livers for transplantation come from cadavers or from living patients, as the liver can regrow itself. The most common reason for transplants in adults is cirrhosis; the most common reason in children is biliary atresia. CPT codes for reporting liver transplant procedures are based on documentation of the lobes being transplanted.

47133 Donor hepatectomy (including cold preservation), from cadaver donor

47135 Liver allotransplantation; orthotopic, partial or whole, from cadaver or living donor, any age

47136 heterotopic, partial or whole, from cadaver or living donor, any age

47140 Donor hepatectomy (including cold preservation), from living donor; left lateral segment only (segments II and III)

47141 total left lobectomy (segments II, III and IV)

47142 total right lobectomy (segments V, VI, VII and VIII)

47143 Backbench standard preparation of cadaver donor whole liver graft prior to allotransplantation, including cholecystectomy, if necessary, and dissection and removal of surrounding soft tissues to prepare the vena cava, portal vein, hepatic artery, and common bile duct for implantation; without trisegment or lobe split

47144 with trisegment split of whole liver graft into 2 partial liver grafts (ie, left lateral segment [segments II and III] and right trisegment [segments I and IV through VIII])

47145 with lobe split of whole liver graft into 2 partial liver grafts (ie, left lobe [segments II, III, and IV] and right lobe [segments I and V through VIII])

47146 Backbench reconstruction of cadaver or living donor liver graft prior to allotransplantation; venous anastomosis, each

47147 arterial anastomosis, each

FIGURE 5-24. Liver Segments and Lobes

The Couinard classification shown in Figure 5-24 describes functional liver anatomy. The system divides the liver into eight independent functional sections, rather than basing classification on the **morphology** of the organ. Each Couinard segment may be **resected** without damaging segments that remain.

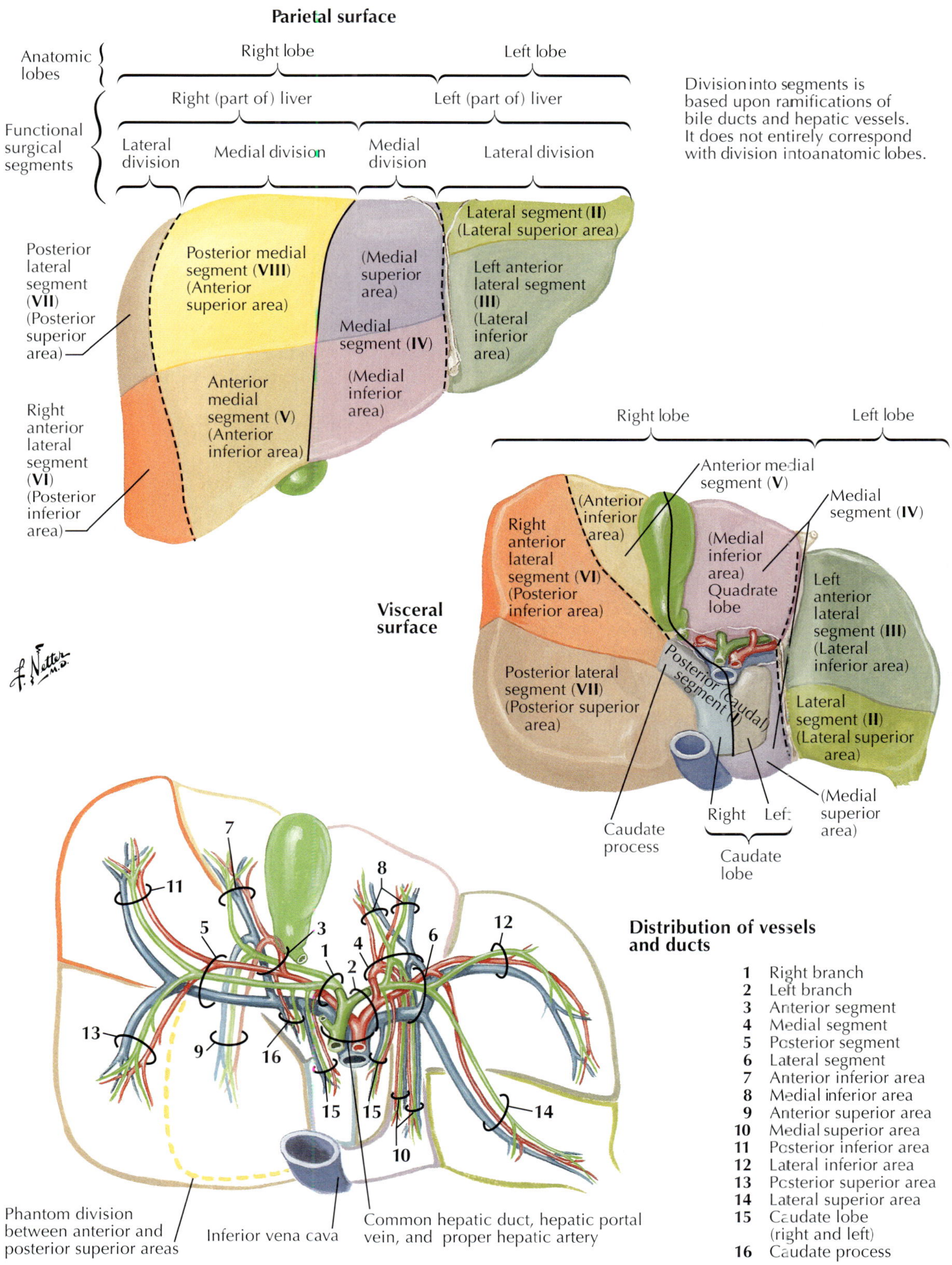

Repair

Coding Atlas

Liver tissue is highly vascularized and very delicate. Abscess of the liver is usually the result of a biliary tract obstruction and infection.

47300 Marsupialization of cyst or abscess of liver

47350 Management of liver hemorrhage; simple suture of liver wound or injury

47360 complex suture of liver wound or injury, with or without hepatic artery ligation

47361 exploration of hepatic wound, extensive debridement, coagulation and/or suture, with or without packing of liver

47362 re-exploration of hepatic wound for removal of packing

Laparoscopy

Coding Atlas

Laparoscopy is a technique developed to reduce risk and recovery time during abdominal surgery. Several small abdominal incisions act as portals for a tiny video camera (laparoscope), light source, and surgical tools. The physician manipulates the surgical tools while viewing the surgical site on a video display screen or through an eyepiece. To enhance visibility, the abdomen may be filled with gas during the procedure. **Radiofrequency ablation** (RFA) of liver tumors is used to destroy targeted tissue. This is done by inserting a needle electrode into the site and applying high-frequency electrical current into the needle to destroy the abnormal cells. Cryosurgery involves use of a freezing probe inserted into the malignant tissue to destroy it.

47370 Laparoscopy, surgical, ablation of 1 or more liver tumor(s); radiofrequency

47371 cryosurgical

47379 Unlisted laparoscopic procedure, liver

Other Procedures

Coding Atlas

In an **open** approach, the physician has **direct visualization** of the liver through an abdominal incision. In a **percutaneous** approach, ultrasound or computed tomography guidance aids the physician in correct placement of the ablation tool through a small percutaneous incision; this is done without direct visualization. **Radiofrequency** ablation (RFA) of liver tumors is used to destroy targeted tissue. This is done by inserting a needle electrode into the site and applying high-frequency electrical current into the needle to destroy the abnormal cells. **Cryosurgery** involves use of a freezing probe inserted into the malignant tissue to destroy it.

47380 Ablation, open, of 1 or more liver tumor(s); radiofrequency

47381 cryosurgical

⊙ **47382** Ablation, 1 or more liver tumor(s), percutaneous, radiofrequency

⊙ **47383** Ablation, 1 or more liver tumor(s), percutaneous, cryoablation

FIGURE 5-25. Laparoscopy

For many digestive procedures, **laparoscopy** has become the treatment of choice. It is considered less invasive, less expensive, and has a shorter recovery time than that for **laparotomy**. In laparoscopy, small incisions are made in the patient's abdomen to provide portals for lighting, tools, and a camera. The image from the camera is projected onto a video display, and the surgeon performs the surgery while watching the video image. In Figure 5-25, the physician is using a laparoscopic approach to biopsy a patient's liver. Note: Tools, implants, and/or equipment depicted in the illustration may be outdated but the procedural approach is valid.

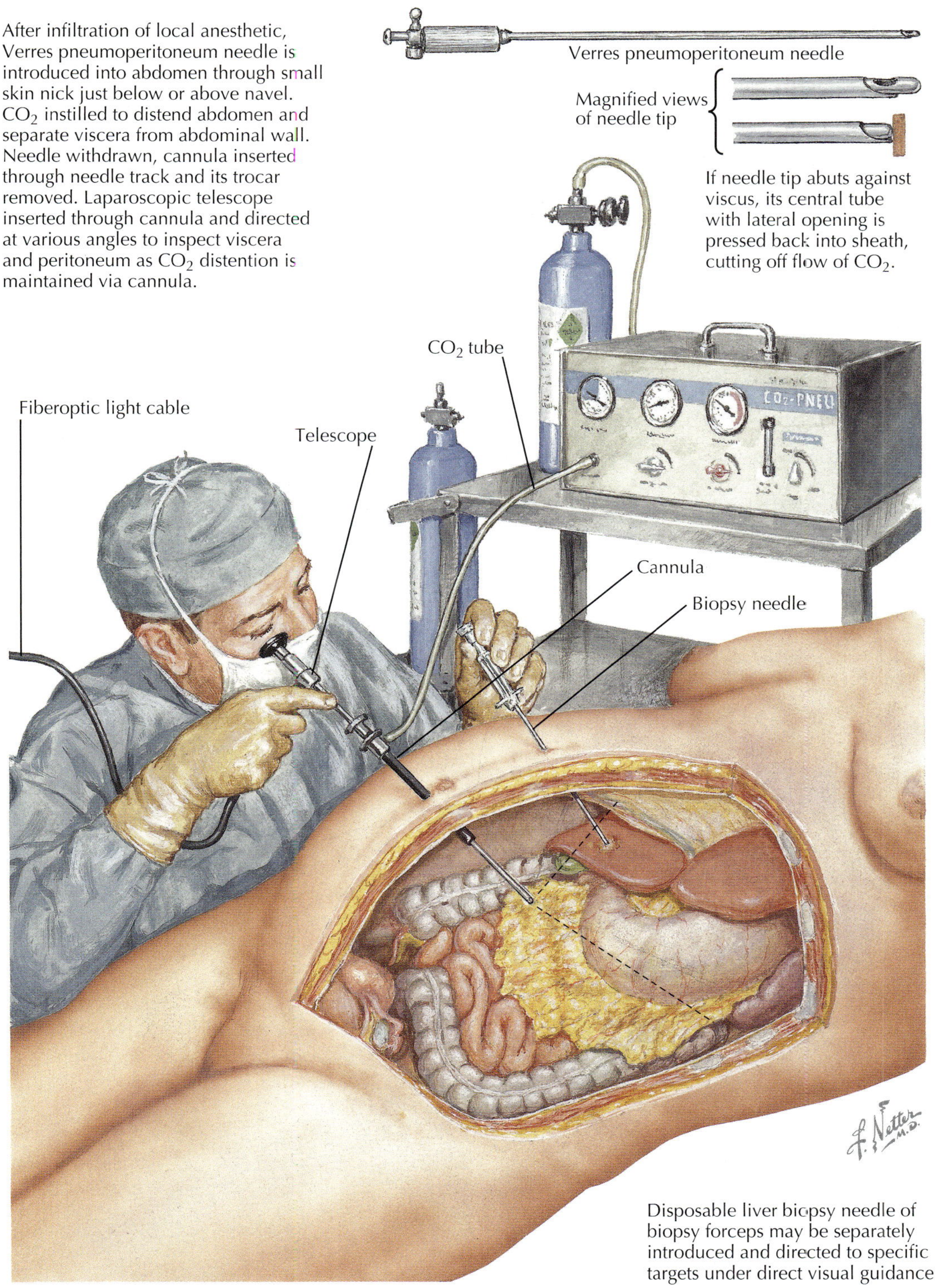

Biliary Tract

Incision

Coding Atlas

In cholelithiasis, **concretions** form from bile salts and fat in the **biliary tract**. The condition may be **benign** and asymptomatic. However, stones (**calculi**) that migrate into the cystic duct or common bile duct (CBD) may cause blockages. The stones may also cause gallbladder inflammation, or **cholecystitis**. **Choledocholithiasis** is the presence of one or more gallstones in the CBD, and **cholangitis** describes infection of the biliary tract.

47400 Hepaticotomy or hepaticostomy with exploration, drainage, or removal of calculus

47420 Choledochotomy or choledochostomy with exploration, drainage, or removal of calculus, with or without cholecystotomy; without transduodenal sphincterotomy or sphincteroplasty

47425 with transduodenal sphincterotomy or sphincteroplasty

47460 Transduodenal sphincterotomy or sphincteroplasty, with or without transduodenal extraction of calculus (separate procedure)

47480 Cholecystotomy or cholecystostomy, open, with exploration, drainage, or removal of calculus (separate procedure)

Introduction

Coding Atlas

Obstruction of the biliary system can be caused by **cholelithiasis**, infection, trauma, **cirrhosis**, or malignancy. The obstruction may be treated with a **stent** to maintain **patency** of the flow of **bile** or by **ostomy** or **catheter** to drain the bile to the skin surface, where it can be collected in a pouch. Percutaneous transhepatic cholangiography is often referred to as PTC.

47490 Cholecystostomy, percutaneous, complete procedure, including imaging guidance, catheter placement, cholecystogram when performed, and radiological supervision and interpretation

47500 Injection procedure for percutaneous transhepatic cholangiography

47505 Injection procedure for cholangiography through an existing catheter (eg, percutaneous transhepatic or T-tube)

47510 Introduction of percutaneous transhepatic catheter for biliary drainage

47511 Introduction of percutaneous transhepatic stent for internal and external biliary drainage

⊙ **47525** Change of percutaneous biliary drainage catheter

47530 Revision and/or reinsertion of transhepatic tube

Endoscopy

Coding Atlas

Many biliary procedures include **endoscopic retrograde cholangiopancreatography** (ERCP) and are reported using codes 43260-43278, which are found in the Esophagus subsection of the CPT code set. Codes in the range 47552-47556 are used to report procedures in which the approach is **percutaneous**, ie, through a T-tube. The top of the hollow T-tube is inserted into the common bile duct, and the stem of the T-tube extends from an incision in the duct to emerge through the skin. The scope and operative tools are inserted through the T-tube.

✚ **47550** Biliary endoscopy, intraoperative (choledochoscopy) (List separately in addition to code for primary procedure)

47552 Biliary endoscopy, percutaneous via T-tube or other tract; diagnostic, with collection of specimen(s) by brushing and/or washing, when performed (separate procedure)

47553 with biopsy, single or multiple

47554 with removal of calculus/calculi

47555 with dilation of biliary duct stricture(s) without stent

47556 with dilation of biliary duct stricture(s) with stent

Laparoscopy

Coding Atlas

Laparoscopy is a technique developed to reduce risk and recovery time during abdominal surgery. Several small abdominal incisions act as portals for a tiny video camera (laparoscope), light source, and surgical tools. The physician manipulates the surgical tools while viewing the surgical site on a video display screen or through an eyepiece. To enhance visibility, the abdomen may be filled with gas (**pneumoperitoneum**) during the procedure.

47560 Laparoscopy, surgical; with guided transhepatic cholangiography, without biopsy

47561 with guided transhepatic cholangiography with biopsy

FIGURE 5-26. The Gallbladder and Extrahepatic Bile Ducts

The gallbladder stores and concentrates **bile**, which is manufactured in the liver. When the walls of the duodenum sense that the nutrients within are high in protein or fat, the duodenum signals for the release of bile from the gallbladder. The bile travels from the gallbladder through the cystic duct and into the common bile duct (CBD) to the duodenum. There, bile salts react with and emulsify the fats. **Cholelithiasis** occurs when the bile salts crystalize with cholesterol to form stones (**calculi**).

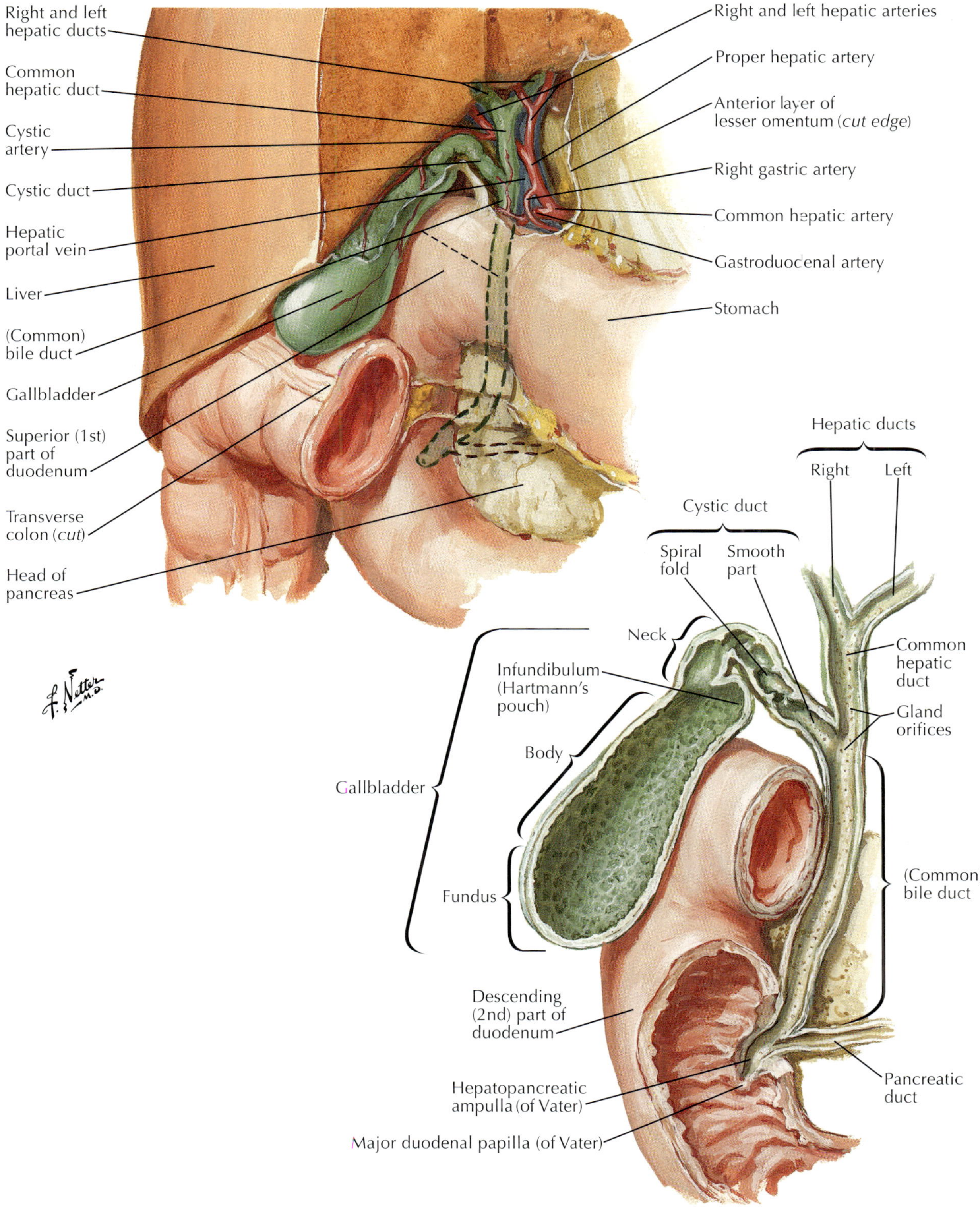

47562 cholecystectomy

47563 cholecystectomy with cholangiography

47564 cholecystectomy with exploration of common duct

47570 cholecystoenterostomy

Excision

Coding Atlas

Patency of the biliary ducts is essential to the health of the pancreas, liver, and gallbladder. Patency may be checked via cholangiography or X ray of the ducts using contrast. In some cases, an open procedure will be required to treat stones, atresia, or a bile duct tumor.

47600 Cholecystectomy;

47605 with cholangiography

47610 Cholecystectomy with exploration of common duct;

47612 with choledochoenterostomy

47620 with transduodenal sphincterotomy or sphincteroplasty, with or without cholangiography

47630 Biliary duct stone extraction, percutaneous via T-tube tract, basket, or snare (eg, Burhenne technique)

47700 Exploration for congenital atresia of bile ducts, without repair, with or without liver biopsy, with or without cholangiography

47701 Portoenterostomy (eg, Kasai procedure)

47711 Excision of bile duct tumor, with or without primary repair of bile duct; extrahepatic

47712 intrahepatic

47715 Excision of choledochal cyst

Repair

Coding Atlas

A communication between the common bile duct and the intestine may be surgically created so that bile can drain into the intestine. This is called choledochoenterostomy.

47720 Cholecystoenterostomy; direct

47721 with gastroenterostomy

47740 Roux-en-Y

47741 Roux-en-Y with gastroenterostomy

47760 Anastomosis, of extrahepatic biliary ducts and gastrointestinal tract

47765 Anastomosis, of intrahepatic ducts and gastrointestinal tract

47780 Anastomosis, Roux-en-Y, of extrahepatic biliary ducts and gastrointestinal tract

47785 Anastomosis, Roux-en-Y, of intrahepatic biliary ducts and gastrointestinal tract

47800 Reconstruction, plastic, of extrahepatic biliary ducts with end-to-end anastomosis

47801 Placement of choledochal stent

47802 U-tube hepaticoenterostomy

47900 Suture of extrahepatic biliary duct for pre-existing injury (separate procedure)

Pancreas

Incision

Coding Atlas

Pancreatitis is an inflammatory disorder in which pancreatic enzymes that usually are transported to the duodenum to digest food remain to erode and "digest" pancreatic tissue. Drains may be placed to aid healing.

48000 Placement of drains, peripancreatic, for acute pancreatitis;

48001 with cholecystostomy, gastrostomy, and jejunostomy

48020 Removal of pancreatic calculus

Excision

Coding Atlas

The ampulla of Vater is formed by the union of the pancreatic duct and the common bile duct. It may also be referred to as the hepatopancreatic ampulla. The proximal pancreas includes the head and uncinate process. The distal end includes the body and tail of the pancreas.

48100 Biopsy of pancreas, open (eg, fine needle aspiration, needle core biopsy, wedge biopsy)

48102 Biopsy of pancreas, percutaneous needle

48105 Resection or debridement of pancreas and peripancreatic tissue for acute necrotizing pancreatitis

48120 Excision of lesion of pancreas (eg, cyst, adenoma)

FIGURE 5-27. The Pancreas

The pancreas is an endocrine gland that contains both endocrine and exocrine components. The head of the pancreas communicates with the duodenum through the pancreatic duct (duct of Wirsung); digestive enzymes flow through this duct to aid in duodenal digestion. The pancreas also contains islets of Langerhans, which are cell clusters that produce insulin. Insulin is taken up by the bloodstream to metabolize sugars in the blood.

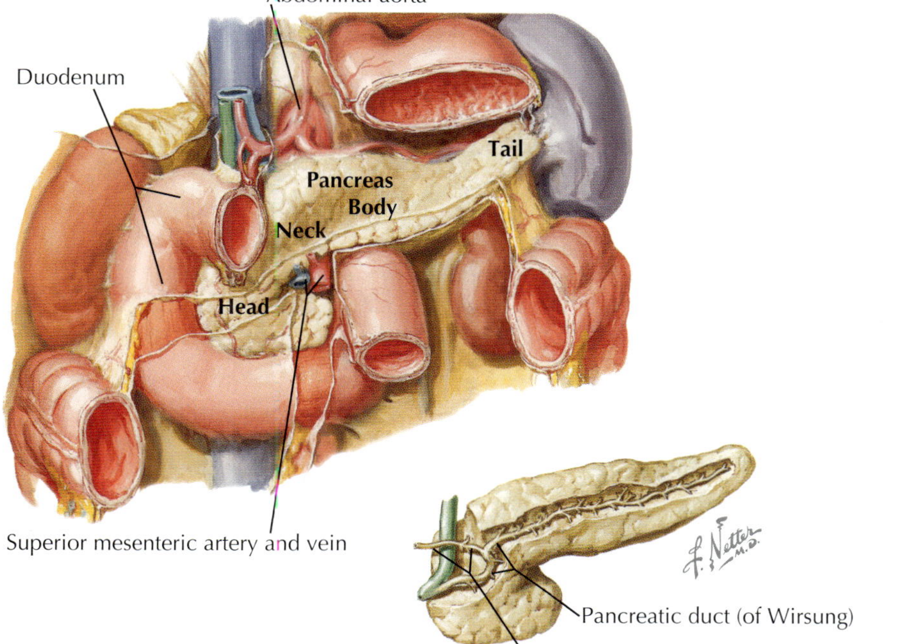

48140	Pancreatectomy, distal subtotal, with or without splenectomy; without pancreaticojejunostomy
48145	with pancreaticojejunostomy
48146	Pancreatectomy, distal, near-total with preservation of duodenum (Child-type procedure)
48148	Excision of ampulla of Vater
48150	Pancreatectomy, proximal subtotal with total duodenectomy, partial gastrectomy, choledochoenterostomy and gastrojejunostomy (Whipple-type procedure); with pancreatojejunostomy
48152	without pancreatojejunostomy
48153	Pancreatectomy, proximal subtotal with near-total duodenectomy, choledochoenterostomy and duodenojejunostomy (pylorus-sparing, Whipple-type procedure); with pancreatojejunostomy
48154	without pancreatojejunostomy
48155	Pancreatectomy, total
48160	Pancreatectomy, total or subtotal, with autologous transplantation of pancreas or pancreatic islet cells

Introduction

✚ 48400	Injection procedure for intraoperative pancreatography (List separately in addition to code for primary procedure)

Repair

Coding Atlas

In **marsupialization**, a **cyst** is unroofed and its edges are sutured so that the cyst's floor becomes continuous with the adjacent surface.

48500	Marsupialization of pancreatic cyst
48510	External drainage, pseudocyst of pancreas, open
48520	Internal anastomosis of pancreatic cyst to gastrointestinal tract; direct
48540	Roux-en-Y
48545	Pancreatorrhaphy for injury

48547 Duodenal exclusion with gastrojejunostomy for pancreatic injury

48548 Pancreaticojejunostomy, side-to-side anastomosis (Puestow-type operation)

Pancreas Transplantation

Coding Atlas

The majority of pancreas transplants involve type 1 diabetes patients who are undergoing concurrent kidney transplant. This is called a simultaneous pancreas-kidney transplant. Some pancreas transplants are performed in patients who have already undergone kidney transplant, while a small number of patients undergo pancreatic transplant without kidney transplant. The donor pancreatic tissue is usually from a cadaver.

48550 Donor pancreatectomy (including cold preservation), with or without duodenal segment for transplantation

48551 Backbench standard preparation of cadaver donor pancreas allograft prior to transplantation, including dissection of allograft from surrounding soft tissues, splenectomy, duodenotomy, ligation of bile duct, ligation of mesenteric vessels, and Y-graft arterial anastomoses from iliac artery to superior mesenteric artery and to splenic artery

48552 Backbench reconstruction of cadaver donor pancreas allograft prior to transplantation, venous anastomosis, each

48554 Transplantation of pancreatic allograft

48556 Removal of transplanted pancreatic allograft

Abdomen, Peritoneum, and Omentum

Incision

Coding Atlas

Abdominal paracentesis may be performed to gather a sample for pathological analysis or as a therapy for ascites, which is the accumulation of fluid in the abdominal cavity. In laparotomy, a midline incision is made in the abdomen so that the organs can be seen by direct visualization.

49000 Exploratory laparotomy, exploratory celiotomy with or without biopsy(s) (separate procedure)

49002 Reopening of recent laparotomy

49010 Exploration, retroperitoneal area with or without biopsy(s) (separate procedure)

49020 Drainage of peritoneal abscess or localized peritonitis, exclusive of appendiceal abscess, open

49040 Drainage of subdiaphragmatic or subphrenic abscess, open

49060 Drainage of retroperitoneal abscess, open

49062 Drainage of extraperitoneal lymphocele to peritoneal cavity, open

49082 Abdominal paracentesis (diagnostic or therapeutic); without imaging guidance

49083 with imaging guidance

49084 Peritoneal lavage, including imaging guidance, when performed

Excision, Destruction

Coding Atlas

Some abdominal tumors do not appear to be attached to a specific organ but rather lie in the connective tissues of the abdomen. The codes used to report biopsy or excision of these tumors are based on anatomical region rather than the specific organ.

49180 Biopsy, abdominal or retroperitoneal mass, percutaneous needle

49203 Excision or destruction, open, intra-abdominal tumors, cysts or endometriomas, 1 or more peritoneal, mesenteric, or retroperitoneal primary or secondary tumors; largest tumor 5 cm diameter or less

49204 largest tumor 5.1-10.0 cm diameter

49205 largest tumor greater than 10.0 cm diameter

49215 Excision of presacral or sacrococcygeal tumor

49220 Staging laparotomy for Hodgkins disease or lymphoma (includes splenectomy, needle or open biopsies of both liver lobes, possibly also removal of abdominal nodes, abdominal node and/or bone marrow biopsies, ovarian repositioning)

49250 Umbilectomy, omphalectomy, excision of umbilicus (separate procedure)

49255 Omentectomy, epiploectomy, resection of omentum (separate procedure)

FIGURE 5-28. The Retroperitoneum

The **retroperitoneum** is the space within the abdominal cavity that lies behind the parietal **peritoneum** and is **anterior** to the fascia and muscle of the flank and lower back. Organs in the retroperitoneum include the kidneys, aorta, and rectum. The peritoneum is the membrane that forms the lining of the abdominal cavity, and the **omentum** is a peritoneal fold that connects organs to the abdominal wall.

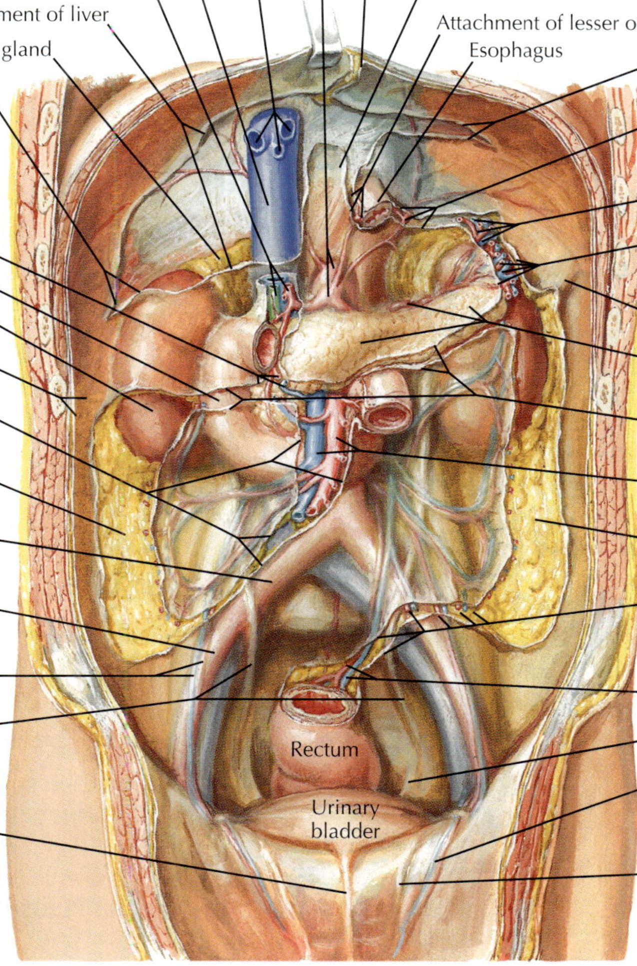

Laparoscopy

Coding Atlas

Laparoscopy is a technique developed to reduce risk and recovery time during abdominal surgery. Several small abdominal incisions act as portals for a tiny video camera (laparoscope), light source, and surgical tools. The physician manipulates the surgical tools while viewing the surgical site on a video display screen or through an eyepiece. To enhance visibility, the abdomen may be filled with gas (**pneumoperitoneum**) during the procedure.

49320 Laparoscopy, abdomen, peritoneum, and omentum, diagnostic, with or without collection of specimen(s) by brushing or washing (separate procedure)

49321 Laparoscopy, surgical; with biopsy (single or multiple)

49322 with aspiration of cavity or cyst (eg, ovarian cyst) (single or multiple)

49323 with drainage of lymphocele to peritoneal cavity

49324 with insertion of tunneled intraperitoneal catheter

49325 with revision of previously placed intraperitoneal cannula or catheter, with removal of intraluminal obstructive material if performed

✚ **49326** with omentopexy (omental tacking procedure) (List separately in addition to code for primary procedure)

✚ **49327** with placement of interstitial device(s) for radiation therapy guidance (eg, fiducial markers, dosimeter), intra-abdominal, intrapelvic, and/or retroperitoneum, including imaging guidance, if performed, single or multiple (List separately in addition to code for primary procedure)

Introduction, Revision, Removal

Coding Atlas

At times during the treatment or recovery of a patient, the continuous **lumen** that is the alimentary canal must be temporarily or permanently disrupted. The disruption may be a blockage, eg, esophageal **malignancy**, or a more generalized problem, eg, malnutrition in a severely weakened patient. The disruption can be bypassed with the creation of a communication from the lumen to the exterior of the body. Nutrition may be provided through this communication. A **gastrostomy**, **duodenostomy**, or **jejunostomy** tube may be inserted percutaneously so that nutrients can be injected, bypassing the mouth, esophagus, and/or stomach proximal to the site. This feeding tube is often referred to as a **G-tube** (gastrostomy tube) or **J-tube** (jejunostomy tube). The tube may also be placed in the duodenum for enteral feeding or in the cecum (**C-tube**) for bowel management in patients with fecal incontinence.

49400 Injection of air or contrast into peritoneal cavity (separate procedure)

49402 Removal of peritoneal foreign body from peritoneal cavity

⊙ **49405** Image-guided fluid collection drainage by catheter (eg, abscess, hematoma, seroma, lymphocele, cyst); visceral (eg, kidney, liver, spleen, lung/mediastinum), percutaneous

⊙ **49406** peritoneal or retroperitoneal, percutaneous

⊙ **49407** peritoneal or retroperitoneal, transvaginal or transrectal

⊙ **49411** Placement of interstitial device(s) for radiation therapy guidance (eg, fiducial markers, dosimeter), percutaneous, intra-abdominal, intra-pelvic (except prostate), and/or retroperitoneum, single or multiple

✚ **49412** Placement of interstitial device(s) for radiation therapy guidance (eg, fiducial markers, dosimeter), open, intra-abdominal, intrapelvic, and/or retroperitoneum, including image guidance, if performed, single or multiple (List separately in addition to code for primary procedure)

⊙ **49418** Insertion of tunneled intraperitoneal catheter (eg, dialysis, intraperitoneal chemotherapy instillation, management of ascites), complete procedure, including imaging guidance, catheter placement, contrast injection when performed, and radiological supervision and interpretation, percutaneous

49419 Insertion of tunneled intraperitoneal catheter, with subcutaneous port (ie, totally implantable)

49421 Insertion of tunneled intraperitoneal catheter for dialysis, open

49422 Removal of tunneled intraperitoneal catheter

49423 Exchange of previously placed abscess or cyst drainage catheter under radiological guidance (separate procedure)

49424 Contrast injection for assessment of abscess or cyst via previously placed drainage catheter or tube (separate procedure)

49425 Insertion of peritoneal-venous shunt

49426 Revision of peritoneal-venous shunt

49427 Injection procedure (eg, contrast media) for evaluation of previously placed peritoneal-venous shunt

49428 Ligation of peritoneal-venous shunt

49429 Removal of peritoneal-venous shunt

✚ **49435** Insertion of subcutaneous extension to intraperitoneal cannula or catheter with remote chest exit site (List separately in addition to code for primary procedure)

49436 Delayed creation of exit site from embedded subcutaneous segment of intraperitoneal cannula or catheter

Initial Placement

⊙ **49440** Insertion of gastrostomy tube, percutaneous, under fluoroscopic guidance including contrast injection(s), image documentation and report

⊙ **49441** Insertion of duodenostomy or jejunostomy tube, percutaneous, under fluoroscopic guidance including contrast injection(s), image documentation and report

⊙ **49442** Insertion of cecostomy or other colonic tube, percutaneous, under fluoroscopic guidance including contrast injection(s), image documentation and report

FIGURE 5-29. The Inguinal Canal

The inguinal canal is a **bilateral** passage in the lower anterior abdomen through which the ilioinguinal nerve and the spermatic cord passes in the male and the ilioinguinal nerve and round ligament passes in the female. Because of its composition and location, the inguinal canal can be a site through which abdominal contents can bulge in what is called an inguinal hernia. Figure 5-29 shows the inguinal canal of a male. Male inguinal canals are larger than those of the female, and the frequency of inguinal hernias is higher in males.

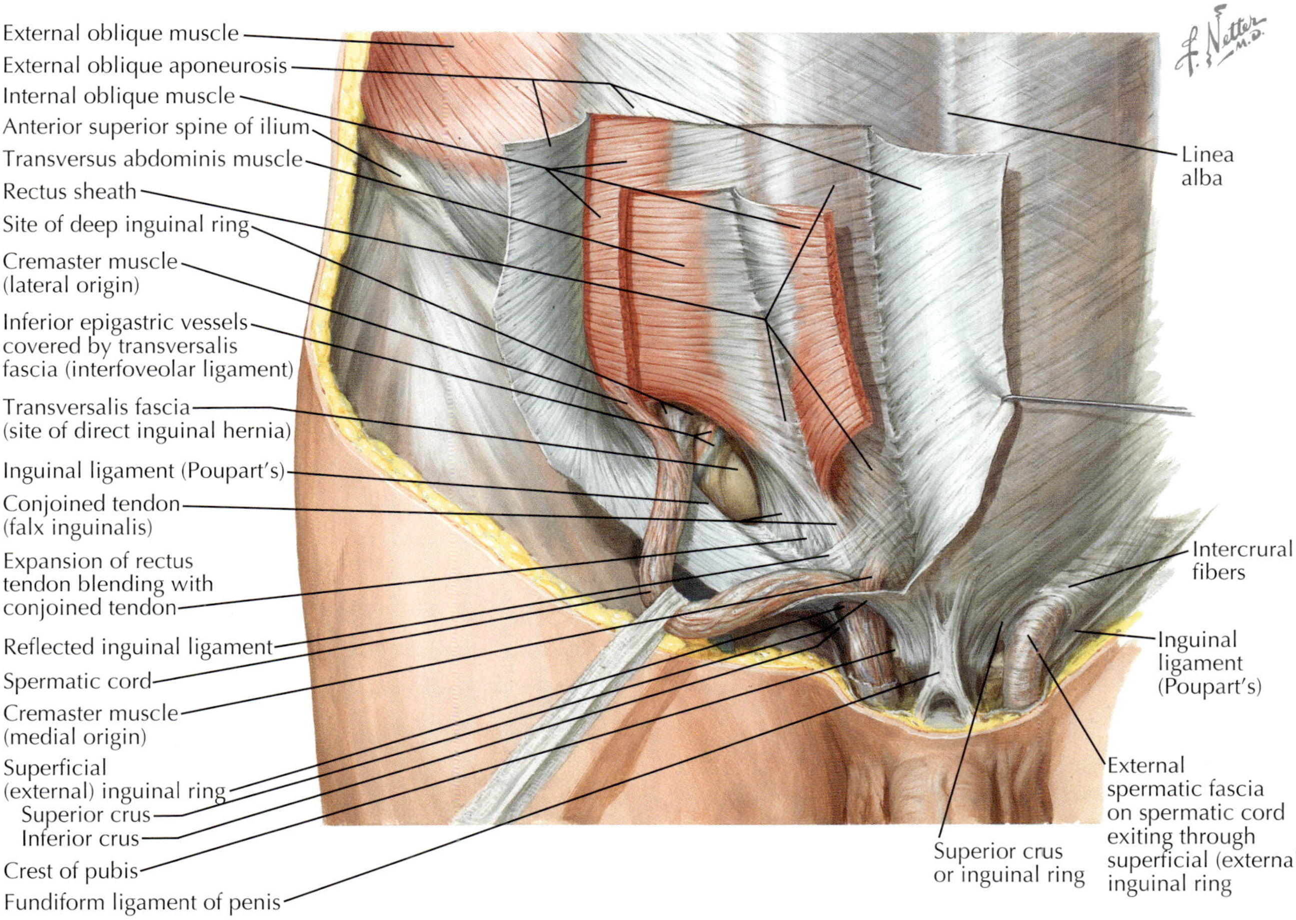

Conversion

⊙ 49446 Conversion of gastrostomy tube to gastro-jejunostomy tube, percutaneous, under fluoroscopic guidance including contrast injection(s), image documentation and report

Replacement

49450 Replacement of gastrostomy or cecostomy (or other colonic) tube, percutaneous, under fluoroscopic guidance including contrast injection(s), image documentation and report

49451 Replacement of duodenostomy or jejunostomy tube, percutaneous, under fluoroscopic guidance including contrast injection(s), image documentation and report

49452 Replacement of gastro-jejunostomy tube, percutaneous, under fluoroscopic guidance including contrast injection(s), image documentation and report

Mechanical Removal of Obstructive Material

49460 Mechanical removal of obstructive material from gastrostomy, duodenostomy, jejunostomy, gastro-jejunostomy, or cecostomy (or other colonic) tube, any method, under fluoroscopic guidance including contrast injection(s), if performed, image documentation and report

Other

49465 Contrast injection(s) for radiological evaluation of existing gastrostomy, duodenostomy, jejunostomy, gastro-jejunostomy, or cecostomy (or other colonic) tube, from a percutaneous approach including image documentation and report

Repair

Coding Atlas

There are many types of hernias. An **inguinal hernia** occurs in the abdomen near the groin area; an **umbilical hernia** occurs close to the belly button; a **ventral hernia** occurs at the site of a previous incision; and a **femoral hernia** occurs in the upper thigh near the groin. Code selection for hernia repair is based on the patient's age, the location of the hernia, whether it is a recurrent hernia, and whether the hernia is strangulated or incarcerated.

Hernioplasty, Herniorrhaphy, Herniotomy

49491 Repair, initial inguinal hernia, preterm infant (younger than 37 weeks gestation at birth), performed from birth up to 50 weeks postconception age, with or without hydrocelectomy; reducible

49492 incarcerated or strangulated

49495 Repair, initial inguinal hernia, full term infant younger than age 6 months, or preterm infant older than 50 weeks postconception age and younger than age 6 months at the time of surgery, with or without hydrocelectomy; reducible

49496 incarcerated or strangulated

49500 Repair initial inguinal hernia, age 6 months to younger than 5 years, with or without hydrocelectomy; reducible

49501 incarcerated or strangulated

49505 Repair initial inguinal hernia, age 5 years or older; reducible

49507 incarcerated or strangulated

49520 Repair recurrent inguinal hernia, any age; reducible

49521 incarcerated or strangulated

49525 Repair inguinal hernia, sliding, any age

49540 Repair lumbar hernia

49550 Repair initial femoral hernia, any age; reducible

49553 incarcerated or strangulated

49555 Repair recurrent femoral hernia; reducible

49557 incarcerated or strangulated

49560 Repair initial incisional or ventral hernia; reducible

49561 incarcerated or strangulated

49565 Repair recurrent incisional or ventral hernia; reducible

49566 incarcerated or strangulated

✚ 49568 Implantation of mesh or other prosthesis for open incisional or ventral hernia repair or mesh for closure of debridement for necrotizing soft tissue infection (List separately in addition to code for the incisional or ventral hernia repair)

49570 Repair epigastric hernia (eg, preperitoneal fat); reducible (separate procedure)

49572 incarcerated or strangulated

49580 Repair umbilical hernia, younger than age 5 years; reducible

49582 incarcerated or strangulated

49585 Repair umbilical hernia, age 5 years or older; reducible

49587 incarcerated or strangulated

49590 Repair spigelian hernia

49600 Repair of small omphalocele, with primary closure

49605 Repair of large omphalocele or gastroschisis; with or without prosthesis

49606 with removal of prosthesis, final reduction and closure, in operating room

49610 Repair of omphalocele (Gross type operation); first stage

49611 second stage

Laparoscopy

49650 Laparoscopy, surgical; repair initial inguinal hernia

49651 repair recurrent inguinal hernia

49652 Laparoscopy, surgical, repair, ventral, umbilical, spigelian or epigastric hernia (includes mesh insertion, when performed); reducible

49653 incarcerated or strangulated

49654 Laparoscopy, surgical, repair, incisional hernia (includes mesh insertion, when performed); reducible

49655 incarcerated or strangulated

49656 Laparoscopy, surgical, repair, recurrent incisional hernia (includes mesh insertion, when performed); reducible

49657 incarcerated or strangulated

Suture

49900 Suture, secondary, of abdominal wall for evisceration or dehiscence

Other Procedures

Coding Atlas

An omental pedicle flap can be key to the reconstruction of some anatomical structures. To create the flap, the physician dissects a portion of **omentum** and rotates the omentum to its new site. This keeps the **flap** connected to its blood supply. In some cases, a **free flap** is used, the severed omentum is secured, and its vessels **anastomosed** at the new site.

49904 Omental flap, extra-abdominal (eg, for reconstruction of sternal and chest wall defects)

✚ **49905** Omental flap, intra-abdominal (List separately in addition to code for primary procedure)

49906 Free omental flap with microvascular anastomosis

FIGURE 5-30. Inguinal Hernias

The most common hernia present at birth is an indirect inguinal hernia. This is the result of an abnormality in the development of the fetus. Inguinal hernias do not spontaneously repair themselves. Because of the risk of **incarceration**, surgical intervention is usually required. In incarceration, abdominal tissue is trapped in the inguinal canal and cannot be manually reduced or returned to the abdomen. A **strangulated** hernia is one to which the blood supply has been compromised. Note: Tools, implants, and/or equipment depicted in the illustration may be outdated but the procedural approach is valid.

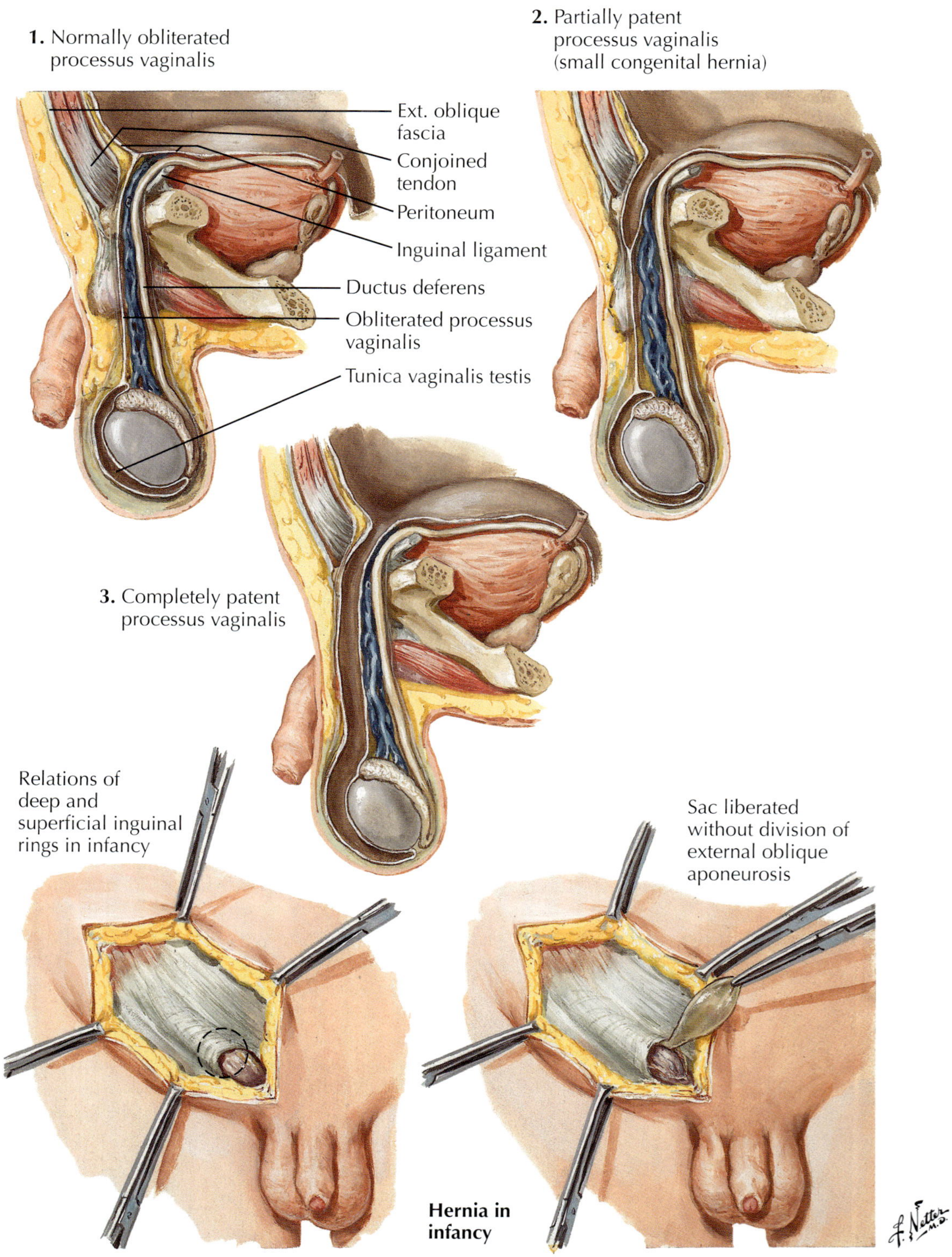

FIGURE 5-31. Omphalocele

An **omphalocele** is a **congenital** defect in which the intestines and other abdominal organs of the newborn are herniated through the navel and covered by a thin sac. The defect can be repaired in stages as the surgeon systematically coaxes the abdominal organs back into place; in time, the entire bulge is reduced. Note: Tools, implants, and/or equipment depicted in the illustration may be outdated but the procedural approach is valid.

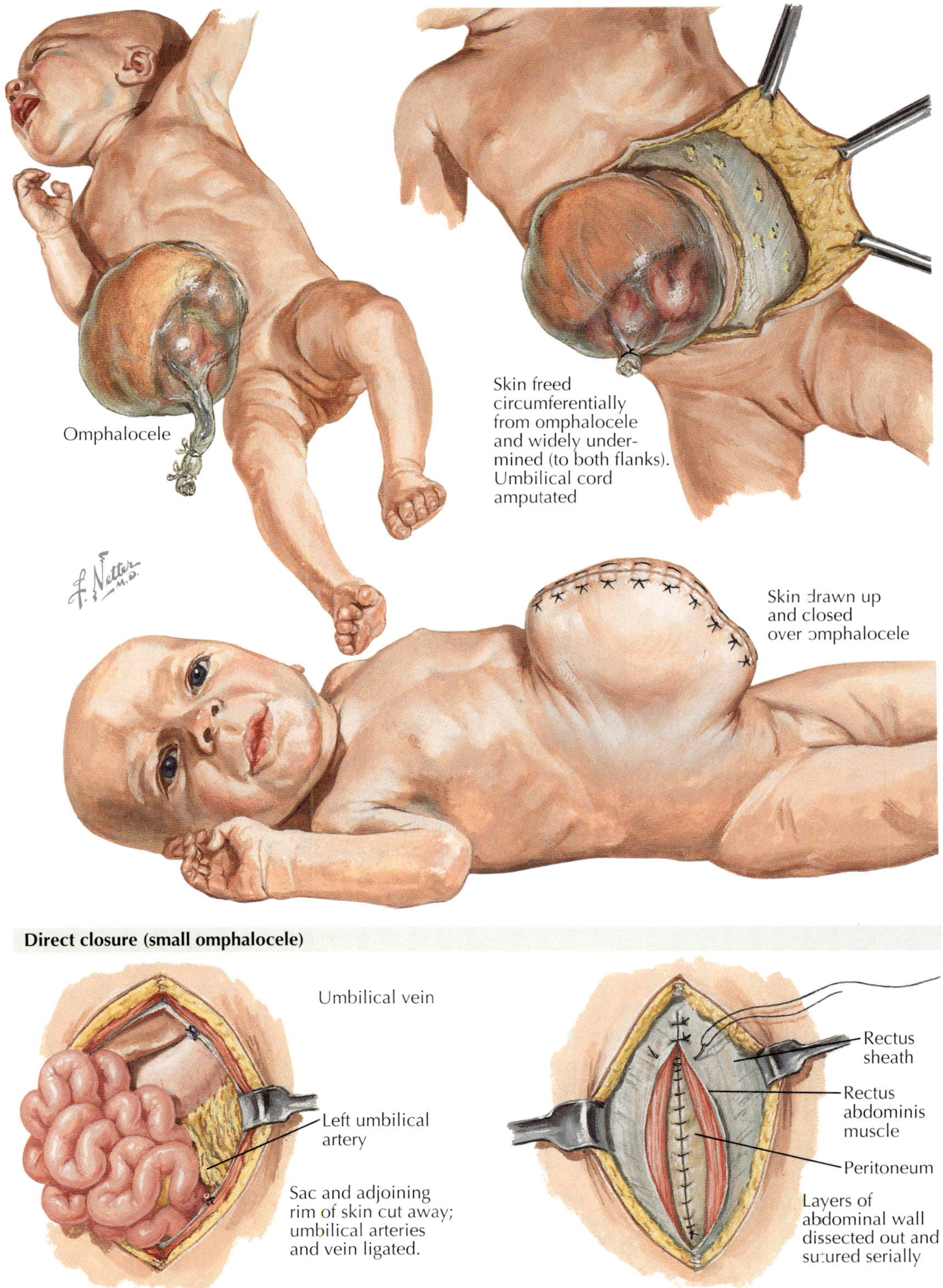

FIGURE 5-32. The Greater Omentum and Abdominal Viscera

The greater omentum is a fatty layer that covers the lower abdomen and supports and covers the **viscera**. Also referred to as the epiploon or gastrocolic omentus, the greater omentum extends from the stomach's **greater curvature** to the lower abdomen. It is secured in place by the gastrocolic and gastrosplenic ligaments.

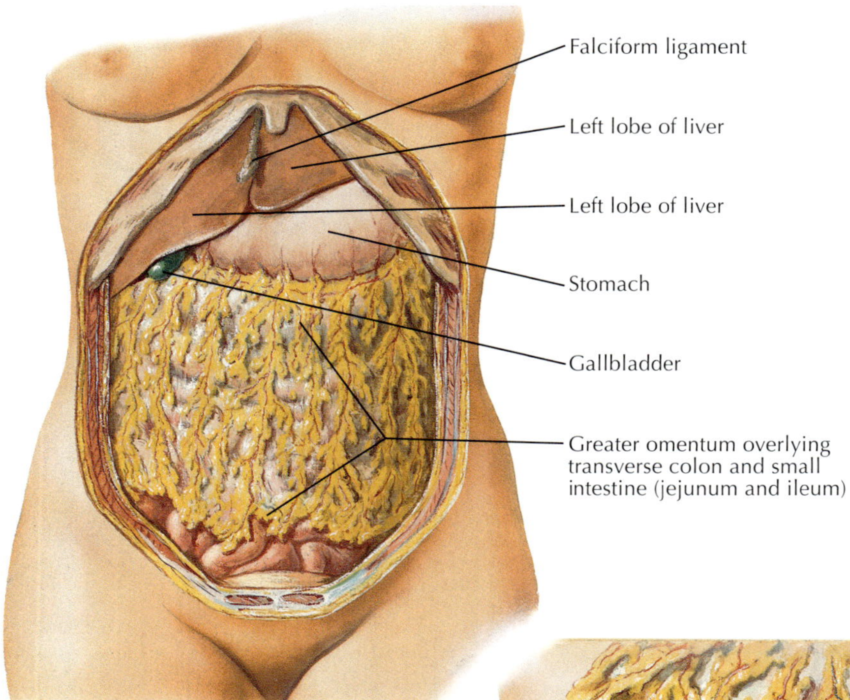

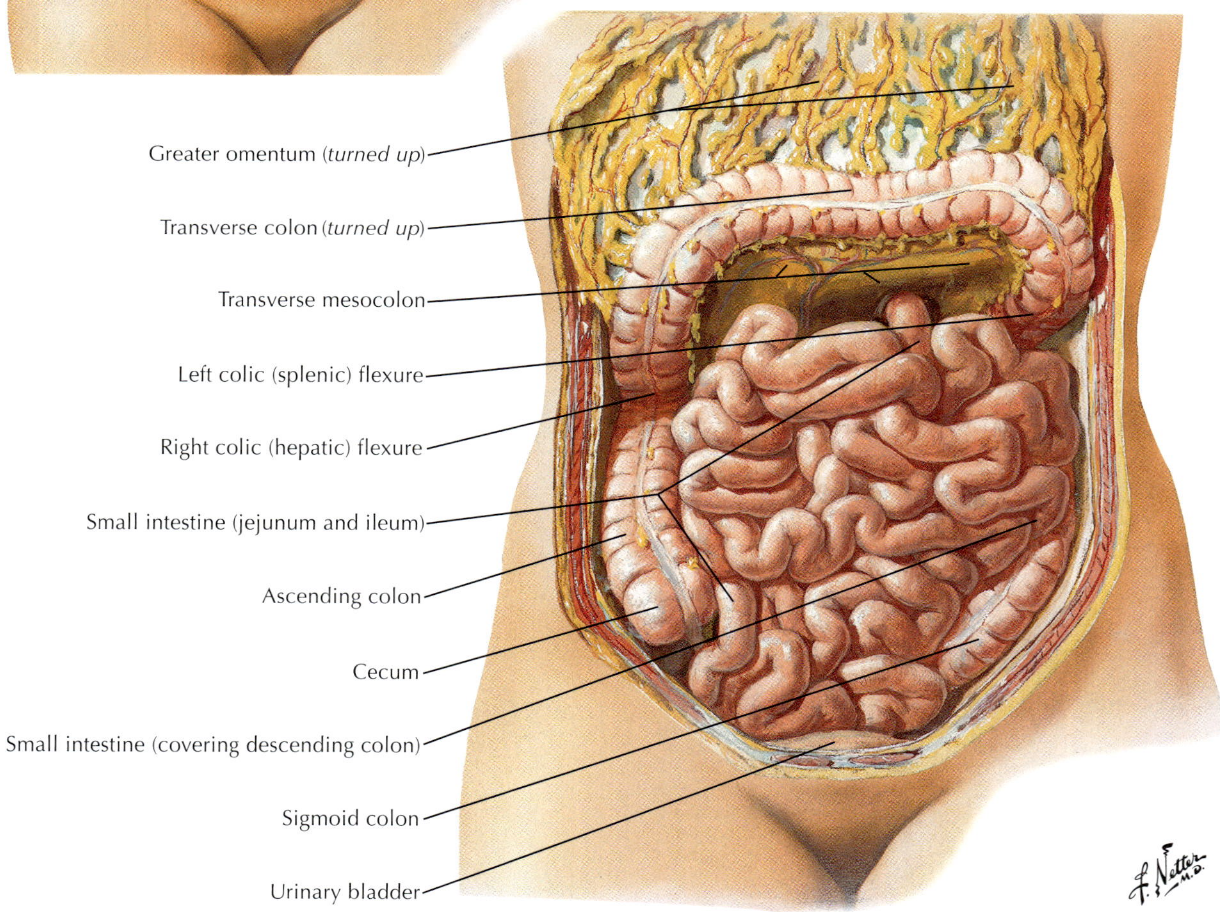

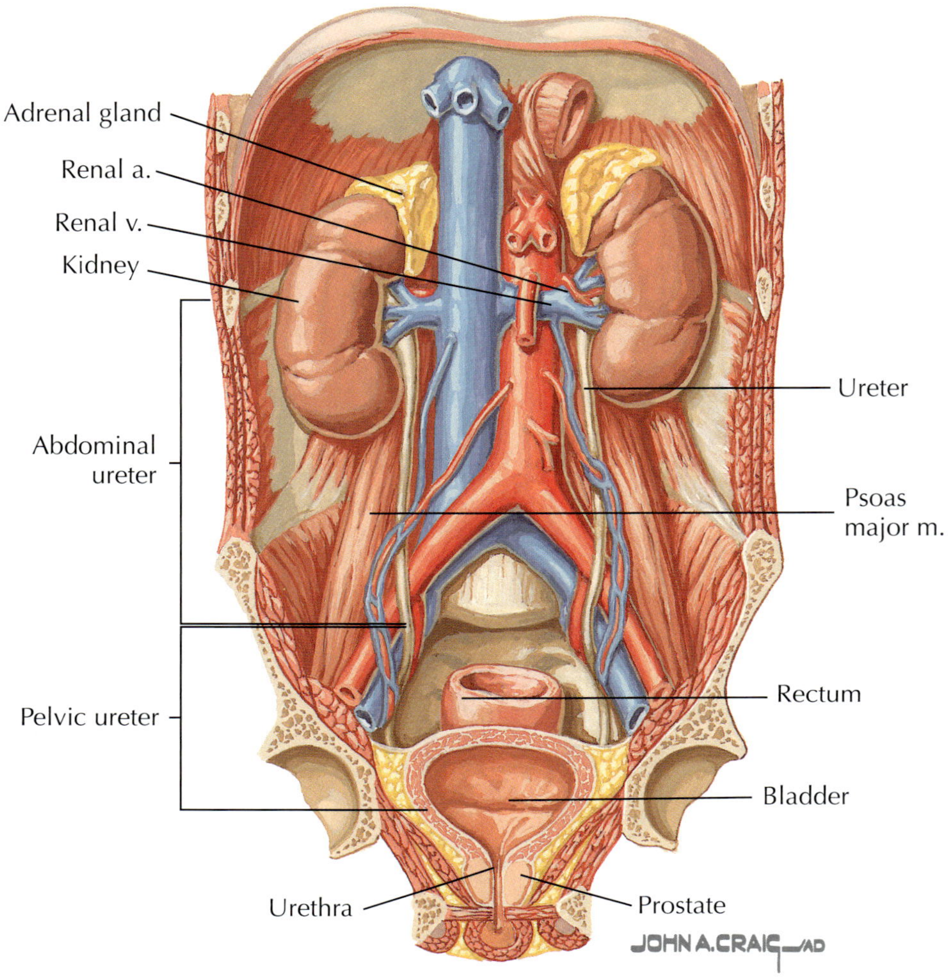
Adrenal gland
Renal a.
Renal v.
Kidney
Abdominal ureter
Pelvic ureter
Ureter
Psoas major m.
Rectum
Bladder
Urethra
Prostate
JOHN A.CRAIG—/AD

◈ CHAPTER 6 ◈

Urinary System

The urinary system consists of the kidneys, ureters, urinary bladder, and urethra. The kidneys filter metabolic wastes, excess ions, and chemicals from the blood to form urine, which is released from the body through **micturition** (urination). The ureters, urinary bladder, and urethra form the urinary tract to drain urine from the kidneys, store it, and then release it during urination. Besides filtering and eliminating wastes from the body, the urinary system also maintains the homeostasis of water, ions (potassium, sodium, calcium, magnesium, phosphate, and chloride ions), pH, blood pressure, and calcium. The glomeruli of the paired kidneys, each attached to a ureter that carries the waste (urine) to the bladder, perform the filtration process.

Each kidney is covered in a protective shell called the renal capsule. Within the capsule, glomerular tubules in the nephrons of the medulla filter and siphon fluids and waste from blood gathered from surrounding blood vessels. Some components are reabsorbed into the bloodstream, while others are diverted to the renal pelvis as waste and then diverted to the ureter.

In glomerular filtration, excess water, small proteins, salts, **glucose**, nitrogenous waste products such as urea, and other drugs or metabolic waste are filtered from the blood. The efficiency of glomerular filtration is called the glomerular filtration rate (**GFR**) and is a benchmark in the diagnosis and management of kidney disease.

Once filtration occurs in the kidney nephrons, the waste fluid converges at the renal pelvis, which narrows to join the ureter, a foot-long **lumen** that drains urine into the bladder. The bladder is a hollow, muscular organ that can stretch to hold up to 400 milliliters of urine. The muscle walls of the bladder sense when the bladder is reaching capacity and signal the need to micturate to the brain. To empty the bladder, urine is released into the hollow urethra and expelled from the body. Two urethral **sphincters** control the release of urine: the internal urinary sphincter (IUS) and external urinary sphincter (EUS). The internal urethral **sphincter** is at the base of the bladder and prevents leakage of urine into the urethra. The external sphincter lies in the tissue just **proximal** to the **perineum**. In males, the urethra may be 11 inches in length, while in females, it is typically about 2 inches in length. In males, the urethra serves a dual purpose: urination and ejaculation.

A common problem in the renal system is urinary **obstruction**. Obstruction may occur anywhere along the urinary pathway: in the kidney, ureter, bladder, or urethra. The obstruction may be a tumor, **stenosis**, or a **congenital** malformation or it may be due to a kidney or ureteral **calculus**. The stones, nephrolithiasis or ureterolithiasis, are likely caused by two factors: high levels of calcium, oxalate, and uric acid in the bloodstream, which lead to the formation of crystals, or calcium plaque that accumulates in the **subepithelial** space of the renal papilla. Obstruction caused by a stone is eliminated if the stone passes spontaneously. When the stone does not pass spontaneously, surgery may be needed, especially if the obstruction is significant or if there is an accompanying infection. A stone may be accessed using a **cystoscope** or through a **percutaneous**, **laparoscopic**, or **open** approach.

The male urethra transverses the prostate gland, which squeezes with the external sphincter to control urination. The prostate gland also contributes fluid to semen and so has both urinary and reproductive functions. While **open** procedures on the prostate are reported using codes from the Male Genital CPT code set, prostate procedures performed using a **transurethral** approach (cystoscope) are reported with codes from the Urinary System section. For reporting an open or laparoscopic approach for prostate surgery, see codes in the ranges 55700-55866 and 55873-55876.

Urinary System

Kidney

Incision

Coding Atlas

The term "pyelo" describes the pelvis of the kidney, while "nephro" is a more general term for kidney. Thus, a **nephrotomy** is an incision into any kidney site, while a **pyelotomy** is an incision into the renal pelvis. The renal pelvis is a collection site for urine produced throughout the kidney. From the renal pelvis, the urine is funneled into the ureter.

50010 Renal exploration, not necessitating other specific procedures

50020 Drainage of perirenal or renal abscess, open

50040 Nephrostomy, nephrotomy with drainage

50045 Nephrotomy, with exploration

50060 Nephrolithotomy; removal of calculus

50065 secondary surgical operation for calculus

50070 complicated by congenital kidney abnormality

50075 removal of large staghorn calculus filling renal pelvis and calyces (including anatrophic pyelolithotomy)

50080 Percutaneous nephrostolithotomy or pyelostolithotomy, with or without dilation, endoscopy, lithotripsy, stenting, or basket extraction; up to 2 cm

50081 over 2 cm

50100 Transection or repositioning of aberrant renal vessels (separate procedure)

50120 Pyelotomy; with exploration

50125 with drainage, pyelostomy

50130 with removal of calculus (pyelolithotomy, pelviolithotomy, including coagulum pyelolithotomy)

50135 complicated (eg, secondary operation, congenital kidney abnormality)

Excision

Coding Atlas

In a patient with renal cell **carcinoma** (RCC), nephron-sparing surgery (NSS) is sometimes an alternative to total **nephrectomy**. In NSS, only a portion of the kidney is removed. In **ablation**, a probe is inserted into a kidney tumor to freeze it after the kidney has been exposed surgically for direct visualization.

⊙ **50200** Renal biopsy; percutaneous, by trocar or needle

50205 by surgical exposure of kidney

50220 Nephrectomy, including partial ureterectomy, any open approach including rib resection;

50225 complicated because of previous surgery on same kidney

50230 radical, with regional lymphadenectomy and/or vena caval thrombectomy

50234 Nephrectomy with total ureterectomy and bladder cuff; through same incision

50236 through separate incision

50240 Nephrectomy, partial

50250 Ablation, open, 1 or more renal mass lesion(s), cryosurgical, including intraoperative ultrasound guidance and monitoring, if performed

50280 Excision or unroofing of cyst(s) of kidney

50290 Excision of perinephric cyst

FIGURE 6-1. Kidney Structure

The kidney is a **bilateral** organ covered in a fibrous capsule. Urine is filtered from blood in the medulla, where the nephrons reside, and then channeled into renal **calices** (calyces), which flow toward the **renal pelvis**. From there, urine is carried into the ureter.

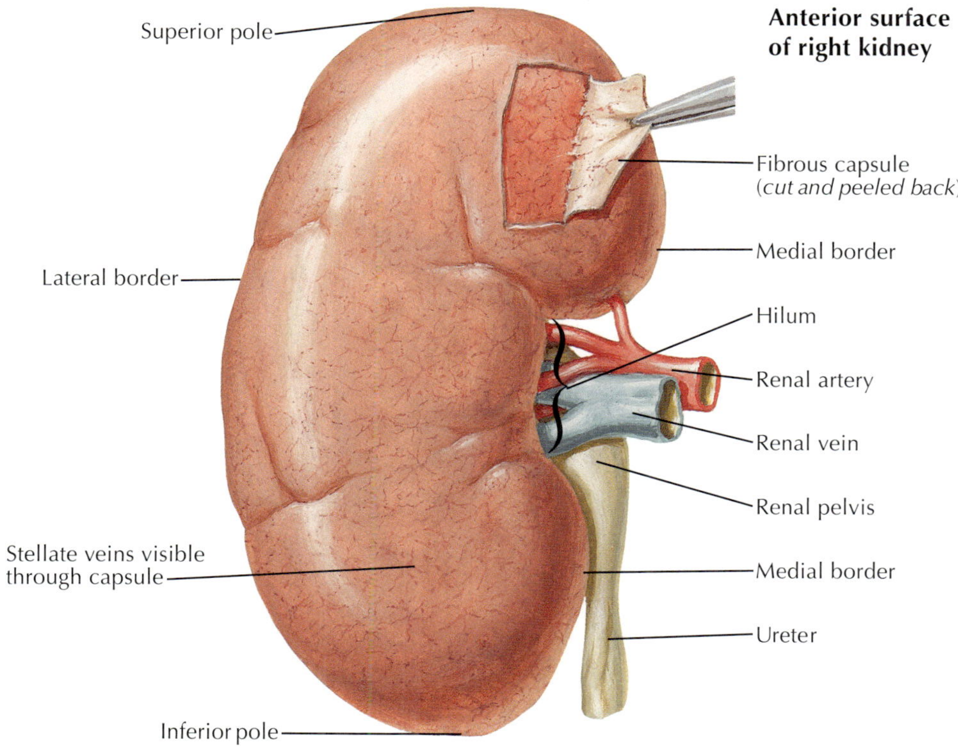

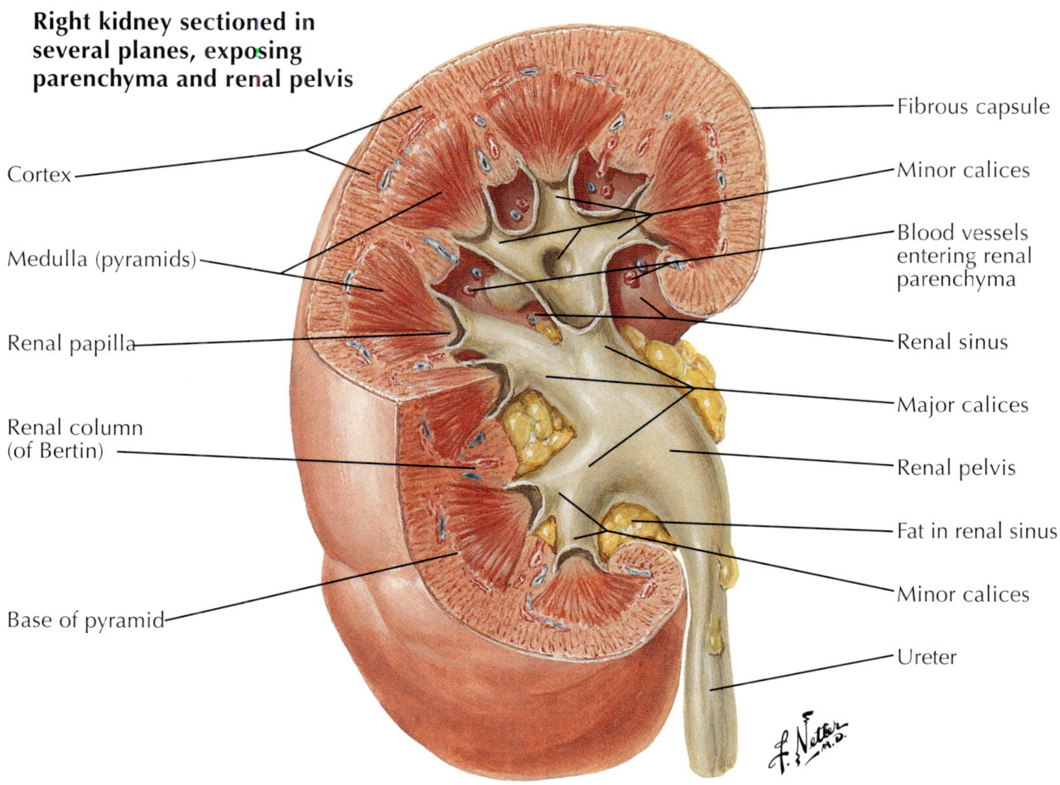

FIGURE 6-2. Kidney In Situ: Posterior View

Because the kidneys are located in the **retroperitoneum**, surgical access is often through the **flank** of the patient's back, in what may be referred to as a **subcostal** (below the ribs) approach. For transplant patients, access to the kidneys may be through a **transabdominal** approach. A **laparoscopic** approach may be retroperitoneal or through the abdomen.

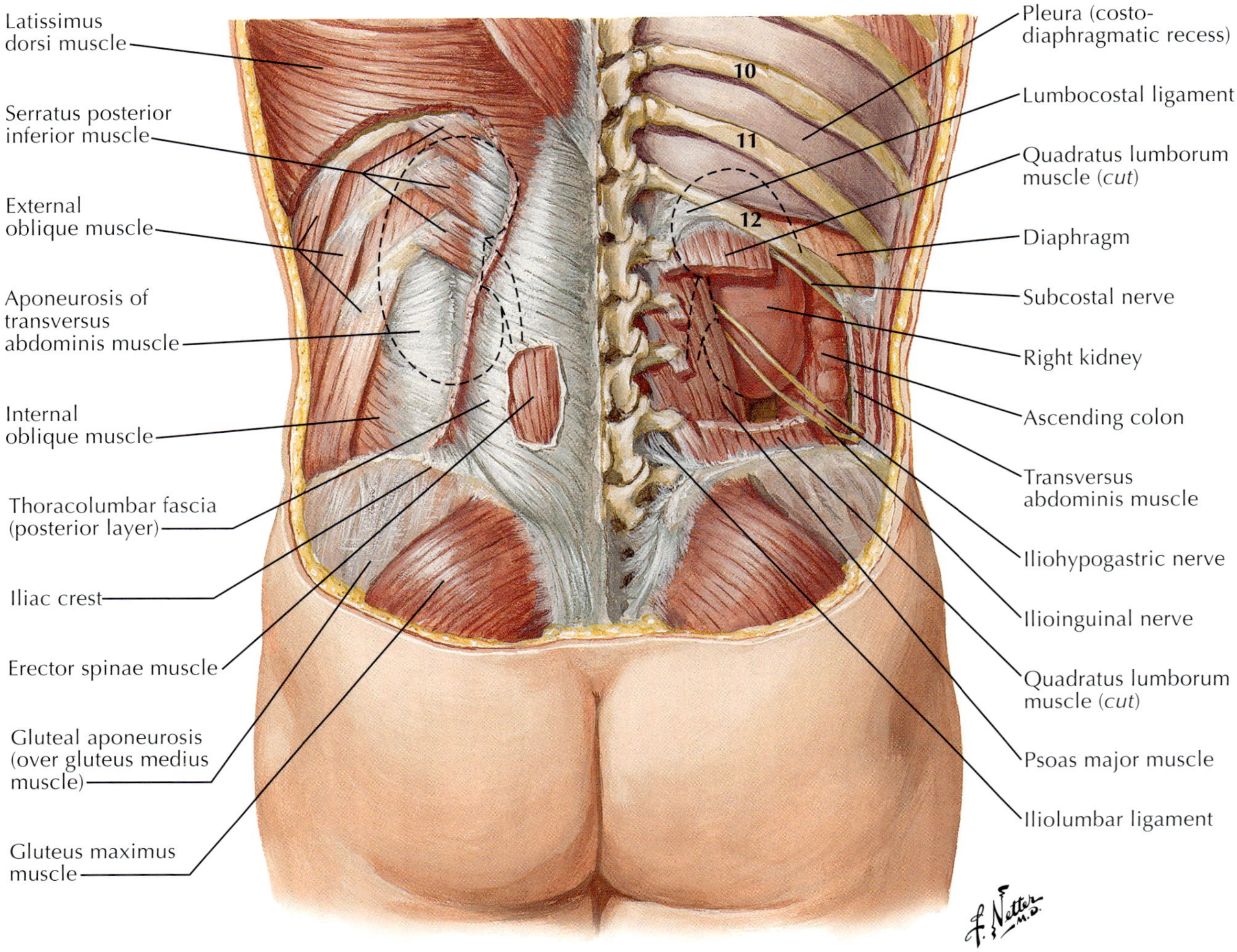

FIGURE 6-3. Renal Biopsy

A renal **biopsy** may be indicated for conditions including renal failure, infection, renal mass, and **hematuria.** The approach for renal biopsy is through the patient's back. In some cases, the biopsy can be performed using a **trocar** or needle (code 50200). In other cases, an incision is made in the skin overlying the kidney, and tissue is removed using an **open** approach (code 50205). Note: Tools, implants, and/or equipment depicted in the illustration may be outdated but the procedural approach is valid.

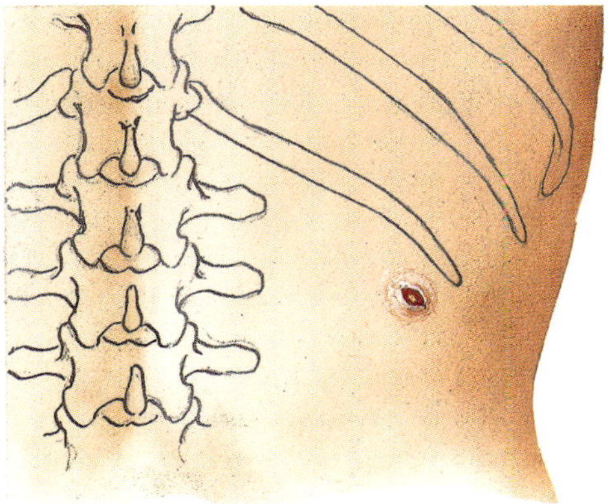

Small skin incision made in wheal at biopsy site

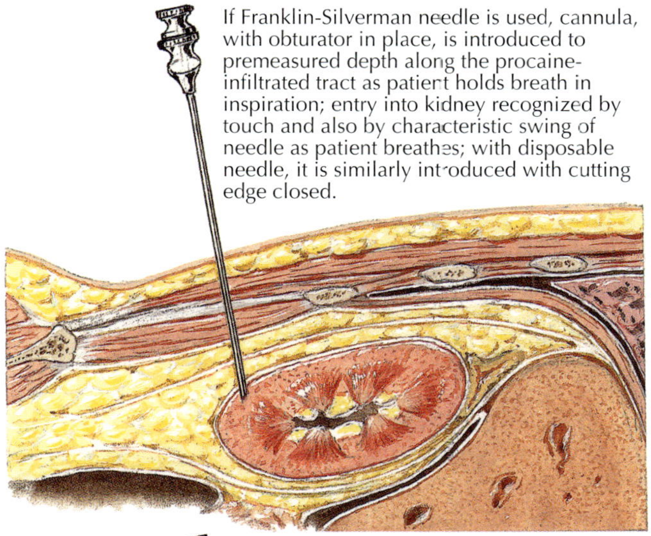

If Franklin-Silverman needle is used, cannula, with obturator in place, is introduced to premeasured depth along the procaine-infiltrated tract as patient holds breath in inspiration; entry into kidney recognized by touch and also by characteristic swing of needle as patient breathes; with disposable needle, it is similarly introduced with cutting edge closed.

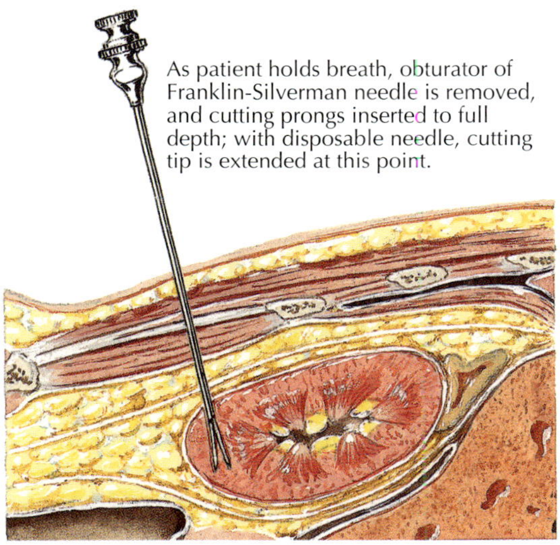

As patient holds breath, obturator of Franklin-Silverman needle is removed, and cutting prongs inserted to full depth; with disposable needle, cutting tip is extended at this point.

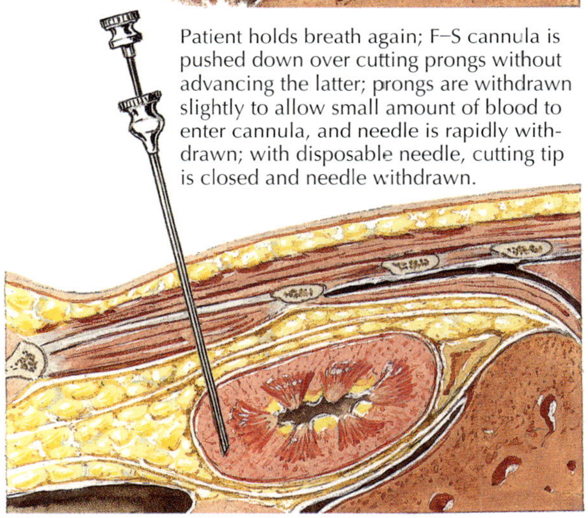

Patient holds breath again; F–S cannula is pushed down over cutting prongs without advancing the latter; prongs are withdrawn slightly to allow small amount of blood to enter cannula, and needle is rapidly withdrawn; with disposable needle, cutting tip is closed and needle withdrawn.

Surgical biopsy

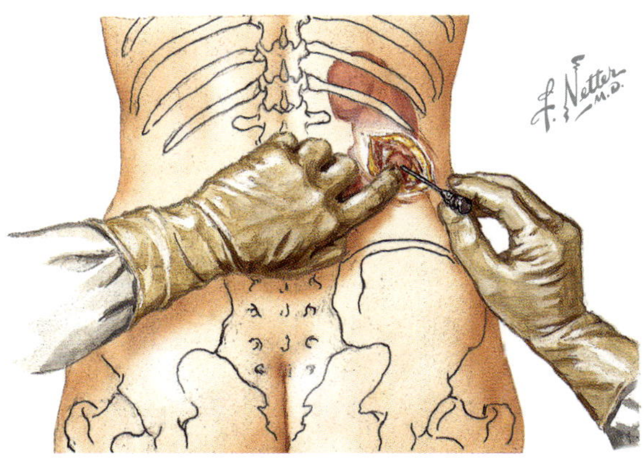

A 2-inch incision is made below outer end of 12th rib; musculature and fascia are penetrated by blunt dissection; lower pole of kidney identified by index finger of left hand which then guides needle into kidney parenchyma; biopsy specimen then taken in usual manner.

Renal Transplantation

Coding Atlas

End-stage renal disease (ESRD) occurs when the kidneys are no longer capable of filtering the body's waste. A kidney transplant can cure this condition. Although the kidneys naturally occur in pairs, a single kidney is capable of performing the filtration necessary for good health. For this reason, living donors for kidney transplants are relatively common. However, cadavers still outnumber live donors as an organ source. For transplant, three procedures are required: harvest of the donor organ, preparation of the donated organ before implant (backbench), and implant of the kidney into the recipient. Often, the existing kidneys remain in situ and the new kidney is inserted in an incision made in the patient's abdomen.

50300 Donor nephrectomy (including cold preservation); from cadaver donor, unilateral or bilateral

50320 open, from living donor

50323 Backbench standard preparation of cadaver donor renal allograft prior to transplantation, including dissection and removal of perinephric fat, diaphragmatic and retroperitoneal attachments, excision of adrenal gland, and preparation of ureter(s), renal vein(s), and renal artery(s), ligating branches, as necessary

50325 Backbench standard preparation of living donor renal allograft (open or laparoscopic) prior to transplantation, including dissection and removal of perinephric fat and preparation of ureter(s), renal vein(s), and renal artery(s), ligating branches, as necessary

50327 Backbench reconstruction of cadaver or living donor renal allograft prior to transplantation; venous anastomosis, each

50328 arterial anastomosis, each

50329 ureteral anastomosis, each

50340 Recipient nephrectomy (separate procedure)

50360 Renal allotransplantation, implantation of graft; without recipient nephrectomy

50365 with recipient nephrectomy

50370 Removal of transplanted renal allograft

50380 Renal autotransplantation, reimplantation of kidney

Introduction

Coding Atlas

Ureteral stents are thin catheters advanced into the ureter for diversion of urine into the bladder (internal) or into a collection system (external). Ureteral stents are removed when they are no longer necessary or when they need to be replaced.

Renal Pelvis Catheter Procedures

Internally Dwelling

⊙ **50382** Removal (via snare/capture) and replacement of internally dwelling ureteral stent via percutaneous approach, including radiological supervision and interpretation

⊙ **50384** Removal (via snare/capture) of internally dwelling ureteral stent via percutaneous approach, including radiological supervision and interpretation

⊙ **50385** Removal (via snare/capture) and replacement of internally dwelling ureteral stent via transurethral approach, without use of cystoscopy, including radiological supervision and interpretation

⊙ **50386** Removal (via snare/capture) of internally dwelling ureteral stent via transurethral approach, without use of cystoscopy, including radiological supervision and interpretation

Externally Accessible

⊙ **50387** Removal and replacement of externally accessible transnephric ureteral stent (eg, external/internal stent) requiring fluoroscopic guidance, including radiological supervision and interpretation

50389 Removal of nephrostomy tube, requiring fluoroscopic guidance (eg, with concurrent indwelling ureteral stent)

Other Introduction Procedures

50390 Aspiration and/or injection of renal cyst or pelvis by needle, percutaneous

50391 Instillation(s) of therapeutic agent into renal pelvis and/or ureter through established nephrostomy, pyelostomy or ureterostomy tube (eg, anticarcinogenic or antifungal agent)

50392 Introduction of intracatheter or catheter into renal pelvis for drainage and/or injection, percutaneous

50393 Introduction of ureteral catheter or stent into ureter through renal pelvis for drainage and/or injection, percutaneous

FIGURE 6-4. Kidney Transplantation

A donor kidney is usually transplanted to the right iliac fossa with the renal artery anastomosed end-to-end to the hypogastric artery. Then, the renal vein end is anastomosed end-to-side to the iliac vein. The ureter is implanted into the bladder. This procedure is called an allotransplant because the donor organ is of the same species as the recipient. Note: Tools, implants, and/or equipment depicted in the illustration may be outdated but the procedural approach is valid.

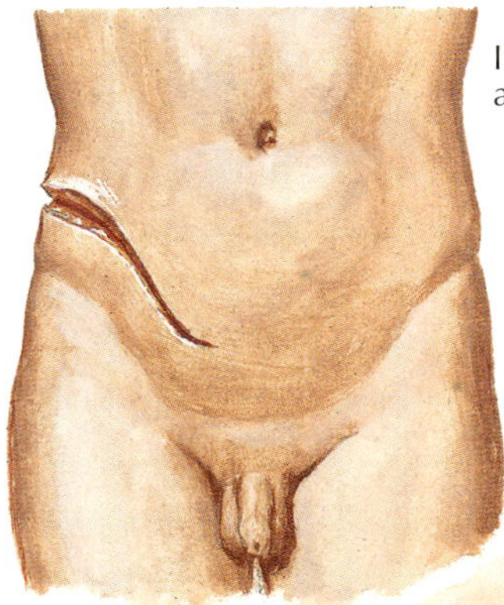

Incision in right lower quadrant and flank through skin, supeficial fat and fascia, muscles, and transversalis fascia, leaving peritoneum intact.

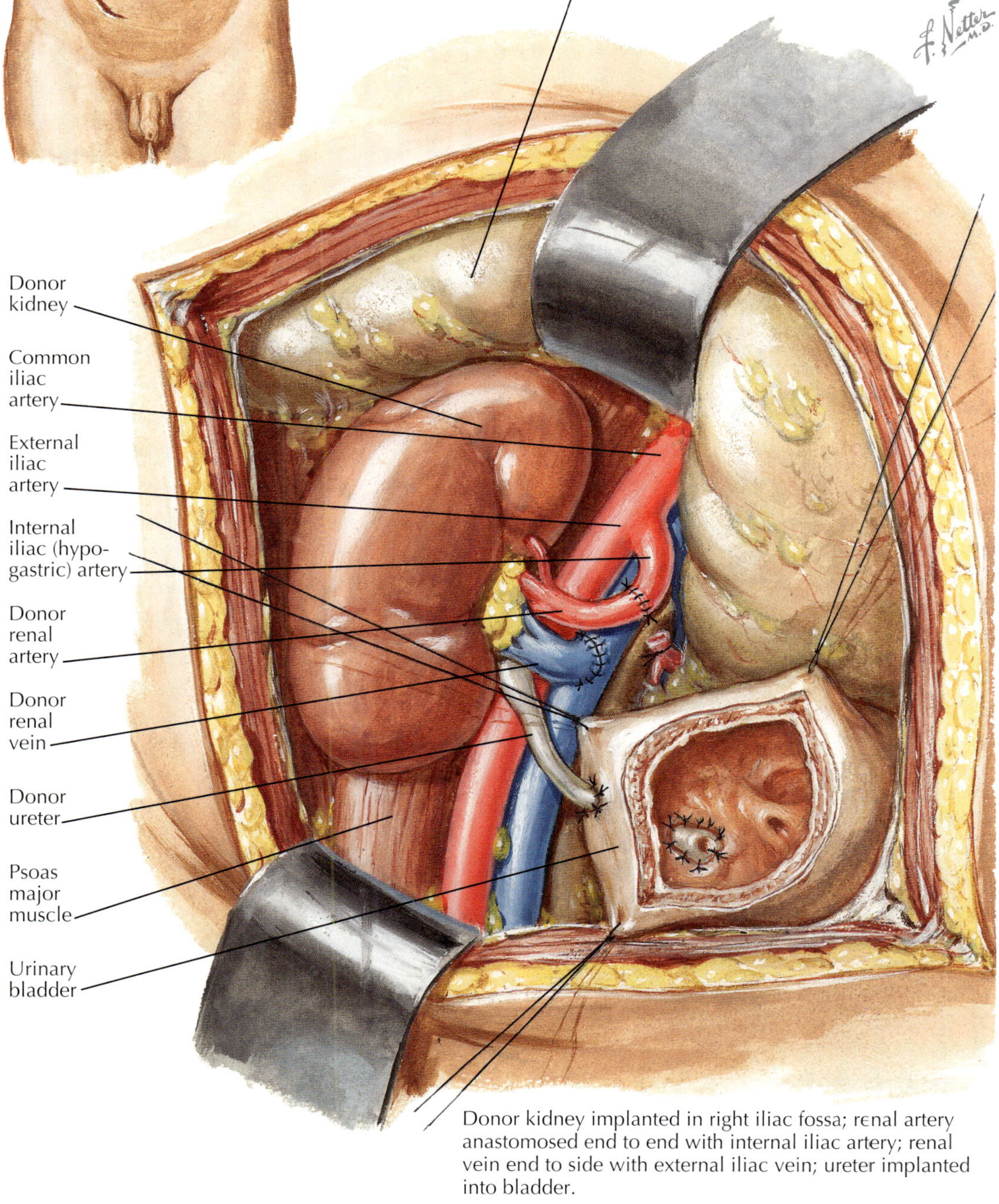

Donor kidney implanted in right iliac fossa; renal artery anastomosed end to end with internal iliac artery; renal vein end to side with external iliac vein; ureter implanted into bladder.

50394 Injection procedure for pyelography (as nephrostogram, pyelostogram, antegrade pyeloureterograms) through nephrostomy or pyelostomy tube, or indwelling ureteral catheter

50395 Introduction of guide into renal pelvis and/or ureter with dilation to establish nephrostomy tract, percutaneous

50396 Manometric studies through nephrostomy or pyelostomy tube, or indwelling ureteral catheter

50398 Change of nephrostomy or pyelostomy tube

Repair

Coding Atlas

A Foley Y-**pyeloplasty** widens the **ureteropelvic junction** (UPJ) by advancing a Y-shaped flap of renal pelvis into a vertical incision in the upper ureter.

50400 Pyeloplasty (Foley Y-pyeloplasty), plastic operation on renal pelvis, with or without plastic operation on ureter, nephropexy, nephrostomy, pyelostomy, or ureteral splinting; simple

50405 complicated (congenital kidney abnormality, secondary pyeloplasty, solitary kidney, calycoplasty)

50500 Nephrorrhaphy, suture of kidney wound or injury

50520 Closure of nephrocutaneous or pyelocutaneous fistula

50525 Closure of nephrovisceral fistula (eg, renocolic), including visceral repair; abdominal approach

50526 thoracic approach

50540 Symphysiotomy for horseshoe kidney with or without pyeloplasty and/or other plastic procedure, unilateral or bilateral (1 operation)

Laparoscopy

Coding Atlas

Laparoscopy is a technique developed to reduce risk and recovery time during abdominal or pelvic surgery. Several small incisions act as portals for a tiny video camera (**laparoscope**), light source, and surgical tools. The physician manipulates the surgical tools while viewing the surgical site on a video display screen or through an eyepiece. To enhance visibility, the abdomen may be filled with gas during the procedure.

50541 Laparoscopy, surgical; ablation of renal cysts

50542 ablation of renal mass lesion(s), including intraoperative ultrasound guidance and monitoring, when performed

50543 partial nephrectomy

50544 pyeloplasty

50545 radical nephrectomy (includes removal of Gerota's fascia and surrounding fatty tissue, removal of regional lymph nodes, and adrenalectomy)

50546 nephrectomy, including partial ureterectomy

50547 donor nephrectomy (including cold preservation), from living donor

50548 nephrectomy with total ureterectomy

Endoscopy

Coding Atlas

A **nephrostomy** is a communication between the kidney and the skin's surface for the diversion of urine. A **pyelostomy** is a communication between the renal pelvis and the skin's surface for the diversion of urine. A **nephrotomy** is an incision into the kidney, and a **pyelotomy** is an incision into the kidney pelvis. An **endoscope** may be advanced through a **stoma** (codes 50551-50562) or an incision (codes 50570-50580) for **diagnostic** or **therapeutic** purposes. Codes are selected based on the type of access and the procedure that is performed through the endoscope.

50551 Renal endoscopy through established nephrostomy or pyelostomy, with or without irrigation, instillation, or ureteropyelography, exclusive of radiologic service;

50553 with ureteral catheterization, with or without dilation of ureter

50555 with biopsy

50557 with fulguration and/or incision, with or without biopsy

50561 with removal of foreign body or calculus

50562 with resection of tumor

50570 Renal endoscopy through nephrotomy or pyelotomy, with or without irrigation, instillation, or ureteropyelography, exclusive of radiologic service;

50572 with ureteral catheterization, with or without dilation of ureter

50574 with biopsy

50575 with endopyelotomy (includes cystoscopy, ureteroscopy, dilation of ureter and ureteral pelvic junction, incision of ureteral pelvic junction and insertion of endopyelotomy stent)

50576 with fulguration and/or incision, with or without biopsy

50580 with removal of foreign body or calculus

FIGURE 6-5. Renal Fusion

Of possible congenital renal malformations, the horseshoe kidney is the most common. In a horseshoe kidney, two functioning kidneys are connected at their lower ends by a segment of renal parenchyma or fibrous tissue. The aberrant kidneys may develop chronic obstruction, calculi, or infection, though some patients with horseshoe kidneys are asymptomatic throughout life.

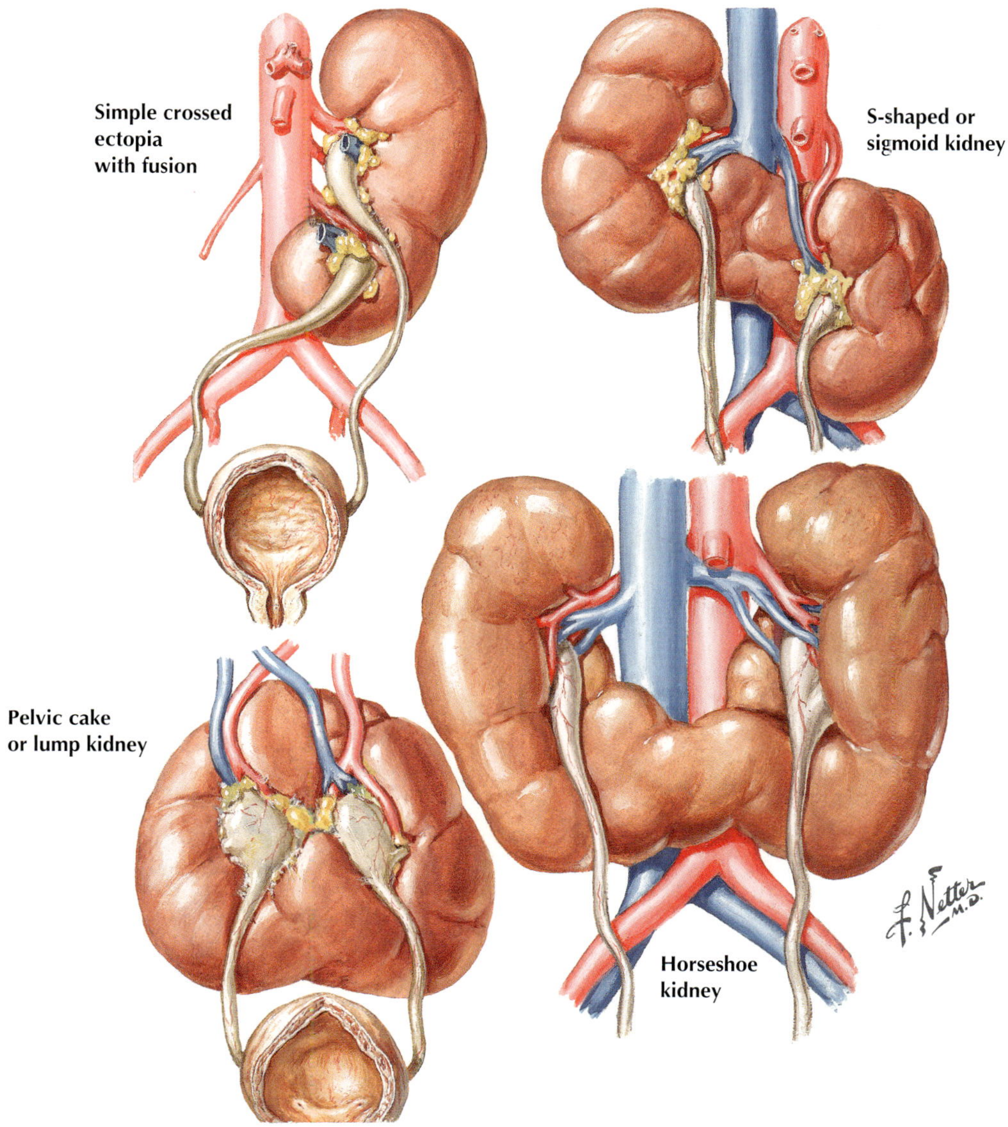

Other Procedures

Coding Atlas

In percutaneous ablation, a thin probe or multiple probes are inserted through a small incision overlying the kidney, and a tumor or tumors are subjected to radiofrequency or cryotherapy.

50590	Lithotripsy, extracorporeal shock wave
⊙ 50592	Ablation, 1 or more renal tumor(s), percutaneous, unilateral, radiofrequency
⊙ 50593	Ablation, renal tumor(s), unilateral, percutaneous, cryotherapy

FIGURE 6-6. Extracorporeal Shock Wave Lithotripsy

Lithotripsy involves the use of focused, high-energy sound waves to break up **calculi** in the kidney, bladder, or ureter so that the resultant pieces can easily move through the urinary tract and be eliminated during urination. During lithotripsy, **fluoroscopy** or **ultrasound** is used to localize the stone so that the sound waves can be focused on it. The patient is placed on water-filled cushions to minimize dissipation of energy from the shock waves as they pass through the skin. Note: Tools, implants, and/or equipment depicted in the illustration may be outdated but the procedural approach is valid.

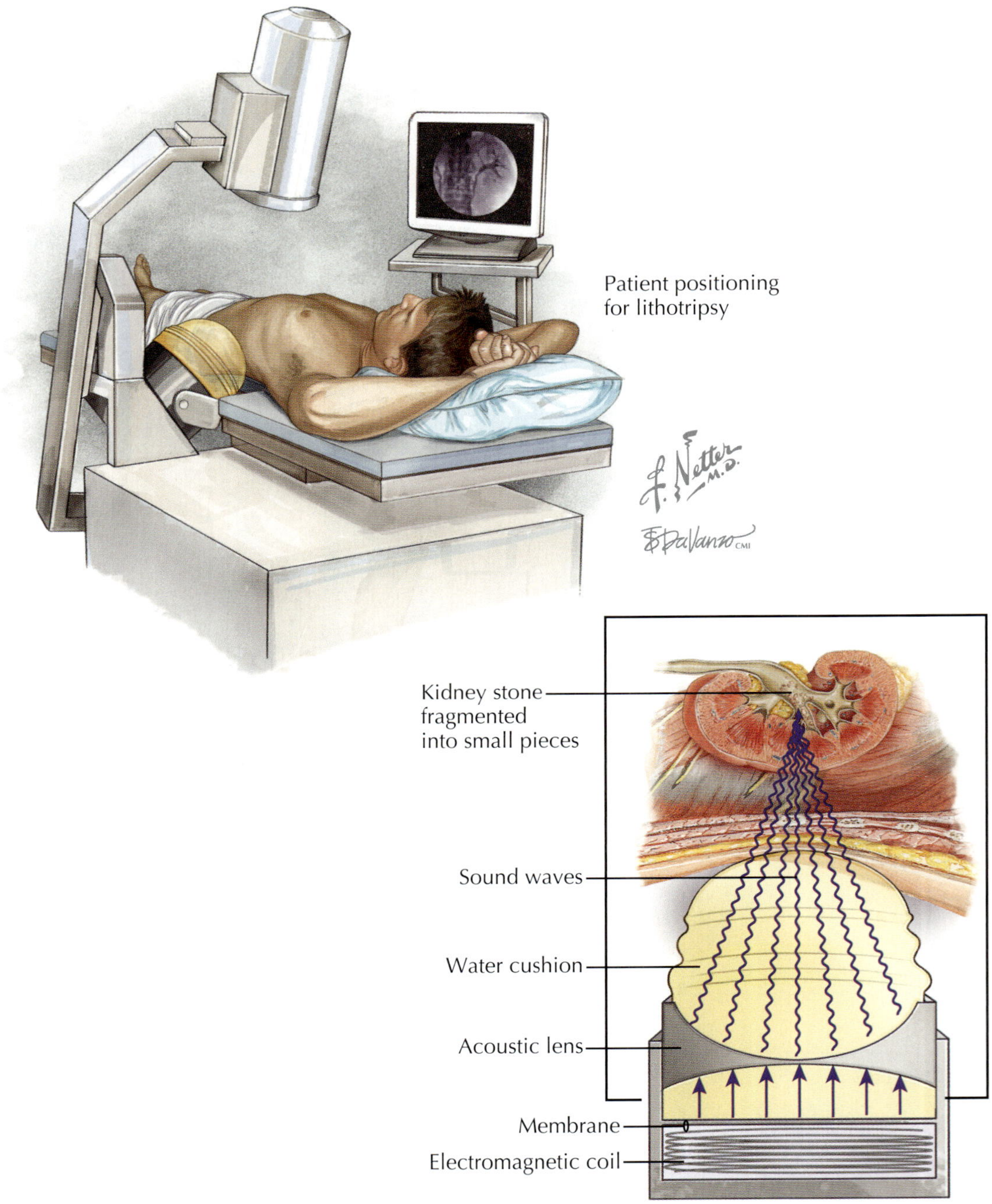

Ureter

Incision

Coding Atlas

Code 50605 is used to report a procedure in which the physician makes an incision in the skin overlying the ureter (open **ureterotomy**) and incises the ureter for the placement of a **stent** under **direct visualization**. This is generally performed when there is an **obstruction** in the ureter that endangers kidney function. The stent acts to open the ureteral obstruction. It would not be appropriate to report code 50605 for a more complex procedure that involves ureteral **anastomosis** or if the physician approaches the stent site from the bladder or the kidney.

50600 Ureterotomy with exploration or drainage (separate procedure)

50605 Ureterotomy for insertion of indwelling stent, all types

50610 Ureterolithotomy; upper one-third of ureter

50620 middle one-third of ureter

50630 lower one-third of ureter

Excision

Coding Atlas

An **ectopic** ureter is a **congenital** anomaly in which a ureter connects to the kidney for urine drainage but does not connect **distally** to the bladder. Instead, it empties into the urethra, vagina, or elsewhere. The ectopic ureter may be a redundant ureter, meaning one kidney has two ureters: one that empties urine into the bladder and one that empties urine elsewhere.

50650 Ureterectomy, with bladder cuff (separate procedure)

50660 Ureterectomy, total, ectopic ureter, combination abdominal, vaginal and/or perineal approach

Introduction

Coding Atlas

Manometry is the measurement of pressure. Code 50686 is used to report the measurement of pressure in the ureter as fluid is infused through a **ureterostomy** or catheter site. This infusion study can be used to identify points of ureteral obstruction.

50684 Injection procedure for ureterography or ureteropyelography through ureterostomy or indwelling ureteral catheter

50686 Manometric studies through ureterostomy or indwelling ureteral catheter

50688 Change of ureterostomy tube or externally accessible ureteral stent via ileal conduit

50690 Injection procedure for visualization of ileal conduit and/or ureteropyelography, exclusive of radiologic service

Repair

Coding Atlas

A **ureteroileal** conduit is a surgical solution for a patient whose bladder has been removed. A portion of **ileum** is excised, and the remaining bowel is reanastamosed end-to-end. The segment of ileum becomes a **neobladder**. One end of this segment is fashioned as a **stoma** site on the skin surface, while the other end is closed to create the neobladder pouch. The ureter is then anastamosed into the side of the pouch. Code 50820 is used to report this procedure. If the second ureter is anastamosed to the pouch, a **bilateral** modifier would be applied to code 50820. If the bladder is removed during the same surgical session, the procedure would be reported with code 51590.

50700 Ureteroplasty, plastic operation on ureter (eg, stricture)

50715 Ureterolysis, with or without repositioning of ureter for retroperitoneal fibrosis

50722 Ureterolysis for ovarian vein syndrome

50725 Ureterolysis for retrocaval ureter, with reanastomosis of upper urinary tract or vena cava

50727 Revision of urinary-cutaneous anastomosis (any type urostomy);

50728 with repair of fascial defect and hernia

50740 Ureteropyelostomy, anastomosis of ureter and renal pelvis

50750 Ureterocalycostomy, anastomosis of ureter to renal calyx

50760 Ureteroureterostomy

50770 Transureteroureterostomy, anastomosis of ureter to contralateral ureter

50780 Ureteroneocystostomy; anastomosis of single ureter to bladder

50782 anastomosis of duplicated ureter to bladder

50783 with extensive ureteral tailoring

50785 with vesico-psoas hitch or bladder flap

FIGURE 6-7. The Ureters

The ureters are paired muscular tubes that begin at the renal pelvis and connect distally to the bladder. The ureters begin in the posterior abdomen and transverse many structures for 25 centimeters to 30 centimeters before terminating at the bladder in the anterior of the pelvis. **Peristalsis** moves the urine in a bolus toward the bladder when the flow is light. When the urine flow is heavier, the ureter opens like a pipe for a free flow of urine.

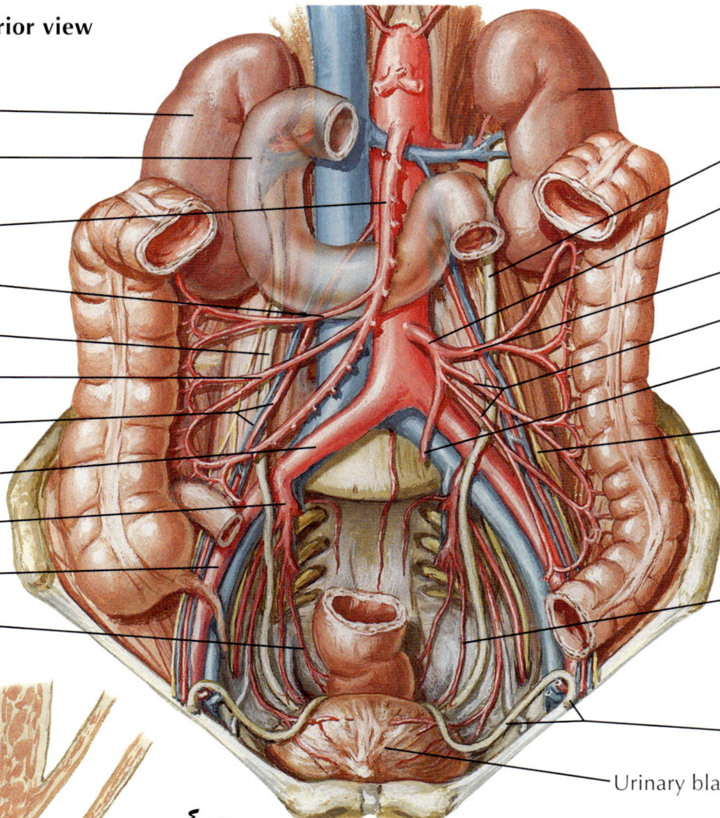

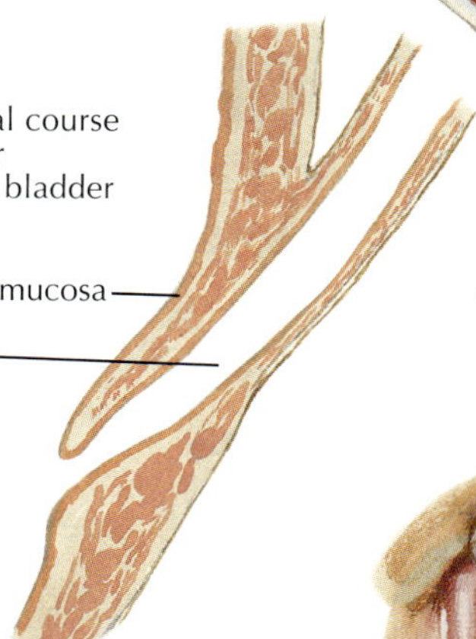

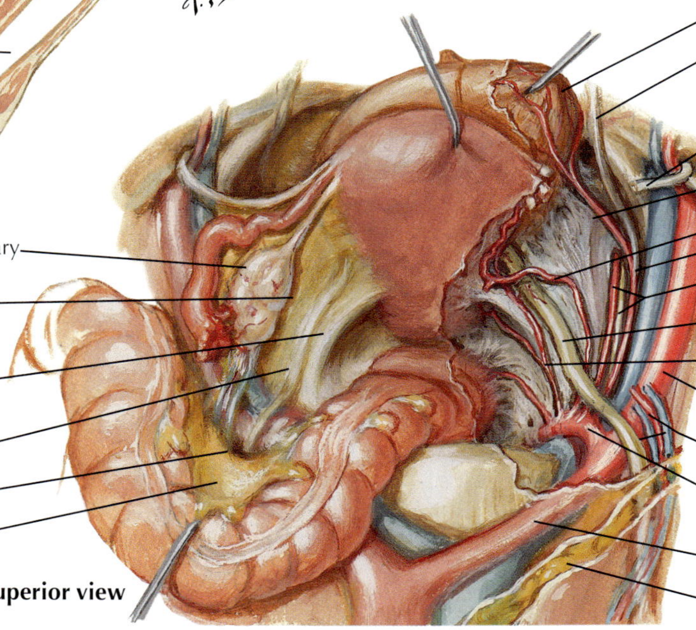

50800 Ureteroenterostomy, direct anastomosis of ureter to intestine

50810 Ureterosigmoidostomy, with creation of sigmoid bladder and establishment of abdominal or perineal colostomy, including intestine anastomosis

50815 Ureterocolon conduit, including intestine anastomosis

50820 Ureteroileal conduit (ileal bladder), including intestine anastomosis (Bricker operation)

50825 Continent diversion, including intestine anastomosis using any segment of small and/or large intestine (Kock pouch or Camey enterocystoplasty)

50830 Urinary undiversion (eg, taking down of ureteroileal conduit, ureterosigmoidostomy or ureteroenterostomy with ureteroureterostomy or ureteroneocystostomy)

50840 Replacement of all or part of ureter by intestine segment, including intestine anastomosis

50845 Cutaneous appendico-vesicostomy

50860 Ureterostomy, transplantation of ureter to skin

50900 Ureterorrhaphy, suture of ureter (separate procedure)

50920 Closure of ureterocutaneous fistula

50930 Closure of ureterovisceral fistula (including visceral repair)

50940 Deligation of ureter

Laparoscopy

Coding Atlas

Laparoscopy is a technique developed to reduce risk and recovery time during abdominal or pelvic surgery. Several small incisions act as portals for a tiny video camera (laparoscope), light source, and surgical tools. The physician manipulates the surgical tools while viewing the surgical site on a video display screen or through an eyepiece. To enhance visibility, the abdomen may be filled with gas (**pneumoperitoneum**) during the procedure.

50945 Laparoscopy, surgical; ureterolithotomy

50947 ureteroneocystostomy with cystoscopy and ureteral stent placement

50948 ureteroneocystostomy without cystoscopy and ureteral stent placement

Endoscopy

Coding Atlas

A **ureterostomy** is a communication between the ureter and the skin's surface. A **ureterotomy** is an incision into the ureter. **Stomas** placed for the diversion of urine (codes 50951-50961) or incisions into the ureter (codes 50970-50980) can each accommodate the advancement of an **endoscope** through the skin and into the ureter for **diagnostic** or **therapeutic** purposes. Codes are selected based on the type of access and the procedure performed through the **endoscope**.

50951 Ureteral endoscopy through established ureterostomy, with or without irrigation, instillation, or ureteropyelography, exclusive of radiologic service;

50953 with ureteral catheterization, with or without dilation of ureter

50955 with biopsy

50957 with fulguration and/or incision, with or without biopsy

50961 with removal of foreign body or calculus

50970 Ureteral endoscopy through ureterotomy, with or without irrigation, instillation, or ureteropyelography, exclusive of radiologic service;

50972 with ureteral catheterization, with or without dilation of ureter

50974 with biopsy

50976 with fulguration and/or incision, with or without biopsy

50980 with removal of foreign body or calculus

Bladder

Incision

Coding Atlas

A cystostomy is a communication between the bladder and the skin's surface. A cystotomy is an incision into the bladder. Transvesical ureterolithotomy is an incision into the ureter with an approach through a skin incision into the bladder. From the bladder, the ureter is incised. Perivesical describes an area near the bladder; prevesical space describes the space of Retzius, which is anterior to the bladder.

51020 Cystotomy or cystostomy; with fulguration and/or insertion of radioactive material

51030 with cryosurgical destruction of intravesical lesion

51040 Cystostomy, cystotomy with drainage

51045 Cystotomy, with insertion of ureteral catheter or stent (separate procedure)

51050 Cystolithotomy, cystotomy with removal of calculus, without vesical neck resection

51060 Transvesical ureterolithotomy

51065 Cystotomy, with calculus basket extraction and/or ultrasonic or electrohydraulic fragmentation of ureteral calculus

51080 Drainage of perivesical or prevesical space abscess

Removal

Coding Atlas

Urine may be aspirated from the bladder for diagnostic or therapeutic purposes using a syringe with a needle, either a trocar or intracatheter. Code 51102 is used to report the percutaneous insertion of a catheter for urinary drainage.

51100 Aspiration of bladder; by needle

51101 by trocar or intracatheter

51102 with insertion of suprapubic catheter

Excision

Coding Atlas

A bilateral pelvic lymphadenectomy (PLND) is often performed in conjunction with complete cystectomy to determine the staging of a malignancy or for therapeutic removal of metastases. After a complete cystectomy is performed, a piece of bowel is fashioned into a pouch to hold urine. The pouch may be continent or incontinent. An ileal conduit is an incontinent diversion, with a stoma (cystostomy) secured at the skin surface. Both the Indiana pouch and orthotopic neobladder are considered continent diversions.

51500 Excision of urachal cyst or sinus, with or without umbilical hernia repair

51520 Cystotomy; for simple excision of vesical neck (separate procedure)

51525 for excision of bladder diverticulum, single or multiple (separate procedure)

51530 for excision of bladder tumor

51535 Cystotomy for excision, incision, or repair of ureterocele

51550 Cystectomy, partial; simple

51555 complicated (eg, postradiation, previous surgery, difficult location)

51565 Cystectomy, partial, with reimplantation of ureter(s) into bladder (ureteroneocystostomy)

51570 Cystectomy, complete; (separate procedure)

51575 with bilateral pelvic lymphadenectomy, including external iliac, hypogastric, and obturator nodes

51580 Cystectomy, complete, with ureterosigmoidostomy or ureterocutaneous transplantations;

51585 with bilateral pelvic lymphadenectomy, including external iliac, hypogastric, and obturator nodes

51590 Cystectomy, complete, with ureteroileal conduit or sigmoid bladder, including intestine anastomosis;

51595 with bilateral pelvic lymphadenectomy, including external iliac, hypogastric, and obturator nodes

51596 Cystectomy, complete, with continent diversion, any open technique, using any segment of small and/or large intestine to construct neobladder

51597 Pelvic exenteration, complete, for vesical, prostatic or urethral malignancy, with removal of bladder and ureteral transplantations, with or without hysterectomy and/or abdominoperineal resection of rectum and colon and colostomy, or any combination thereof

FIGURE 6-8. Male and Female Bladder: Lateral View

The bladder lies posterior to the pubic **symphysis** in the anterior pelvis. The space between the bladder and the pubic symphysis is called the space of Retzius or retropubic space. The bladder is surrounded by extraperitoneal fat and connective tissue and is held in place by the external urethral **sphincter**, **ligaments**, and muscles.

Paramedian (sagittal) dissection: Male

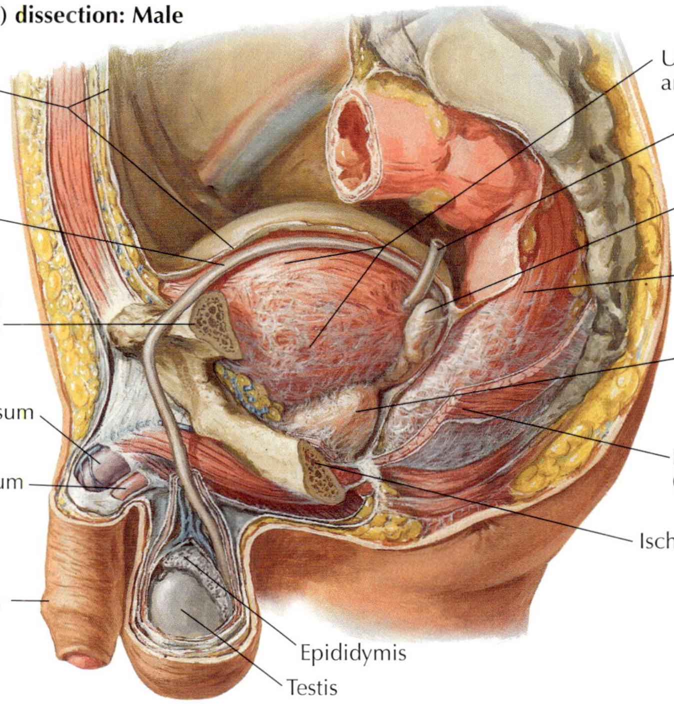

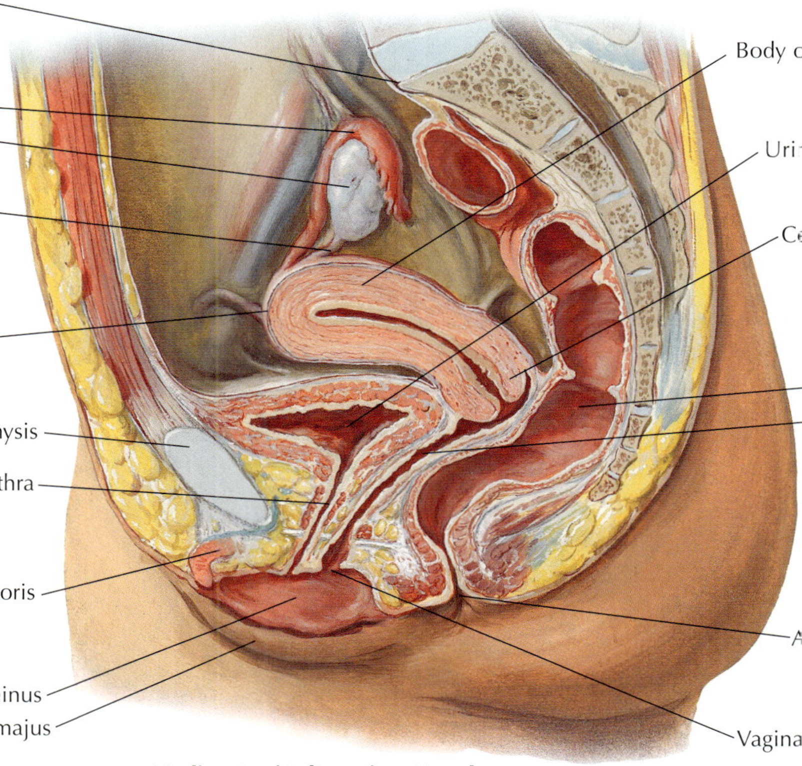

Median (sagittal) section: Female

FIGURE 6-9. Male and Female Bladder: Anterior View

The bladder greatly increases in size as it fills with urine. The **trigone** of the bladder is an imaginary triangle of interior bladder surface formed by the connection of three points: the two ureteric **orifices** on the **posterior** wall of the bladder and the bladder neck, where the **proximal** urethra connects. The trigone is very sensitive to expansion and signals the brain of the need for **micturition** as the bladder fills.

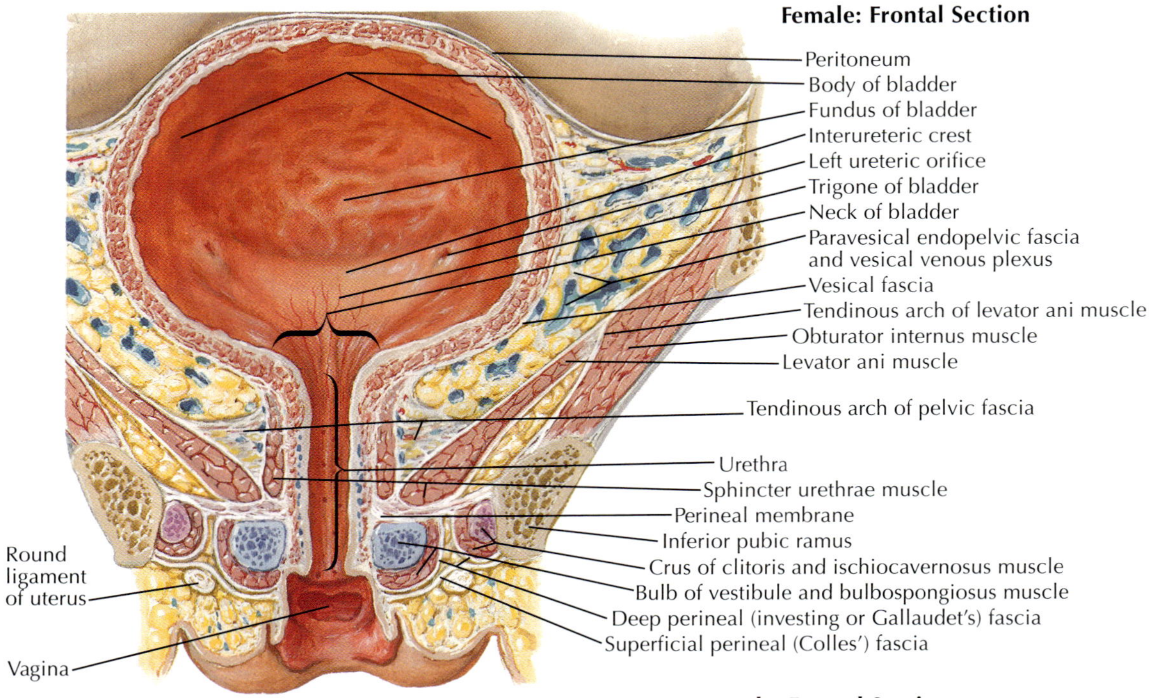

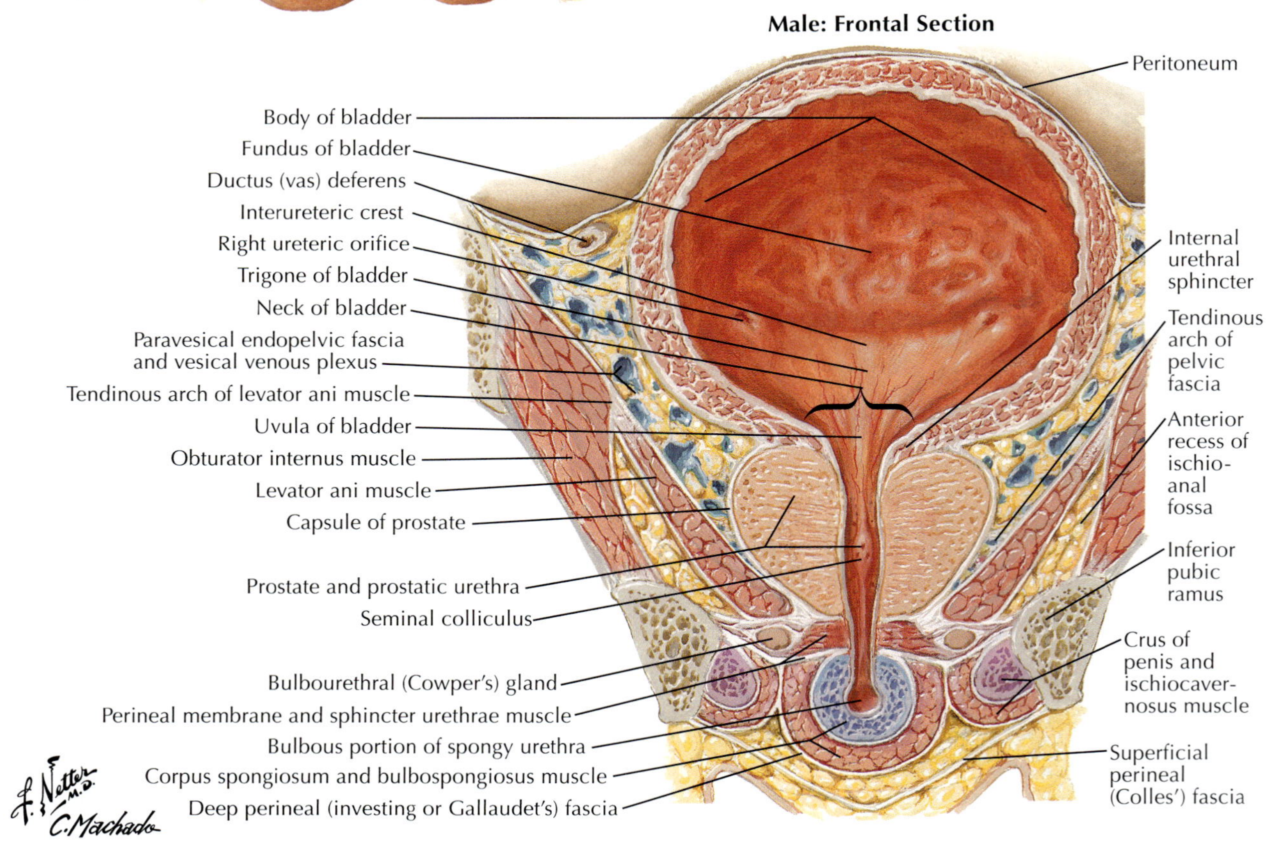

FIGURE 6-10. Diverticula of the Bladder

Bladder **diverticula** may be acquired or **congenital** and appear as herniations of the bladder **mucosa** through the muscular bladder wall. Diverticula may be solitary or multiple; they may be small or larger than the bladder. These **herniations** may cause **obstructions**, vesicoureteral **reflux**, and poor bladder emptying. Diverticula of the bladder may contain **calculi**.

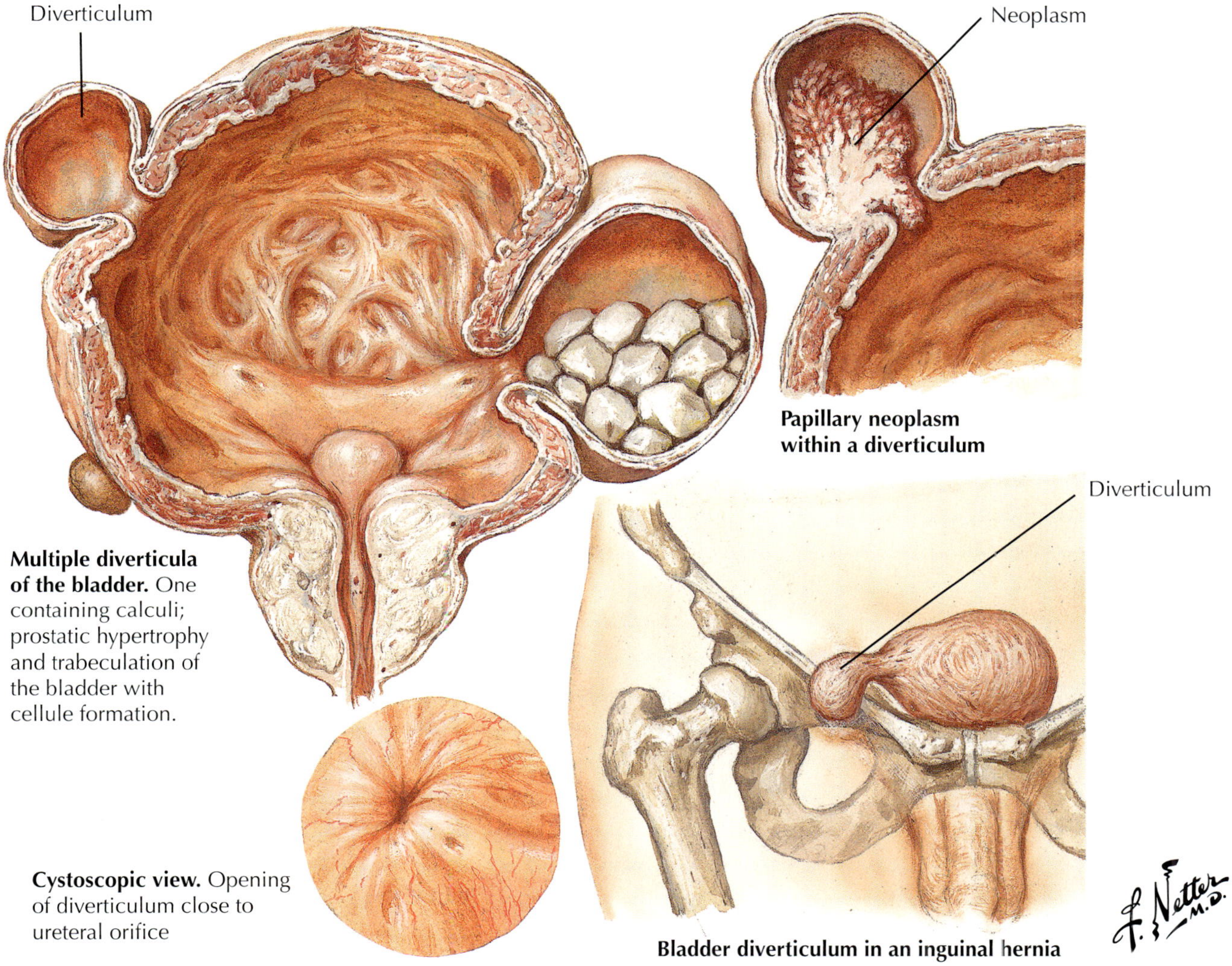

FIGURE 6-11. Cystometrography

Urodynamics describes the relationship of pressure and flow between the bladder and the urethra, and testing this relationship provides information that can lead to a definitive diagnosis. A simple cystometrography (CMG) assesses the patient's sensations associated with bladder filling and may be documented as a single-channel CMG. Note: Tools, implants, and/or equipment depicted in the illustration may be outdated but the procedural approach is valid.

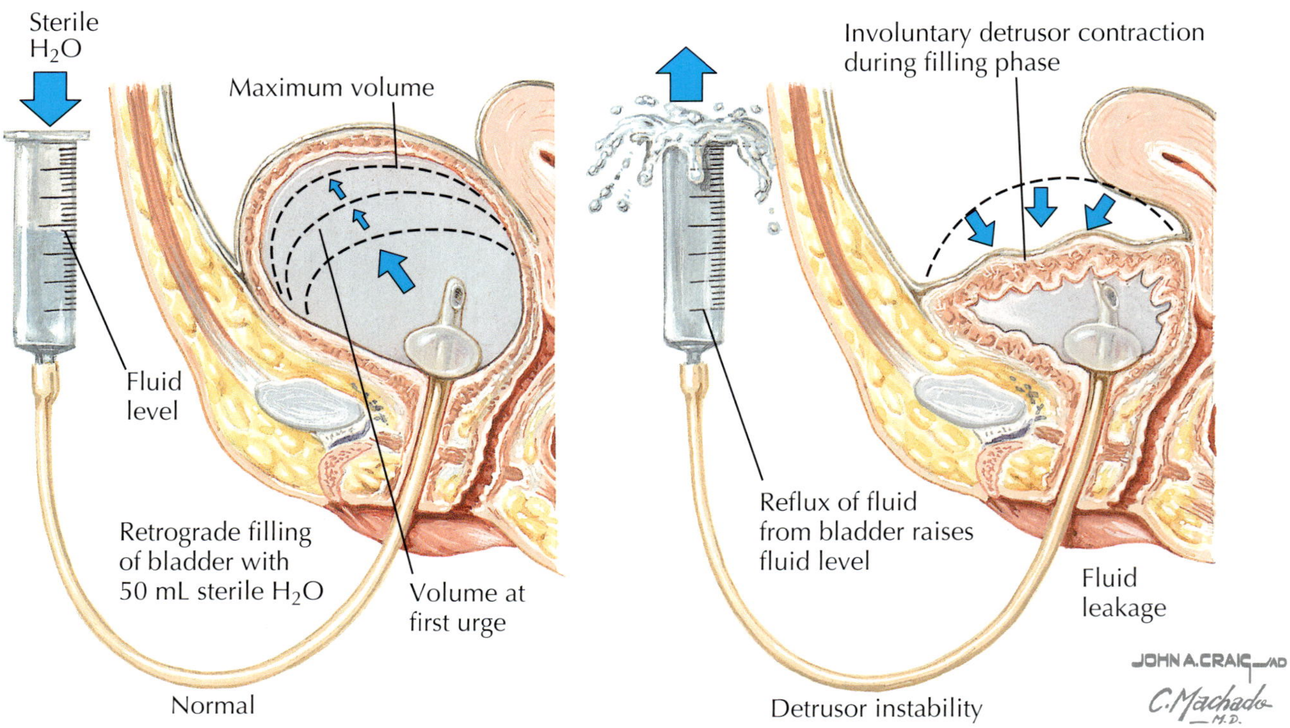

Introduction

Coding Atlas

Code 51702 is used to report the routine insertion of an indwelling bladder catheter (Foley) for urinary drainage in patients with chronic problems, eg, neurogenic bladder, or acute problems, eg, urinary retention. Non-indwelling describes a catheter that is immediately removed after bladder evacuation or urine sampling.

51600 Injection procedure for cystography or voiding urethrocystography

51605 Injection procedure and placement of chain for contrast and/or chain urethrocystography

51610 Injection procedure for retrograde urethrocystography

51700 Bladder irrigation, simple, lavage and/or instillation

51701 Insertion of non-indwelling bladder catheter (eg, straight catheterization for residual urine)

51702 Insertion of temporary indwelling bladder catheter; simple (eg, Foley)

51703 complicated (eg, altered anatomy, fractured catheter/balloon)

51705 Change of cystostomy tube; simple

51710 complicated

51715 Endoscopic injection of implant material into the submucosal tissues of the urethra and/or bladder neck

51720 Bladder instillation of anticarcinogenic agent (including retention time)

Urodynamics

Coding Atlas

A **cystourethrogram**, which is a recording of urinary bladder pressure at varying volumes, is performed to differentiate among possible voiding dysfunctions in a symptomatic patient. A **transurethral** catheter is necessary for any cystourethrogram. **Voiding** pressure (VP) measures the pressure and flow during the emptying of the bladder and may include measurement of abdominal pressure as well as **intravesical** pressure. The amount of urine remaining after voiding is measured using a post-voiding residual (PVR) study.

51725 Simple cystometrogram (CMG) (eg, spinal manometer)

51726 Complex cystometrogram (ie, calibrated electronic equipment);

51727 with urethral pressure profile studies (ie, urethral closure pressure profile), any technique

51728 with voiding pressure studies (ie, bladder voiding pressure), any technique

51729 with voiding pressure studies (ie, bladder voiding pressure) and urethral pressure profile studies (ie, urethral closure pressure profile), any technique

#✚ **51797** Voiding pressure studies, intra-abdominal (ie, rectal, gastric, intraperitoneal) (List separately in addition to code for primary procedure)

51736 Simple uroflowmetry (UFR) (eg, stop-watch flow rate, mechanical uroflowmeter)

51741 Complex uroflowmetry (eg, calibrated electronic equipment)

51784 Electromyography studies (EMG) of anal or urethral sphincter, other than needle, any technique

51785 Needle electromyography studies (EMG) of anal or urethral sphincter, any technique

51792 Stimulus evoked response (eg, measurement of bulbocavernosus reflex latency time)

51797 Code is out of numerical sequence. See 51725-51798

51798 Measurement of post-voiding residual urine and/or bladder capacity by ultrasound, non-imaging

Repair

Coding Atlas

In a patient with stress urinary incontinence (SUI), the urethra is hypermobile or the urethral **sphincter** is deficient. Both problems arise in the **urethral vesicular junction** (UVJ). Surgical fixation of the urethra can eliminate or reduce SUI. Both the Burch and Marshall-Marchetti-Krantz (MMK) procedures can be used to accomplish this goal. For the **laparoscopic** approach to Burch or MMK procedures, see codes 51990, 51992.

51800 Cystoplasty or cystourethroplasty, plastic operation on bladder and/or vesical neck (anterior Y-plasty, vesical fundus resection), any procedure, with or without wedge resection of posterior vesical neck

51820 Cystourethroplasty with unilateral or bilateral ureteroneocystostomy

51840 Anterior vesicourethropexy, or urethropexy (eg, Marshall-Marchetti-Krantz, Burch); simple

51841 complicated (eg, secondary repair)

51845 Abdomino-vaginal vesical neck suspension, with or without endoscopic control (eg, Stamey, Raz, modified Pereyra)

51860 Cystorrhaphy, suture of bladder wound, injury or rupture; simple

51865 complicated

51880 Closure of cystostomy (separate procedure)

51900 Closure of vesicovaginal fistula, abdominal approach

51920 Closure of vesicouterine fistula;

51925 with hysterectomy

51940 Closure, exstrophy of bladder

51960 Enterocystoplasty, including intestinal anastomosis

51980 Cutaneous vesicostomy

FIGURE 6-12. Exstrophy of Bladder

Exstrophy of the bladder is a **congenital** malformation in which the bladder is exposed and outside of the body and has not closed to form a continent sac. Urine from the kidneys drains through the ureters into the bladder orifice and out of the abdomen. Exstrophy is the result of failure of the abdominal wall to close during fetal development; it can be corrected surgically. The condition is more common in males than females.

Exstrophy of bladder in male

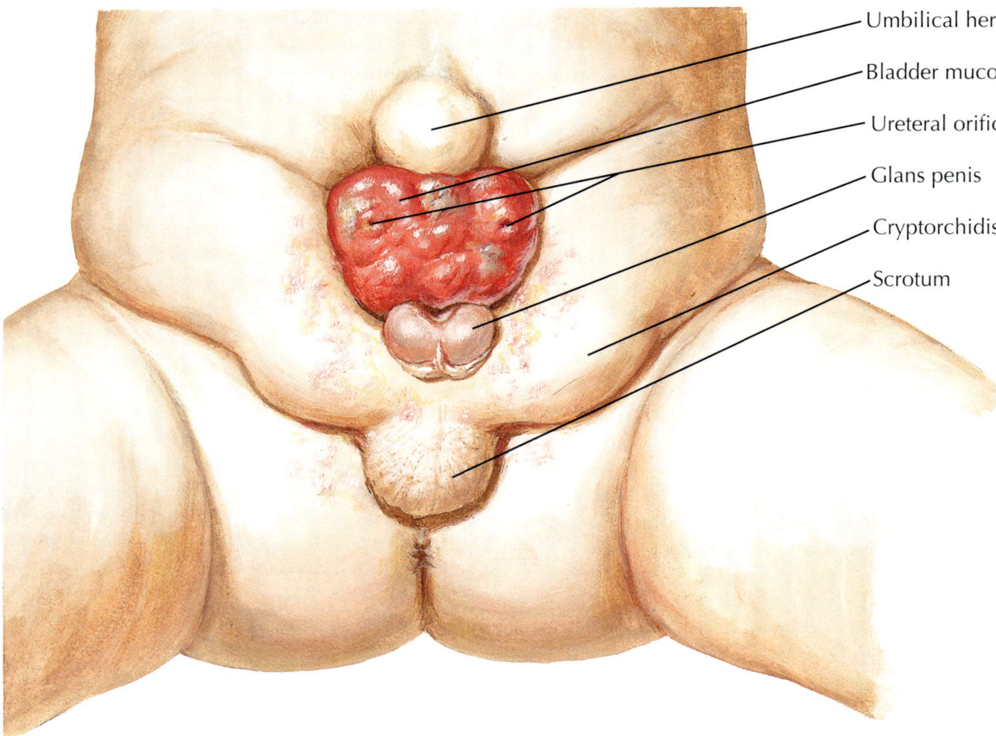

Exstrophy of bladder in female

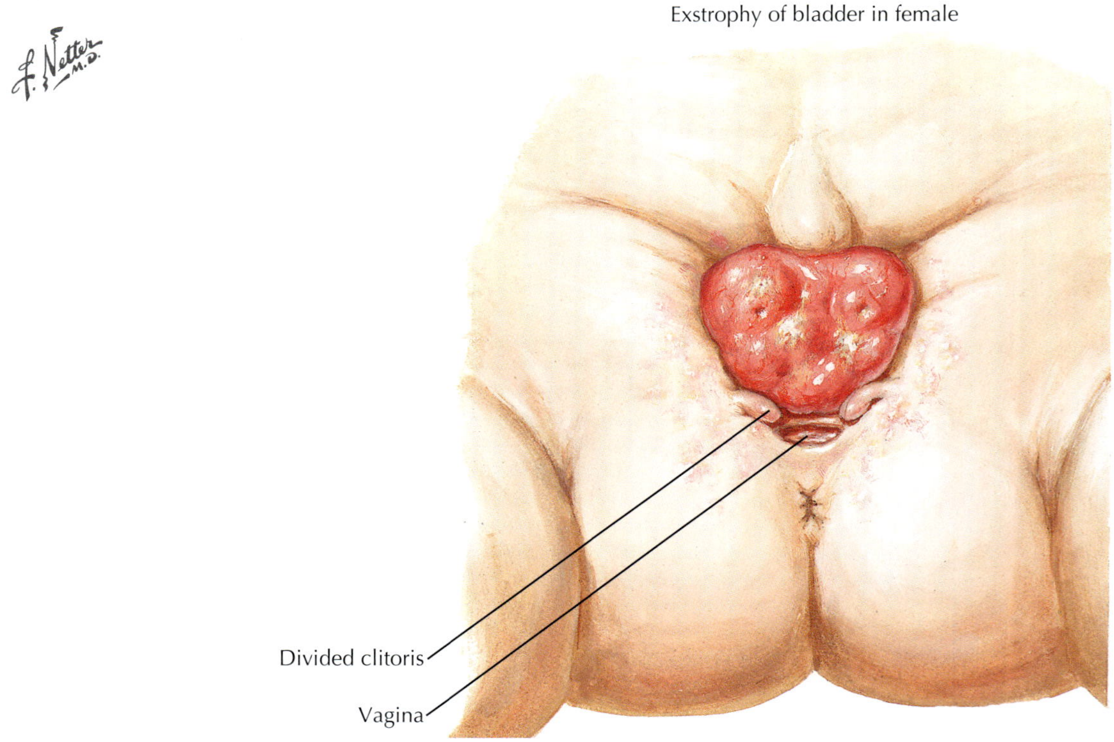

Laparoscopy

Coding Atlas

In a patient with stress urinary incontinence (SUI), the urethra is hypermobile or the urethral sphincter is deficient. Both problems arise in the urethral vesicular junction (UVJ). Surgical fixation of the urethra can eliminate or reduce SUI. Both the Burch and Marshall-Marchetti-Krantz (MMK) procedures accomplish this goal. Code 51990 or 51992 is reported when the laparoscopic approach is used for these procedures, depending on the technique. For the open approach to Burch or MMK procedures, see codes 51840 and 51841.

51990 Laparoscopy, surgical; urethral suspension for stress incontinence

51992 sling operation for stress incontinence (eg, fascia or synthetic)

Endoscopy—Cystoscopy, Urethroscopy, Cystourethroscopy

Coding Atlas

Cystourethroscopy enables the physician to visually inspect and also treat the urinary tract. This is done using a camera that projects an image onto a video display or by viewing sites within the urinary system through an eyepiece. The thin scope is inserted through the urethra and advanced so that the urinary system can be examined and/or irrigated. In addition, a therapeutic or diagnostic fluid may be administered through the scope.

52000 Cystourethroscopy (separate procedure)

52001 Cystourethroscopy with irrigation and evacuation of multiple obstructing clots

52005 Cystourethroscopy, with ureteral catheterization, with or without irrigation, instillation, or ureteropyelography, exclusive of radiologic service;

52007 with brush biopsy of ureter and/or renal pelvis

52010 Cystourethroscopy, with ejaculatory duct catheterization, with or without irrigation, instillation, or duct radiography, exclusive of radiologic service

Transurethral Surgery

Coding Atlas

Cystourethroscopy enables the physician to visually inspect and also treat the urinary tract. This is done using a camera that projects an image onto a video display or by viewing a site in the urinary system through an eyepiece. The thin scope is inserted through the urethra and advanced to the targeted site. The scope can be threaded through the urethra to the bladder and into the ureter and pelvis of the kidney. Tools can be fed through the scope to the site of a defect, and the defect can be examined, sampled, or treated. Cystourethroscopy, cystoscopy, urinary endoscopy, and urethroscopy each describe an intraluminal, transurethral approach to the urinary system.

Urethra and Bladder

52204 Cystourethroscopy, with biopsy(s)

52214 Cystourethroscopy, with fulguration (including cryosurgery or laser surgery) of trigone, bladder neck, prostatic fossa, urethra, or periurethral glands

52224 Cystourethroscopy, with fulguration (including cryosurgery or laser surgery) or treatment of MINOR (less than 0.5 cm) lesion(s) with or without biopsy

52234 Cystourethroscopy, with fulguration (including cryosurgery or laser surgery) and/or resection of; SMALL bladder tumor(s) (0.5 up to 2.0 cm)

52235 MEDIUM bladder tumor(s) (2.0 to 5.0 cm)

52240 LARGE bladder tumor(s)

52250 Cystourethroscopy with insertion of radioactive substance, with or without biopsy or fulguration

52260 Cystourethroscopy, with dilation of bladder for interstitial cystitis; general or conduction (spinal) anesthesia

52265 local anesthesia

52270 Cystourethroscopy, with internal urethrotomy; female

52275 male

52276 Cystourethroscopy with direct vision internal urethrotomy

52277 Cystourethroscopy, with resection of external sphincter (sphincterotomy)

52281 Cystourethroscopy, with calibration and/or dilation of urethral stricture or stenosis, with or without meatotomy, with or without injection procedure for cystography, male or female

FIGURE 6-13. Urinary Fistulas

A urinary **fistula** may be a late effect of radiation treatment, hysterectomy, or obstetrical complication in females, and is typically the result of tissue **ischemia** following a repair or injury. The fistula may lead from the bladder to the vagina (vesicovaginal), the bladder to the urethra (vesicourethral), or the bladder to the uterus (vesicouterine). The condition may present as urinary incontinence.

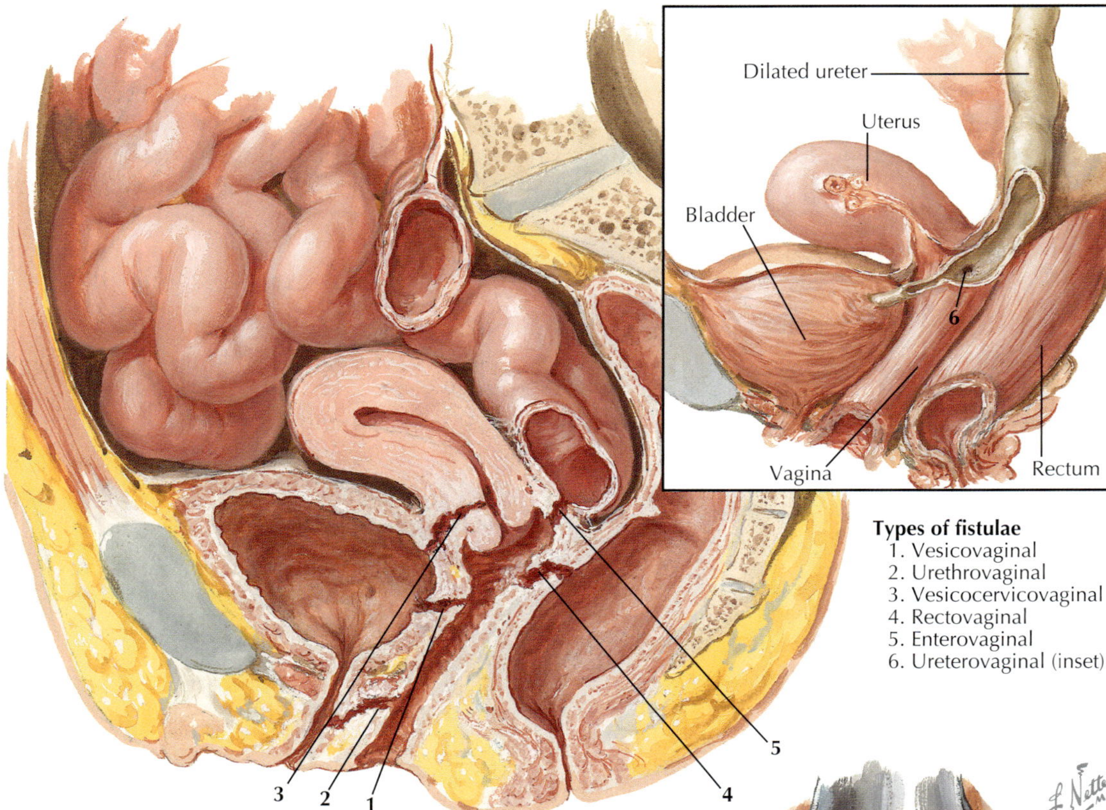

Types of fistulae
1. Vesicovaginal
2. Urethrovaginal
3. Vesicocervicovaginal
4. Rectovaginal
5. Enterovaginal
6. Ureterovaginal (inset)

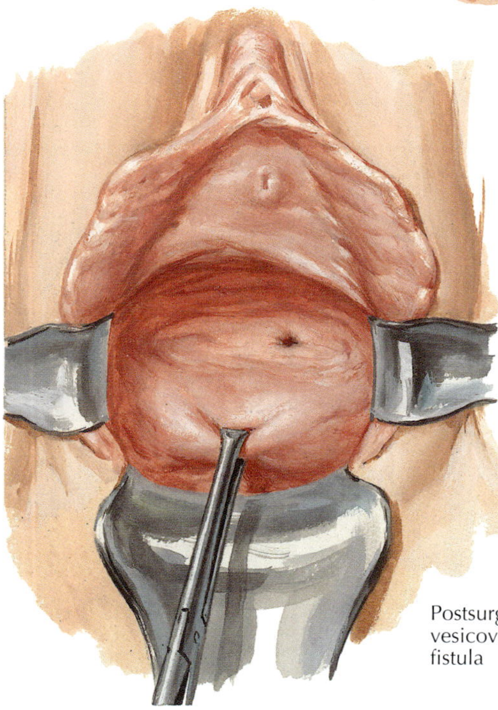

Postsurgical vesicovaginal fistula

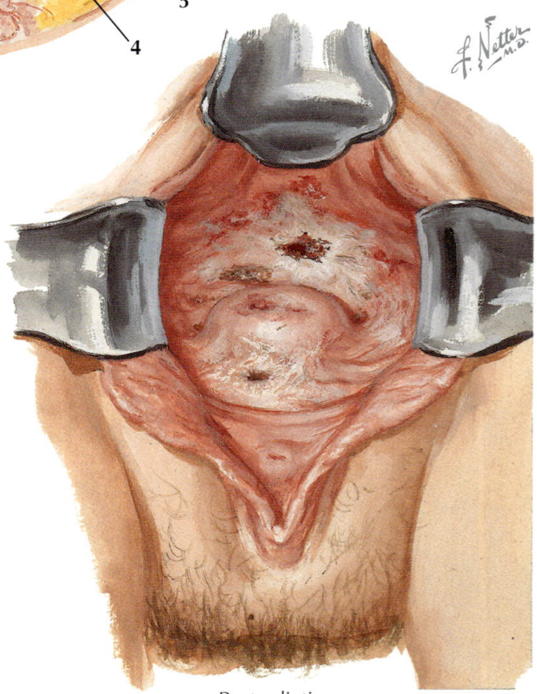

Postradiation vesicorectovaginal fistula (patient in knee-chest position)

FIGURE 6-14. Bladder Tumor Approaches

Bladder **tumors** may be treated **endoscopically** or by use of an **open** approach, depending on the size and type of **lesion**. In the top portion of Figure 6-14, a rigid **cystourethroscope** is used to remove small **papillomas** of the bladder. Urothelial papillomas are **benign** but may recur. **Open** procedures, as seen in the bottom portion of Figure 6-14, provide the physician with **direct visualization** of a **malignancy**, which may be excised with a margin of healthy bladder tissue. Note: Tools, implants, and/or equipment depicted in the illustration may be outdated but the procedural approach is valid.

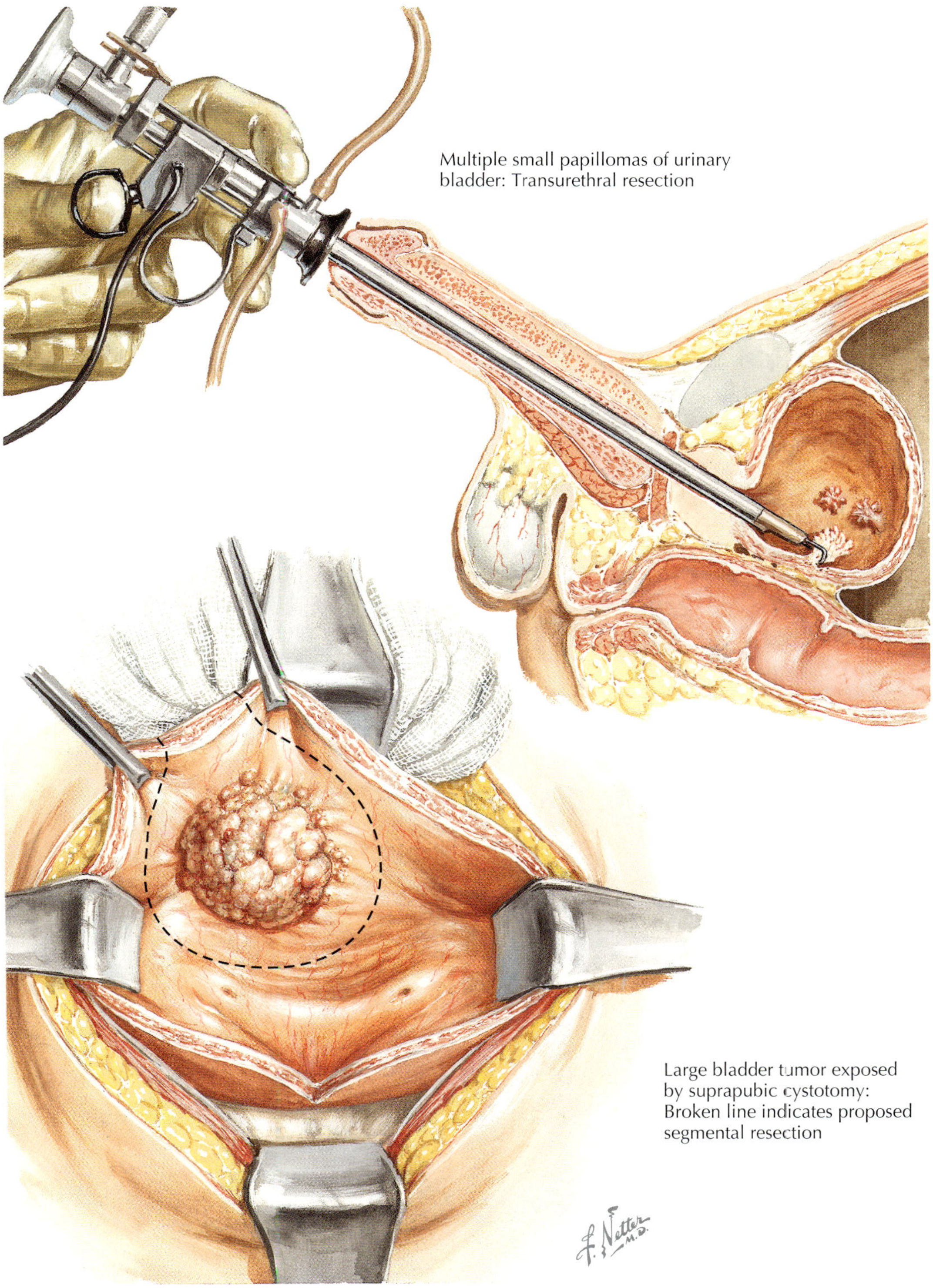

52282 Cystourethroscopy, with insertion of permanent urethral stent

52283 Cystourethroscopy, with steroid injection into stricture

52285 Cystourethroscopy for treatment of the female urethral syndrome with any or all of the following: urethral meatotomy, urethral dilation, internal urethrotomy, lysis of urethrovaginal septal fibrosis, lateral incisions of the bladder neck, and fulguration of polyp(s) of urethra, bladder neck, and/or trigone

52287 Cystourethroscopy, with injection(s) for chemodenervation of the bladder

52290 Cystourethroscopy; with ureteral meatotomy, unilateral or bilateral

52300 with resection or fulguration of orthotopic ureterocele(s), unilateral or bilateral

52301 with resection or fulguration of ectopic ureterocele(s), unilateral or bilateral

52305 with incision or resection of orifice of bladder diverticulum, single or multiple

52310 Cystourethroscopy, with removal of foreign body, calculus, or ureteral stent from urethra or bladder (separate procedure); simple

52315 complicated

52317 Litholapaxy: crushing or fragmentation of calculus by any means in bladder and removal of fragments; simple or small (less than 2.5 cm)

52318 complicated or large (over 2.5 cm)

Ureter and Pelvis

52320 Cystourethroscopy (including ureteral catheterization); with removal of ureteral calculus

52325 with fragmentation of ureteral calculus (eg, ultrasonic or electro-hydraulic technique)

52327 with subureteric injection of implant material

52330 with manipulation, without removal of ureteral calculus

52332 Cystourethroscopy, with insertion of indwelling ureteral stent (eg, Gibbons or double-J type)

52334 Cystourethroscopy with insertion of ureteral guide wire through kidney to establish a percutaneous nephrostomy, retrograde

52341 Cystourethroscopy; with treatment of ureteral stricture (eg, balloon dilation, laser, electrocautery, and incision)

52342 with treatment of ureteropelvic junction stricture (eg, balloon dilation, laser, electrocautery, and incision)

52343 with treatment of intra-renal stricture (eg, balloon dilation, laser, electrocautery, and incision)

52344 Cystourethroscopy with ureteroscopy; with treatment of ureteral stricture (eg, balloon dilation, laser, electrocautery, and incision)

52345 with treatment of ureteropelvic junction stricture (eg, balloon dilation, laser, electrocautery, and incision)

52346 with treatment of intra-renal stricture (eg, balloon dilation, laser, electrocautery, and incision)

52351 Cystourethroscopy, with ureteroscopy and/or pyeloscopy; diagnostic

52352 with removal or manipulation of calculus (ureteral catheterization is included)

52353 with lithotripsy (ureteral catheterization is included)

52356 with lithotripsy including insertion of indwelling ureteral stent (eg, Gibbons or double-J type)

52354 with biopsy and/or fulguration of ureteral or renal pelvic lesion

52355 with resection of ureteral or renal pelvic tumor

52356 Code is out of numerical sequence. See 52320-52355

Vesical Neck and Prostate

Coding Atlas

The bladder neck is contiguous with the prostate in males and, together, they function as the internal urethral sphincter. Benign prostatic hyperplasia (BPH) is the most common cause of bladder outlet obstruction in men. Codes 52400-52700 are used to report a cystoscopic approach to treatment of the bladder neck and prostate. For alternative approaches to the prostate, see codes 55700-55876.

52400 Cystourethroscopy with incision, fulguration, or resection of congenital posterior urethral valves, or congenital obstructive hypertrophic mucosal folds

52402 Cystourethroscopy with transurethral resection or incision of ejaculatory ducts

52441 Cystourethroscopy, with insertion of permanent adjustable transprostatic implant; single implant

✚ **52442** each additional permanent adjustable transprostatic implant (List separately in addition to code for primary procedure)

52450 Transurethral incision of prostate

52500 Transurethral resection of bladder neck (separate procedure)

52601 Transurethral electrosurgical resection of prostate, including control of postoperative bleeding, complete (vasectomy, meatotomy, cystourethroscopy, urethral calibration and/or dilation, and internal urethrotomy are included)

FIGURE 6-15. Ureterocele

A **ureterocele** is an anomalous pouching of the **distal** ureter. It may occur with **congenital** anomalies such as **orthotopic** or **ectopic** ureters. Ureteroceles are clinically significant because they can obstruct the flow of urine from the kidney to the bladder, leading to kidney damage. Also, ureteroceles can allow vesicoureteral **reflux** (VUR), ie, the backward flow of urine from the bladder into the ureter, which is associated with chronic urinary tract infection (UTI).

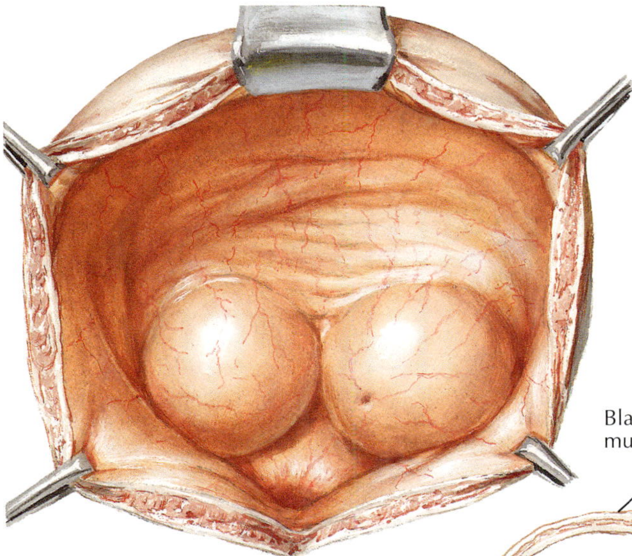

Bilateral ureteroceles: Orifice of right ureterocele not visible because it is on undersurface of the cyst

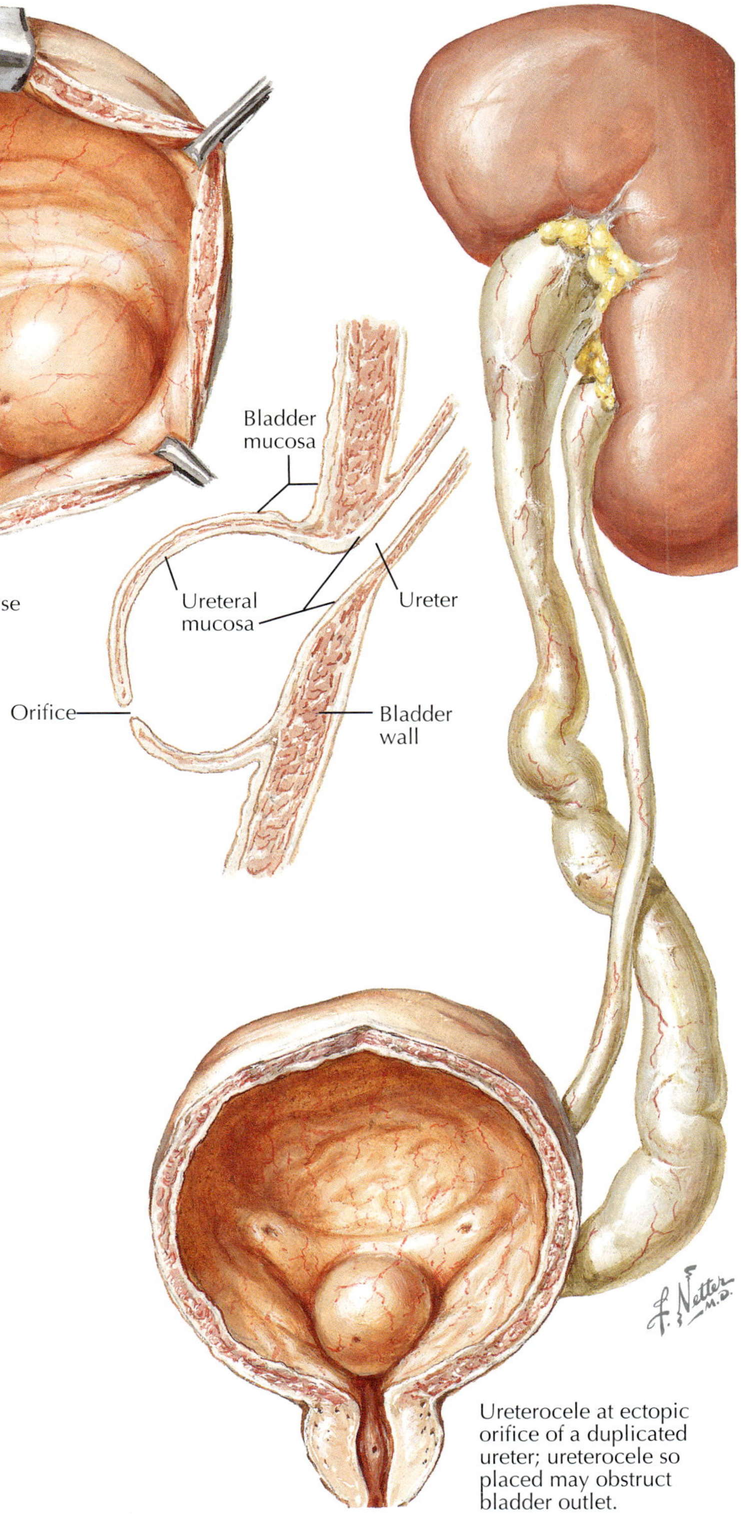

Ureterocele at ectopic orifice of a duplicated ureter; ureterocele so placed may obstruct bladder outlet.

FIGURE 6-16. Transurethral Resection of Prostate

Benign prostatic hyperplasia (BPH), which is common in aging males, is a condition in which the prostate volume increases. The urethra's path transects the prostate, so prostatic **hyperplasia** may encroach on the urethra as well as on the vesical neck. This may cause obstruction and urinary symptoms. The hypertrophic tissue may be resected using a **transurethral** approach, as illustrated in Figure 6-16, along with possible complications of transurethral prostatectomy. Note: Tools, implants, and/or equipment depicted in the illustration may be outdated but the procedural approach is valid.

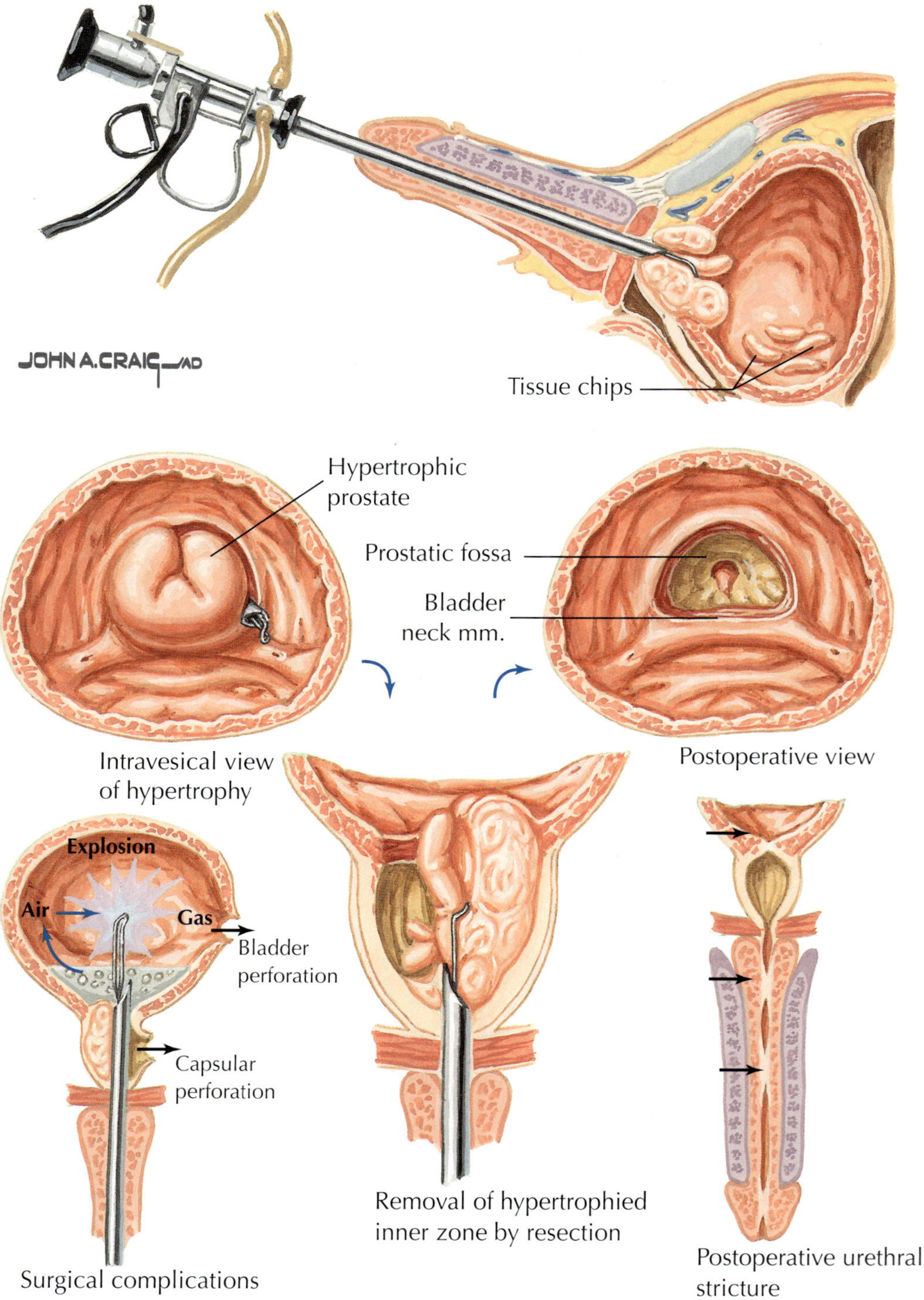

52630 Transurethral resection; residual or regrowth of obstructive prostate tissue including control of postoperative bleeding, complete (vasectomy, meatotomy, cystourethroscopy, urethral calibration and/or dilation, and internal urethrotomy are included)

52640 of postoperative bladder neck contracture

52647 Laser coagulation of prostate, including control of postoperative bleeding, complete (vasectomy, meatotomy, cystourethroscopy, urethral calibration and/or dilation, and internal urethrotomy are included if performed)

52648 Laser vaporization of prostate, including control of postoperative bleeding, complete (vasectomy, meatotomy, cystourethroscopy, urethral calibration and/or dilation, internal urethrotomy and transurethral resection of prostate are included if performed)

52649 Laser enucleation of the prostate with morcellation, including control of postoperative bleeding, complete (vasectomy, meatotomy, cystourethroscopy, urethral calibration and/or dilation, internal urethrotomy and transurethral resection of prostate are included if performed)

52700 Transurethral drainage of prostatic abscess

Urethra

Incision

Coding Atlas

The male spongy (penile) urethra is divided into two parts: the bulbar urethra, which is located at the base of the penis, and the pendulous urethra, which runs along the length of the penis from the bulbar urethra up to and including the **navicular fossa** in the glans penis.

53000 Urethrotomy or urethrostomy, external (separate procedure); pendulous urethra

53010 perineal urethra, external

53020 Meatotomy, cutting of meatus (separate procedure); except infant

53025 infant

53040 Drainage of deep periurethral abscess

53060 Drainage of Skene's gland abscess or cyst

53080 Drainage of perineal urinary extravasation; uncomplicated (separate procedure)

53085 complicated

Excision

Coding Atlas

Cowper's glands, also known as bulbourethral glands, are located below the apex of the prostate in the **penile urethra**. These glands produce a clear lubricant during male sexual arousal. The lubricant is transported through the urethra to the **glans penis**. Skene's glands are found at the base of the female urethra and produce urethral lubricant. Bartholin's glands in females are considered the equivalent of Cowper's glands in males.

53200 Biopsy of urethra

53210 Urethrectomy, total, including cystostomy; female

53215 male

53220 Excision or fulguration of carcinoma of urethra

53230 Excision of urethral diverticulum (separate procedure); female

53235 male

53240 Marsupialization of urethral diverticulum, male or female

53250 Excision of bulbourethral gland (Cowper's gland)

53260 Excision or fulguration; urethral polyp(s), distal urethra

53265 urethral caruncle

53270 Skene's glands

53275 urethral prolapse

FIGURE 6-17. The Male Urethra

The male urethra is between 17 centimeters and 20 centimeters in length. The male urethra can be divided into three segments: prostatic, membranous, and spongy urethras. The prostatic urethra is so named because it is surrounded by prostate that is just **distal** to the bladder. The membranous urethra begins at the distal prostate and extends to the perineal membrane. It contains the external urethral **sphincter**. The spongy urethra runs through the corpus spongiosum of the penis and is the longest segment.

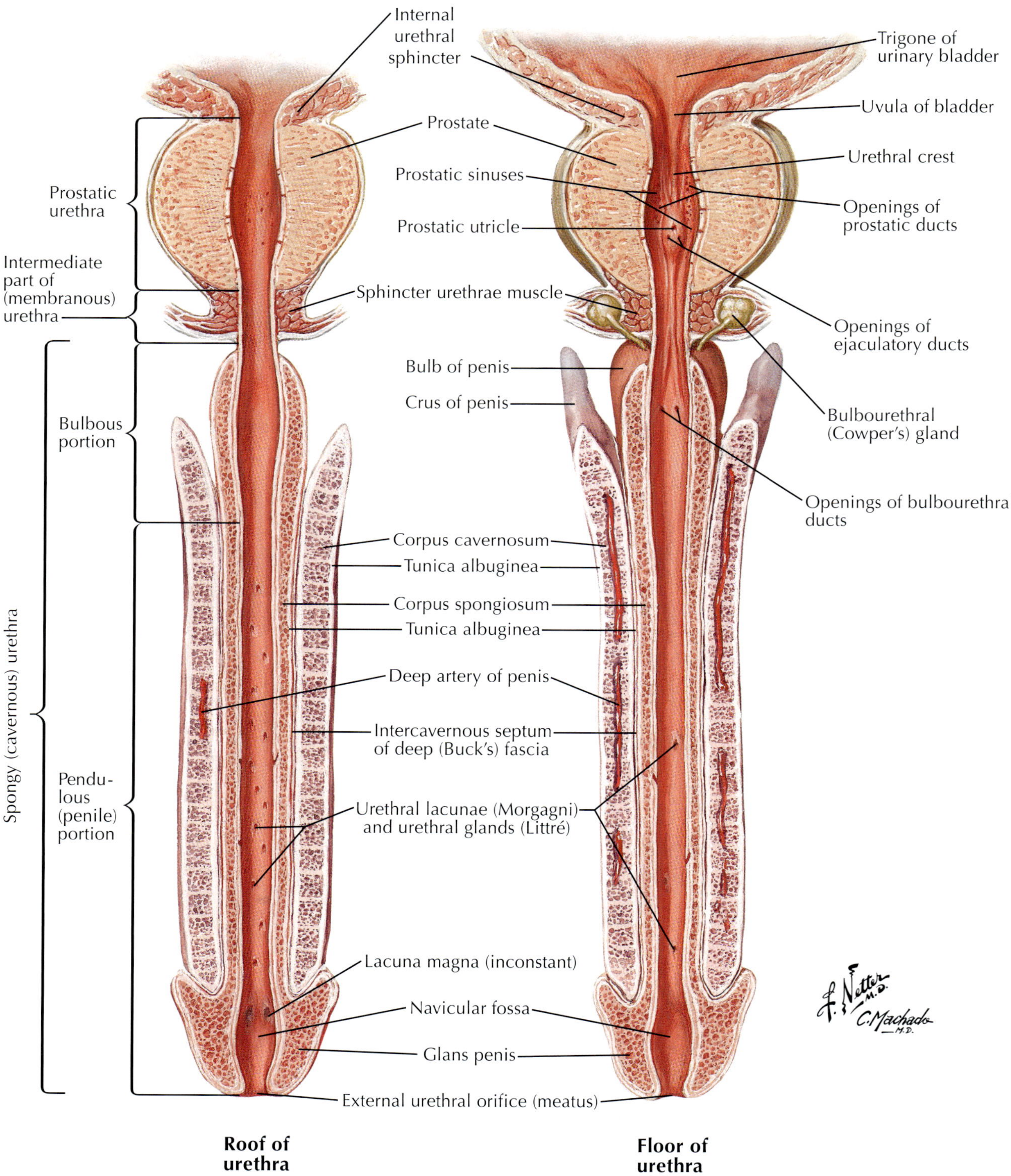

FIGURE 6-18. The Female Urethra

The female urethra is approximately 4 centimeters in length. Its **proximal** end is connected to the vesical neck; the **distal** meatus ends at the vaginal vestibule. Paraurethral Skene's glands empty into two paired ducts on either side of the external urethral **meatus**. The Skene's glands produce lubrication.

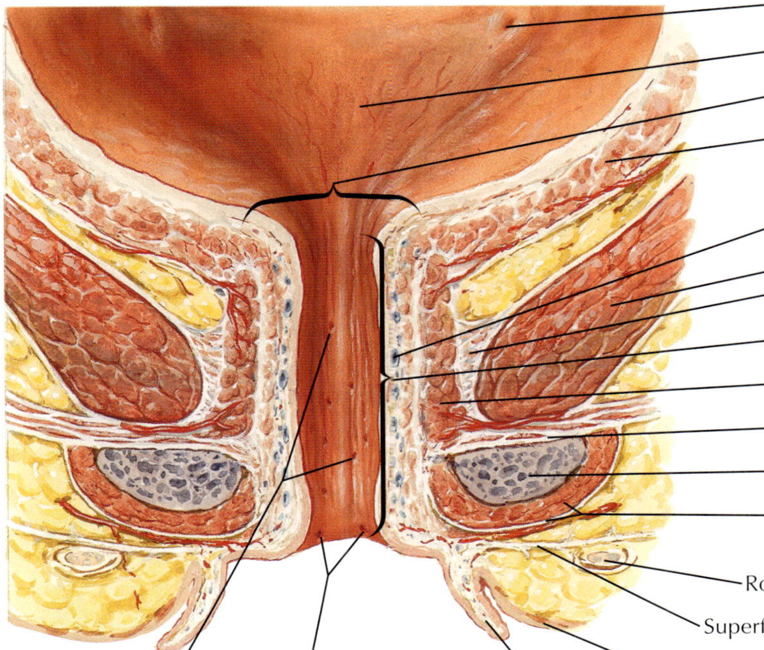

Repair

Coding Atlas

Sphincters are anatomical gatekeepers, and urinary sphincters act to retain urine in the bladder until the brain receives a signal to void. An inflatable urinary sphincter is a medical device designed to provide bladder control in an otherwise **incontinent** patient. The system has three components: an inflatable cuff that fits around the urethra, a reservoir connected to the cuff, and a pump that transfers volume from the reservoir to the cuff and back again. When the cuff is empty, the urethra is open and voiding occurs. When the cuff is full, the urethra is crimped so that urine may not escape. The reservoir and pump are implanted under the skin.

53400 Urethroplasty; first stage, for fistula, diverticulum, or stricture (eg, Johannsen type)

53405 second stage (formation of urethra), including urinary diversion

53410 Urethroplasty, 1-stage reconstruction of male anterior urethra

53415 Urethroplasty, transpubic or perineal, 1-stage, for reconstruction or repair of prostatic or membranous urethra

53420 Urethroplasty, 2-stage reconstruction or repair of prostatic or membranous urethra; first stage

53425 second stage

53430 Urethroplasty, reconstruction of female urethra

53431 Urethroplasty with tubularization of posterior urethra and/or lower bladder for incontinence (eg, Tenago, Leadbetter procedure)

53440 Sling operation for correction of male urinary incontinence (eg, fascia or synthetic)

53442 Removal or revision of sling for male urinary incontinence (eg, fascia or synthetic)

53444 Insertion of tandem cuff (dual cuff)

53445 Insertion of inflatable urethral/bladder neck sphincter, including placement of pump, reservoir, and cuff

53446 Removal of inflatable urethral/bladder neck sphincter, including pump, reservoir, and cuff

53447 Removal and replacement of inflatable urethral/bladder neck sphincter including pump, reservoir, and cuff at the same operative session

53448 Removal and replacement of inflatable urethral/bladder neck sphincter including pump, reservoir, and cuff through an infected field at the same operative session including irrigation and debridement of infected tissue

53449 Repair of inflatable urethral/bladder neck sphincter, including pump, reservoir, and cuff

53450 Urethromeatoplasty, with mucosal advancement

53460 Urethromeatoplasty, with partial excision of distal urethral segment (Richardson type procedure)

53500 Urethrolysis, transvaginal, secondary, open, including cystourethroscopy (eg, postsurgical obstruction, scarring)

53502 Urethrorrhaphy, suture of urethral wound or injury, female

53505 Urethrorrhaphy, suture of urethral wound or injury; penile

53510 perineal

53515 prostatomembranous

53520 Closure of urethrostomy or urethrocutaneous fistula, male (separate procedure)

Manipulation

Coding Atlas

In urethral **dilation**, rods of increasing diameter are inserted into the urethral **meatus** to increase its diameter. **The filiform and follower** technique involves insertion of a small catheter through the urethral opening and into the bladder and attachment of a larger-diameter follower to the distal tip of the filiform. The follower is fed through the length of the urethra and then extracted. A larger follower replaces the first one, and the process is repeated until the urethral diameter is sufficiently enlarged. Codes in the range 53600-53665 are used to report these services based on the procedure and the sex of the patient.

53600 Dilation of urethral stricture by passage of sound or urethral dilator, male; initial

53601 subsequent

53605 Dilation of urethral stricture or vesical neck by passage of sound or urethral dilator, male, general or conduction (spinal) anesthesia

53620 Dilation of urethral stricture by passage of filiform and follower, male; initial

53621 subsequent

53660 Dilation of female urethra including suppository and/or instillation; initial

53661 subsequent

53665 Dilation of female urethra, general or conduction (spinal) anesthesia

Other Procedures

Coding Atlas

Transurethral microwave thermotherapy (TUMT; code 53850) and transurethral needle ablation (TUNA; code 53852) are used to destroy prostatic tissue by causing heat **necrosis**. The use of **radiofrequency** to reduce stress urinary incontinence (SUI) in women involves nonablative levels of energy that shrink and stabilize local **fascia**.

53850 Transurethral destruction of prostate tissue; by microwave thermotherapy

53852 by radiofrequency thermotherapy

53855 Insertion of a temporary prostatic urethral stent, including urethral measurement

53860 Transurethral radiofrequency micro-remodeling of the female bladder neck and proximal urethra for stress urinary incontinence

FIGURE 6-19. Urinary Extravasation

Urinary **extravasation** occurs when the urethra ruptures and urine escapes the urinary tract to pool elsewhere in the pelvis. Extravasation may be a complication of injury, infection, **calculus**, or urethral **stricture**. The extravasation may include blood, depending on the injury. Compartments that contain urine are incised to drain the urine that has extravasated.

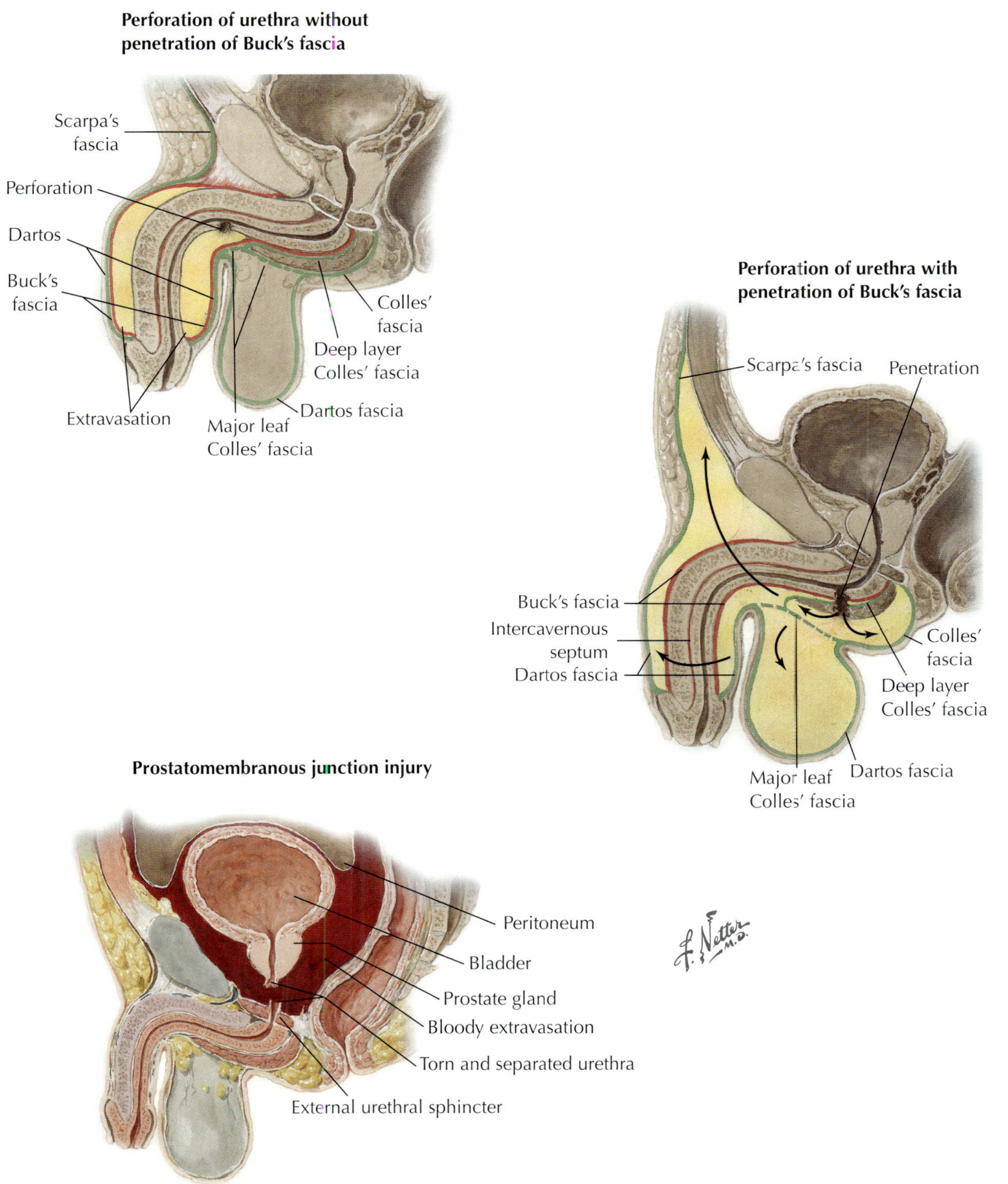

FIGURE 6-20. The Prostate

The role of the prostate gland is to secrete a milky fluid that combines with semen during ejaculation. This fluid helps neutralize acidity in order to prolong the life of acid-sensitive spermatozoa. The fluid from the prostate also nourishes the sperm. During ejaculation, **smooth muscle** in the prostate contracts to propel the semen through the urethra.

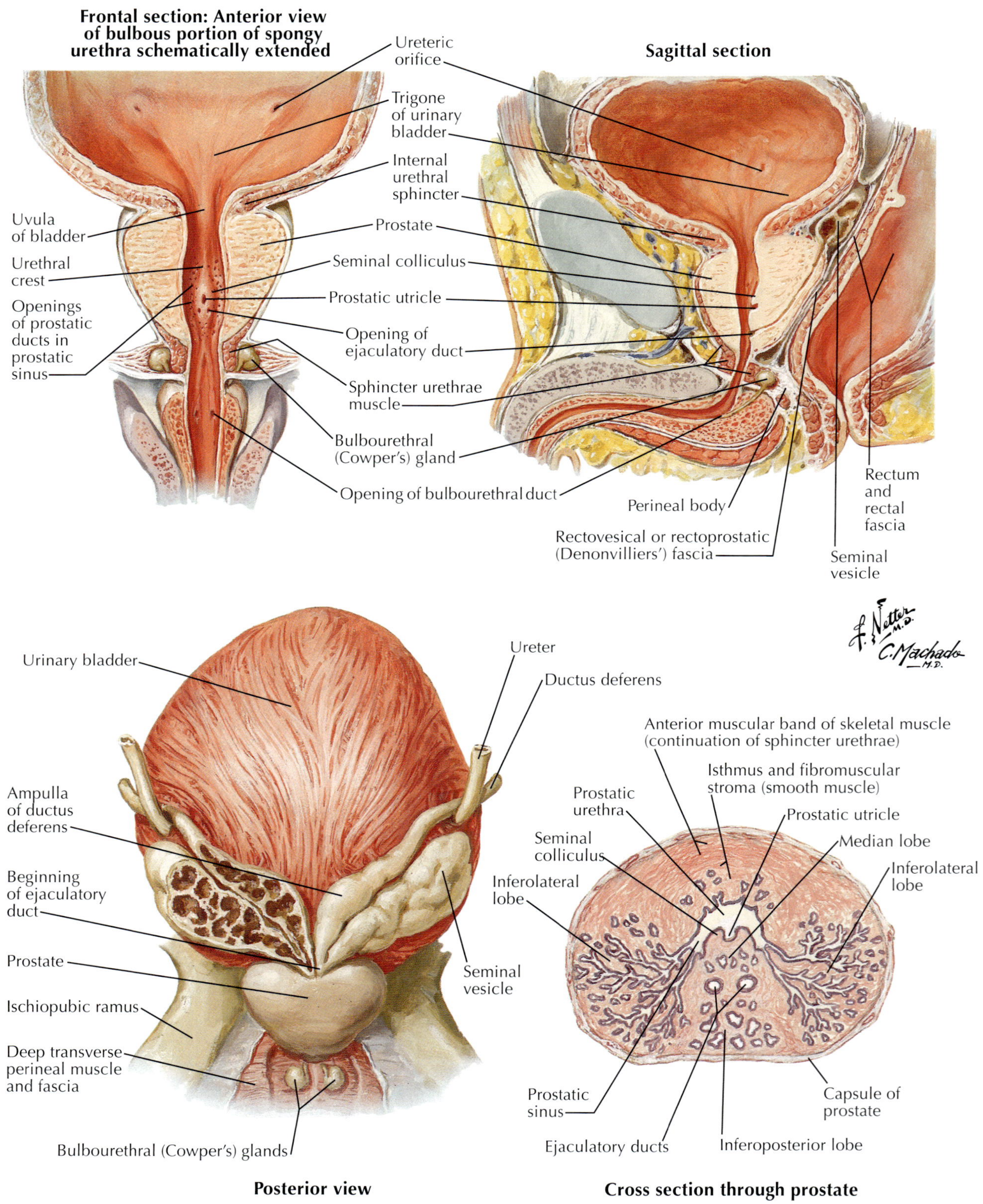

Median (sagittal) section

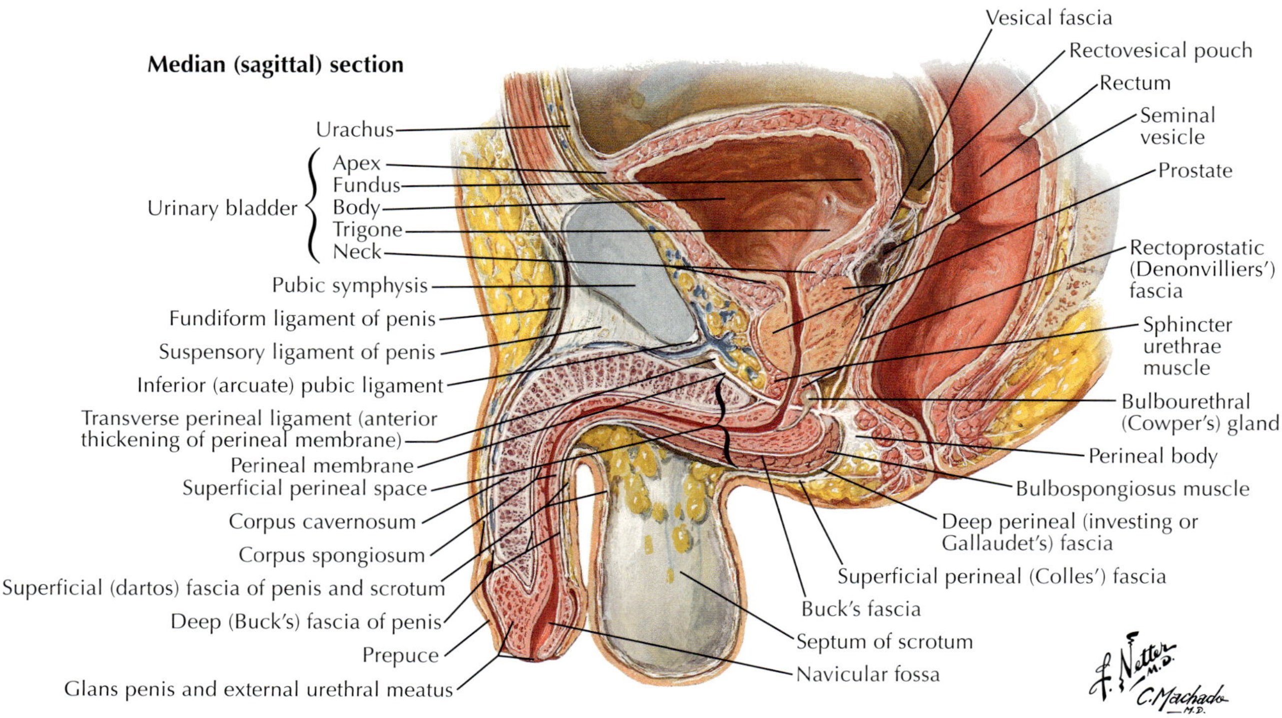

◈ CHAPTER 7 ◈

Male Genital System

The male genital system is the network of internal and external organs and **ducts** that produce, store, and deliver spermatozoa for sexual reproduction.

The scrotum and penis are external organs of the male genital system. The scrotum is a muscular skin pouch with a central **raphe** that divides it into two separate sacs. Each sac houses a testicle (testis). Spermatozoa and the **hormone** testosterone are manufactured in the testes. The scrotum lies **posterior** to the penis to maximize protection of and regulate the temperature of the testes because sperm production is best when the testes are cooler than the core body temperature. Scrotal tissue relaxes, allowing the testes to be further from the body when temperatures rise.

The spermatic cord suspends the testis in the scrotum. The cord is a bundle of structures that stretch from each testis to the deep **inguinal ring**. The bundle contains the vas deferens, tunica vaginalis, and numerous lymphatic, neural, and vascular structures. The vas deferens is the conduit by which spermatozoa are transported from the epididymis, where spermatozoa are matured and stored, to the ejaculatory ducts, where they enter the penile urethra as a component of ejaculate.

The penis is divided into three parts: the bulb, at the base where it attaches to the trunk; the shaft; and the head, or glans penis. The shaft contains three tubular chambers: two corpora cavernosa and one corpus spongiosum. These chambers contain multiple blood vessels and cavities. During sexual arousal, the cavities become engorged with blood in which the blood vessels are dilated and the blood flow is raised, which is a parasympathetic response. On the other hand, ejaculation is a sympathetic response in which the blood vessels are constricted and blood flow is lowered. The urethra runs through the length of the corpus spongiosum.

Procedures on the urethra are considered urinary procedures in the CPT code set. However, the urethra also serves as the pathway for delivery of semen.

Numerous secretions contribute to semen. Spermatozoa, manufactured in the testis, are only a small component. Paired Cowper's glands (bulbourethral glands) at the base of the prostate produce a clear lubricant that is secreted into the urethra. The lubricant lines the urethra to ease the passage of semen and to neutralize the urethra's acidity. Secretions from the Cowper's glands are sometimes referred to as pre-ejaculate.

The prostate gland is the second greatest contributor to the composition of semen. The prostate secretions provide nutrition to the sperm and also contain **enzymes** that help break down the viscous fluid at ejaculation so that the spermatozoa can move more freely. The prostate contains the ejaculatory duct for sperm from the vas deferens, releasing the sperm and prostatic fluid into the urethra. This is followed by the secretions from the seminal vesicles.

Most procedures for the prostate are reported with codes that appear in the Male Genital section of the CPT code set. However, **transurethral** procedures of the prostate are reported with codes from the Urinary System code set.

Seminal vesicles occur **bilaterally** at the base of the bladder. They are **excretory** glands responsible for manufacturing the majority of the fluid found in semen. Many components within the fluid contributed by the seminal vesicles are designed to provide nutrition and protection to the spermatozoa.

Structures described in this section of the CPT code set are bilateral structures, with the exception of the penis and prostate. However, CPT codes in this section report unilateral procedures, unless their descriptions state otherwise.

Penis

Incision

Coding Atlas

Prepuce is a synonym for foreskin, a redundant fold of skin and **mucous membrane** that covers the glans penis. The foreskin may be slit if it cannot be retracted from the glans penis.

54000 Slitting of prepuce, dorsal or lateral (separate procedure); newborn

54001 except newborn

54015 Incision and drainage of penis, deep

Destruction

Coding Atlas

Condylomas, papilloma, molluscum contagiosum, and herpes are usually sexually transmitted. **Destruction** of these lesions is **therapeutic** and may not be curative; the patient will no longer have the wart but may still carry the underlying **virus**.

54050 Destruction of lesion(s), penis (eg, condyloma, papilloma, molluscum contagiosum, herpetic vesicle), simple; chemical

54055 electrodesiccation

54056 cryosurgery

54057 laser surgery

54060 surgical excision

54065 Destruction of lesion(s), penis (eg, condyloma, papilloma, molluscum contagiosum, herpetic vesicle), extensive (eg, laser surgery, electrosurgery, cryosurgery, chemosurgery)

Excision

Coding Atlas

Peyronie disease describes the formation of a **benign** plaque in the tunica albuginea surrounding the corpus cavernosum. The **plaque** may cause pain or may cause the penis to bend when erect, making **coitus** difficult. The plaque may be surgically excised. When a **graft** is performed, procurement of the **donor** tissue may be a separately reportable procedure, if the graft is obtained through a separate incision.

54100 Biopsy of penis; (separate procedure)

54105 deep structures

54110 Excision of penile plaque (Peyronie disease);

54111 with graft to 5 cm in length

54112 with graft greater than 5 cm in length

54115 Removal foreign body from deep penile tissue (eg, plastic implant)

54120 Amputation of penis; partial

54125 complete

54130 Amputation of penis, radical; with bilateral inguinofemoral lymphadenectomy

54135 in continuity with bilateral pelvic lymphadenectomy, including external iliac, hypogastric and obturator nodes

54150 Circumcision, using clamp or other device with regional dorsal penile or ring block

54160 Circumcision, surgical excision other than clamp, device, or dorsal slit; neonate (28 days of age or less)

54161 older than 28 days of age

54162 Lysis or excision of penile post-circumcision adhesions

54163 Repair incomplete circumcision

54164 Frenulotomy of penis

FIGURE 7-1. Penile Structures

From the bulb of the penis, the corpus spongiosum continues along the penile underside until it forms the glans penis. The urethra travels through corpus spongiosum; the meatus is at the tip of the glans penis. The corpora cavernosa are **bilateral** chambers that form the remainder of the penis's circumference. The corpora cavernosa is covered in tunica albuginea, a **fascial** sheath. The corpora cavernosa and corpus spongiosum, as well as blood and nerve supplies, all reside within **Buck's fascia**.

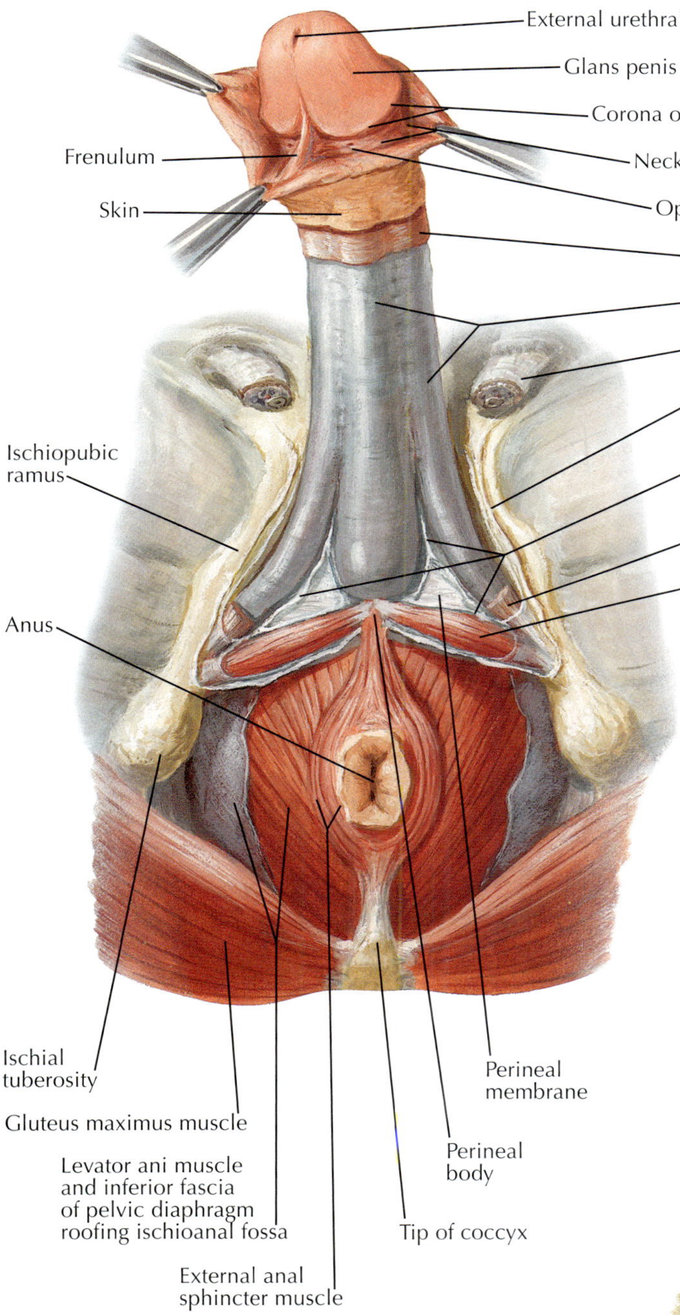

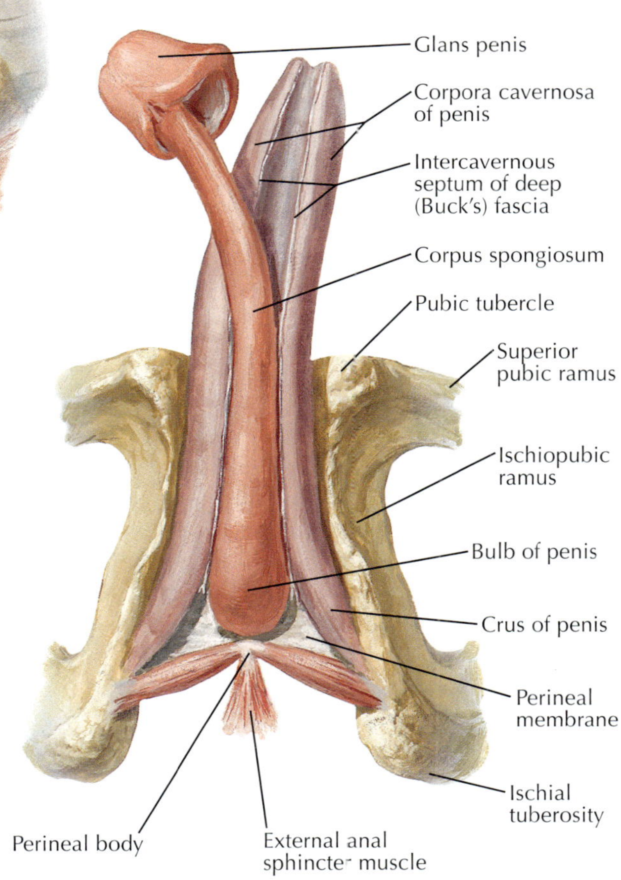

FIGURE 7-2. Lateral View of the Penis

The male urethra shares urinary and reproductive functions. From the bladder, the urethra traverses the prostate and the entire length of the penis. During urination, the urinary **sphincter** releases urine, which is expelled from the urethral **meatus**. During sexual arousal, the urethra is converted into a corridor for the propulsion of semen from **ducts** in the **proximal** penile urethra and out the urethral meatus. The **pH** of semen is alkaline in order to neutralize the urethra, which is made acidic by urine.

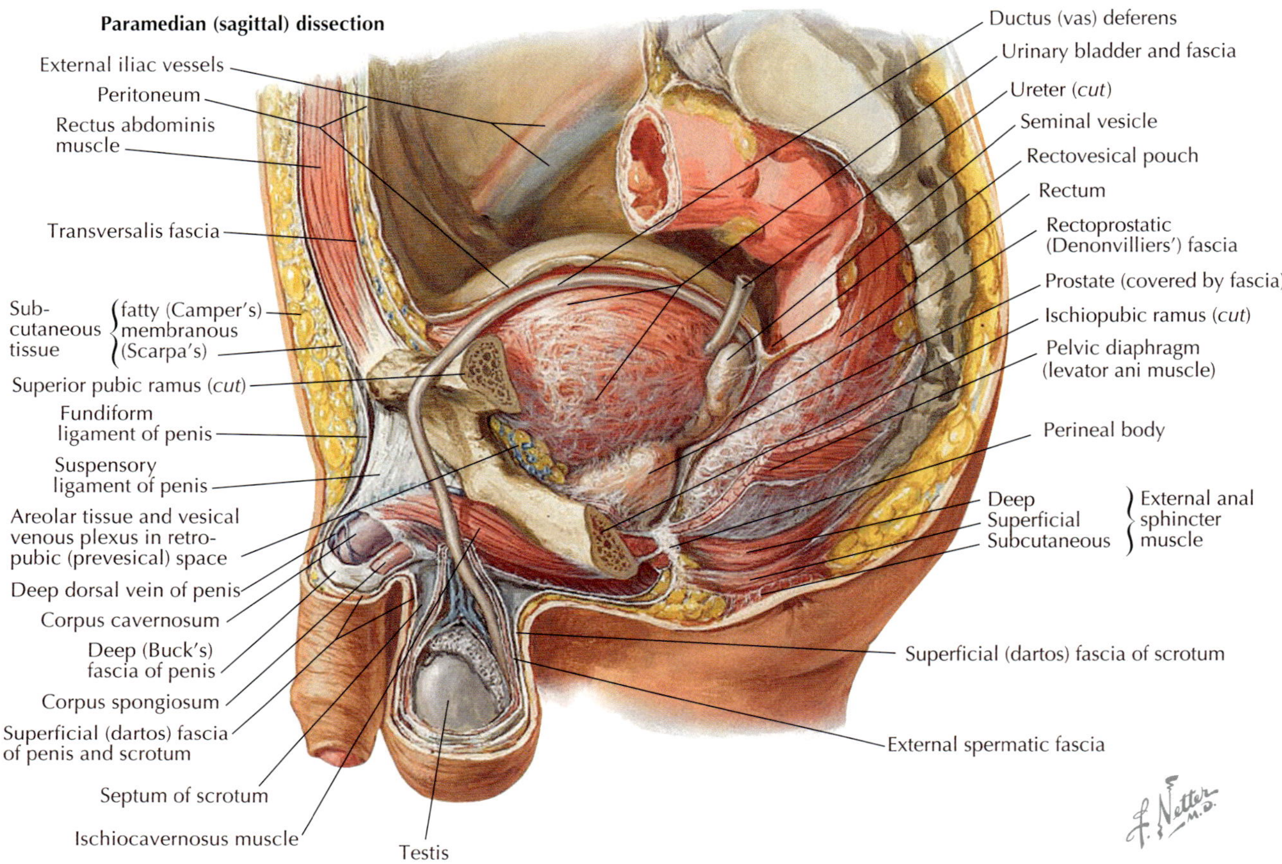

Introduction

Coding Atlas

Priapism describes a persistent penile erection in the absence of arousal. In most cases, priapism involves corpus cavernosum but not corpus spongiosum. **Nocturnal penile tumescence** (NPT) testing is performed to determine whether a patient with erectile dysfunction (ED) is having erections during sleep, which is a normal physiologic occurrence. NPT may rule out a physical cause for the ED.

54200 Injection procedure for Peyronie disease;

54205 with surgical exposure of plaque

54220 Irrigation of corpora cavernosa for priapism

54230 Injection procedure for corpora cavernosography

54231 Dynamic cavernosometry, including intracavernosal injection of vasoactive drugs (eg, papaverine, phentolamine)

54235 Injection of corpora cavernosa with pharmacologic agent(s) (eg, papaverine, phentolamine)

54240 Penile plethysmography

54250 Nocturnal penile tumescence and/or rigidity test

FIGURE 7-3. Foreskin Disorders

Phimosis describes a condition in which the distal foreskin cannot be retracted over the glans penis. Phimosis may be a physiologic condition that occurs naturally at birth and resolves by puberty or a pathologic condition secondary to foreskin (preputial) scarring. In either case, the foreskin is adherent to the glans penis. Manipulation of the foreskin to relieve phimosis is reported with code 54450.

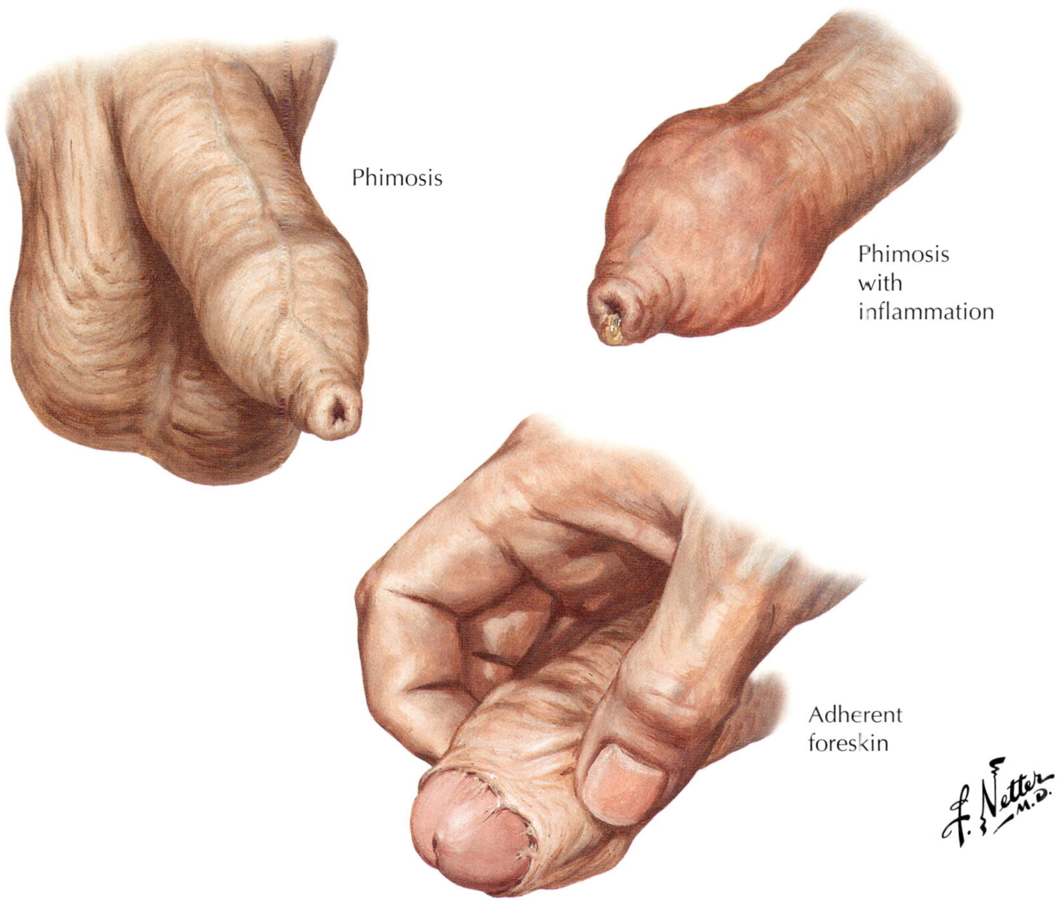

Repair

Coding Atlas

A penile **prosthesis** is an implantable device that provides a surgical solution for patients with erectile dysfunction (ED) who wish to be sexually active. Codes for implant procedures are selected based on whether the implant consists of a pair of malleable rods or a hydraulic, inflatable implant system with a separately implanted pump. The inflatable system has three components: the pump, reservoir, and implant chambers. When the pump is activated, fluid from the reservoir fills the implanted chambers in the penis. To deflate the chambers, the pump returns the fluid to the reservoir.

54300 Plastic operation of penis for straightening of chordee (eg, hypospadias), with or without mobilization of urethra

54304 Plastic operation on penis for correction of chordee or for first stage hypospadias repair with or without transplantation of prepuce and/or skin flaps

54308 Urethroplasty for second stage hypospadias repair (including urinary diversion); less than 3 cm

54312 greater than 3 cm

54316 Urethroplasty for second stage hypospadias repair (including urinary diversion) with free skin graft obtained from site other than genitalia

54318 Urethroplasty for third stage hypospadias repair to release penis from scrotum (eg, third stage Cecil repair)

FIGURE 7-4. Longitudinal and Cross-Section of the Penis

The male urethra is divided into three segments: prostatic, membranous, and spongy. Pre-ejaculate created in the bulbourethral gland is released through **ducts** in the **proximal** spongy urethra during arousal. Components of semen are generated in the prostate gland, seminal vesicles, and testes. During ejaculation, spermatozoa and fluid from the seminal vesicles are released from the ejaculatory ducts, and fluid from the prostate is released through the prostatic ducts to mix in the prostatic urethra. These two fluids together form semen.

Longitudinal section

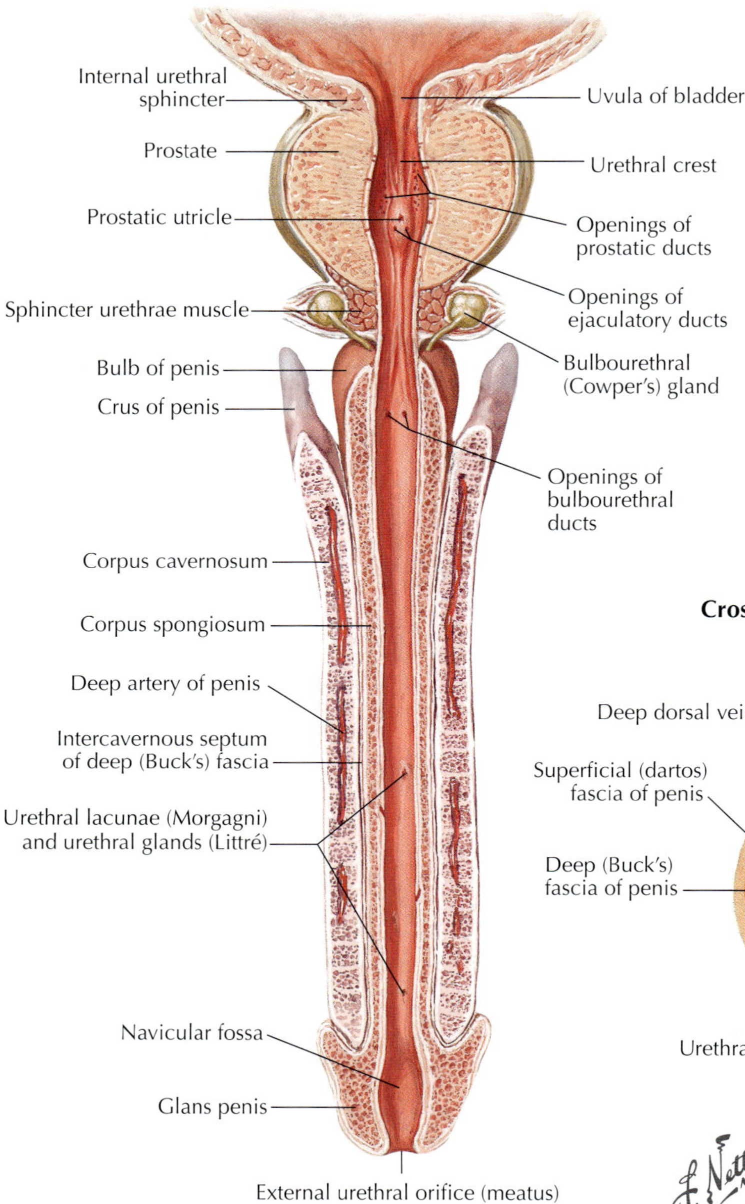

Cross section through body of penis

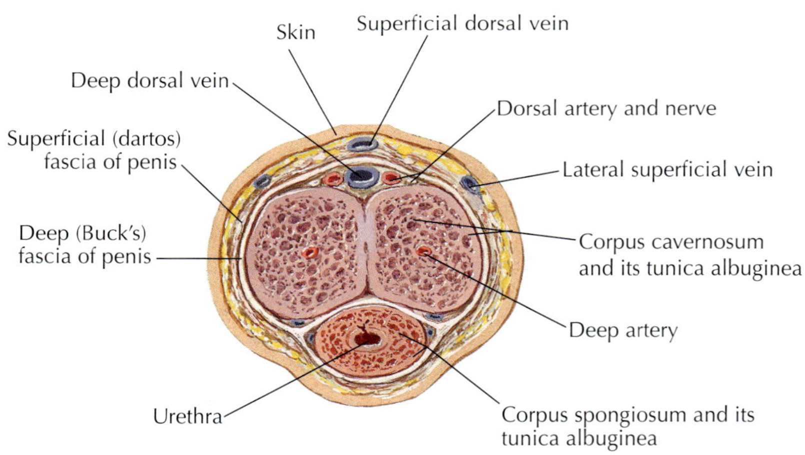

54322 1-stage distal hypospadias repair (with or without chordee or circumcision); with simple meatal advancement (eg, Magpi, V-flap)

54324 with urethroplasty by local skin flaps (eg, flip-flap, prepucial flap)

54326 with urethroplasty by local skin flaps and mobilization of urethra

54328 with extensive dissection to correct chordee and urethroplasty with local skin flaps, skin graft patch, and/or island flap

54332 1-stage proximal penile or penoscrotal hypospadias repair requiring extensive dissection to correct chordee and urethroplasty by use of skin graft tube and/or island flap

54336 1-stage perineal hypospadias repair requiring extensive dissection to correct chordee and urethroplasty by use of skin graft tube and/or island flap

54340 Repair of hypospadias complications (ie, fistula, stricture, diverticula); by closure, incision, or excision, simple

54344 requiring mobilization of skin flaps and urethroplasty with flap or patch graft

54348 requiring extensive dissection and urethroplasty with flap, patch or tubed graft (includes urinary diversion)

54352 Repair of hypospadias cripple requiring extensive dissection and excision of previously constructed structures including re-release of chordee and reconstruction of urethra and penis by use of local skin as grafts and island flaps and skin brought in as flaps or grafts

54360 Plastic operation on penis to correct angulation

54380 Plastic operation on penis for epispadias distal to external sphincter;

54385 with incontinence

54390 with exstrophy of bladder

54400 Insertion of penile prosthesis; non-inflatable (semi-rigid)

54401 inflatable (self-contained)

54405 Insertion of multi-component, inflatable penile prosthesis, including placement of pump, cylinders, and reservoir

54406 Removal of all components of a multi-component, inflatable penile prosthesis without replacement of prosthesis

54408 Repair of component(s) of a multi-component, inflatable penile prosthesis

54410 Removal and replacement of all component(s) of a multi-component, inflatable penile prosthesis at the same operative session

54411 Removal and replacement of all components of a multi-component inflatable penile prosthesis through an infected field at the same operative session, including irrigation and debridement of infected tissue

54415 Removal of non-inflatable (semi-rigid) or inflatable (self-contained) penile prosthesis, without replacement of prosthesis

54416 Removal and replacement of non-inflatable (semi-rigid) or inflatable (self-contained) penile prosthesis at the same operative session

54417 Removal and replacement of non-inflatable (semi-rigid) or inflatable (self-contained) penile prosthesis through an infected field at the same operative session, including irrigation and debridement of infected tissue

54420 Corpora cavernosa-saphenous vein shunt (priapism operation), unilateral or bilateral

54430 Corpora cavernosa-corpus spongiosum shunt (priapism operation), unilateral or bilateral

54435 Corpora cavernosa-glans penis fistulization (eg, biopsy needle, Winter procedure, rongeur, or punch) for priapism

54440 Plastic operation of penis for injury

Manipulation

54450 Foreskin manipulation including lysis of preputial adhesions and stretching

FIGURE 7-5. Hypospadias and Chordee

Hypospadias is a congenital anomaly in which the urethral meatus is not at its normal centered position on the tip of the glans penis. It is located somewhere proximal to that location along the length of the shaft, at the base of the scrotum, or on the perineum. Chordee is a condition in which the penis is curved due to abnormalities in the fascial tissues and/or corpus spongiosum. These conditions often occur together, and each is surgically correctable.

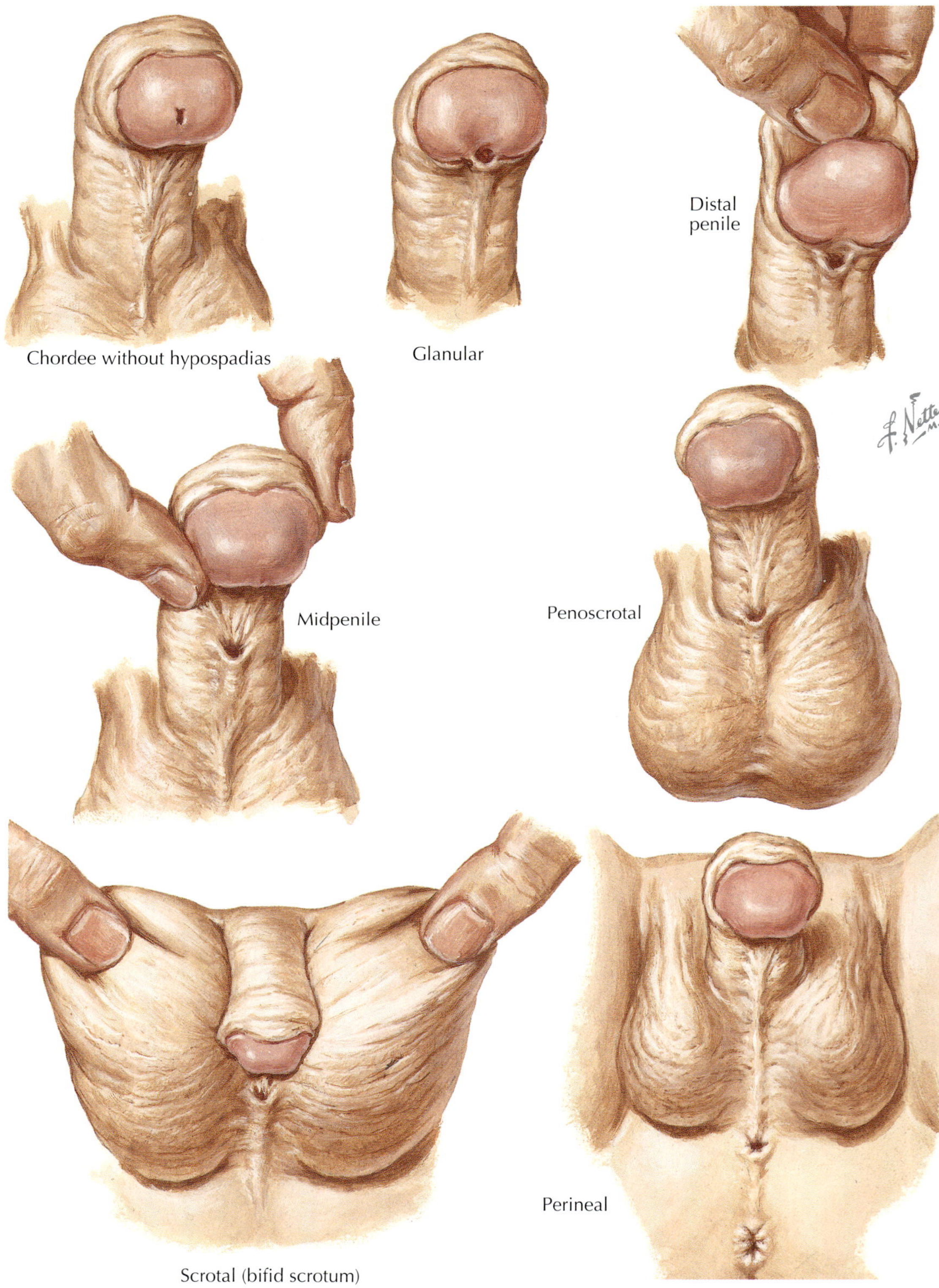

FIGURE 7-6. The Scrotum and Spermatic Cord

The scrotum contains the testes. Each testis is suspended by a spermatic cord, which stretches from the testis to the deep **inguinal ring**. The spermatic cord contains the vas deferens, arteries (testicular, cremastertic, and ductus deferens), a network of small veins called the pampiniform **plexus**, nerves (genital branch of the genitofemoral nerve and sympathetic nerve fibers), and **lymphatics**. It has multiple layers of protective **fascia**.

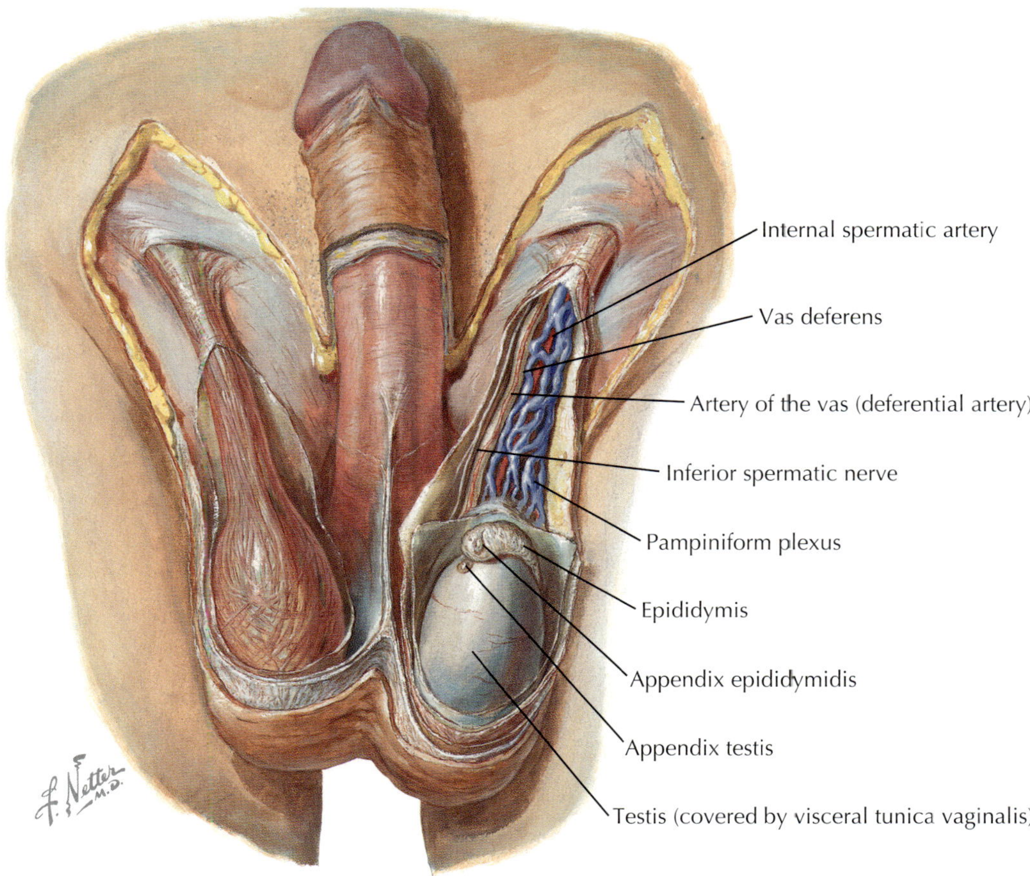

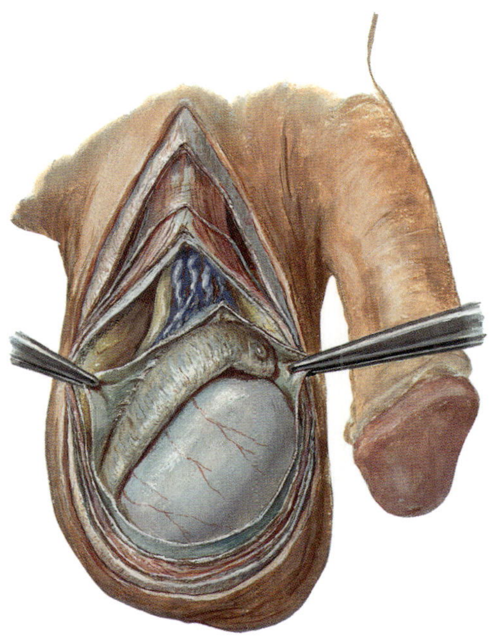

Testis

Excision

Coding Atlas

Orchiectomy, also called orchidectomy, describes the **excision** of an entire testis.

54500 Biopsy of testis, needle (separate procedure)

54505 Biopsy of testis, incisional (separate procedure)

54512 Excision of extraparenchymal lesion of testis

54520 Orchiectomy, simple (including subcapsular), with or without testicular prosthesis, scrotal or inguinal approach

54522 Orchiectomy, partial

54530 Orchiectomy, radical, for tumor; inguinal approach

54535 with abdominal exploration

Exploration

Coding Atlas

No **excision** or **orchiopexy** is performed during procedures reported with CPT codes 54550 or 54560, which describe **unilateral** exploration for undescended testis only.

54550 Exploration for undescended testis (inguinal or scrotal area)

54560 Exploration for undescended testis with abdominal exploration

Repair

Coding Atlas

Torsion of testis describes a twisting of the spermatic cord, which contains the vas deferens, lymphatics, nerve pathways, and blood supply to the testis. The twisting compromises the blood supply to the testis and scrotum and may lead to **edema** and/or **ischemia**. Torsion may be due to a congenital twist, the result of an injury, or caused by a deficiency in the anchoring tissue between the testis and the scrotum (bell clapper deformity).

54600 Reduction of torsion of testis, surgical, with or without fixation of contralateral testis

54620 Fixation of contralateral testis (separate procedure)

54640 Orchiopexy, inguinal approach, with or without hernia repair

54650 Orchiopexy, abdominal approach, for intra-abdominal testis (eg, Fowler-Stephens)

54660 Insertion of testicular prosthesis (separate procedure)

54670 Suture or repair of testicular injury

54680 Transplantation of testis(es) to thigh (because of scrotal destruction)

Laparoscopy

Coding Atlas

Laparoscopy is a technique developed to reduce risk and recovery time during abdominal or pelvic surgery. Several small abdominal or pelvic incisions act as portals for a tiny video camera (laparoscope), light source, and surgical tools. The physician manipulates the surgical tools while viewing the surgical site on a video display screen. To enhance visibility, the abdomen or pelvis may be filled with gas during the procedure.

54690 Laparoscopy, surgical; orchiectomy

54692 orchiopexy for intra-abdominal testis

FIGURE 7-7. The Testis, Epididymis, and Ductus Deferens

Spermatozoa are manufactured in seminiferous tubules of the testes. Immature spermatozoa are transferred to the epididymis. Initially, immature sperm are stored in the head of the epididymis until they are ready for maturation. These sperm are then transferred to the body of the epididymis where they mature, a process that takes about a week. Mature sperm then advance into the tail of the epididymis. From there, they are transported via the ductus deferens (vas deferens) during arousal in the first step toward ejaculation.

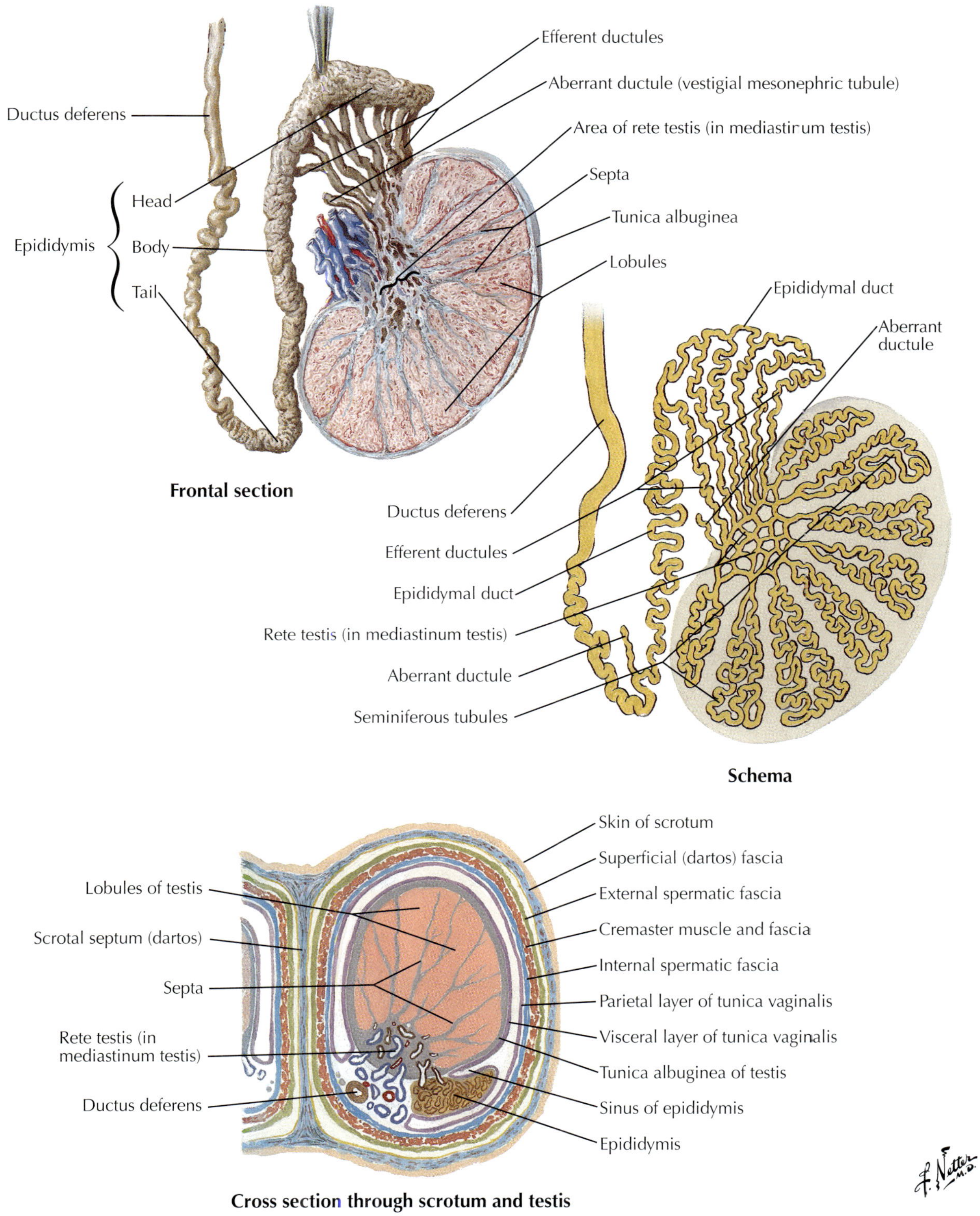

FIGURE 7-8. Descent of the Testes

Testes originate in the fetal abdomen and normally descend into the scrotum before birth. In the scrotum, testes remain cool when core body temperature rises. The spermatozoa in undescended testes may not develop normally due to increased temperatures. Up to 20% of premature infants and 3% to 5% of all males are born with undescended testes, diagnosed upon discovery of empty scrotal sacs. Most testes spontaneously descend in the first three months after birth. Other cases may be corrected surgically.

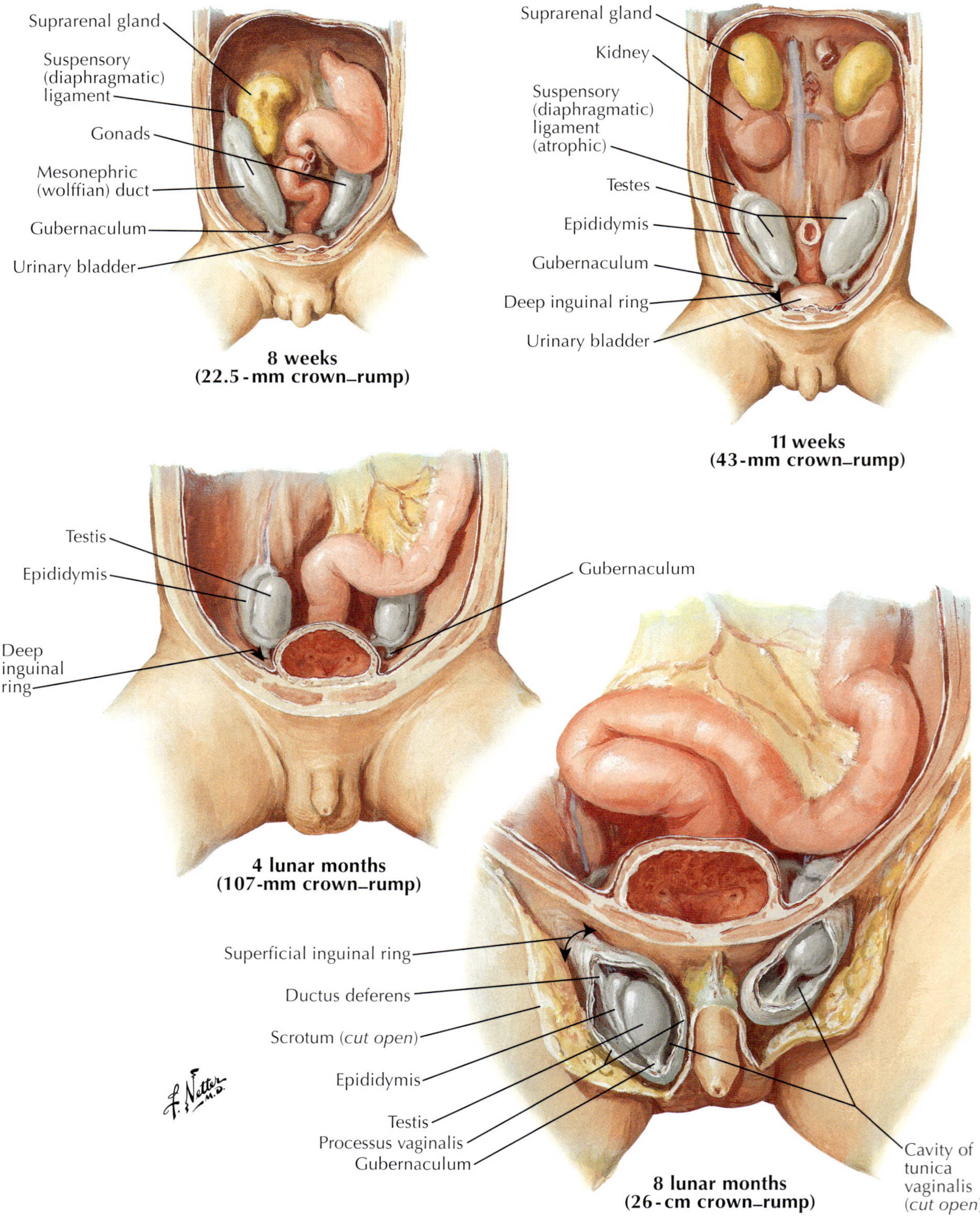

Epididymis

Incision

54700 Incision and drainage of epididymis, testis and/or scrotal space (eg, abscess or hematoma)

Excision

Coding Atlas

The epididymis is a tightly wound tubular structure that rises from the posterior border of the testis. In the epididymis, immature spermatozoa are received from the testis, matured, and released into the vas deferens in preparation of ejaculation. The entire structure is only about 5 centimeters long. However, if the epididymis were to be unbundled into a single tube, it would be approximately 20 feet in length. A spermatocele is a benign cyst arising from the head of the epididymis and containing an accumulation of sperm.

54800 Biopsy of epididymis, needle

54830 Excision of local lesion of epididymis

54840 Excision of spermatocele, with or without epididymectomy

54860 Epididymectomy; unilateral

54861 bilateral

Exploration

54865 Exploration of epididymis, with or without biopsy

Repair

Coding Atlas

Epididymovasostomy describes the reconstruction of the spermatic duct system that has an obstruction. It is performed to restore the patency of the tubule and, in turn, restore fertility; it is most commonly done as a reversal of a vasectomy procedure. In epididymovasostomy, the vas deferens is anastomosed to the epididymis. Microsurgical anastomosis that requires an operating microscope would be reported in addition to the main procedure using CPT code 69990.

54900 Epididymovasostomy, anastomosis of epididymis to vas deferens; unilateral

54901 bilateral

Tunica Vaginalis

Incision

55000 Puncture aspiration of hydrocele, tunica vaginalis, with or without injection of medication

Excision

Coding Atlas

When a hydrocele is excised in conjunction with a hernia repair, reported using a code from the range 49505-49507, the hydrocele excision code would be reported in addition to the hernia repair code.

55040 Excision of hydrocele; unilateral

55041 bilateral

Repair

Coding Atlas

The tunica vaginalis is a pouch of serous membrane covering the testis and epididymis.

55060 Repair of tunica vaginalis hydrocele (Bottle type)

FIGURE 7-9. Hydrocele and Spermatocele

A **hydrocele** is an accumulation of **peritoneal** fluid between the **parietal** and **visceral** layers of the tunica vaginalis within the scrotum or along the spermatic cord. The hydrocele may be a **congenital** or **acquired** defect. A **spermatocele** is a benign **cyst** arising from the head of the epididymis and containing an accumulation of sperm.

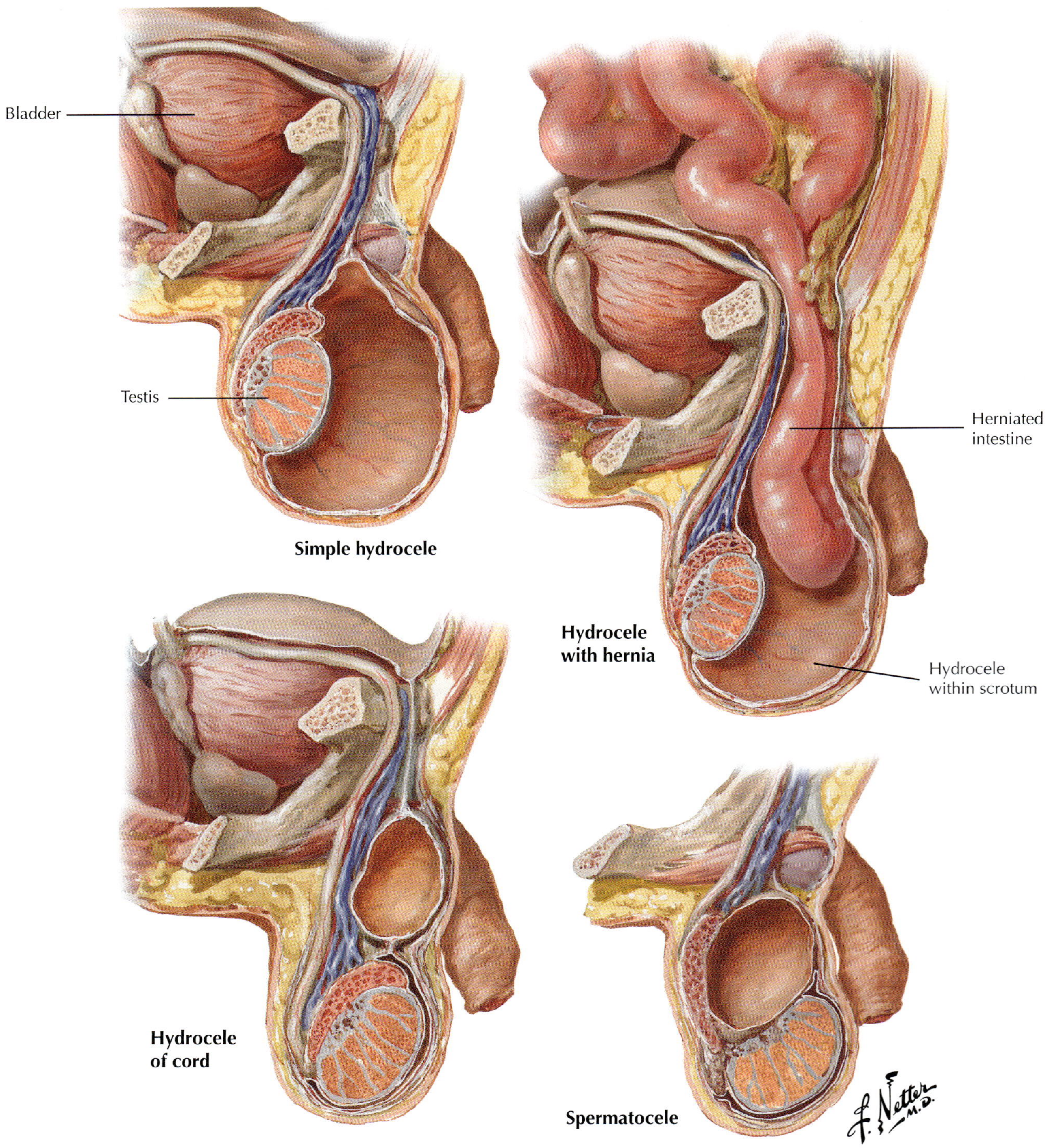

Scrotum

Incision

Coding Atlas

The scrotum is a sac of skin and muscle located **posterior** to the penis and **anterior** to the anus. Involuntary contractions of the muscle fibers in the dartos fascia of the scrotum cause the scrotum to thicken and ascend closer to the perineum. This occurs when the scrotum is exposed to cool temperatures. Warm temperatures cause the dartos fascia to relax. The testes within the scrotum are thus protected from extreme temperatures. Sperm production is optimal when the testes are cooler than the core body temperature. Procedures on the scrotum involve the layers of the scrotal sac or the space between the inner scrotal wall and its contents (testes, epididymis, spermatic cord).

55100 Drainage of scrotal wall abscess

55110 Scrotal exploration

55120 Removal of foreign body in scrotum

Excision

Coding Atlas

Excision of a local skin lesion on the scrotum would be reported using a code from the Integumentary System code set.

55150 Resection of scrotum

Repair

Coding Atlas

Scrotoplasty describes the **plastic repair** of the scrotum. Usually, it is associated with injury or a postsurgical defect but may also be performed due to a **congenital** malformation.

55175 Scrotoplasty; simple

55180 complicated

Vas Deferens

Incision

Coding Atlas

The vas deferens, also known as the ductus deferens, is a muscular tube that connects to the epididymis. As a component of the spermatic cord, the vas deferens passes through the **inguinal canal**, enters the abdomen, and redirects back into the pelvic cavity where it forms the ejaculatory **duct** with the seminal vesicle. Its purpose is to deliver spermatozoa during ejaculation.

55200 Vasotomy, cannulization with or without incision of vas, unilateral or bilateral (separate procedure)

Excision

55250 Vasectomy, unilateral or bilateral (separate procedure), including postoperative semen examination(s)

Introduction

55300 Vasotomy for vasograms, seminal vesiculograms, or epididymograms, unilateral or bilateral

Repair

55400 Vasovasostomy, vasovasorrhaphy

Suture

55450 Ligation (percutaneous) of vas deferens, unilateral or bilateral (separate procedure)

FIGURE 7-10. Vasectomy

In a vasectomy, the vas deferens is severed or occluded as a form of permanent birth control, thus preventing spermatozoa from reaching the seminal vesicle during coitus. It may be performed using an open technique, as illustrated and reported using code 55250, or by performing a no scalpel vasectomy (NSV), which exposes the vas deferens using a percutaneous technique, reported using code 55450. Note: Tools, implants, and/or equipment depicted in the illustration may be outdated but the procedural approach is valid.

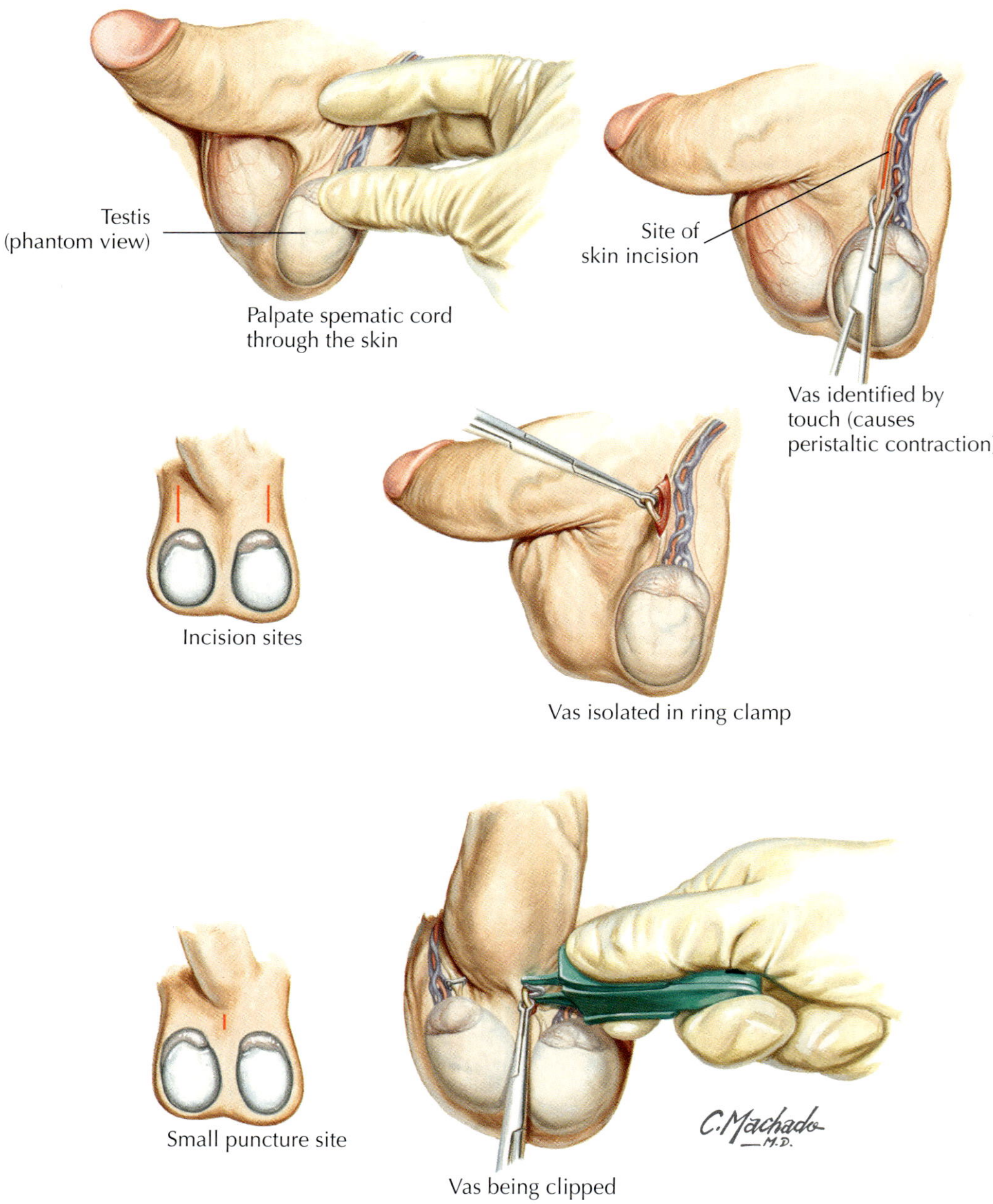

Spermatic Cord

Excision

Coding Atlas

A varicocele forms in the spermatic cord when valves inside the pampiniform venous plexus fail, causing backflow of blood, congestion, and expansion of the vein that is a component of the spermatic cord. The condition may be treated with varicocelectomy or ligation, reported using codes 55530-55540. If the varicocele is treated by embolization using transcatheter methodology, the procedure is reported using code 37241.

55500 Excision of hydrocele of spermatic cord, unilateral (separate procedure)

55520 Excision of lesion of spermatic cord (separate procedure)

55530 Excision of varicocele or ligation of spermatic veins for varicocele; (separate procedure)

55535 abdominal approach

55540 with hernia repair

Laparoscopy

55550 Laparoscopy, surgical, with ligation of spermatic veins for varicocele

Seminal Vesicles

Incision

Coding Atlas

Vesiculotomy is surgical incision into the seminal vesicle.

55600 Vesiculotomy;

55605 complicated

Excision

Coding Atlas

A Mullerian duct cyst is a remnant of fetal development and is usually located in the middle of the posterior bladder wall. The cyst may cause urinary symptoms and require excision if it enlarges due to fluid accumulation.

55650 Vesiculectomy, any approach

55680 Excision of Mullerian duct cyst

Prostate

Incision

Coding Atlas

The differences between a standard prostate needle biopsy, reported using code 55700, and guided saturation sampling, reported using code 55706, are many. The standard prostate needle biopsy can be performed under local anesthesia and may include between 6 and 12 core samples. It is performed transanally. Stereotactic guided saturation sampling is performed under general anesthesia, and between 35 and 60 core samples are collected using a transperineal approach and a template grid that organizes the collection sites systematically.

55700 Biopsy, prostate; needle or punch, single or multiple, any approach

55705 incisional, any approach

55706 Biopsies, prostate, needle, transperineal, stereotactic template guided saturation sampling, including imaging guidance

55720 Prostatotomy, external drainage of prostatic abscess, any approach; simple

55725 complicated

FIGURE 7-11. Approaches to Seminal Vesicles

The seminal vesicles are paired organs situated adjacent to the **posterior** bladder and posterior prostate. Because the seminal vesicles lie deep in the pelvis, several approaches may be considered for surgery. Possible incision sites include the abdomen, perineum, or gluteal cleft. For procedures on the seminal vesicle(s), the approach is not a component for proper CPT code selection. Note: Tools, implants, and/or equipment depicted in the illustration may be outdated but the procedural approach is valid.

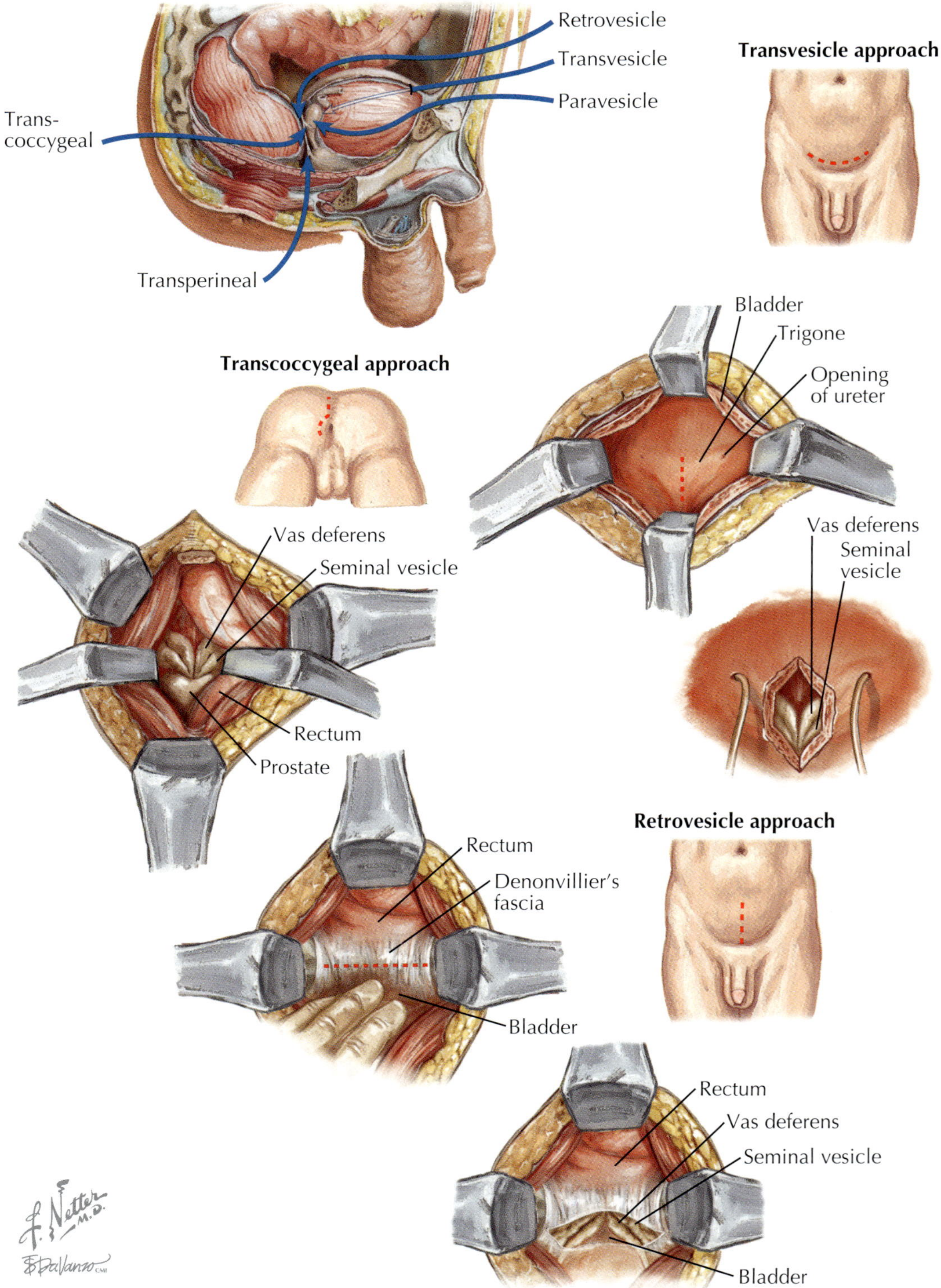

FIGURE 7-12. The Prostate, Bladder, Seminal Vesicles, and Vas (Ductus) Deferens

The vas deferens and seminal vesicles sit **bilaterally** atop the prostate at the **posterior** bladder. From this position, fluids from the vas deferens and seminal vesicles flow into the ejaculatory **ducts** in the urethra. The prostate contributes fluid through the prostatic duct and, with the other secretions, forms semen. The proximity of the vas deferens and seminal vesicles means that surgery on the prostate may impact future sexual function and **fertility**.

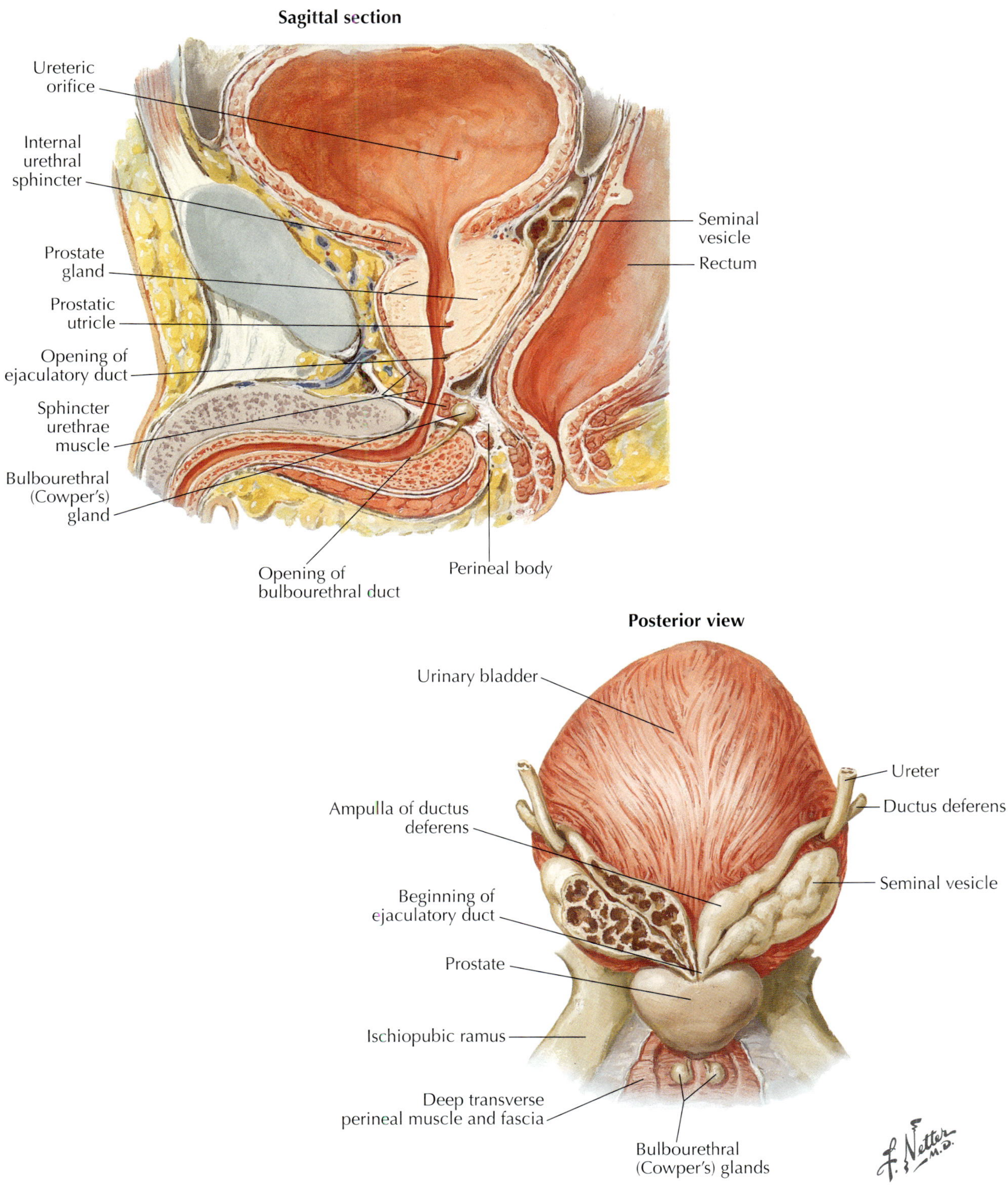

FIGURE 7-13. Radical Prostatectomy

Radical prostatectomy describes removal of the entire prostate, seminal vesicles, and **periprostatic** tissues. The approach may be retropubic (radical **retropubic** prostatectomy [RRP]) or perineal (radical **perineal** prostatectomy [RPP]) for an open procedure. Laparoscopic radical prostatectomy (LRP) may be performed using a retropubic approach. Note: Tools, implants, and/or equipment depicted in the illustration may be outdated but the procedural approach is valid.

Anatomical position of the prostate. The prostate is located within the pelvis between the bladder and urethra, adjacent to the rectum, surrounded by a venous plexus and neurovascular bundles.

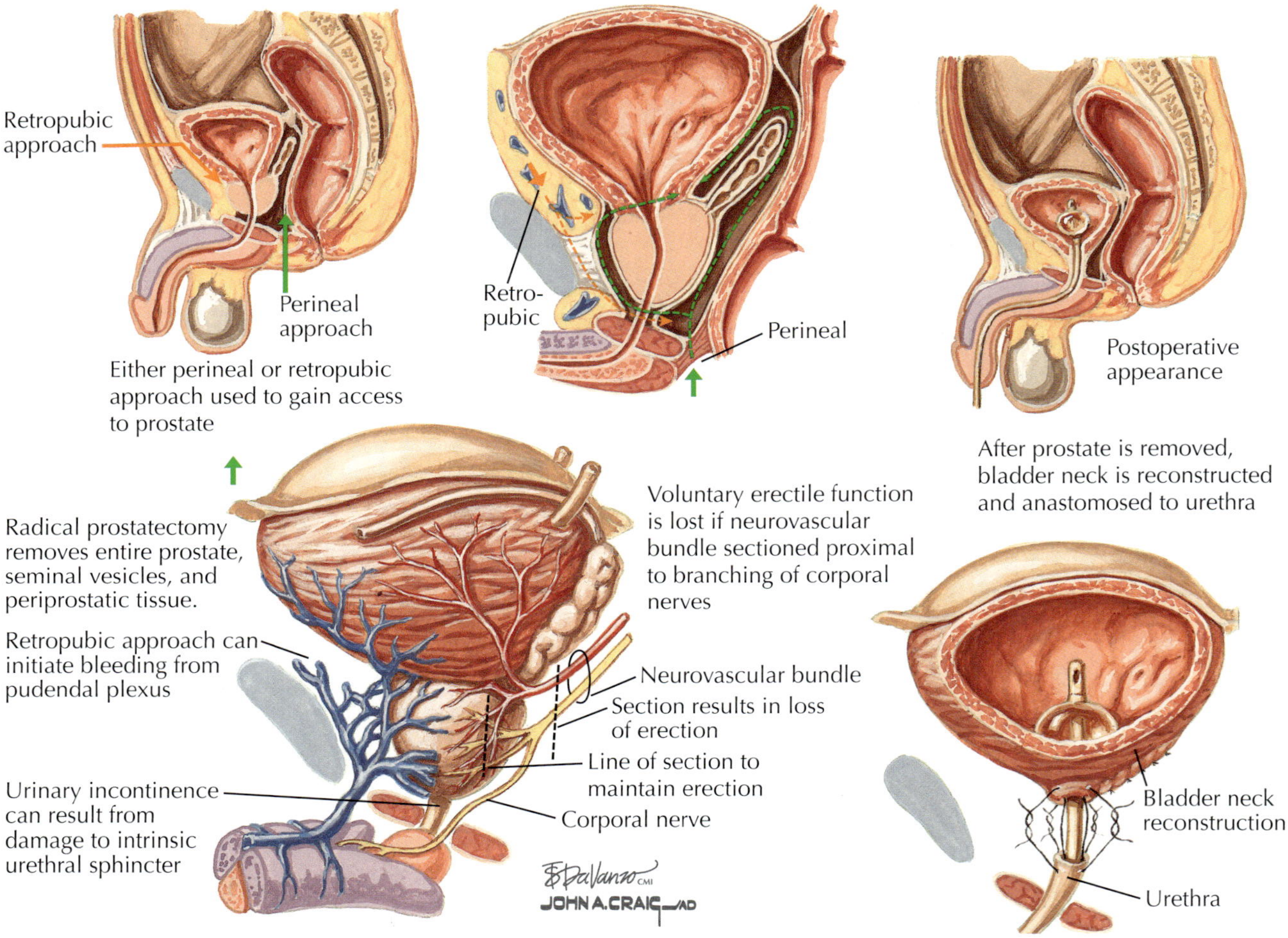

Excision

Coding Atlas

Benign prostatic hyperplasia (BPH) commonly affects men who are 60 and older. The enlarged prostate may encroach on the urethra and cause urinary obstruction. In many cases, a transurethral therapy may be recommended for BPH. Transurethral prostate procedures are reported with codes from the Urinary System section of the CPT code set. Some malignancies also respond well to transurethral approaches. Direct visualization of the prostate may be desired during excision of some cancers, eg, adenocarcinoma. Codes 55801-55845 are used to report open procedures that provide a more visual approach to treatment.

55801 Prostatectomy, perineal, subtotal (including control of postoperative bleeding, vasectomy, meatotomy, urethral calibration and/or dilation, and internal urethrotomy)

55810 Prostatectomy, perineal radical;

55812 with lymph node biopsy(s) (limited pelvic lymphadenectomy)

55815 with bilateral pelvic lymphadenectomy, including external iliac, hypogastric and obturator nodes

55821 Prostatectomy (including control of postoperative bleeding, vasectomy, meatotomy, urethral calibration and/or dilation, and internal urethrotomy); suprapubic, subtotal, 1 or 2 stages

55831 retropubic, subtotal

55840 Prostatectomy, retropubic radical, with or without nerve sparing;

55842 with lymph node biopsy(s) (limited pelvic lymphadenectomy)

55845 with bilateral pelvic lymphadenectomy, including external iliac, hypogastric, and obturator nodes

55860 Exposure of prostate, any approach, for insertion of radioactive substance;

55862 with lymph node biopsy(s) (limited pelvic lymphadenectomy)

55865 with bilateral pelvic lymphadenectomy, including external iliac, hypogastric and obturator nodes

Laparoscopy

55866 Laparoscopy, surgical prostatectomy, retropubic radical, including nerve sparing, includes robotic assistance, when performed

Other Procedures

Coding Atlas

Ejaculation can be induced by electrical stimulation. For patients with neurological impairment who wish to procreate, electroejaculation (EEJ) provides a method for harvesting semen that can be used for artificial insemination.

55870 Electroejaculation

55873 Cryosurgical ablation of the prostate (includes ultrasonic guidance and monitoring)

55875 Transperineal placement of needles or catheters into prostate for interstitial radioelement application, with or without cystoscopy

55876 Placement of interstitial device(s) for radiation therapy guidance (eg, fiducial markers, dosimeter), prostate (via needle, any approach), single or multiple

Reproductive System Procedures

55920 Placement of needles or catheters into pelvic organs and/or genitalia (except prostate) for subsequent interstitial radioelement application

Intersex Surgery

55970 Intersex surgery; male to female

55980 female to male

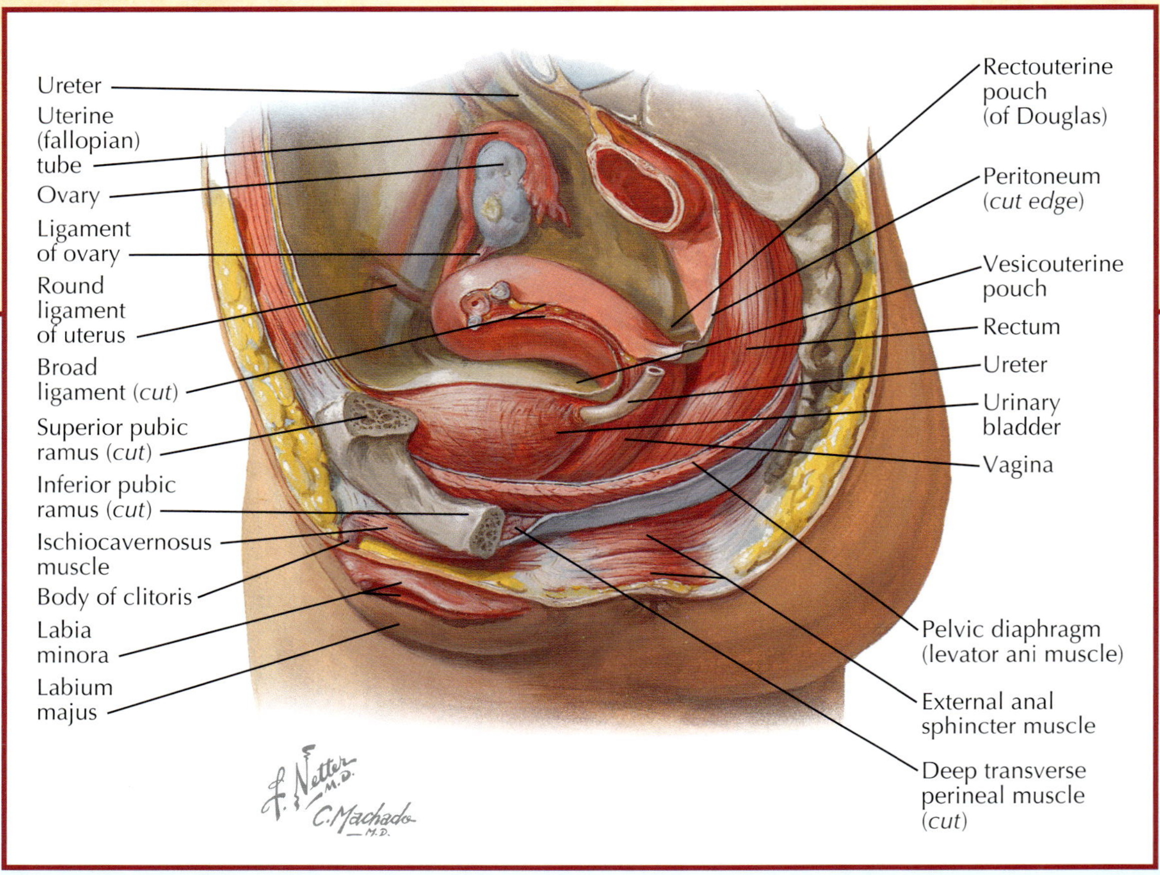
Ureter
Uterine (fallopian) tube
Ovary
Ligament of ovary
Round ligament of uterus
Broad ligament (cut)
Superior pubic ramus (cut)
Inferior pubic ramus (cut)
Ischiocavernosus muscle
Body of clitoris
Labia minora
Labium majus
Rectouterine pouch (of Douglas)
Peritoneum (cut edge)
Vesicouterine pouch
Rectum
Ureter
Urinary bladder
Vagina
Pelvic diaphragm (levator ani muscle)
External anal sphincter muscle
Deep transverse perineal muscle (cut)
F. Netter M.D.
C. Machado M.D.

CHAPTER 8

Female Genital System

The biological function of the female reproductive system is to accept spermatozoa from the male and provide an environment for the manufacture and fertilization of an ovum, the **gestation** of a fetus, and the vaginal delivery of a neonate.

External female genitalia include the contents of the vulva: perineum, mons pubis, clitoris, labia majora and minora, vestibule, hymen, Bartholin's gland, and the **periurethral** area. The external genitalia may be called the pudendum or vulva. It is bordered by the mons pubis **anteriorly** and the rectum **posteriorly** and by the crease of the thigh (**genitocrural fold**) bilaterally. The internal genitalia include the vagina, uterus, cervix, fallopian tubes, and ovaries. All internal female genitalia lie within the pelvis.

The **bilateral** ovaries secrete two groups of sex hormones, which are estrogen and progesterone. These secretions, along with secretions from the **hypothalamus** and pituitary glands, regulate the menstrual cycle (consists of ovarian and uterine cycles), which is crucial to reproduction. The ovarian cycle has three phases: follicular, ovulation, and luteal. During the follicular phase, a Graafian follicle within the ovary develops a mature egg (**ovum**). At the same time, the lining of the endometrium of the uterus proliferates in preparation for **embryo** implantation (uterine cycle). The follicle ruptures at about day 14 in the follicular phase, and an ovum is released (ovulation). The luteal phase begins at that point. The luteal phase also lasts about 14 days. During the first half of the luteal phase, the ovum is swept by **fimbriae** into the fallopian tube and advances into the uterus. A fertilized egg—one that has united with a sperm from the male—may embed successfully in the endometrial lining. If this does not occur, the endometrial lining begins to slough off (menstruation). Following the completion of **menses**, the follicular phase begins again. The first day of menstruation is considered day 1 of the menstrual cycle.

Spermatozoa travel through the vagina and cervical os into the uterus and then into the fallopian tube. Fertilization occurs in the fallopian tube, and the fertilized egg (**zygote**) migrates into the uterus. By this phase, the zygote has begun cell division, and the cluster of cells (**blastocyst**) implants itself in the nutrient-rich endometrial lining.

A normal pregnancy is 40 weeks long. However, pregnancy is measured from the last menstrual period (LMP). Ovulation does not occur until two weeks after the LMP, and implantation generally occurs a week after ovulation. So, the actual length of a pregnancy is 37 weeks once implantation occurs.

The growing fetus is suspended in the amniotic sac, which is filled with amniotic fluid. The fetal **umbilicus** connects the baby's future belly-button site and fetal circulatory system to the placenta, an organ of pregnancy that draws maternal blood away from the uterus. The fetus is nourished and oxygenated by this maternal blood until birth.

Labor and delivery usually begin with contractions that function to open the cervix and push the fetus into the birth canal. After the neonate is born, contractions continue until the placenta is delivered (afterbirth). Within a month or two, the uterus returns to its normal size, ie, the size of a pear.

Surgical encounters associated with the female genital system are often related to pregnancy or fertility, irregular menses, **incontinence**, **hernias** of the genital system, and neoplasms. Many procedures on the internal female genitalia may be performed using a vaginal or laparoscopic approach; an open surgical approach may be used when **direct visualization** is desired or in the case of a cesarean section.

Vulva, Perineum, and Introitus

Incision

Coding Atlas

The Bartholin's glands are **bilateral** glands at the base of the labia minora with **ducts** that drain into the vestibule. The glands supply lubrication to the vaginal opening (introitus) during sexual arousal. In **marsupialization**, a **cyst** is unroofed and the edges are sutured so that the cyst's floor becomes continuous with the adjacent surface. This may be performed on a Bartholin's gland cyst in order to prevent future infections.

56405 Incision and drainage of vulva or perineal abscess

56420 Incision and drainage of Bartholin's gland abscess

56440 Marsupialization of Bartholin's gland cyst

56441 Lysis of labial adhesions

56442 Hymenotomy, simple incision

Destruction

Coding Atlas

CPT codes 56501 and 56515 are used to report **destruction** of any type of lesion on external female genitalia. Condyloma, papilloma, molluscum contagiosum, and herpes are usually sexually transmitted. Destruction of a lesion is **therapeutic** but may not be curative; the patient will no longer have the wart but may still carry the underlying **virus**. Destruction of lesions of the vagina is reported with CPT codes 57061 and 57065.

56501 Destruction of lesion(s), vulva; simple (eg, laser surgery, electrosurgery, cryosurgery, chemosurgery)

56515 extensive (eg, laser surgery, electrosurgery, cryosurgery, chemosurgery)

Excision

Coding Atlas

A **vulvectomy** is a surgical treatment that is usually performed for a malignancy of the external female genitalia. A simple vulvectomy is the removal of skin and superficial fat and **subcutaneous** tissue. In a partial vulvectomy, less than 80% of the vulvar area is removed, while in a complete vulvectomy, more than 80% is removed. A radical vulvectomy involves removal of skin and deep subcutaneous tissue as well.

56605 Biopsy of vulva or perineum (separate procedure); 1 lesion

✚ **56606** each separate additional lesion (List separately in addition to code for primary procedure)

56620 Vulvectomy simple; partial

56625 complete

56630 Vulvectomy, radical, partial;

56631 with unilateral inguinofemoral lymphadenectomy

56632 with bilateral inguinofemoral lymphadenectomy

56633 Vulvectomy, radical, complete;

56634 with unilateral inguinofemoral lymphadenectomy

56637 with bilateral inguinofemoral lymphadenectomy

56640 Vulvectomy, radical, complete, with inguinofemoral, iliac, and pelvic lymphadenectomy

56700 Partial hymenectomy or revision of hymenal ring

56740 Excision of Bartholin's gland or cyst

FIGURE 8-1. The Vulva, Perineum, and Introitus

In its entirety, external female genitalia may be referred to as the vulva or the pudendum. The vulva includes the mons pubis, labia minor (labium minus) and majora (majus), clitoris, vestibule, urethral **meatus**, Skene's and Bartholin's glands, vaginal orifice, and hymen. The vaginal orifice may be referred to as the introitus. The vestibule describes the area between the introitus and the labia minor.

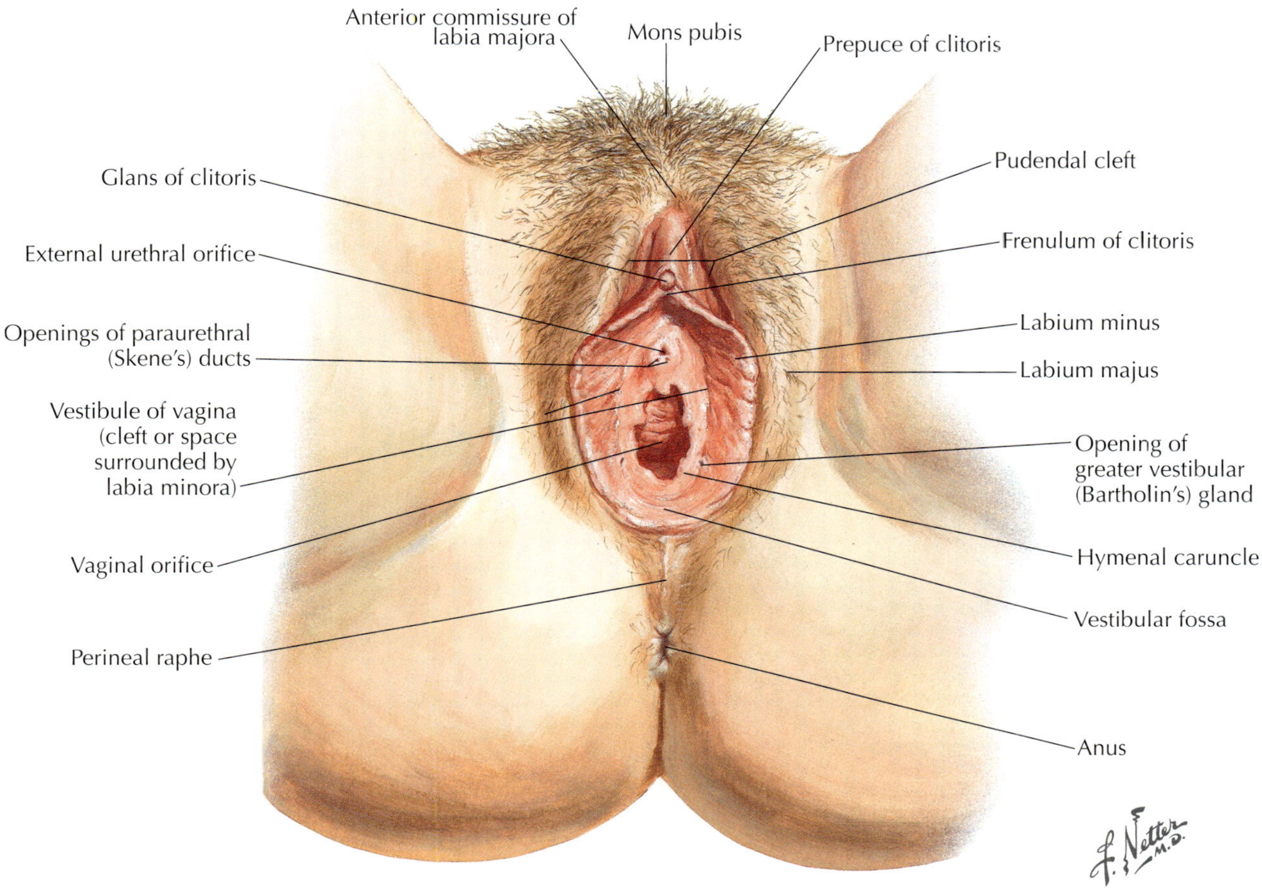

Repair

Coding Atlas

The opening of the vagina into the perineum is called the introitus. In **plastic repair** of the introitus (**introitoplasty**), the vaginal opening is altered to correct a defect. In **perineoplasty**, the perineum between the vagina and anus, including the perineal body, is repaired or strengthened. Perineoplasty may also be referred to as perineorrhaphy.

56800 Plastic repair of introitus

56805 Clitoroplasty for intersex state

56810 Perineoplasty, repair of perineum, nonobstetrical (separate procedure)

Endoscopy

Coding Atlas

Colposcopy (culposcopy) involves the use of a light and low-powered microscope to examine the vulva. The procedure is performed with the patient's feet in stirrups and the colposcope positioned over the vulva. In procedures reported with codes 56820 and 56821, the vulva is examined and may be painted with 5% acetic acid stain to highlight lesions associated with the human papilloma virus (HPV) or vulvar intraepithelial neoplasia (VIN). A colposcope may also be used to examine the vagina or cervix, and codes specific to those anatomical sites should be chosen if they are the target of the exam.

56820 Colposcopy of the vulva;

56821 with biopsy(s)

FIGURE 8-2. Dissection Exposing the Perineal Body

The perineal body describes a fibromuscular convergence of **pelvic floor** muscles, fascia, and fibrous tissue in the **medial** plane of the perineum between the vagina and anus. Essential to the integrity of the pelvic floor, the perineal body may be damaged during vaginal delivery, predisposing women to **prolapse** involving the uterus, bladder, and/or rectum. Damage to the perineal body may also result in urinary or fecal **incontinence**.

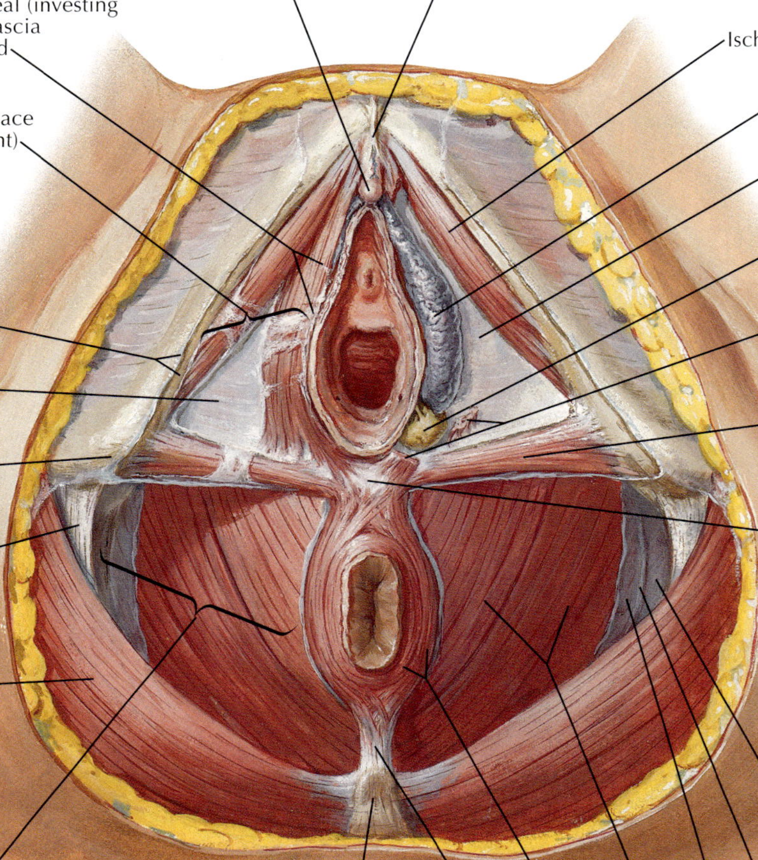

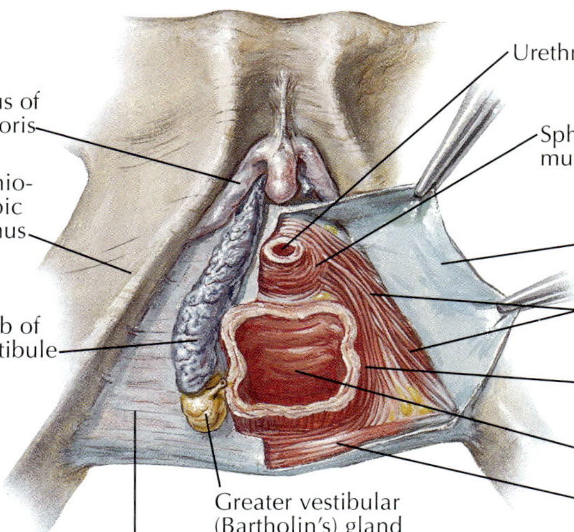

Vagina

Incision

Coding Atlas

Colpotomy is an incision into the vaginal wall. Colpotomy may also be documented as culpotomy or vaginotomy. In **colpocentesis** (culdocentesis), an aspirating syringe needle is inserted through the vaginal wall for collection of fluid from the recto-uterine cul-de-sac (pouch of Douglas). This pouch is the lowest site in the **intraperitoneal** space, and free fluids, including blood and pus, will pool there, creating a good site for diagnostic **aspiration** of peritoneal fluid.

57000 Colpotomy; with exploration

57010 with drainage of pelvic abscess

57020 Colpocentesis (separate procedure)

57022 Incision and drainage of vaginal hematoma; obstetrical/postpartum

57023 non-obstetrical (eg, post-trauma, spontaneous bleeding)

Destruction

Coding Atlas

Destruction of a **lesion** involves breaking down the lesion tissue using heat, cold, or chemicals. The lesion may be burned or frozen to destroy individual cells. Destruction is a common method for treating vaginal warts.

57061 Destruction of vaginal lesion(s); simple (eg, laser surgery, electrosurgery, cryosurgery, chemosurgery)

57065 extensive (eg, laser surgery, electrosurgery, cryosurgery, chemosurgery)

Excision

Coding Atlas

A complete **vaginectomy** includes removal of the entire vaginal wall and the vascular connective tissues supporting the vagina. Partial vaginectomy includes partial excision of the vaginal wall, usually the upper or lower half. Vaginectomy may be referred to as **colpectomy**. Pelvic **lymphadenectomy** may be referred to as pelvic lymph node dissection (PLND).

57100 Biopsy of vaginal mucosa; simple (separate procedure)

57105 extensive, requiring suture (including cysts)

57106 Vaginectomy, partial removal of vaginal wall;

57107 with removal of paravaginal tissue (radical vaginectomy)

57109 with removal of paravaginal tissue (radical vaginectomy) with bilateral total pelvic lymphadenectomy and para-aortic lymph node sampling (biopsy)

57110 Vaginectomy, complete removal of vaginal wall;

57111 with removal of paravaginal tissue (radical vaginectomy)

57112 with removal of paravaginal tissue (radical vaginectomy) with bilateral total pelvic lymphadenectomy and para-aortic lymph node sampling (biopsy)

57120 Colpocleisis (Le Fort type)

57130 Excision of vaginal septum

57135 Excision of vaginal cyst or tumor

FIGURE 8-3. The Vagina and Other Internal Genitalia

The vagina extends from the introitus of the vulva to the cervix. While the vagina in Figure 8-3 appears to have a substantial diameter, vaginas do not normally contain space. Rather, vaginal walls will stretch considerably during coitus, childbirth, or the insertion of a speculum during a medical exam, but otherwise are flattened tubes. The cervix uteri connects the vagina to the body of the uterus. The **mucosa**-lined vagina is **anterior** to the rectum and **posterior** to the bladder.

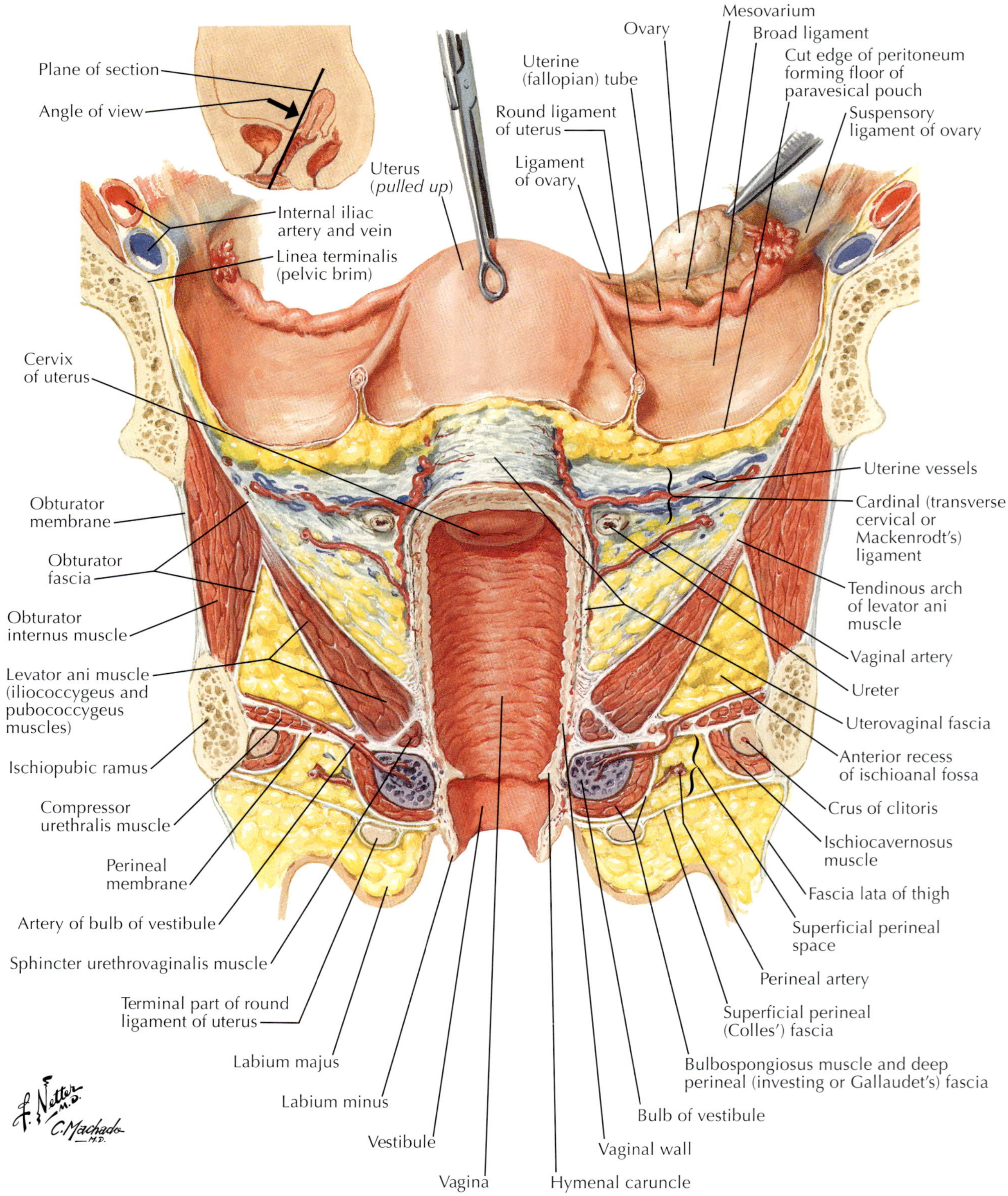

FIGURE 8-4. Pessary Therapy

The insertion of a vaginal pessary to support the uterus and vagina offers the least invasive solution to symptoms of pelvic organ **prolapse** (POP). Pessaries are manufactured in a number of shapes and sizes, and a **pessary** is selected and fitted based on lifestyle and symptoms. POP describes a condition in which the muscles and **fascia** that support the pelvic floor become damaged, affecting the bladder, uterus, vagina, small bowel, and/or rectum. This may lead to urinary symptoms including urinary incontinence or to fecal **incontinence**.

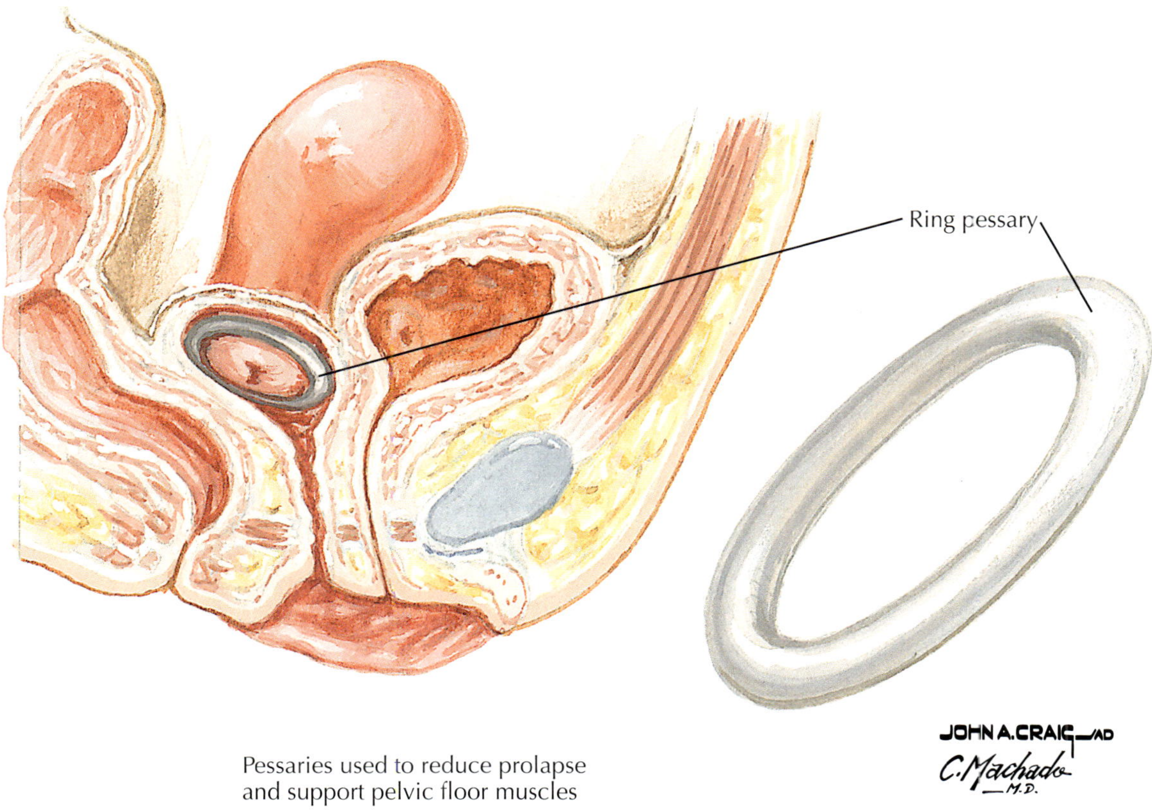

Pessaries used to reduce prolapse and support pelvic floor muscles

Introduction

Coding Atlas

To treat some malignancies of the female genitalia, pelvic **irradiation** may be achieved using an **intracavitary** delivery device in a treatment known as **brachytherapy**. An irradiated object may be secured in the vagina or uterus so that the object delivers a constant dose of irradiation (code 57155). Another method for brachytherapy is the use of an **afterloading** device (code 57156). The device is secured in the vagina and then attached to an applicator that delivers a radiation source into the device. For **Heyman capsule** brachytherapy, see code 58346.

57150	**Irrigation** of vagina and/or application of medicament for treatment of bacterial, parasitic, or fungoid disease
⊙ **57155**	Insertion of uterine **tandem** and/or vaginal **ovoids** for clinical **brachytherapy**
57156	Insertion of a vaginal radiation **afterloading** apparatus for clinical brachytherapy
57160	Fitting and insertion of **pessary** or other intravaginal support device
57170	Diaphragm or **cervical cap** fitting with instructions
57180	Introduction of any hemostatic agent or pack for spontaneous or traumatic **nonobstetrical** vaginal **hemorrhage** (separate procedure)

FIGURE 8-5. Rectocele, Enterocele

Weakness in the pelvic floor and vaginal wall may cause the rectum or small intestines to bulge against the vaginal wall. In **rectocele**, the rectum **prolapses** and pushes against the **posterior** wall of the vagina and pelvic floor. Rectocele may cause difficulties with bowel evacuation. **Enterocele** is a **herniation** in which a segment of small bowel drops into the **pouch of Douglas** and presses against the posterior wall of the vagina and the pelvic floor. Enteroceles may be asymptomatic or cause symptoms of vaginal discomfort and low back pain. Note: Tools, implants, and/or equipment depicted in the illustration may be outdated but the procedural approach is valid.

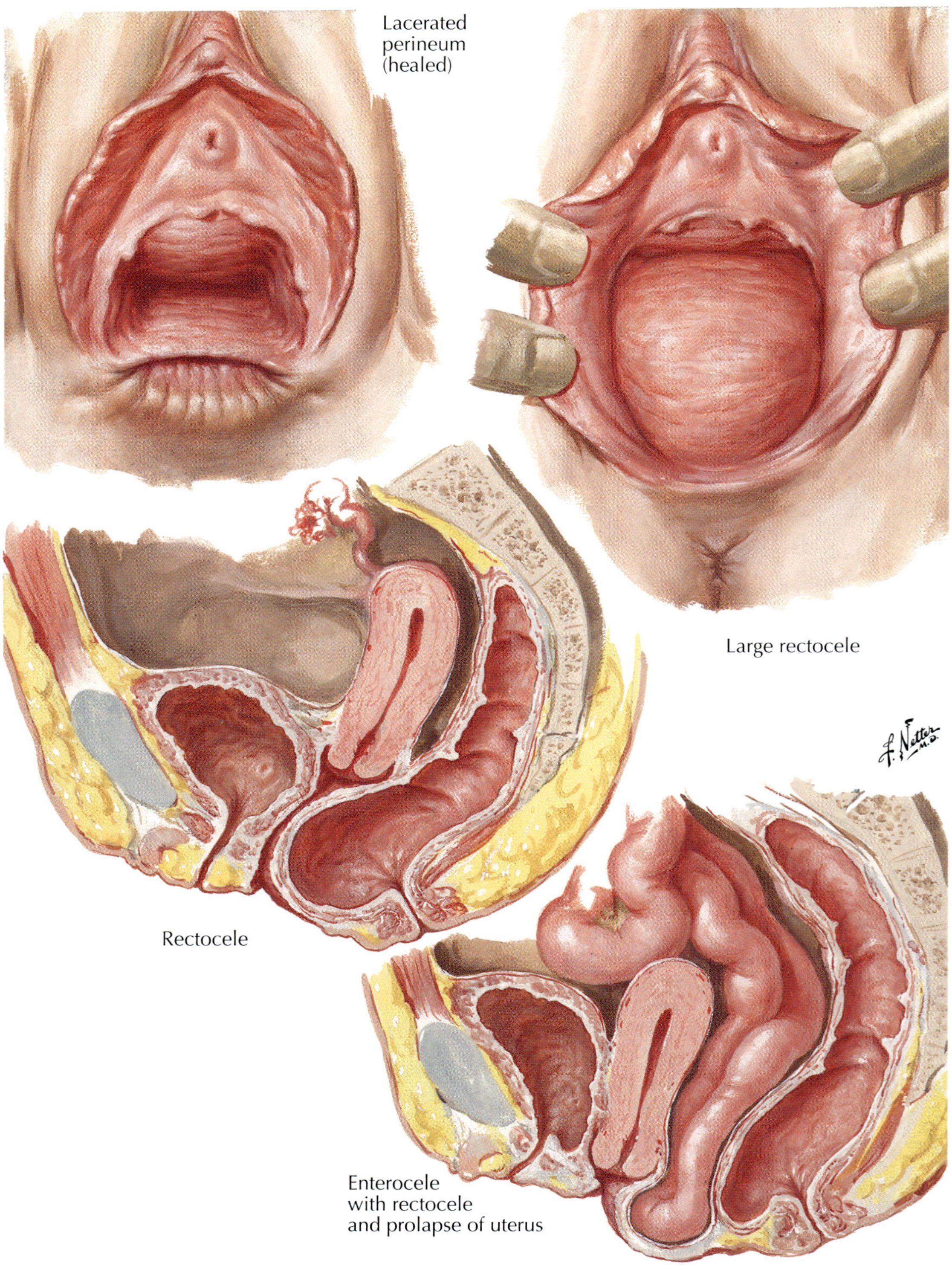

Repair

Coding Atlas

Colpopexy (vaginopexy, culpopexy, vaginofixation) corrects **prolapse** of the vagina. Colpopexy may also benefit a patient who has uterine prolapse (UP) since correcting the position of the vagina also affects the uterus. Vaginal prolapse is most commonly seen in women who have undergone a hysterectomy or as a result of menopause or childbirth. Colpopexy may be performed **transabdominally** or **transvaginally**.

57200 Colporrhaphy, suture of injury of vagina (nonobstetrical)

57210 Colpoperineorrhaphy, suture of injury of vagina and/or perineum (nonobstetrical)

57220 Plastic operation on urethral sphincter, vaginal approach (eg, Kelly urethral plication)

57230 Plastic repair of urethrocele

57240 Anterior colporrhaphy, repair of cystocele with or without repair of urethrocele

57250 Posterior colporrhaphy, repair of rectocele with or without perineorrhaphy

57260 Combined anteroposterior colporrhaphy;

57265 with enterocele repair

✚ **57267** Insertion of mesh or other prosthesis for repair of pelvic floor defect, each site (anterior, posterior compartment), vaginal approach (List separately in addition to code for primary procedure)

57268 Repair of enterocele, vaginal approach (separate procedure)

57270 Repair of enterocele, abdominal approach (separate procedure)

57280 Colpopexy, abdominal approach

57282 Colpopexy, vaginal; extra-peritoneal approach (sacrospinous, iliococcygeus)

57283 intra-peritoneal approach (uterosacral, levator myorrhaphy)

57284 Paravaginal defect repair (including repair of cystocele, if performed); open abdominal approach

57285 vaginal approach

57287 Removal or revision of sling for stress incontinence (eg, fascia or synthetic)

57288 Sling operation for stress incontinence (eg, fascia or synthetic)

57289 Pereyra procedure, including anterior colporrhaphy

57291 Construction of artificial vagina; without graft

57292 with graft

57295 Revision (including removal) of prosthetic vaginal graft; vaginal approach

57296 open abdominal approach

57300 Closure of rectovaginal fistula; vaginal or transanal approach

57305 abdominal approach

57307 abdominal approach, with concomitant colostomy

57308 transperineal approach, with perineal body reconstruction, with or without levator plication

57310 Closure of urethrovaginal fistula;

57311 with bulbocavernosus transplant

57320 Closure of vesicovaginal fistula; vaginal approach

57330 transvesical and vaginal approach

57335 Vaginoplasty for intersex state

Manipulation

Coding Atlas

A patient's psychological or physical condition sometimes requires the use of anesthesia services for minor pelvic procedures. Codes 57400-57415 are used to report these circumstances.

57400 Dilation of vagina under anesthesia (other than local)

57410 Pelvic examination under anesthesia (other than local)

57415 Removal of impacted vaginal foreign body (separate procedure) under anesthesia (other than local)

FIGURE 8-6. Cystocele, Urethrocele

Weakness in the pelvic floor and vaginal wall may cause the bladder or urethra to bulge against the vaginal wall. In **cystocele**, the bladder presses against the **anterior** wall of the vagina. In **urethrocele**, the urethra prolapses against the **distal** anterior vaginal wall. In **cystourethrocele**, both a cystocele and urethrocele are present. Note: Tools, implants, and/or equipment depicted in the illustration may be outdated but the procedural approach is valid.

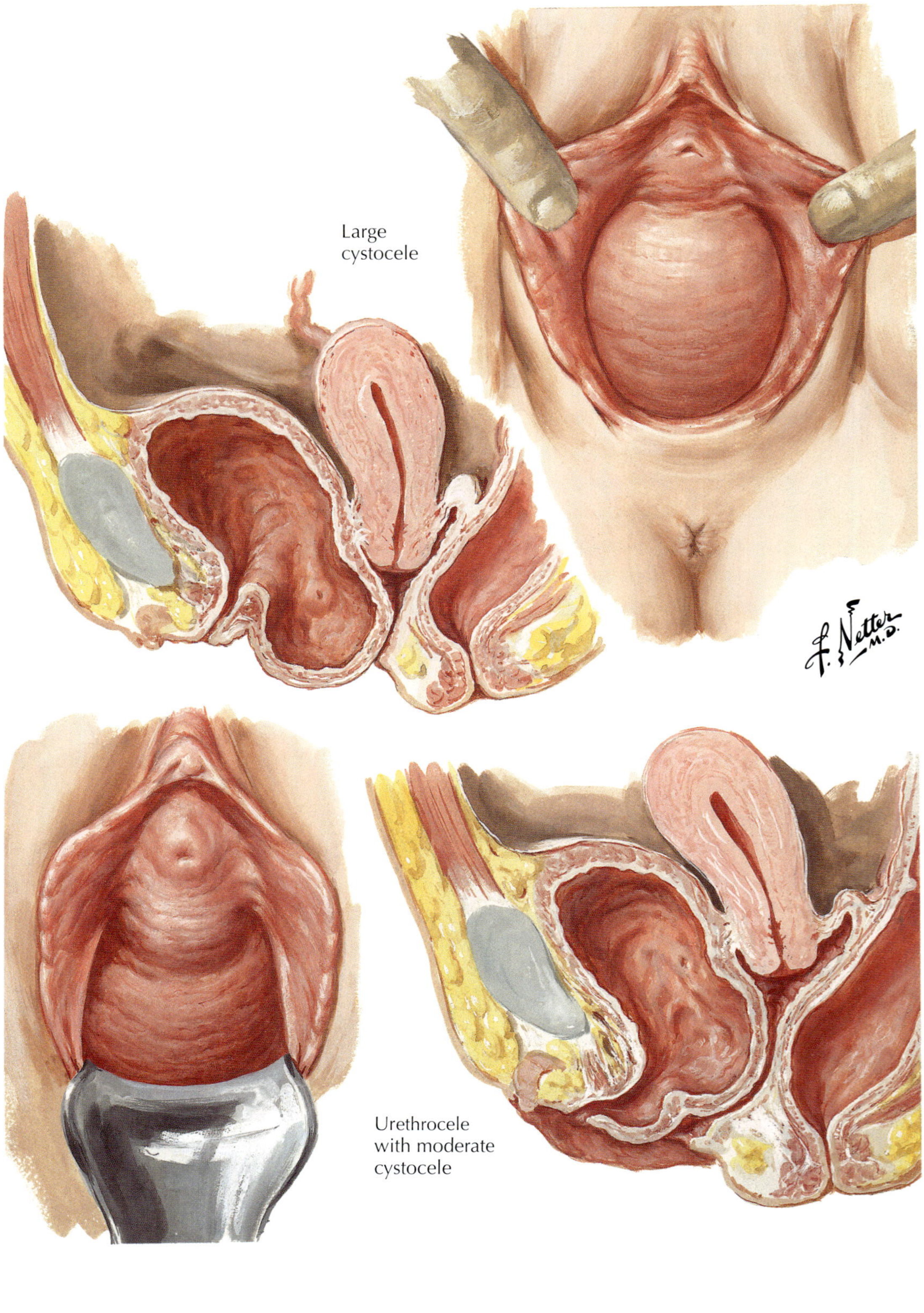

FIGURE 8-7. Colposcopy

Colposcopy involves the use of a light and low-powered microscope to examine the vulva, vagina, and/or cervix. Colposcopy is performed with the patient's feet in stirrups and the colposcope positioned over the vulva. Tissue being examined may be painted with 5% acetic acid stain to highlight lesions associated with the human papilloma virus (HPV) or vulvar/vaginal/cervical intraepithelial neoplasia (VIN, VAIN, CIN). When the vagina or cervix is being examined, a **speculum** is inserted into the vagina. Note: Tools, implants, and/or equipment depicted in the illustration may be outdated but the procedural approach is valid.

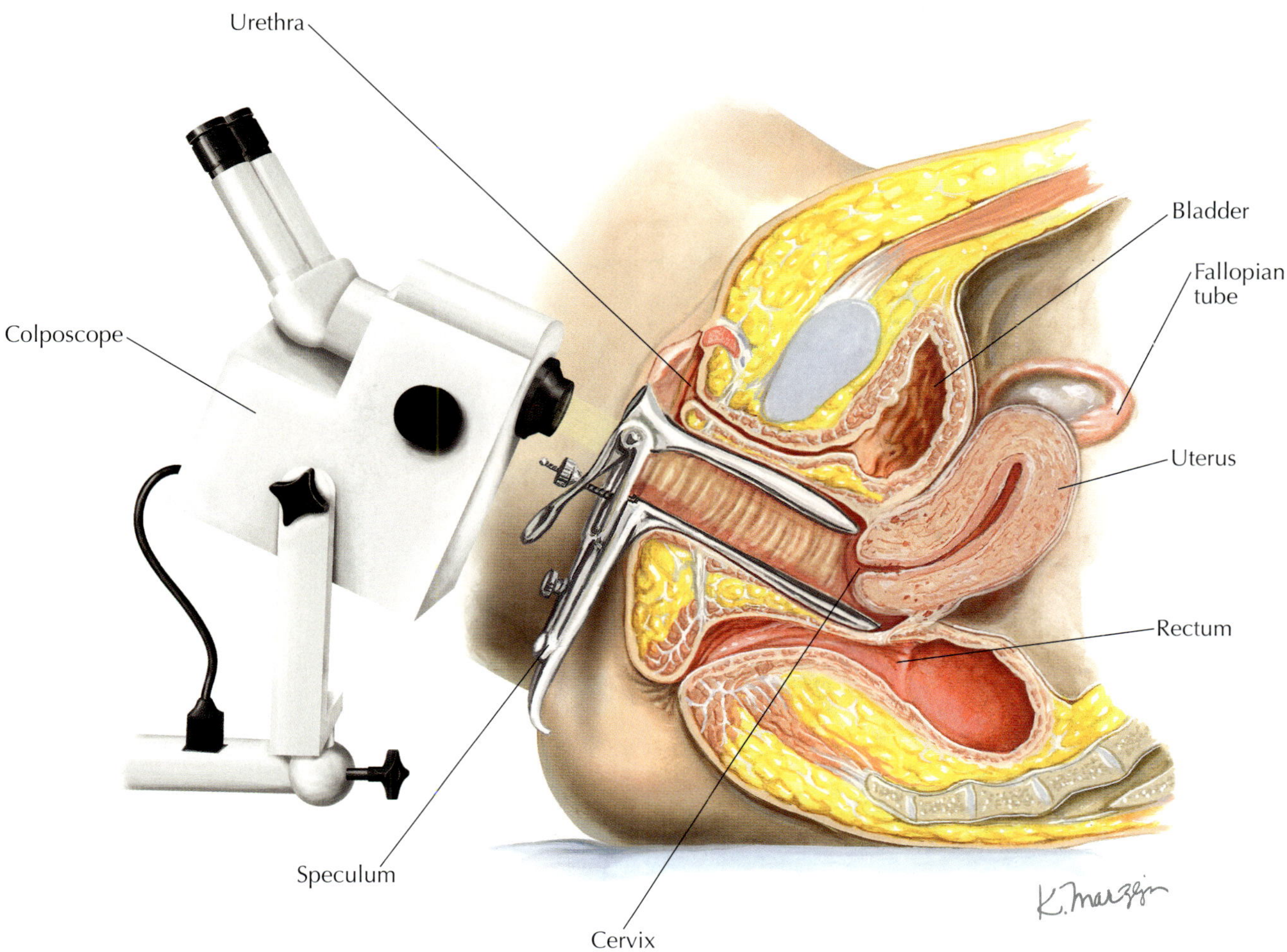

Endoscopy/Laparoscopy

Coding Atlas

Laparoscopy is a technique developed to reduce risk and recovery time during abdominal or pelvic surgery. Several small abdominal incisions act as portals for a tiny video camera (laparoscope), light source, and surgical tools. The physician manipulates the surgical tools while viewing the surgical site on a video display screen or through an eyepiece. To enhance visibility, the abdomen or pelvis may be filled with gas (**pneumoperitoneum**) during the procedure.

57420 Colposcopy of the entire vagina, with cervix if present;

57421 with biopsy(s) of vagina/cervix

57423 Paravaginal defect repair (including repair of cystocele, if performed), laparoscopic approach

57425 Laparoscopy, surgical, colpopexy (suspension of vaginal apex)

57426 Revision (including removal) of prosthetic vaginal graft, laparoscopic approach

FIGURE 8-8. The Internal Female Genitalia: Sagittal View

The cervix separates the uterine body from the vagina. A midline cervical canal (os) allows the passage of semen into the uterus, as well as the passage of the products of menses and of conception from the uterus into the vagina. The **distal** canal (external os) opens into the vagina, and the **proximal** canal (internal os) opens into the endometrial cavity of the uterus. The tissue lining the canal is called the endocervix. The portion of the cervix that extends into the vagina is called the ectocervix.

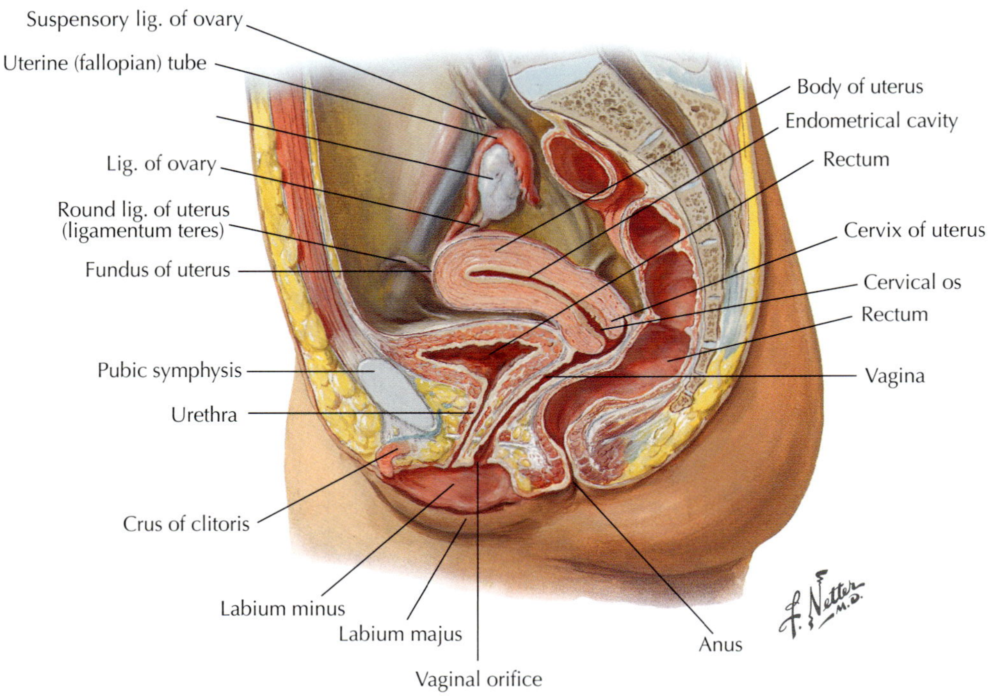

Cervix Uteri

Endoscopy

Coding Atlas

In cervical conization, a cone-shaped portion of the cervix, including the external os, is excised, usually to treat **dysplasia**. This may be performed as a loop electrical excision procedure (LEEP), also called a large loop excision of the transformation zone (LLETZ), which is reported with CPT code 57461. In LEEP, tissue is removed **en bloc**. Other techniques for conization are reported using CPT codes 57520 and 57522.

57452 Colposcopy of the cervix including upper/adjacent vagina;

57454 with biopsy(s) of the cervix and endocervical curettage

57455 with biopsy(s) of the cervix

57456 with endocervical curettage

57460 with loop electrode biopsy(s) of the cervix

57461 with loop electrode conization of the cervix

Excision

Coding Atlas

Trachelectomy (cervicectomy) describes the surgical excision of the cervix uteri. Excision of the cervical stump describes the surgical removal of all or a portion of the cervix that remains following a previous subtotal hysterectomy.

57500 Biopsy of cervix, single or multiple, or local excision of lesion, with or without fulguration (separate procedure)

57505 Endocervical curettage (not done as part of a dilation and curettage)

57510 Cautery of cervix; electro or thermal

57511 cryocautery, initial or repeat

57513 laser ablation

57520 Conization of cervix, with or without fulguration, with or without dilation and curettage, with or without repair; cold knife or laser

57522 loop electrode excision

57530 Trachelectomy (cervicectomy), amputation of cervix (separate procedure)

57531 Radical trachelectomy, with bilateral total pelvic lymphadenectomy and para-aortic lymph node sampling biopsy, with or without removal of tube(s), with or without removal of ovary(s)

57540 Excision of cervical stump, abdominal approach;

57545 with pelvic floor repair

57550 Excision of cervical stump, vaginal approach;

57555 with anterior and/or posterior repair

57556 with repair of enterocele

57558 Dilation and curettage of cervical stump

Repair

Coding Atlas

A nonobstetrical cerclage of the cervix uteri is performed using a vaginal approach and is performed in order to prepare a patient's historically incompetent cervix for a future pregnancy. Cervical cerclage on a patient who is already pregnant would be reported with CPT code 59320 for a vaginal approach or 59325 for an abdominal approach.

57700 Cerclage of uterine cervix, nonobstetrical

57720 Trachelorrhaphy, plastic repair of uterine cervix, vaginal approach

Manipulation

57800 Dilation of cervical canal, instrumental (separate procedure)

Corpus Uteri

Excision

Coding Atlas

Total abdominal hysterectomy describes the removal of the uterus and cervix through an abdominal incision. Supracervical or subtotal hysterectomy describes the removal of most of the uterus, with the sparing of the cervix (cervical stump), using an abdominal approach. Radical hysterectomy is more extensive and includes lymphadenectomy as well as excision of mesentery associated with the uterus in addition to other surrounding tissue. In vaginal hysterectomy, the cervix and uterus are removed through the vagina. Repairs related to pelvic organ prolapse (POP) may be performed with any hysterectomy. For some cases, combination codes are used to report both aspects.

58100 Endometrial sampling (biopsy) with or without endocervical sampling (biopsy), without cervical dilation, any method (separate procedure)

✚ 58110 Endometrial sampling (biopsy) performed in conjunction with colposcopy (List separately in addition to code for primary procedure)

58120 Dilation and curettage, diagnostic and/or therapeutic (nonobstetrical)

58140 Myomectomy, excision of fibroid tumor(s) of uterus, 1 to 4 intramural myoma(s) with total weight of 250 g or less and/or removal of surface myomas; abdominal approach

58145 vaginal approach

58146 Myomectomy, excision of fibroid tumor(s) of uterus, 5 or more intramural myomas and/or intramural myomas with total weight greater than 250 g, abdominal approach

Hysterectomy Procedures

58150 Total abdominal hysterectomy (corpus and cervix), with or without removal of tube(s), with or without removal of ovary(s);

58152 with colpo-urethrocystopexy (eg, Marshall-Marchetti-Krantz, Burch)

58180 Supracervical abdominal hysterectomy (subtotal hysterectomy), with or without removal of tube(s), with or without removal of ovary(s)

58200 Total abdominal hysterectomy, including partial vaginectomy, with para-aortic and pelvic lymph node sampling, with or without removal of tube(s), with or without removal of ovary(s)

FIGURE 8-9. The Uterus, Fallopian Tubes, and Ovaries

The uterus, fallopian tubes, and ovaries lie between layers mesometrium, mesosalpinx, and mesovarium, which are the **mesentery** layers that help secure the uterus, tubes, and ovaries to the walls and floor of the pelvis. The mesometrium, mesosalpinx, and mesovarian are essentially a continuous fold of peritoneum and together may be referred to as the broad ligament of the uterus.

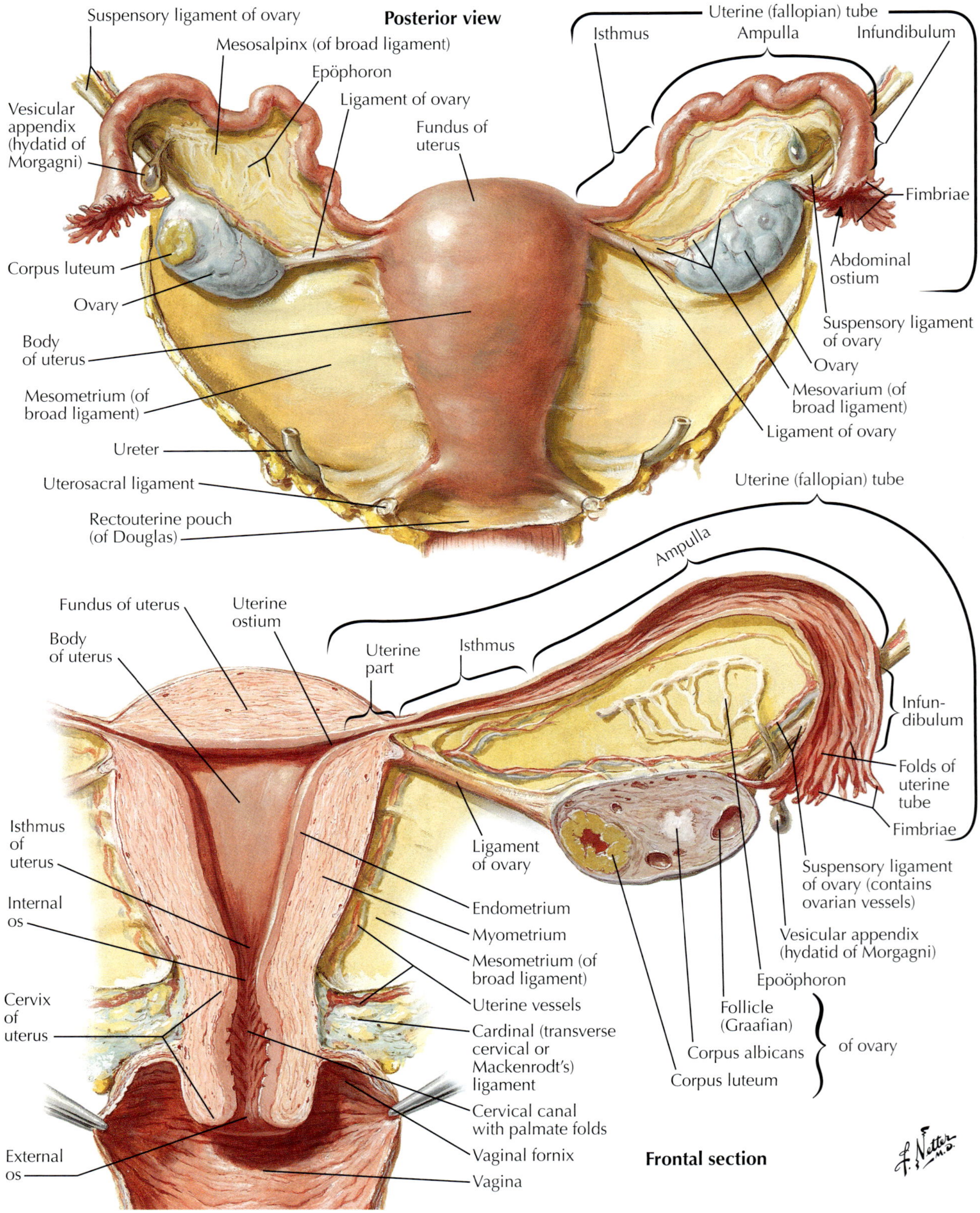

FIGURE 8-10. Uterine Leiomyomas

Uterine myomas (leiomyomas) are **benign** neoplasms that can arise from the smooth muscle (myometrium) of the uterus. They may be referred to as uterine **fibroids**. Myomas can develop on the surface of the uterine lining (**submucosal**), within the uterine muscle wall (**intramural** or **interstitial**), or on the outer surface of the uterus (**subserosal**). Procedures for surgical excision of leiomyomas are based on the approach (abdominal, vaginal, or laparoscopic), the site (intramural or submucosal/subserosal), and, when intramural, the number and total weight of tumors excised.

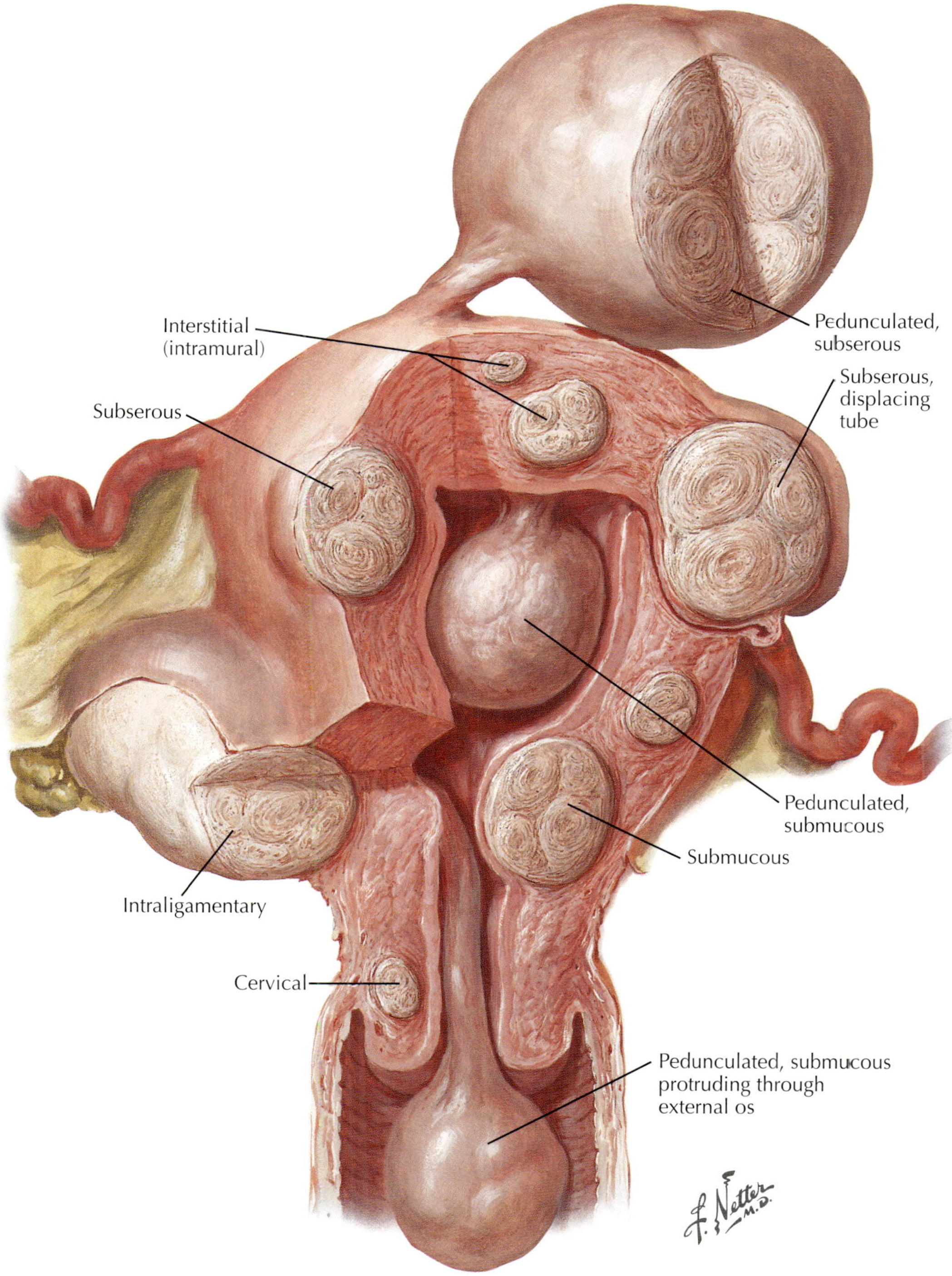

58210 Radical abdominal hysterectomy, with bilateral total pelvic lymphadenectomy and para-aortic lymph node sampling (biopsy), with or without removal of tube(s), with or without removal of ovary(s)

58240 Pelvic exenteration for gynecologic malignancy, with total abdominal hysterectomy or cervicectomy, with or without removal of tube(s), with or without removal of ovary(s), with removal of bladder and ureteral transplantations, and/or abdominoperineal resection of rectum and colon and colostomy, or any combination thereof

58260 Vaginal hysterectomy, for uterus 250 g or less;

58262 with removal of tube(s), and/or ovary(s)

58263 with removal of tube(s), and/or ovary(s), with repair of enterocele

58267 with colpo-urethrocystopexy (Marshall-Marchetti-Krantz type, Pereyra type) with or without endoscopic control

58270 with repair of enterocele

58275 Vaginal hysterectomy, with total or partial vaginectomy;

58280 with repair of enterocele

58285 Vaginal hysterectomy, radical (Schauta type operation)

58290 Vaginal hysterectomy, for uterus greater than 250 g;

58291 with removal of tube(s) and/or ovary(s)

58292 with removal of tube(s) and/or ovary(s), with repair of enterocele

58293 with colpo-urethrocystopexy (Marshall-Marchetti-Krantz type, Pereyra type) with or without endoscopic control

58294 with repair of enterocele

Introduction

Coding Atlas

In **chromotubation**, a dyed sterile solution is pushed by syringe through the cervix and fallopian tubes in order to evaluate the patency of the fallopian tubes. A concurrent laparoscopy allows the physician to monitor the ends of the tubes for appearance of the dye. Spillage of dye indicates **patent** tubes. In this scenario, it would be appropriate to report the chromotubation with a diagnostic laparoscopy.

58300 Insertion of intrauterine device (IUD)

58301 Removal of intrauterine device (IUD)

58321 Artificial insemination; intra-cervical

58322 intra-uterine

58323 Sperm washing for artificial insemination

58340 Catheterization and introduction of saline or contrast material for saline infusion sonohysterography (SIS) or hysterosalpingography

58345 Transcervical introduction of fallopian tube catheter for diagnosis and/or re-establishing patency (any method), with or without hysterosalpingography

58346 Insertion of Heyman capsules for clinical brachytherapy

58350 Chromotubation of oviduct, including materials

58353 Endometrial ablation, thermal, without hysteroscopic guidance

58356 Endometrial cryoablation with ultrasonic guidance, including endometrial curettage, when performed

Repair

Coding Atlas

The round **ligaments** of the uterus extend from the sides of the uterus and curve upward and **laterally** to enter the inguinal canal and terminate in the tissue of the mons pubis. The sacrouterine (rectouterine) ligaments are a paired set of ligaments that arise from the base of the uterus and attach to the **anterior** aspect of the sacrum. Both sets of ligaments help fix the uterus in place.

58400 Uterine suspension, with or without shortening of round ligaments, with or without shortening of sacrouterine ligaments; (separate procedure)

58410 with presacral sympathectomy

58520 Hysterorrhaphy, repair of ruptured uterus (nonobstetrical)

58540 Hysteroplasty, repair of uterine anomaly (Strassman type)

Laparoscopy/Hysteroscopy

Coding Atlas

Laparoscopic hysterectomy procedures vary greatly, and codes have been created to describe these different circumstances. In some cases, a vaginal approach is used in combination with the laparoscopic approach. This method allows for **en bloc** removal of the uterus through the vagina. In a hysterectomy that is exclusively laparoscopic, the uterus must be **morcellated** before it can be removed through laparoscopy **portals**. The weight of the uterus plays a role in code assignment, as does whether the hysterectomy includes the entire uterus or spares the cervix (supracervical). It is also necessary to look for documentation as to whether the ovaries and fallopian tubes are excised. For open procedures, there is no coding distinction between a hysterectomy that includes removal of tubes and ovaries and one that does not. However, codes for laparoscopic hysterectomy differentiate between procedures with removal of **adnexa** and those without removal of adnexa.

58541 Laparoscopy, surgical, supracervical hysterectomy, for uterus 250 g or less;

58542 with removal of tube(s) and/or ovary(s)

58543 Laparoscopy, surgical, supracervical hysterectomy, for uterus greater than 250 g;

58544 with removal of tube(s) and/or ovary(s)

58545 Laparoscopy, surgical, myomectomy, excision; 1 to 4 intramural myomas with total weight of 250 g or less and/or removal of surface myomas

58546 5 or more intramural myomas and/or intramural myomas with total weight greater than 250 g

58548 Laparoscopy, surgical, with radical hysterectomy, with bilateral total pelvic lymphadenectomy and para-aortic lymph node sampling (biopsy), with removal of tube(s) and ovary(s), if performed

58550 Laparoscopy, surgical, with vaginal hysterectomy, for uterus 250 g or less;

58552 with removal of tube(s) and/or ovary(s)

58553 Laparoscopy, surgical, with vaginal hysterectomy, for uterus greater than 250 g;

58554 with removal of tube(s) and/or ovary(s)

58555 Hysteroscopy, diagnostic (separate procedure)

58558 Hysteroscopy, surgical; with sampling (biopsy) of endometrium and/or polypectomy, with or without D & C

58559 with lysis of intrauterine adhesions (any method)

58560 with division or resection of intrauterine septum (any method)

58561 with removal of leiomyomata

58562 with removal of impacted foreign body

58563 with endometrial ablation (eg, endometrial resection, electrosurgical ablation, thermoablation)

58565 with bilateral fallopian tube cannulation to induce occlusion by placement of permanent implants

58570 Laparoscopy, surgical, with total hysterectomy, for uterus 250 g or less;

58571 with removal of tube(s) and/or ovary(s)

58572 Laparoscopy, surgical, with total hysterectomy, for uterus greater than 250 g;

58573 with removal of tube(s) and/or ovary(s)

FIGURE 8-11. Hysteroscopy

A **hysteroscopy** allows the physician to view the interior surface of the uterus with a scope that enters through the vagina and cervical os. The scope contains a light source and may contain an eyepiece for **direct visualization** of the endometrial tissue or it may contain a camera that can broadcast the image on a video screen. In some cases, **media** is infused into the uterus to distend the endometrial cavity for panoramic viewing. In other cases, the scope may be in contact with the endometrium for maximum magnification of a targeted site. Note: Tools, implants, and/or equipment depicted in the illustration may be outdated but the procedural approach is valid.

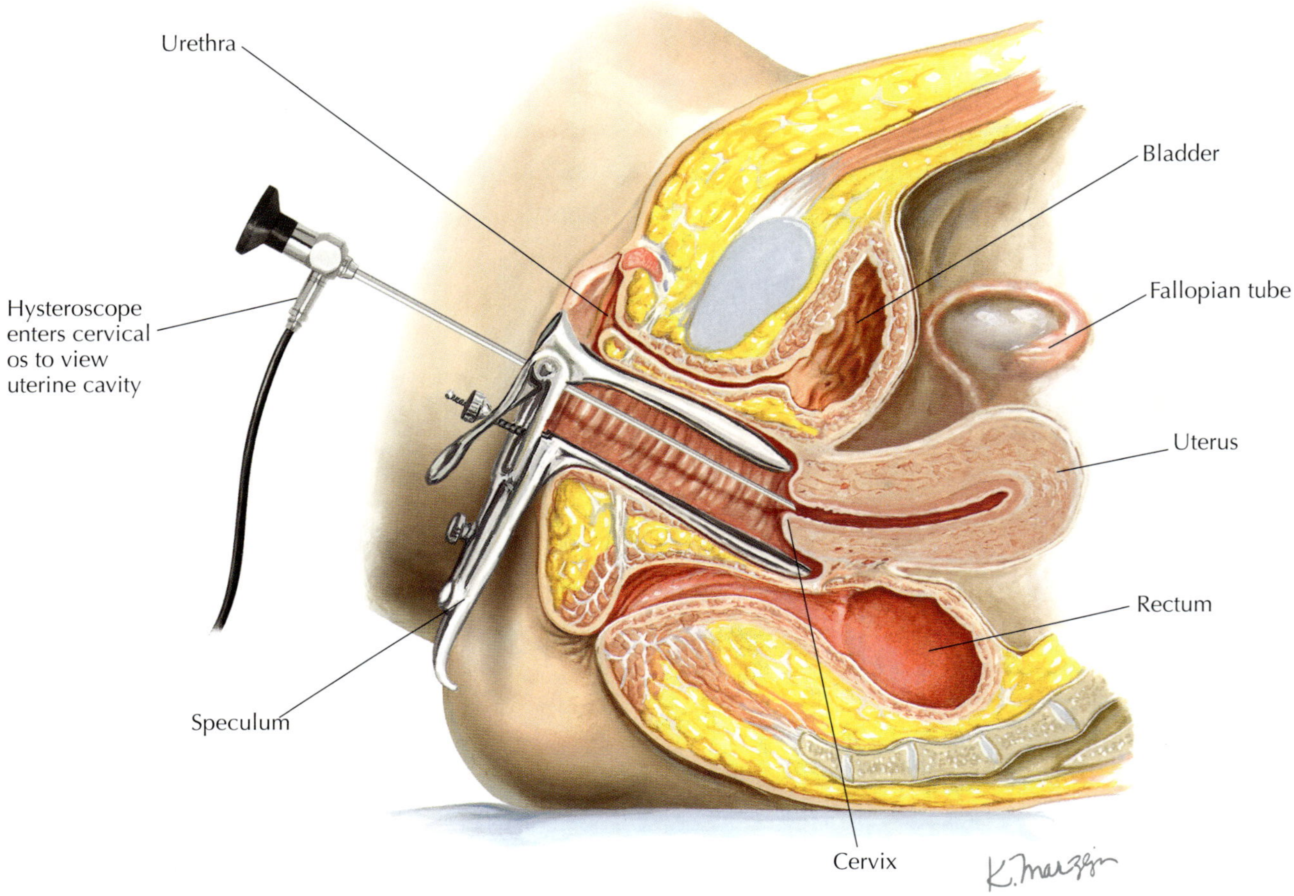

FIGURE 8-12. The Fallopian Tube

Each **bilateral** fallopian tube is between 10 cm and 12 cm in length and together are the **lumen** through which the ovum travels from the ovary to the uterus. **Fimbriae** of the fallopian tube are cilia that draw the **ovum** into the fallopian tube. The **infundibulum** of the fallopian tube is the funnel-shaped lumen that terminates at the fimbriae. The ampulla continues to narrow the lumen until it is very narrow at the **isthmus**, at which point it enters the uterine **fundus**.

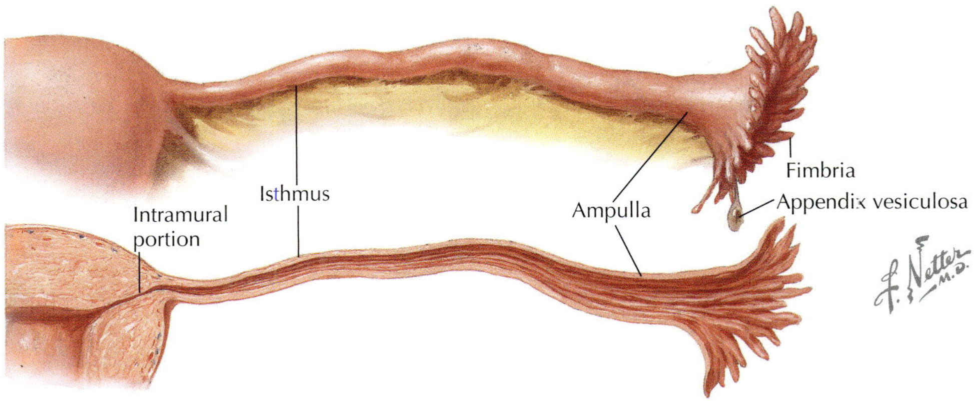

Oviduct/Ovary

Incision

Coding Atlas

Ligation or **occlusion** of the fallopian tubes is performed in order to prevent spermatozoa from reaching the ovum. The fallopian lumen is crimped or severed and each end is sealed, cutting off communication between the ovary and the uterus. Tubal ligation effectively sterilizes the patient without affecting her hormone secretions or requiring other medication or treatment. Codes 58600-58615 are used to report tubal ligation that is achieved with an open incision into the pelvis with **direct visualization** of the fallopian tube. Laparoscopic ligation, reported with codes from the range 58670-58671, is the most common approach for tubal ligation or occlusion in the United States.

58600 Ligation or transection of fallopian tube(s), abdominal or vaginal approach, unilateral or bilateral

58605 Ligation or transection of fallopian tube(s), abdominal or vaginal approach, postpartum, unilateral or bilateral, during same hospitalization (separate procedure)

✚ **58611** Ligation or transection of fallopian tube(s) when done at the time of cesarean delivery or intra-abdominal surgery (not a separate procedure) (List separately in addition to code for primary procedure)

58615 Occlusion of fallopian tube(s) by device (eg, band, clip, Falope ring) vaginal or suprapubic approach

Laparoscopy

Coding Atlas

Laparoscopic **salpingolysis** and **ovariolysis** involve endoscopic inspection and evaluation of the abdomen and pelvis, with **lysis** of **adhesions** of structures adjacent to the uterus (uterine **adnexa**).

58660 Laparoscopy, surgical; with lysis of adhesions (salpingolysis, ovariolysis) (separate procedure)

58661 with removal of adnexal structures (partial or total oophorectomy and/or salpingectomy)

58662 with fulguration or excision of lesions of the ovary, pelvic viscera, or peritoneal surface by any method

58670 with fulguration of oviducts (with or without transection)

58671 with occlusion of oviducts by device (eg, band, clip, or Falope ring)

58672 with fimbrioplasty

58673 with salpingostomy (salpingoneostomy)

Excision

Coding Atlas

Codes 58700 and 58720 are used to report excision of the fallopian tube and/or ovary in a patient who is not experiencing a current ectopic pregnancy. Surgical treatment of a tubal pregnancy that requires excision of the fallopian tube is reported with code 59120.

58700 Salpingectomy, complete or partial, unilateral or bilateral (separate procedure)

58720 Salpingo-oophorectomy, complete or partial, unilateral or bilateral (separate procedure)

Repair

Coding Atlas

Fimbrioplasty describes reconstructive surgery designed to correct infertility. It is done by restoring the function and patency of the fimbriae at the distal fallopian tube.

58740 Lysis of adhesions (salpingolysis, ovariolysis)

58750 Tubotubal anastomosis

58752 Tubouterine implantation

58760 Fimbrioplasty

58770 Salpingostomy (salpingoneostomy)

Ovary

Incision

Coding Atlas

An ovarian cyst is a sac filled with fluid or semiliquid material that arises from the ovary. Ovarian cysts are usually benign but may cause abdominal pain, interfere with bowel movements or urination, or cause symptoms related to menses. They may appear as a single cyst on one ovary or as multiple cysts bilaterally. Codes 58800-58822 are used to report open procedures in which the ovary is accessed transabdominally or transvaginally.

58800 Drainage of ovarian cyst(s), unilateral or bilateral (separate procedure); vaginal approach

58805 abdominal approach

58820 Drainage of ovarian abscess; vaginal approach, open

58822 abdominal approach

58825 Transposition, ovary(s)

Excision

Coding Atlas

While some open surgical procedures performed on patients with adnexal malignancies are intended to remove the entire malignancy (resection), others are performed to reduce the tumor load in the patient's pelvis and abdomen or to reduce tumor size and prevent or reverse obstructions that result from the tumors. Typically, the goal in these "debulking" procedures is to remove tumors that are larger than 1 centimeter.

58900 Biopsy of ovary, unilateral or bilateral (separate procedure)

58920 Wedge resection or bisection of ovary, unilateral or bilateral

58925 Ovarian cystectomy, unilateral or bilateral

58940 Oophorectomy, partial or total, unilateral or bilateral;

58943 for ovarian, tubal or primary peritoneal malignancy, with para-aortic and pelvic lymph node biopsies, peritoneal washings, peritoneal biopsies, diaphragmatic assessments, with or without salpingectomy(s), with or without omentectomy

58950 Resection (initial) of ovarian, tubal or primary peritoneal malignancy with bilateral salpingo-oophorectomy and omentectomy;

58951 with total abdominal hysterectomy, pelvic and limited para-aortic lymphadenectomy

58952 with radical dissection for debulking (ie, radical excision or destruction, intra-abdominal or retroperitoneal tumors)

58953 Bilateral salpingo-oophorectomy with omentectomy, total abdominal hysterectomy and radical dissection for debulking;

58954 with pelvic lymphadenectomy and limited para-aortic lymphadenectomy

58956 Bilateral salpingo-oophorectomy with total omentectomy, total abdominal hysterectomy for malignancy

58957 Resection (tumor debulking) of recurrent ovarian, tubal, primary peritoneal, uterine malignancy (intra-abdominal, retroperitoneal tumors), with omentectomy, if performed;

58958 with pelvic lymphadenectomy and limited para-aortic lymphadenectomy

58960 Laparotomy, for staging or restaging of ovarian, tubal, or primary peritoneal malignancy (second look), with or without omentectomy, peritoneal washing, biopsy of abdominal and pelvic peritoneum, diaphragmatic assessment with pelvic and limited para-aortic lymphadenectomy

FIGURE 8-13. Staging Laparotomy

In **staging** a **laparotomy** for gynecological cancer, the physician explores the abdominopelvic cavity and performs multiple random and targeted **biopsies** to determine the extent of the **malignancy**. A midline incision provides the physician with **direct visualization** of pelvic and abdominal organs. Ovarian cancer is often first diagnosed when it is in advanced stages, with omental caking, **ascites**, or a large pelvic mass. In some cases, a separately reportable total abdominal hysterectomy (TAH) with **bilateral** salpingectomy/oophorectomy (BSO) may be performed during the same encounter. Note: Tools, implants, and/or equipment depicted in the illustration may be outdated but the procedural approach is valid.

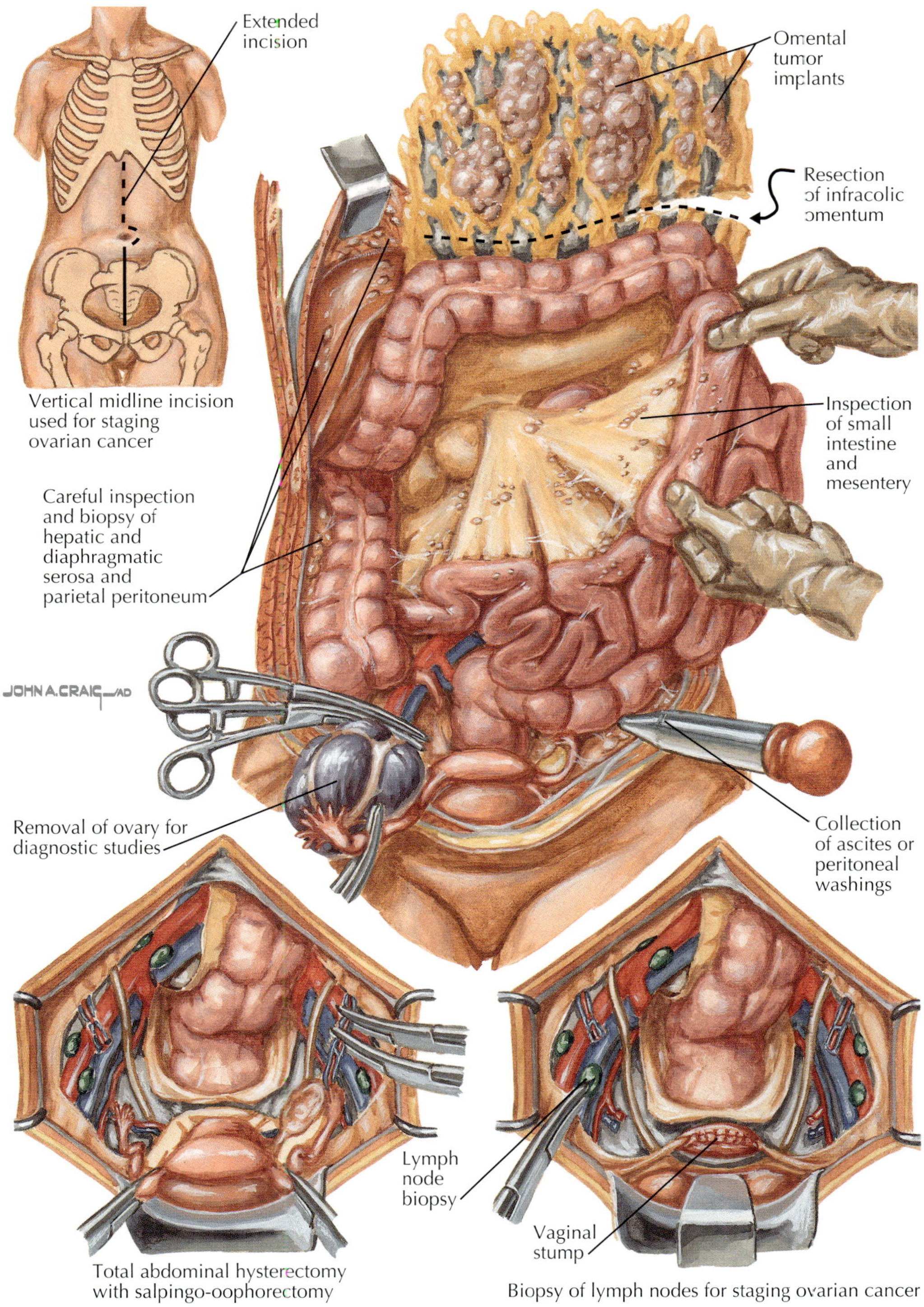

FIGURE 8-14. Gamete/Zygote Intrafallopian Transfer

Gamete intrafallopian transfer (GIFT) and zygote intrafallopian transfer (ZIFT) are two methods of assisted reproductive technology (ART). In GIFT, multiple ova are placed in a catheter with spermatozoa. The eggs and spermatozoa are injected into the fallopian tubes. In ZIFT, in vitro fertilization (IVF) occurs first, and the fertilized eggs are then placed in a catheter and injected into the uterus. Note: Tools, implants, and/or equipment depicted in the illustration may be outdated but the procedural approach is valid.

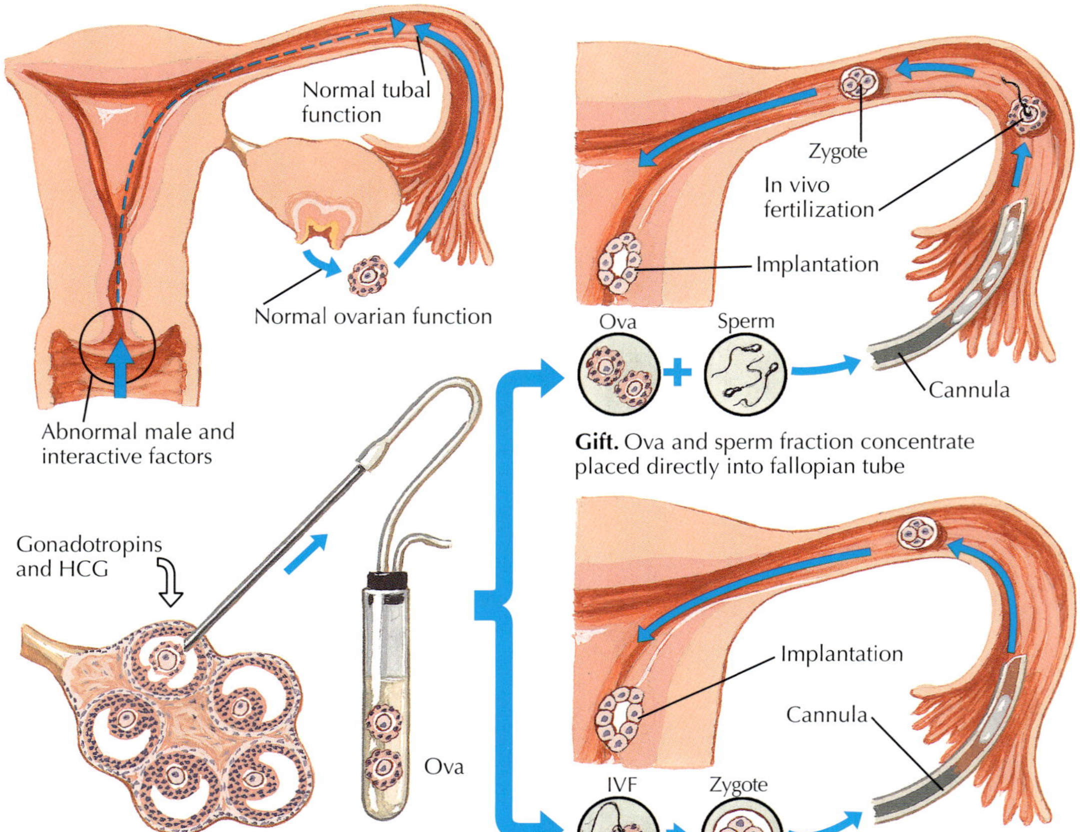

Superovulation induced with gonadotropins and HCG. Ova aspirated from mature follicles for intrafallopian transfer techniques.

Gift. Ova and sperm fraction concentrate placed directly into fallopian tube

Zift. Ova fertilized in itro (IVF); resulting zygotes placed directly into fallopian tube.

In Vitro Fertilization

Coding Atlas

The goal of oocyte retrieval (OCR) is to puncture the ovary in order to obtain a mature egg (ovum) that can be used in an in vitro fertilization. Any approach may be reported using code 58970. A common approach is transvaginal oocyte retrieval (TVOR), during which a needle is guided through the vaginal wall to the site of the follicle. Other approaches include laparoscopic and transabdominal aspiration. Multiple ova may be aspirated during a single encounter.

58970 Follicle puncture for oocyte retrieval, any method

58974 Embryo transfer, intrauterine

58976 Gamete, zygote, or embryo intrafallopian transfer, any method

FIGURE 8-15. Amniocentesis

In **amniocentesis**, amniotic fluid from the amniotic sac is removed using a needle that is inserted through the abdomen and into the uterus. Amniocentesis may be performed for **therapeutic** purposes in a patient with excessive amniotic fluid (**polyhydramnios**). More commonly, amniocentesis is performed for **diagnostic** purposes, as cells from the fluid can be examined to evaluate fetal lung maturity (FLM) and **alloimmunization**. Amniotic fluid can also be tested for genetic anomalies or signs of infection (**chorioamnionitis**). Note: Tools, implants, and/or equipment depicted in the illustration may be outdated but the procedural approach is valid.

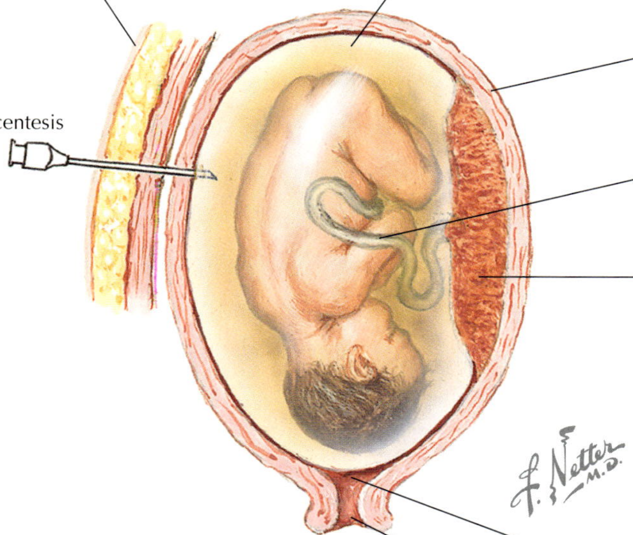

Maternity Care and Delivery

Antepartum and Fetal Invasive Services

Coding Atlas

Chorionic villus sampling (CVS) allows for first-trimester risk assessment and diagnosis of fetal chromosomal anomalies. In CVS, a sample of tissue is obtained from the placenta using a small **catheter** and a transabdominal or, less commonly, transcervical or transvaginal approach. In fetal umbilical cord occlusion (code 59072), the objective is to terminate the pregnancy.

59000 Amniocentesis; diagnostic

59001 therapeutic amniotic fluid reduction (includes ultrasound guidance)

59012 Cordocentesis (intrauterine), any method

59015 Chorionic villus sampling, any method

59020 Fetal contraction stress test

59025 Fetal non-stress test

59030 Fetal scalp blood sampling

59050 Fetal monitoring during labor by consulting physician (ie, non-attending physician) with written report; supervision and interpretation

59051 interpretation only

59070 Transabdominal amnioinfusion, including ultrasound guidance

59072 Fetal umbilical cord occlusion, including ultrasound guidance

FIGURE 8-16. Fetal Contraction Stress Test

During the third trimester of a pregnancy, assessment of fetal well-being may be appropriate. In a contraction stress test (CST), the fetal heart rate's response to contractions is monitored via **ultrasonography** or electrodes. The contractions are induced with **oxytocin** and measured and recorded on a **tocodynamometer** (TOCO). Stressors including uteroplacental insufficiency, cord compression, or **hypoxia** will produce measurable results in the fetal heart rate and contribute to the care plan for delivery. Note: Tools, implants, and/or equipment depicted in the illustration may be outdated but the procedural approach is valid.

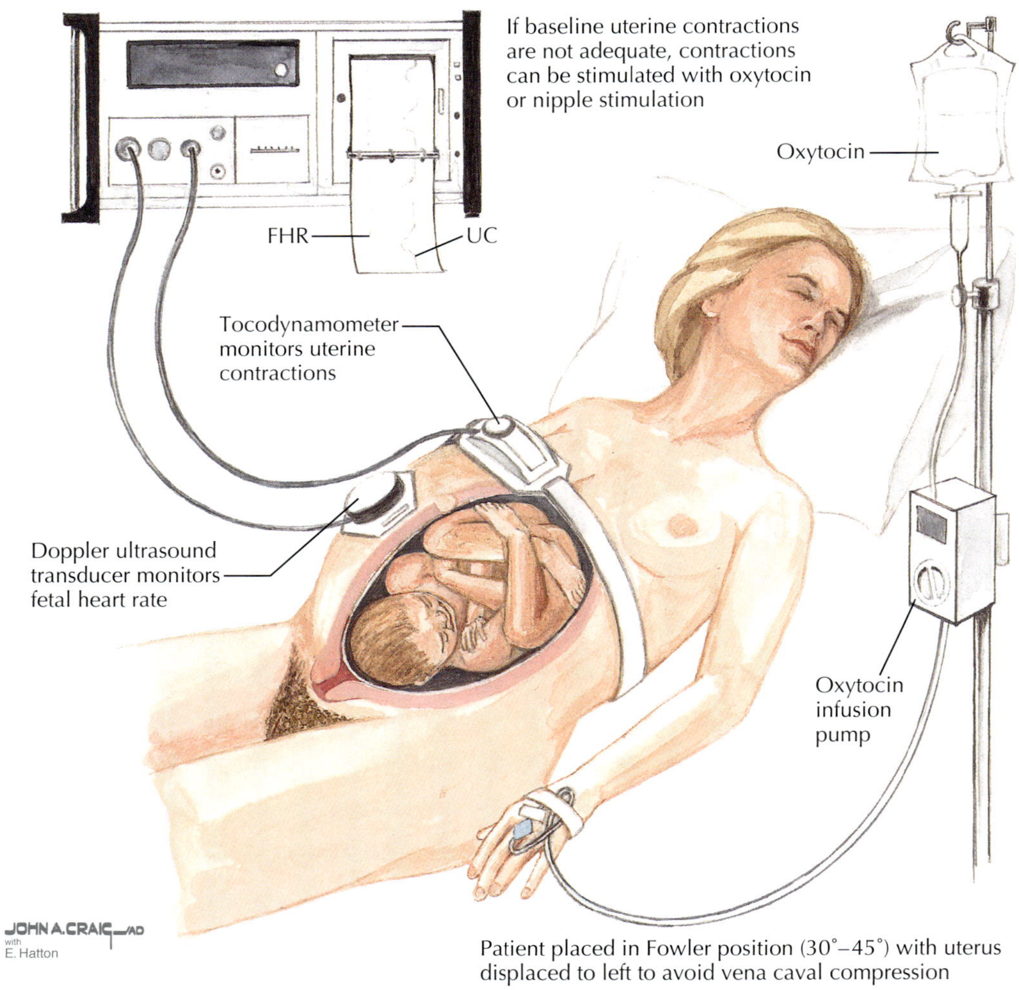

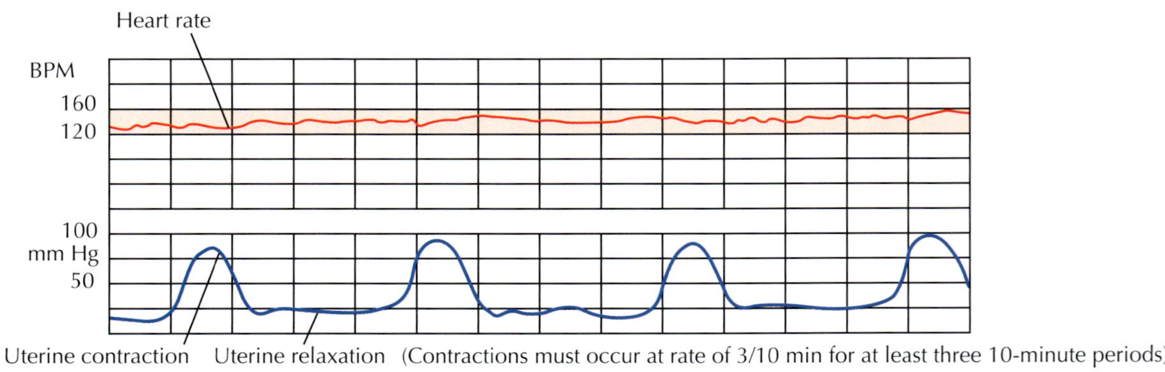

Portion of a "normal" (negative) contraction stress test exhibiting absence of heart rate decelerations following uterine contractions BPM, beats per minute; FHR, fetal heart rate; UC, uterine contractions.

FIGURE 8-17. Fetal Nonstress Test

Fetal nonstress tests (NSTs) are **noninvasive** procedures for evaluating the health of the fetus. The fetal heart rate is monitored via **ultrasonography** or electrodes placed on the mother's abdomen, and a **tocodynamometer** (TOCO) records any uterine contractions. The mother may also press a button to indicate when the fetus is moving. The impact of movement or contractions on the fetal heart rate is evaluated. An NST is a component of the **fetal biophysical profile** (BPP). Note: Tools, implants, and/or equipment depicted in the illustration may be outdated but the procedural approach is valid.

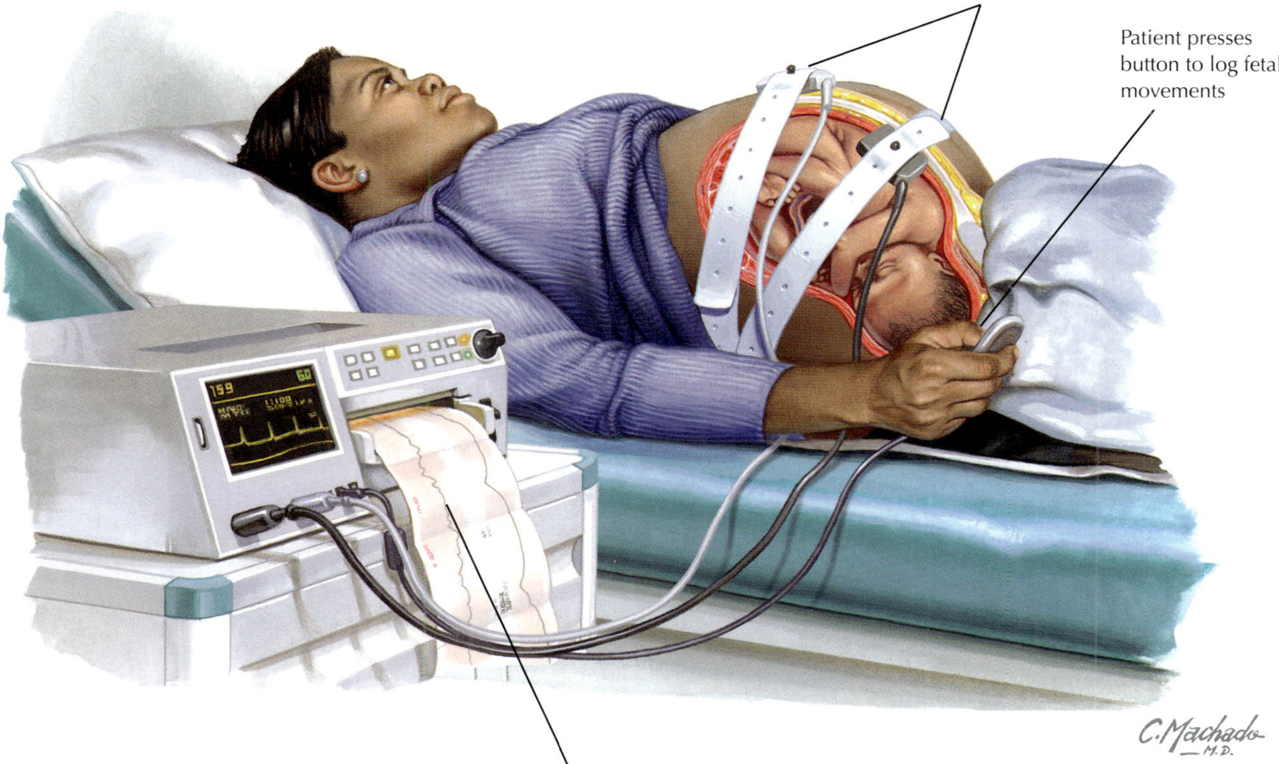

59074 Fetal fluid drainage (eg, vesicocentesis, thoracocentesis, paracentesis), including ultrasound guidance

59076 Fetal shunt placement, including ultrasound guidance

Excision

Coding Atlas

A hydatidiform mole is a gestational trophoblastic disease (GTD), meaning it originates in the placenta. In hysterotomy, the mole is excised through an abdominal incision into the uterus. If the hydatidiform mole is removed using curettage and a vaginal approach, code 59870 is reported.

59100 Hysterotomy, abdominal (eg, for hydatidiform mole, abortion)

59120 Surgical treatment of ectopic pregnancy; tubal or ovarian, requiring salpingectomy and/or oophorectomy, abdominal or vaginal approach

59121 tubal or ovarian, without salpingectomy and/or oophorectomy

59130 abdominal pregnancy

59135 interstitial, uterine pregnancy requiring total hysterectomy

59136 interstitial, uterine pregnancy with partial resection of uterus

59140 cervical, with evacuation

59150 Laparoscopic treatment of ectopic pregnancy; without salpingectomy and/or oophorectomy

59151 with salpingectomy and/or oophorectomy

59160 Curettage, postpartum

Introduction

59200 Insertion of cervical dilator (eg, laminaria, prostaglandin) (separate procedure)

Repair

Coding Atlas

An episiotomy is a surgical incision that begins at the introitus and advances posteriorly into the perineum as prophylaxis against laceration during the birthing process. Repair of an episiotomy or of a vaginal laceration is considered inherent to the obstetrical care package. In some instances, delivery is unattended and the patient seeks medical care after giving birth. In other instances, the physician who delivers the infant is unavailable for the repair of the perineum. In these situations, the repair of the episiotomy/laceration would be reported with CPT code 59300.

59300 Episiotomy or vaginal repair, by other than attending

59320 Cerclage of cervix, during pregnancy; vaginal

59325 abdominal

59350 Hysterorrhaphy of ruptured uterus

FIGURE 8-18. Ectopic Pregnancy

An **ectopic** pregnancy occurs when the fertilized **ova** fails to follow the normal pathway to implantation in the uterine endometrium and instead becomes established somewhere else in the abdomen or pelvis. The most common site for an ectopic pregnancy is the fallopian tube. A tubal pregnancy may be surgically treated with incision into the fallopian tube to remove the pregnancy tissue (**salpingotomy**) or with excision of the tube (**salpingectomy**) when the tube has ruptured or is otherwise not able to be repaired. **Laparoscopic** treatment of an ectopic pregnancy is reported with codes 59150 and 59151.

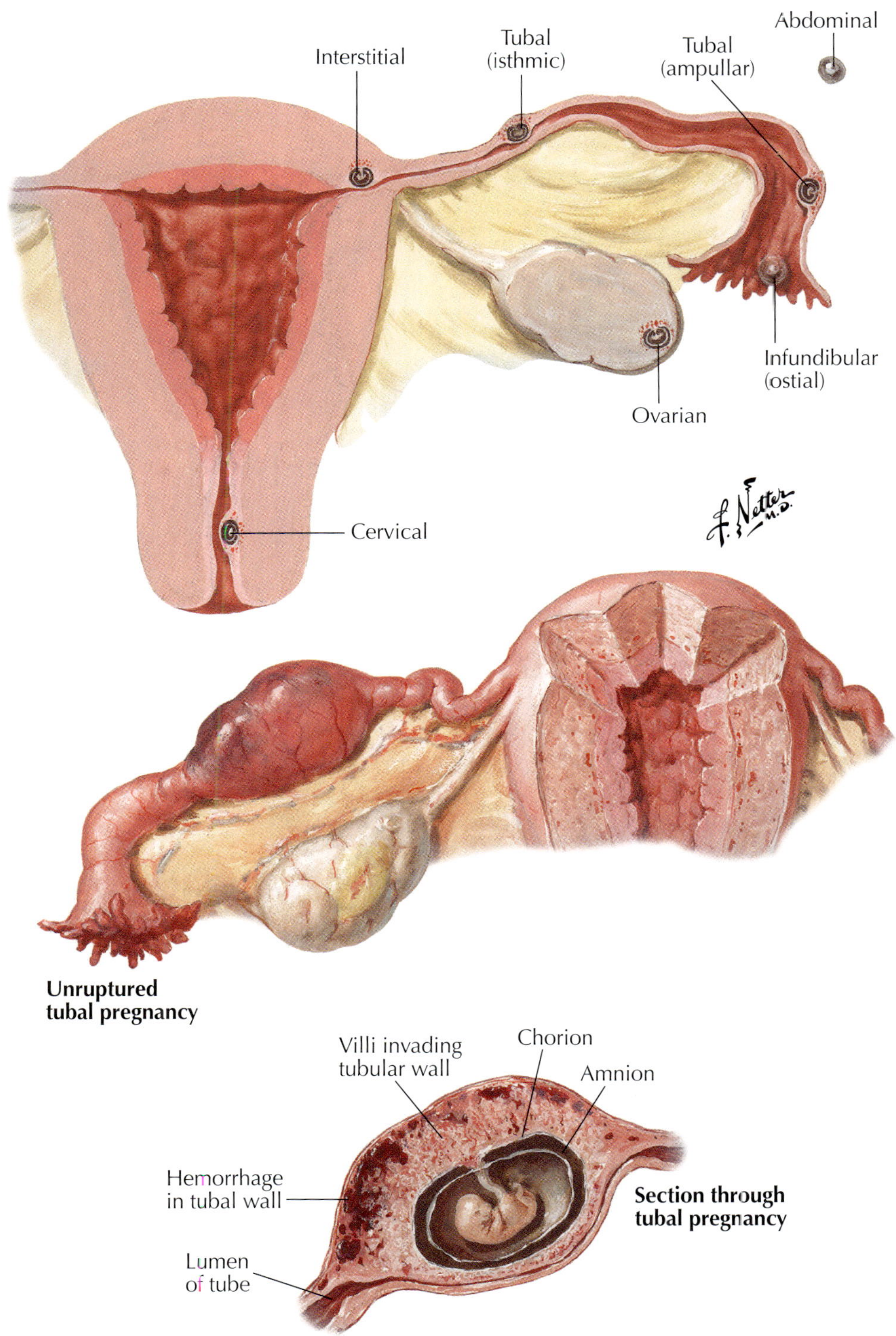

FIGURE 8-19. Cerclage

Cerclage is performed to prevent or delay premature rupture of membranes (PROM) or premature labor in a patient with a history of miscarriage or preterm labor. It may be performed transvaginally or transabdominally. In transvaginal cerclage, a McDonald or Shiradkor procedure is performed. In the McDonald cerclage, shown in Figure 8-19, a suture is cinched down tightly to close the cervix. In Shiradkor cerclage, fascia excised from the thigh is used to close off the internal os. Note: Tools, implants, and/or equipment depicted in the illustration may be outdated but the procedural approach is valid.

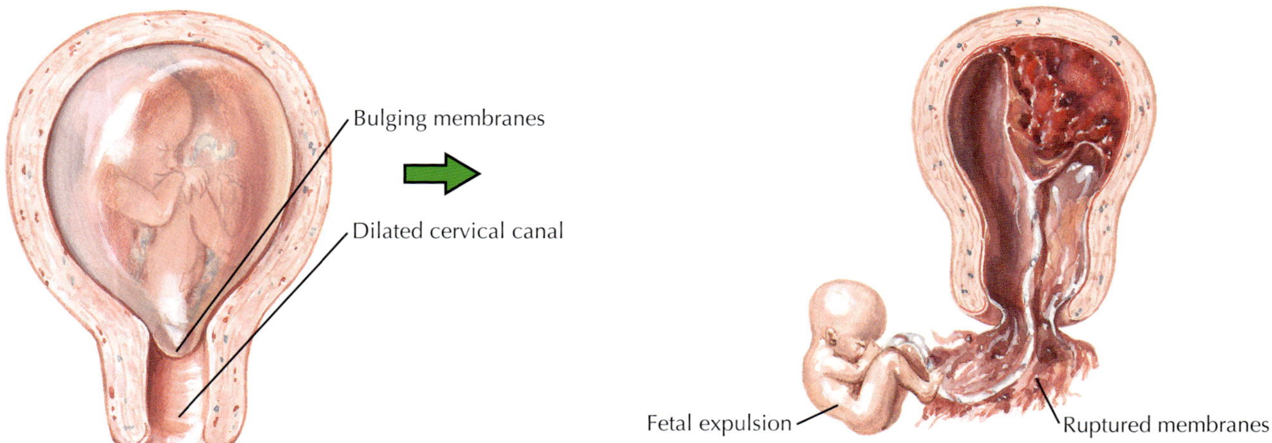

Cervical incompetence becomes manifest in second trimester as dilation of cervical canal

If left untreated, the dilated cervical canal may result in rupture of membranes and/or fetal expulsion.

Surgical Management of Cervical Incompetence (Cerclage)

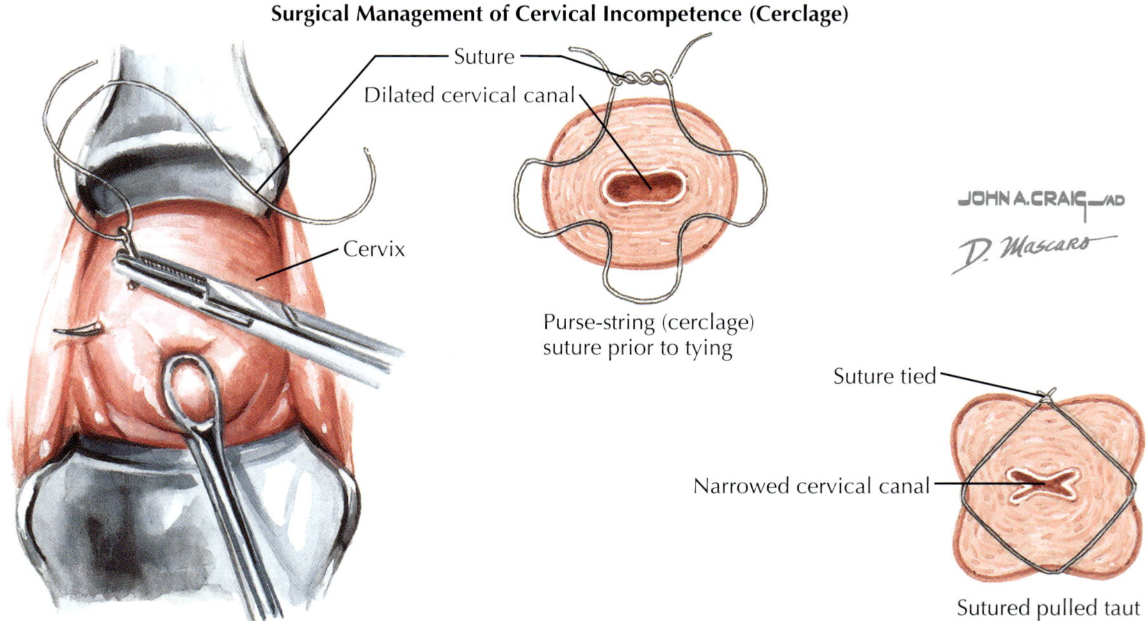

Purse-string (cerclage) suture prior to tying

Nonabsorbable purse-string suture placed around cervix at level of internal os

Sutured pulled taut and tied, narrowing cervical canal.

Vaginal Delivery, Antepartum and Postpartum Care

Coding Atlas

Services normally included in routine **antepartum** care include the initial prenatal history and physical followed by monthly exams with recordings of weight, blood pressure, fetal heart tone, and routine urinalysis until the patient reaches 28 weeks. At that point, the normal care increases to visits every other week, until 36 weeks, at which time the visits become weekly. If additional services are performed during the antepartum period, they should be coded separately. Delivery services include admission to the hospital, history and physical, management of uncomplicated labor, and vaginal delivery.

59400 Routine obstetric care including **antepartum** care, vaginal delivery (with or without episiotomy, and/or forceps) and **postpartum** care

59409 Vaginal delivery only (with or without **episiotomy** and/or **forceps**);

59410 including postpartum care

59412 **External cephalic version**, with or without **tocolysis**

59414 Delivery of placenta (separate procedure)

59425 Antepartum care only; 4-6 visits

59426 7 or more visits

59430 Postpartum care only (separate procedure)

Cesarean Delivery

Coding Atlas

If multiple neonates are delivered by **cesarean** birth, the appropriate code for the cesarean delivery should be reported only once because only one delivery was performed. The global package (code 59510) is reported when a physician from a solo practice or the same physician group practice provides the **antepartum** care, delivery, and **postpartum** care.

59510 Routine obstetric care including **antepartum** care, **cesarean** delivery, and **postpartum** care

59514 Cesarean delivery only;

59515 including postpartum care

✚ 59525 Subtotal or total **hysterectomy** after cesarean delivery (List separately in addition to code for primary procedure)

Delivery After Previous Cesarean Delivery

Coding Atlas

Because a previous **cesarean** birth carries a small risk of uterine rupture into a subsequent pregnancy, patients who have had a cesarean delivery are carefully monitored. Vaginal birth after cesarean (VBAC) or cesarean delivery may result from trial of labor after a cesarean birth (TOLAC). The global package is reported when a physician from a solo practice or the same physician group practice provides the antepartum care, delivery, and postpartum care.

59610 Routine obstetric care including **antepartum** care, vaginal delivery (with or without episiotomy, and/or forceps) and **postpartum** care, after previous **cesarean** delivery

59612 Vaginal delivery only, after previous cesarean delivery (with or without episiotomy and/or forceps);

59614 including postpartum care

59618 Routine obstetric care including antepartum care, cesarean delivery, and postpartum care, following attempted vaginal delivery after previous cesarean delivery

59620 Cesarean delivery only, following attempted vaginal delivery after previous cesarean delivery;

59622 including postpartum care

FIGURE 8-20. Normal Vaginal Birth

The second stage of labor culminates with delivery of the neonate. The following six movements occur during this second stage:

1. The head engages in the pelvis.
2. Flexion of the head puts the occiput in presenting position.
3. The neonate descends into the pelvis.
4. The vertex rotates to maneuver past the lateral ischial spines.
5. The head extends to pass beneath the maternal symphysis.
6. The head emerges and rotates to accommodate shoulder delivery.

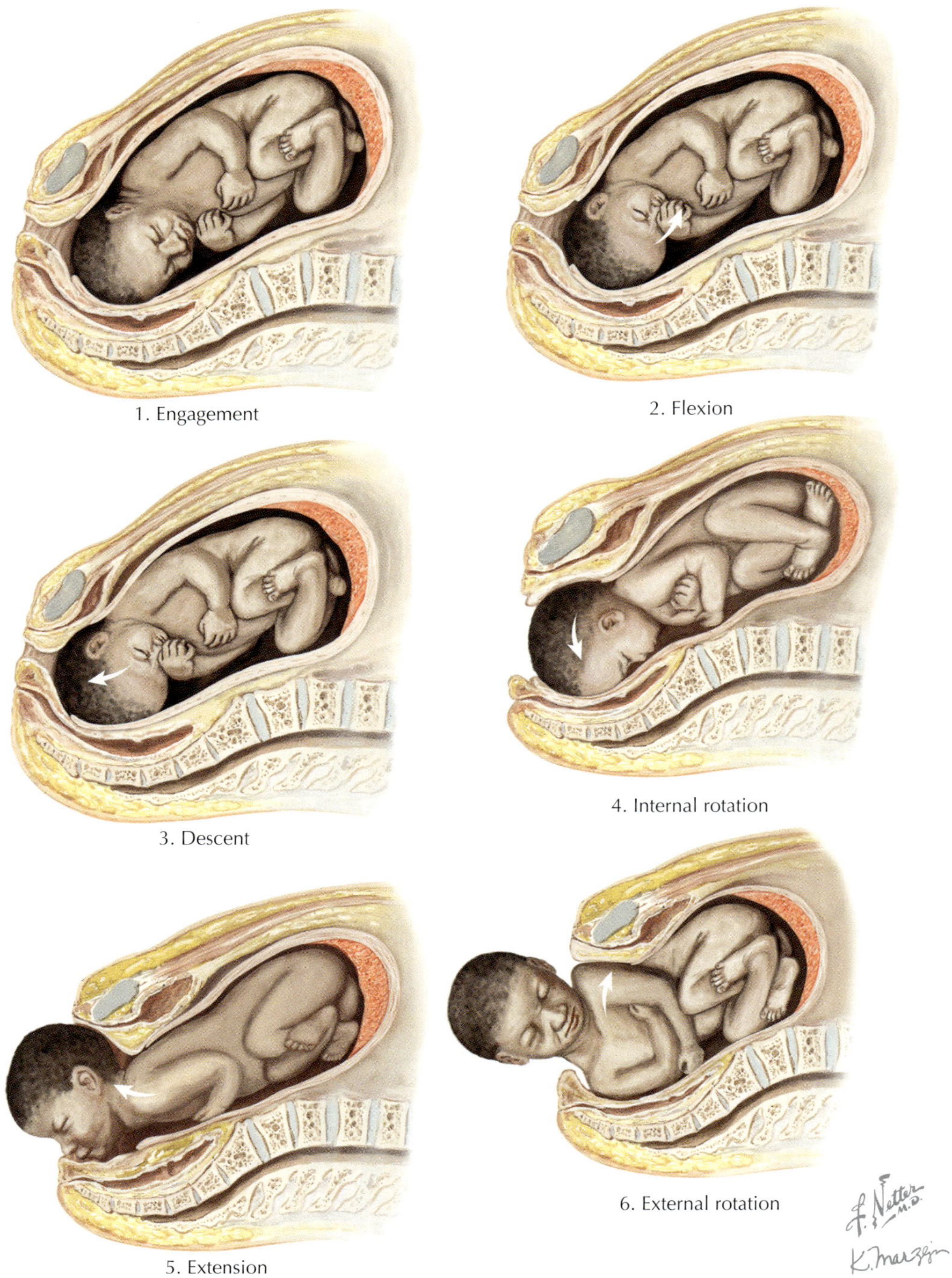

1. Engagement

2. Flexion

3. Descent

4. Internal rotation

5. Extension

6. External rotation

FIGURE 8-21. The Placenta

The **placenta** is the organ that provides the fetus with **bloodborne** nutrients and oxygen and removes waste via the two umbilical arteries and a single umbilical vein. **Percutaneous** umbilical blood sampling (PUBS) can contribute to fetal assessment. The placenta has both maternal and fetal components. The placenta occupies about a third of the uterine wall and is covered with amnion, with the umbilical cord centrally attached.

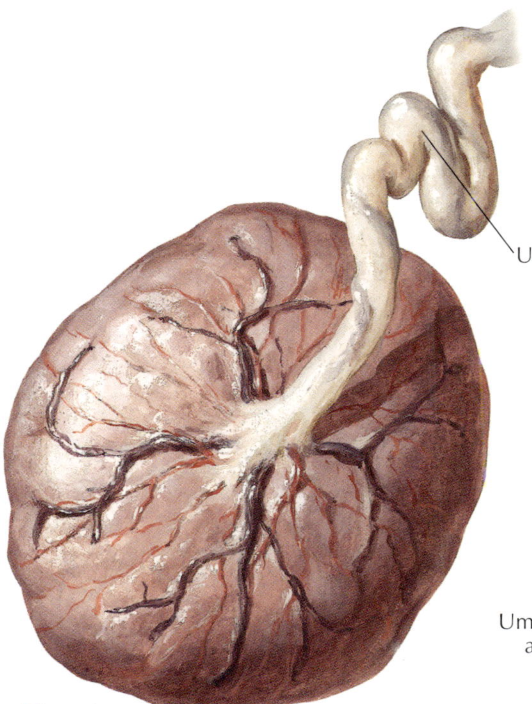

Placenta: Fetal aspect

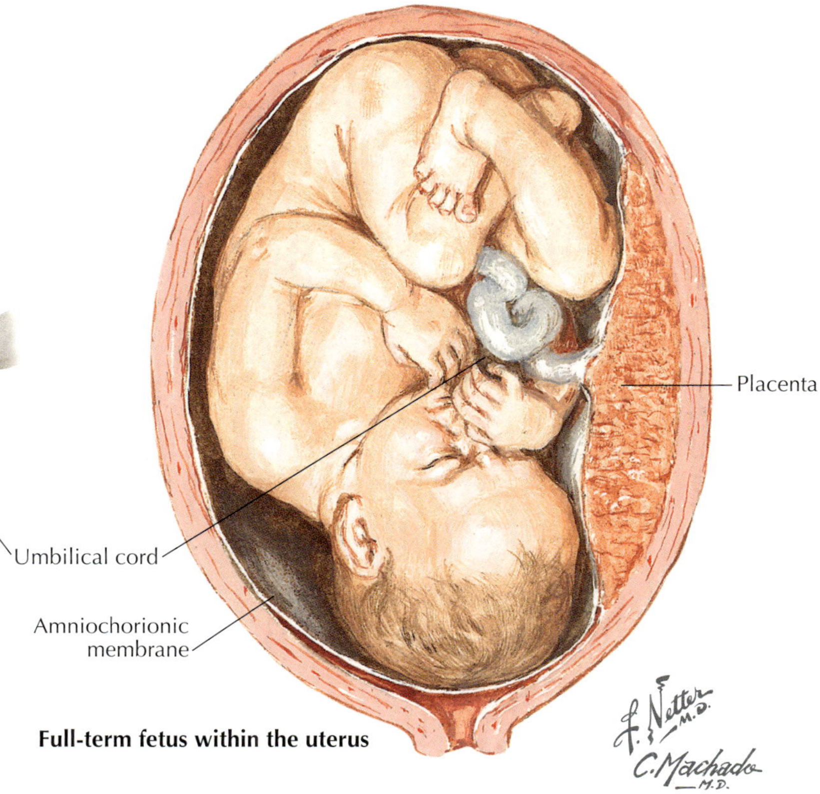

Full-term fetus within the uterus

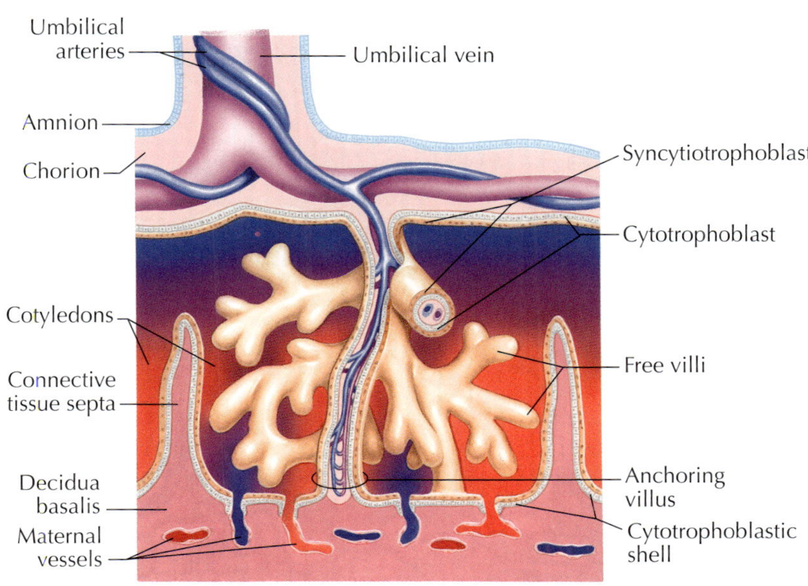

Development of the placenta: Chorionic villi

FIGURE 8-22. Cesarean Birth

In cesarean delivery, a **midline**, **infraumbilical**, **vertical**, or **transverse** incision in the abdomen is followed by an incision in the uterus. The anatomy of the fetus is identified, and the fetus is delivered either head first, as illustrated in Figure 8-22, or as a **breech**. The placenta is usually delivered manually. The leading indications for cesarean deliveries are previous cesarean, breech presentation, **dystocia**, and fetal distress. Note: Tools, implants, and/or equipment depicted in the illustration may be outdated but the procedural approach is valid.

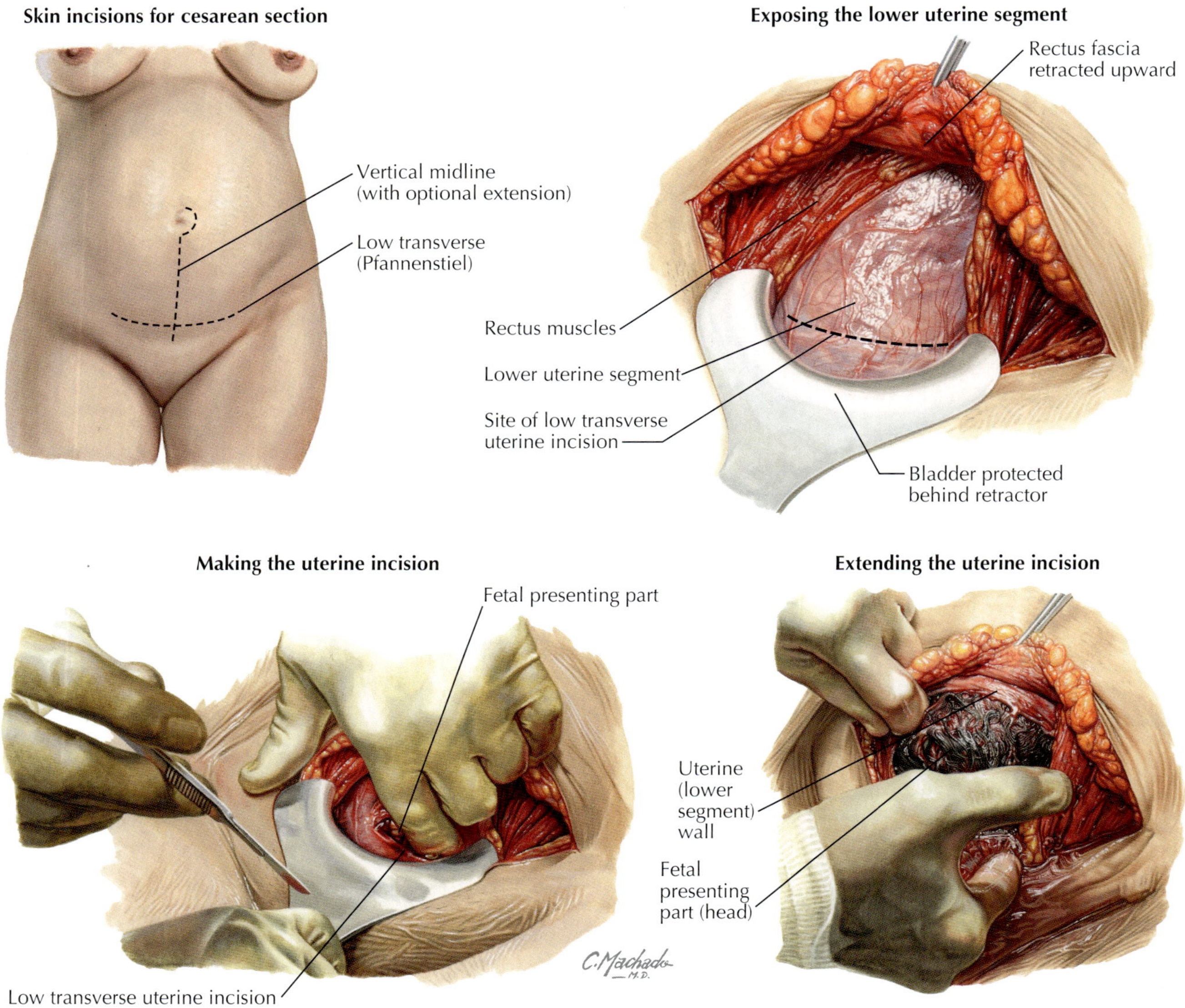

Continued on next page

FIGURE 8-22. Cesarean Birth *(continued)*

Delivering the fetal head

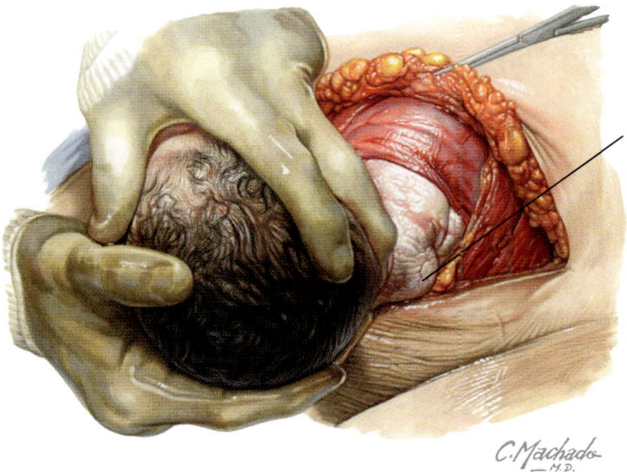

Delivering the placenta

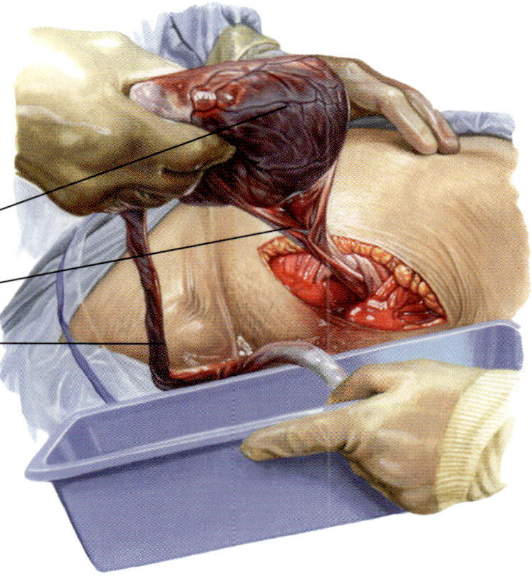

Exploring the uterine cavity (Uterus exteriorized through skin incision)

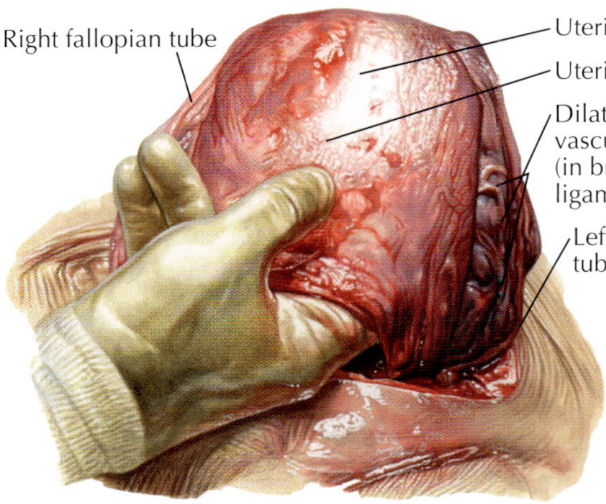

Closing the uterine incision (Uterus exteriorized through incision)

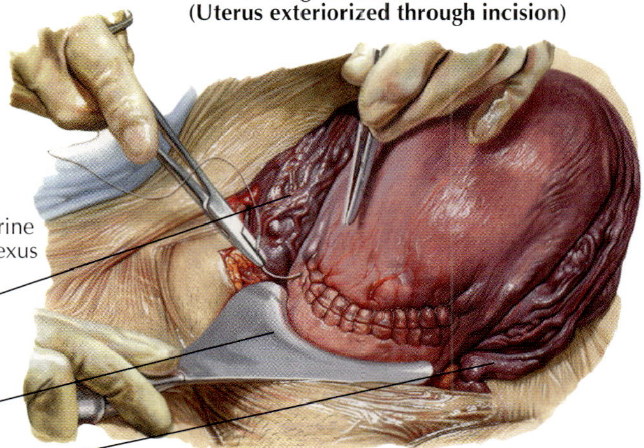

Abortion

Coding Atlas

A **missed abortion** describes a condition in which fetal demise does not result in the natural expulsion of products of conception (miscarriage). An **incomplete abortion** describes a spontaneous abortion (miscarriage) that fails to purge all of the products of conception. A **septic abortion** describes a spontaneous abortion (miscarriage) that occurs due to uterine infection. An **induced abortion** describes medical intervention to end a pregnancy.

59812 Treatment of incomplete abortion, any trimester, completed surgically

59820 Treatment of missed abortion, completed surgically; first trimester

59821 second trimester

59830 Treatment of septic abortion, completed surgically

59840 Induced abortion, by dilation and curettage

59841 Induced abortion, by dilation and evacuation

59850 Induced abortion, by 1 or more intra-amniotic injections (amniocentesis-injections), including hospital admission and visits, delivery of fetus and secundines;

59851 with dilation and curettage and/or evacuation

59852 with hysterotomy (failed intra-amniotic injection)

59855 Induced abortion, by 1 or more vaginal suppositories (eg, prostaglandin) with or without cervical dilation (eg, laminaria), including hospital admission and visits, delivery of fetus and secundines;

59856 with dilation and curettage and/or evacuation

59857 with hysterotomy (failed medical evacuation)

Other Procedures

Coding Atlas

Multifetal pregnancies are often the result of **assisted reproductive technology** (ART) and carry with them increased risk. Some patients elect to undergo fetal reduction, which can be accomplished by injecting potassium chloride into or occluding the umbilical cord of a selected fetus. CPT code 59072 is used to report occlusion of the fetal umbilical cord as a means to terminate a pregnancy. In fetal reduction, the pregnancy continues but with fewer fetuses.

59866 Multifetal pregnancy reduction(s) (MPR)

59870 Uterine evacuation and curettage for hydatidiform mole

59871 Removal of cerclage suture under anesthesia (other than local)

Endocrine System

Thyroid Gland

Incision

60000 Incision and drainage of thyroglossal duct cyst, infected

Excision

Coding Atlas

A **fine needle aspiration** of the thyroid gland using imaging guidance is reported with CPT code 10022. Code 60100 is used to report a **percutaneous core needle biopsy**.

60100 Biopsy thyroid, percutaneous core needle

60200 Excision of cyst or adenoma of thyroid, or transection of isthmus

60210 Partial thyroid lobectomy, unilateral; with or without isthmusectomy

60212 with contralateral subtotal lobectomy, including isthmusectomy

60220 Total thyroid lobectomy, unilateral; with or without isthmusectomy

60225 with contralateral subtotal lobectomy, including isthmusectomy

60240 Thyroidectomy, total or complete

60252 Thyroidectomy, total or subtotal for malignancy; with limited neck dissection

60254 with radical neck dissection

60260 Thyroidectomy, removal of all remaining thyroid tissue following previous removal of a portion of thyroid

60270 Thyroidectomy, including substernal thyroid; sternal split or transthoracic approach

60271 cervical approach

60280 Excision of thyroglossal duct cyst or sinus;

60281 recurrent

Removal

60300 Aspiration and/or injection, thyroid cyst

FIGURE 8-23. The Thyroid and Parathyroid Glands

While thyroid and parathyroid glands share similar names and occur in the neck, the functions of the glands are completely different. The thyroid manufactures hormones that regulate the body's **metabolism**. It consists of two lobes and an **isthmus** joining the two lobes. The parathyroid glands produce hormones that regulate calcium and phosphorus in the body. Paired inferior and superior glands are found on or near the surface of the thyroid gland.

Anterior view

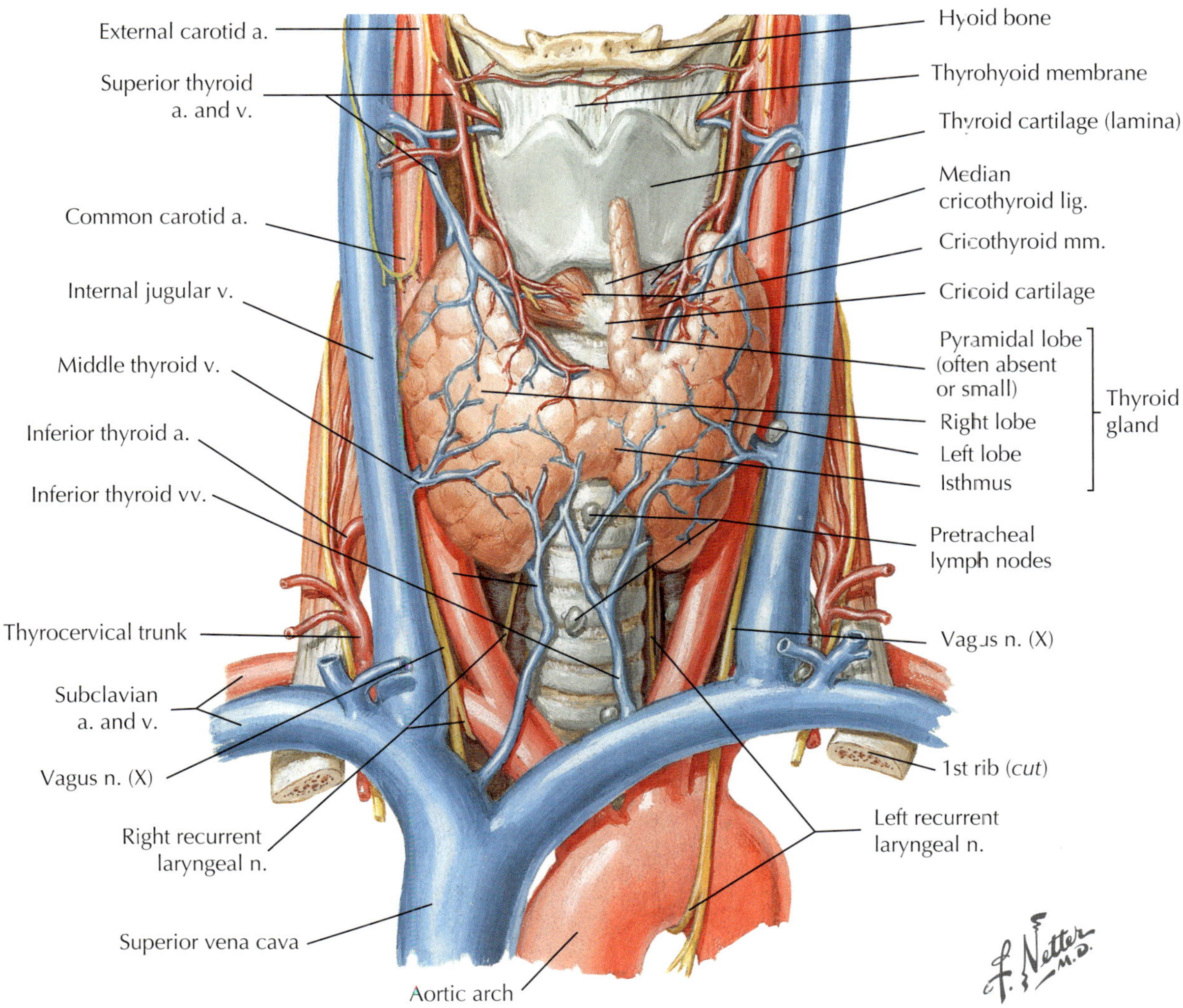

Right lateral view

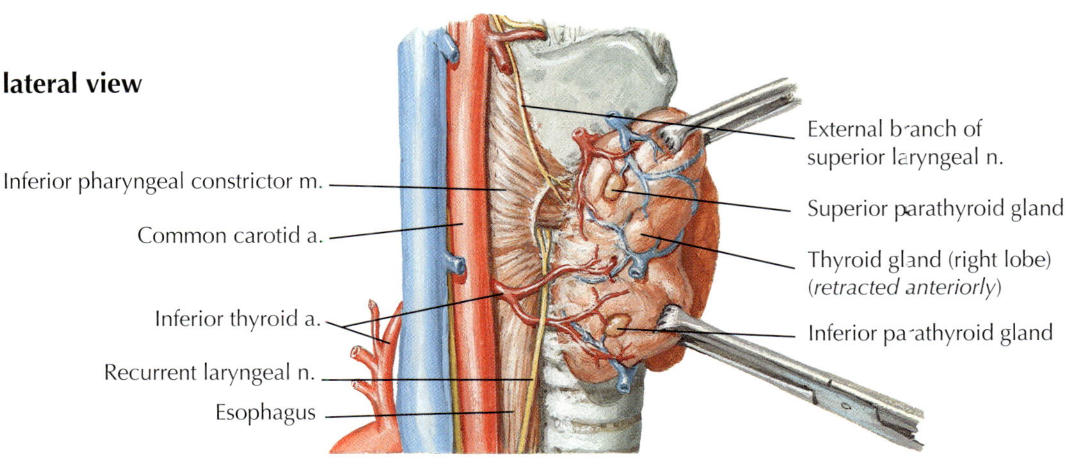

Parathyroid, Thymus, Adrenal Glands, Pancreas, and Carotid Body

Excision

Coding Atlas

The carotid body (carotid glomus; glomus caroticum) is a cluster of **chemoreceptors** that monitor **arterial blood gas**, temperature, and **pH**, contributing to the regulation of breathing. The carotid body is adjacent to the **bifurcation** of the carotid artery in the neck.

60500 Parathyroidectomy or exploration of parathyroid(s);

60502 re-exploration

60505 with mediastinal exploration, sternal split or transthoracic approach

✚ **60512** Parathyroid autotransplantation (List separately in addition to code for primary procedure)

60520 Thymectomy, partial or total; transcervical approach (separate procedure)

60521 sternal split or transthoracic approach, without radical mediastinal dissection (separate procedure)

60522 sternal split or transthoracic approach, with radical mediastinal dissection (separate procedure)

60540 Adrenalectomy, partial or complete, or exploration of adrenal gland with or without biopsy, transabdominal, lumbar or dorsal (separate procedure);

60545 with excision of adjacent retroperitoneal tumor

60600 Excision of carotid body tumor; without excision of carotid artery

60605 with excision of carotid artery

Laparoscopy

60650 Laparoscopy, surgical, with adrenalectomy, partial or complete, or exploration of adrenal gland with or without biopsy, transabdominal, lumbar or dorsal

FIGURE 8-24. The Thymus

During childhood, the thymus is composed of two **lobes** of primarily **lymphatic** tissue; in adulthood, it is composed of fat and fibrous tissue. The thymus gland produces thymosin, a hormone that stimulates the development of **T cells**. The thymus also works to prevent **autoimmunity** errors. The thymus gland is positioned directly behind the sternum and anterior to the heart. **Thymomas** and **lymphomas** can originate in the thymus.

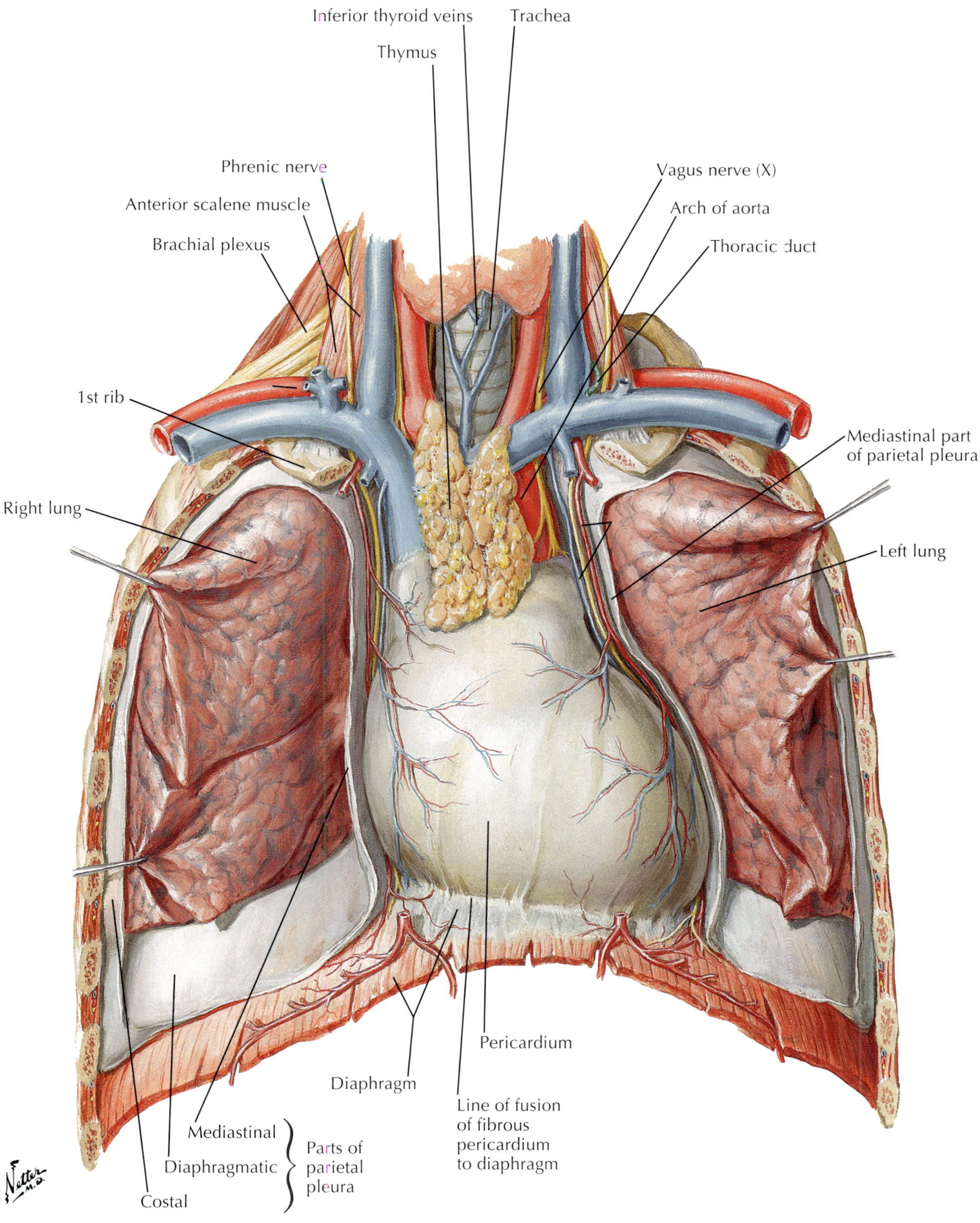

FIGURE 8-25. The Pancreas

The pancreas performs both **endocrine** and **exocrine** functions. Surgical procedures on the pancreas are reported with codes from the Gastrointestinal System code set. The pancreas is included in the Endocrine System because code 60669 would be used to report unlisted laparoscopic procedures of the endocrine system. The **endocrine** portion includes the islets of Langerhans, which secrete **insulin** and **glucagon**. Pancreatic **exocrine** glands secrete **enzymes** that contribute to digestion.

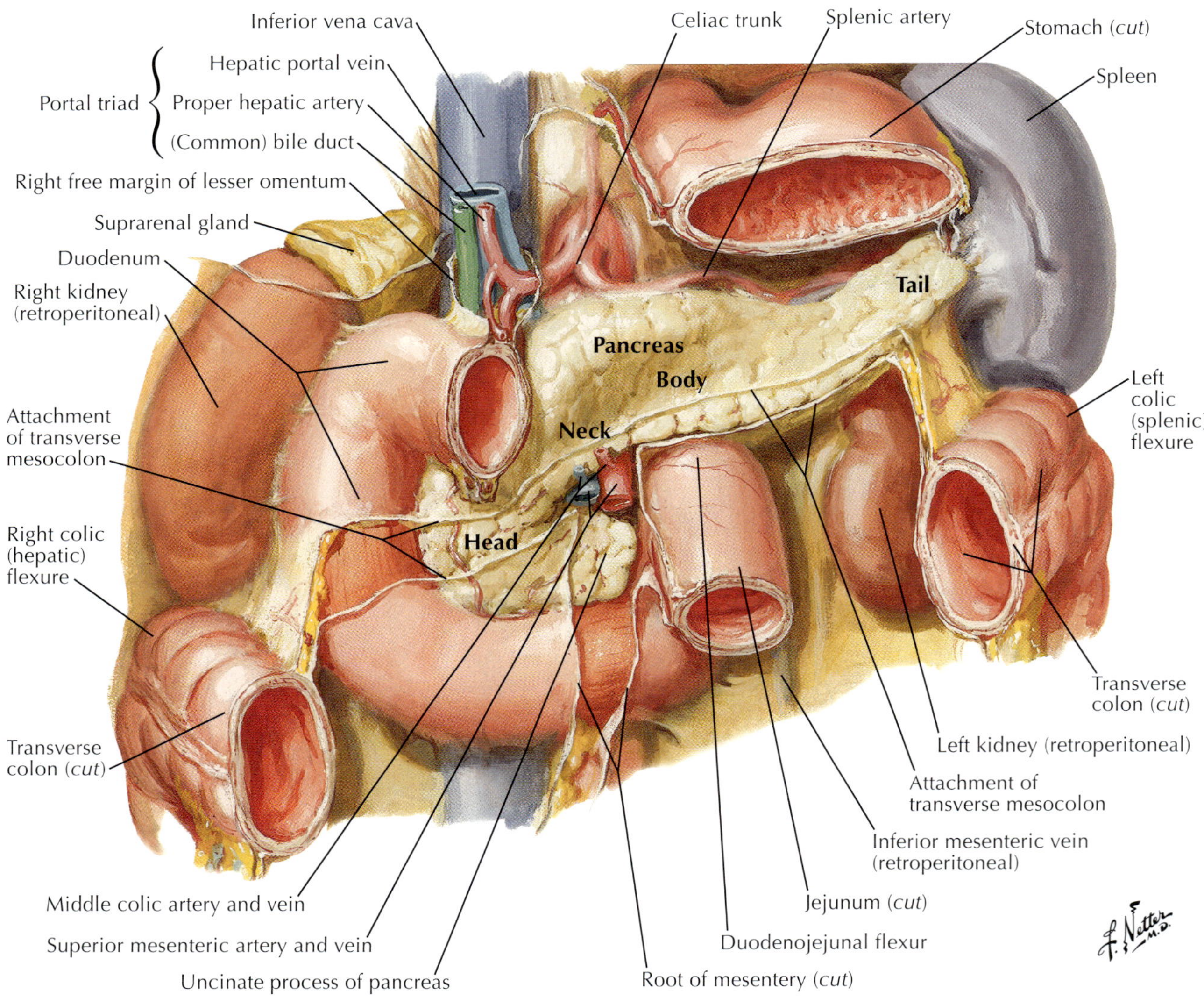

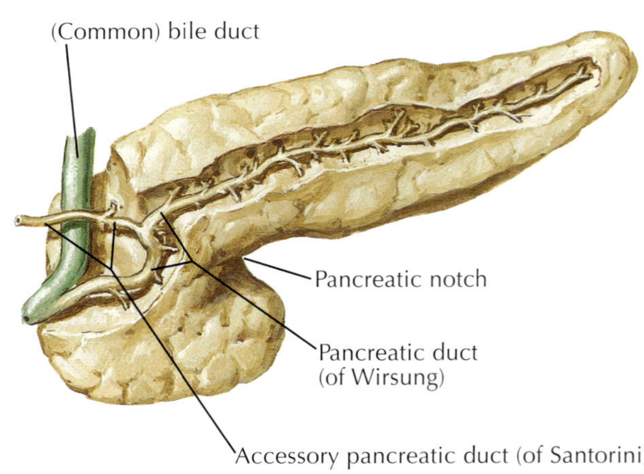

FIGURE 8-26. The Adrenal Glands

The paired adrenal glands lie in the Gerota fascia at the **superior** poles of the kidneys. Each gland contains an adrenal **cortex** and adrenal **medulla**. The adrenal cortex secretes **hormones**, the most important of which are aldosterone, cortisol, and adrenal antigen. The medulla produces epinephrine and norepinephrine, which increase **cardiac output** and **vascular resistance**; these stress hormones are known as adrenaline. Adrenal glands are also called suprarenal glands.

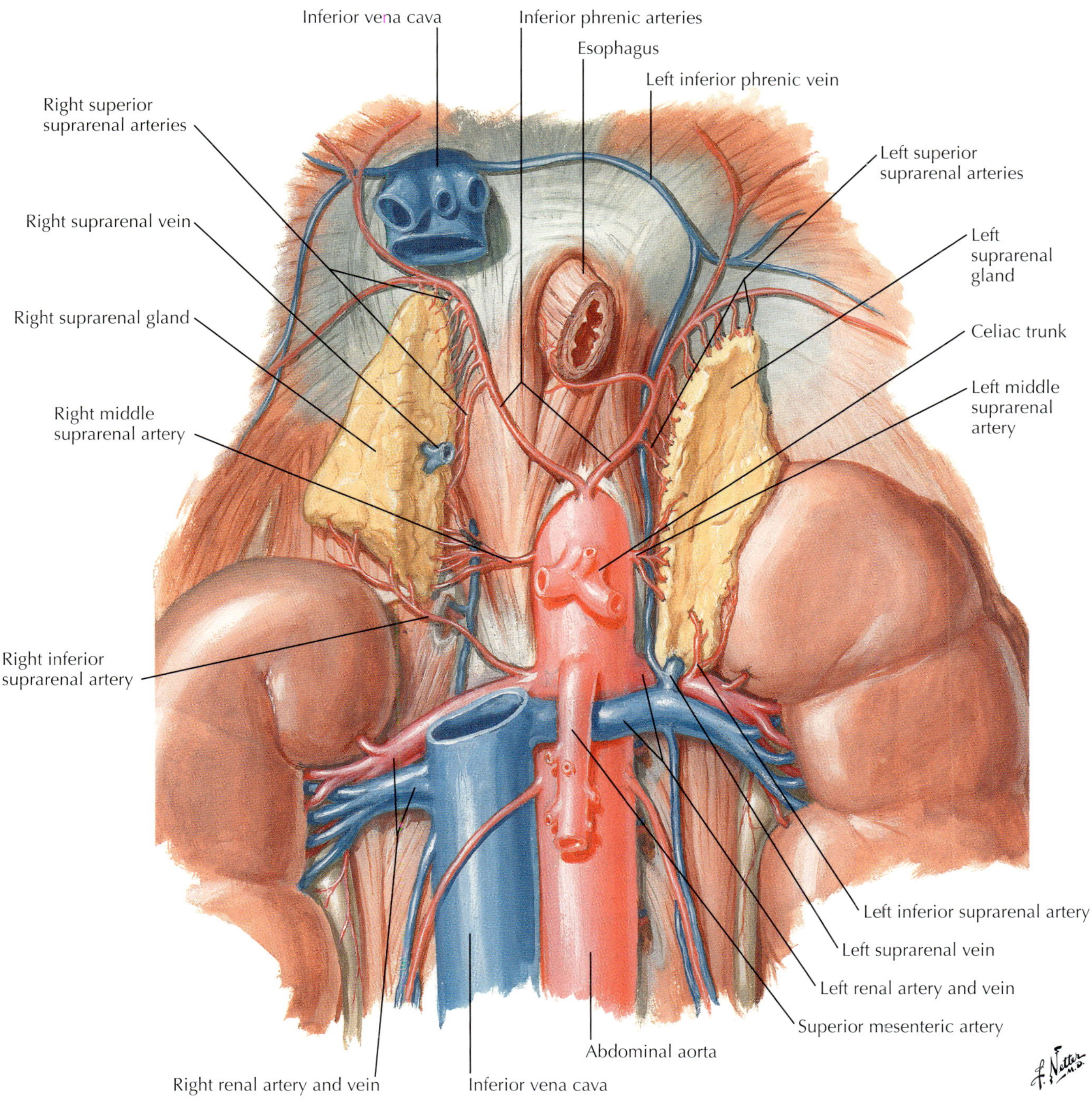

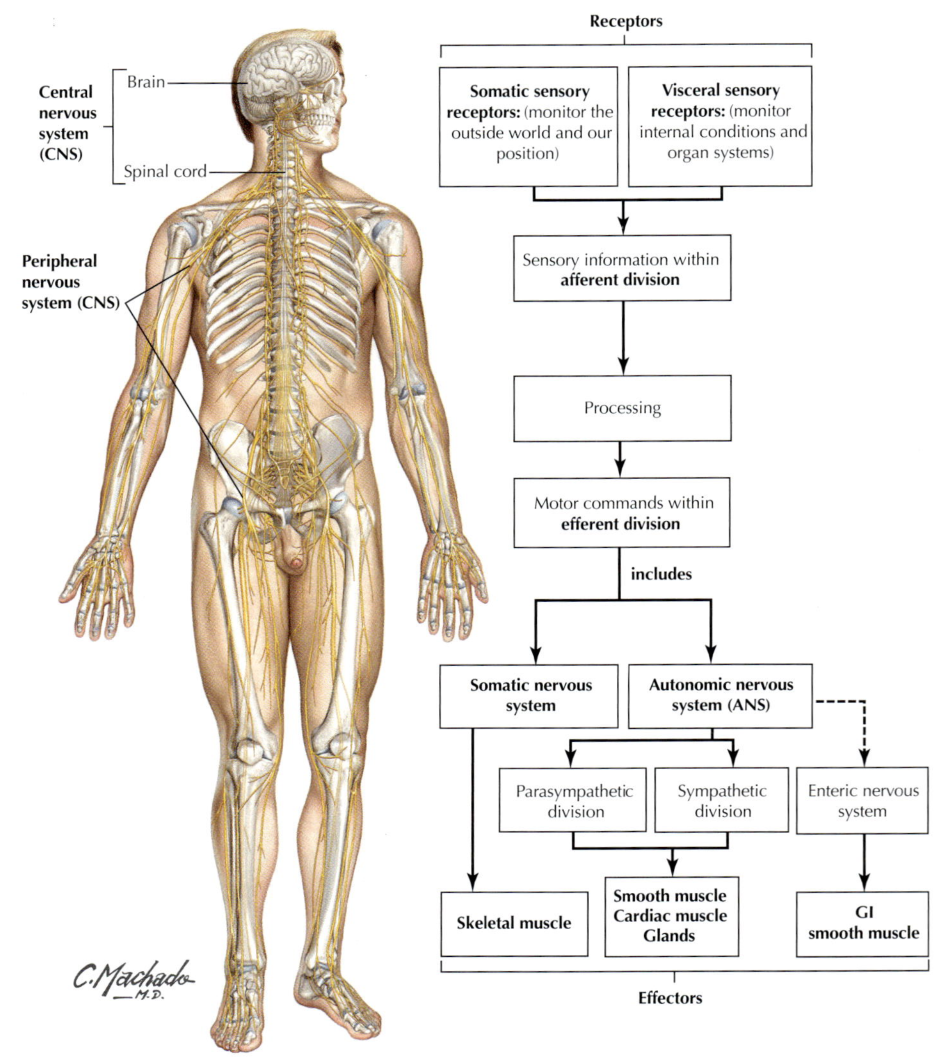
Central nervous system (CNS)
Brain
Spinal cord
Peripheral nervous system (CNS)
C.Machado M.D.
Receptors
Somatic sensory receptors: (monitor the outside world and our position)
Visceral sensory receptors: (monitor internal conditions and organ systems)
Sensory information within afferent division
Processing
Motor commands within efferent division
includes
Somatic nervous system
Autonomic nervous system (ANS)
Parasympathetic division
Sympathetic division
Enteric nervous system
Skeletal muscle
Smooth muscle
Cardiac muscle
Glands
GI
smooth muscle
Effectors

CHAPTER 9

Nervous System

The nervous system contains two major divisions: the **central nervous system** (CNS), which is the body's control center, and the **peripheral nervous system** (PNS), composed of cranial and spinal nerves and ganglia, which senses **physiologic** and **environmental** stimuli, sends the information to the CNS, and reacts according to directives from the CNS.

The CNS includes the spinal cord, the cerebrum, the cerebellum, the diencephalon, and the brain stem and is all contained within membranes called meninges. The meninges are filled with cerebrospinal fluid (CSF). The brain and spinal cord are housed within the skull and bony vertebra for protection. The CSF provides a protective cushion and circulates to provide **nutrients** and remove waste from the brain and spinal cord.

The cerebrum regulates higher-level thinking and has two hemispheres. Each hemisphere controls the **contralateral** body, eg, damage to the right side of the brain may cause weakness in the left side of the body. Each hemisphere is divided into four lobes and is responsible for specific body functions: frontal—motor control, learning, planning, and some speech; parietal—somatic and voluntary sensory function; occipital—vision; and temporal—hearing and some speech.

The cerebellum plays a role in **sensory** perception, motor output, **equilibrium**, and posture. The brain stem includes the midbrain, pons, and medulla oblongata and controls involuntary functions, such as respiration and digestion. The diencephalon contains the hypothalamus, thalamus, and epithalamus and is primarily responsible for visceral activities and the **anatomic nervous system** (ANS).

Four ventricles, or hollow chambers, lie within the brain: one **lateral** ventricle in each hemisphere, a third ventricle that is central and **anterior**, and a fourth ventricle in the **posterior** brain. The choroid plexus of the ventricles manufactures CSF by extracting and modifying fluid from blood. CSF is constantly refreshed with new infusions, and old CSF is cycled back into the bloodstream through the choroid plexus.

The spinal cord lies within the vertebral canal. A site on the spinal cord is identified by the immediately adjacent and **superior** vertebra. The spinal cord is the information conduit between the CNS and PNS. Nerves that join the PNS to the spinal cord or brain are called **nerve roots**. Twelve pairs of nerve roots emerge from the brain stem and the highest level of the spinal cord. The rest of the spinal cord has 31 pairs of nerve roots.

The PNS can be divided into two systems: **afferent** and **efferent**. Afferent nerves are nerves that carry messages from the PNS to the brain, and efferent nerves are nerves that carry messages from the brain to muscles and other tissue. Other divisions within the PNS include the ANS and the **somatic nervous system** (SNS).

The ANS is also known as the visceral or involuntary nervous system as it controls functions performed without conscious effort, such as heartbeat, breathing, and **peristalsis**.The ANS also controls blood pressure, pupillary movement, and male erection. **Parasympathetic** nervous reactions of the ANS create a rest/digest reaction to stress, slowing the heart rate and relaxing muscles. The sympathetic nervous reactions of the ANS promote a fight-or-flight response, raising blood pressure and heart rate and constricting blood vessels.

Any disruption on the neural pathway may result in dysfunction in sensory and/or motor abilities. These disruptions may be small, eg, a compressed medial nerve in the wrist, resulting in tingling in the fingers, or they may be major, eg, a vertebral fracture, causing an injury to the spinal column at the second cervical vertebra and resulting in incontinence and an inability to move or feel sensations in the trunk, arms, or legs.

FIGURE 9-1. Cerebrum In Situ

The cerebrum is the largest section of the brain. It contains right and left cerebral hemispheres joined by the corpus callosum, which is a collection of white matter fibers. The outermost layer of the cerebrum is the cortex; it is covered in a corrugated pattern of grooves (sulcus) and folds (gyrus). The sulci and gyri increase the amount of surface area in the brain, which in turn increases the amount of cerebral cortex, or gray matter.

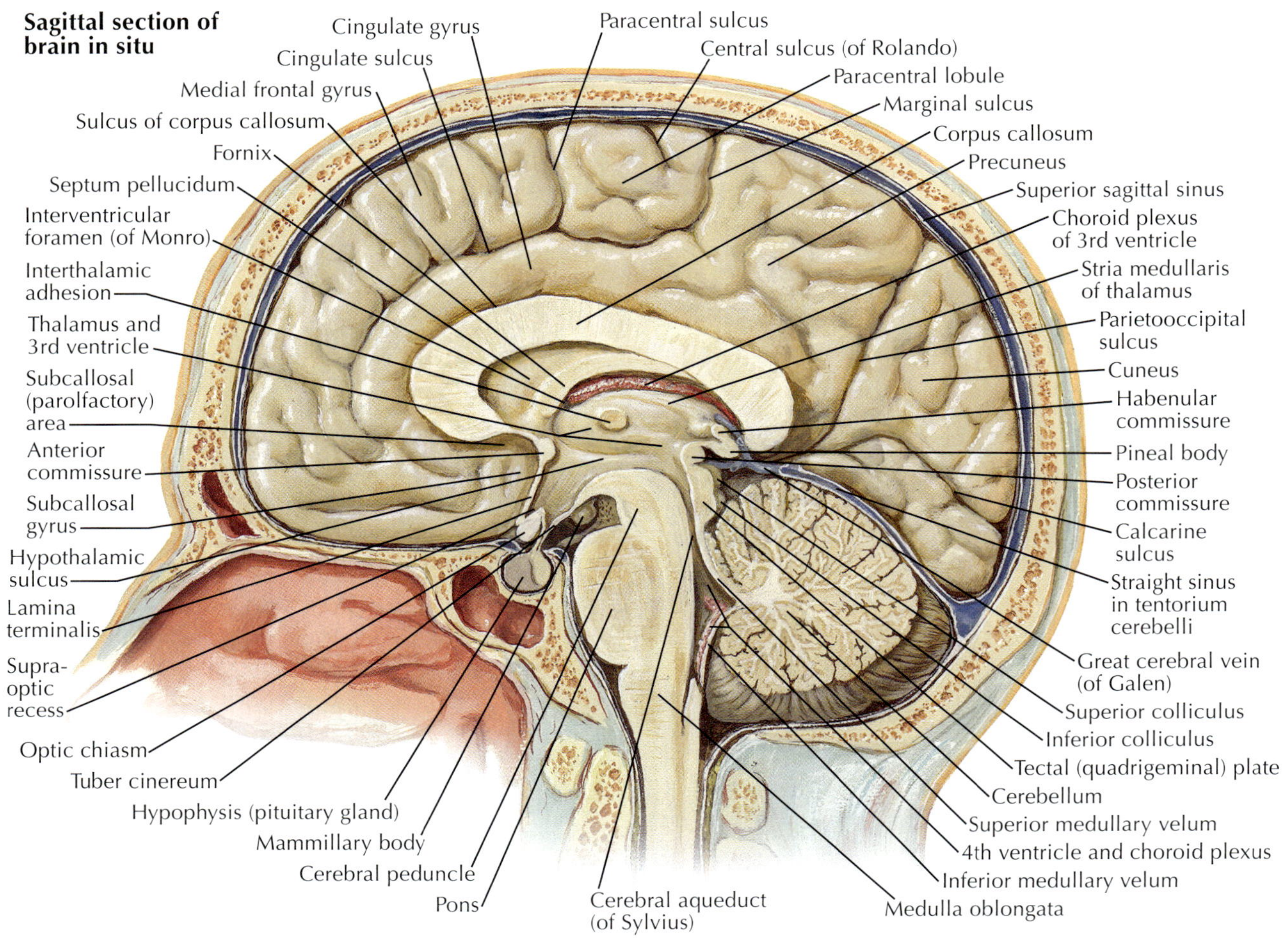

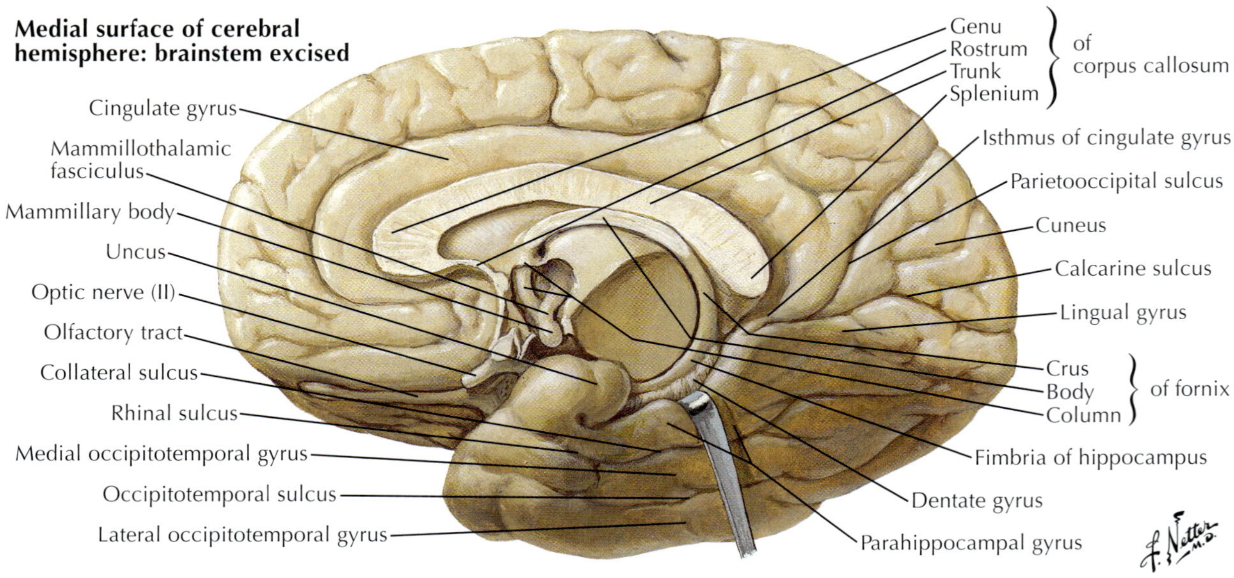

FIGURE 9-2. The Brain Stem

The major parts of the brain stem are the medulla oblongata (myelencephalon), pons (part of the metencephalon), and midbrain. The medulla oblongata is **distal** to the pons and continuous with the cervical spinal cord. The pons lies between the medulla and the midbrain (mesencephalon). The midbrain is proximal to the pons and controls basic **involuntary** body functions including breathing, consciousness, swallowing, and heart rate. Ten of 12 cranial **motor** and **sensory** nerves connect along the brainstem.

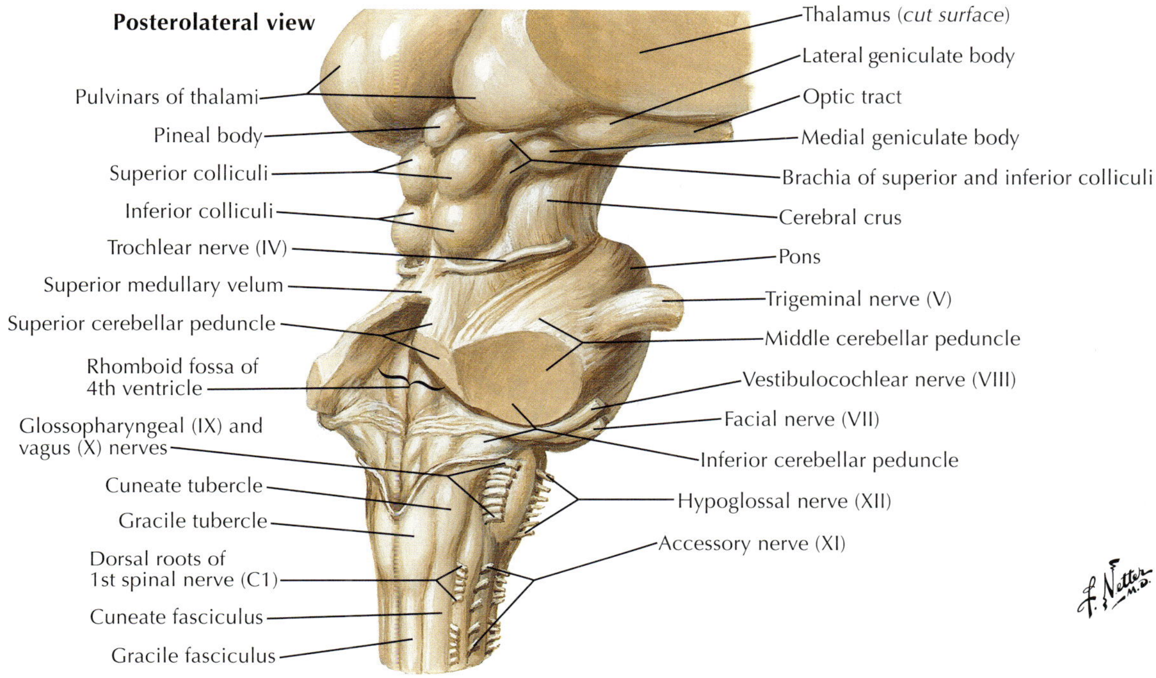

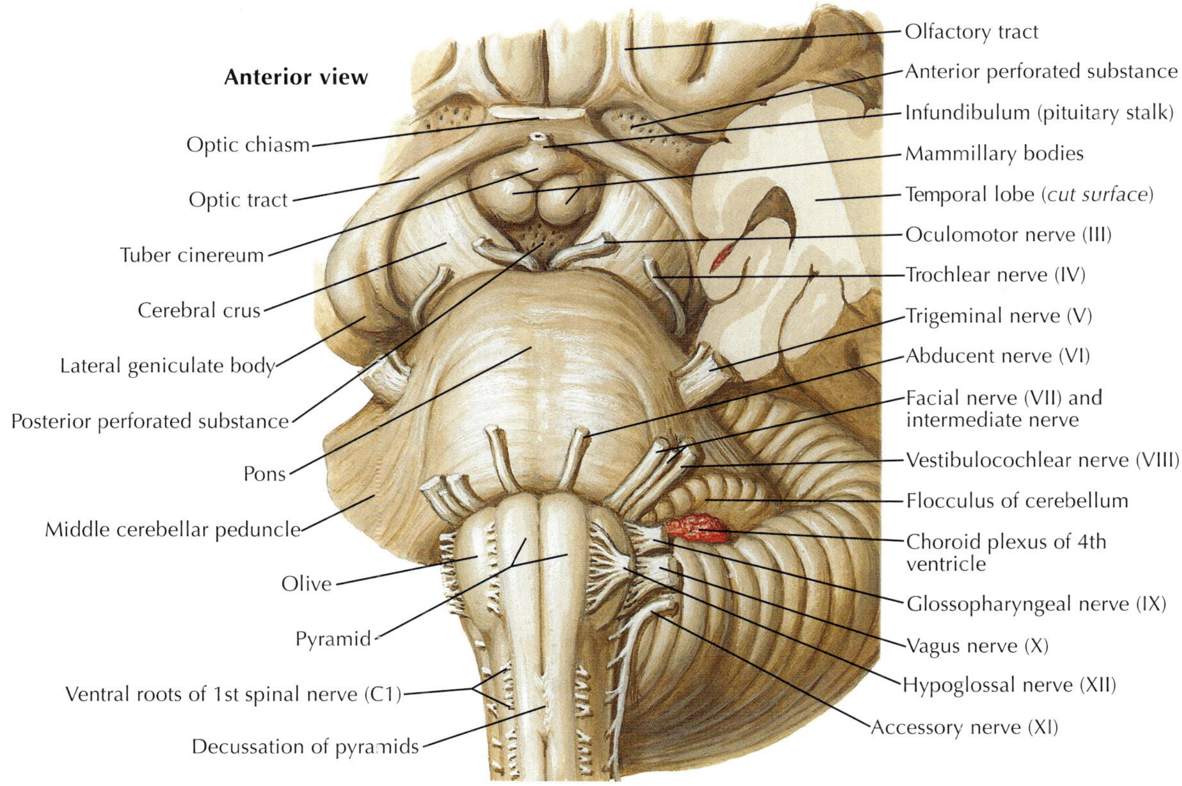

FIGURE 9-3. Ventricles of the Brain

Blood plasma entering the membrane of the choroid plexus within the ventricles is filtered to create cerebrospinal fluid (CFS). The CSF circulates from the lateral ventricles in the cerebrum into the third and fourth ventricles, the subarachnoid space, and the central canal of the spinal cord. CSF is returned to the bloodstream through the arachnoid villi located in the dura sinuses of the meninges.

Left lateral phantom view

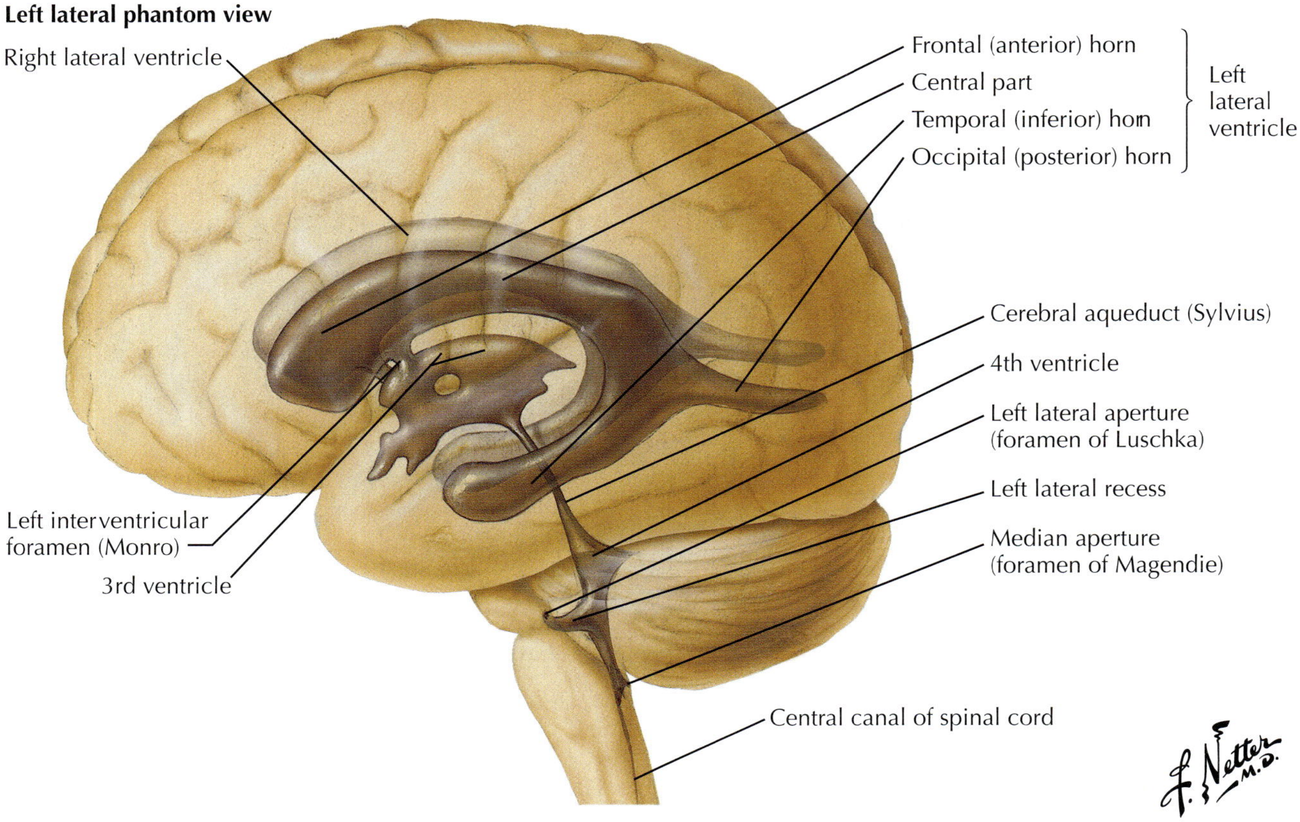

Skull, Meninges, and Brain

Injection, Drainage, or Aspiration

Coding Atlas

Ventricular puncture describes a procedure in which cerebrospinal fluid (CSF) is **aspirated** via a needle inserted through a **burr hole** or other access site into the skull, directly into a ventricle of the brain. A cisternal puncture describes a procedure in which CSF is aspirated via a needle inserted below the occipital bone into the back of the skull at C1-C2 to access the posterior cerebellomedullary cistern, a small pool of CSF at the base of the cerebellum. This site may be referred to as the cisterna magna.

61000 Subdural tap through fontanelle, or suture, infant, unilateral or bilateral; initial

61001 subsequent taps

61020 Ventricular puncture through previous burr hole, fontanelle, suture, or implanted ventricular catheter/reservoir; without injection

61026 with injection of medication or other substance for diagnosis or treatment

61050 Cisternal or lateral cervical (C1-C2) puncture; without injection (separate procedure)

61055 with injection of medication or other substance for diagnosis or treatment

61070 Puncture of shunt tubing or reservoir for aspiration or injection procedure

FIGURE 9-4. Meninges of the Brain and Spinal Cord

The pia mater is the innermost layer of meninges; it follows the folds of the brain and tightly covers the brain and spinal cord. Beyond the pia mater is subarachnoid space and then arachnoid mater, which does not follow the folds of the brain but skims the brain surface. Cerebrospinal fluid (CSF) flows in subarachnoid space between pia mater and arachnoid mater. The outermost layer of the meninges is dura mater, which lines the skull's interior and the spinal cord's exterior.

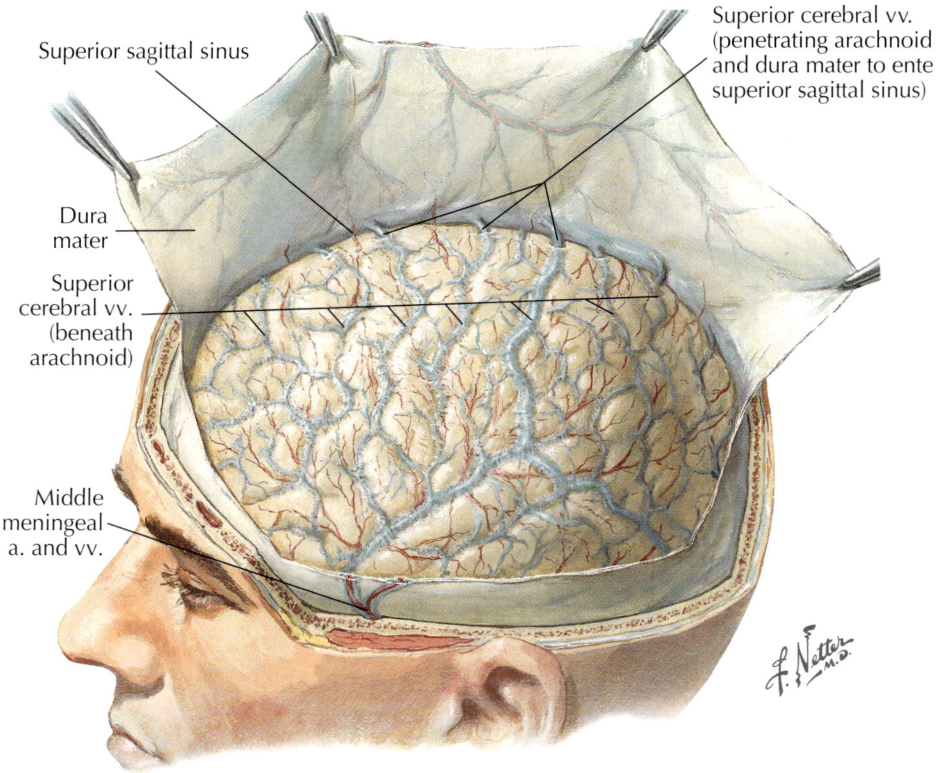

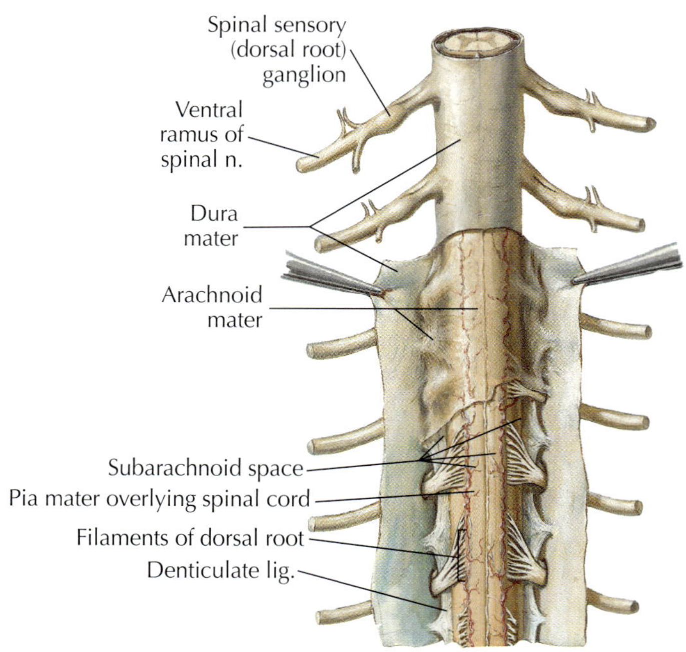

FIGURE 9-5. Subdural Tap and Catheter Placement

A subdural **hematoma** (SDH) may cause increased intracranial pressure. **Aspiration** of a hematoma may be performed through a newborn's fontanelle to relieve symptoms associated with pressure, as illustrated in the bottom portion of Figure 9-5. The subdural space lies beneath the dura, or outermost layer of the lining of the brain (meninges). Aspirated subdural fluid may be blood or cerebrospinal fluid (CSF). A tap may be **therapeutic**, **diagnostic**, or both. In other cases, a **burr hole** and **catheter** may be placed for drainage. Note: Tools, implants, and/or equipment depicted in the illustration may be outdated but the procedural approach is valid.

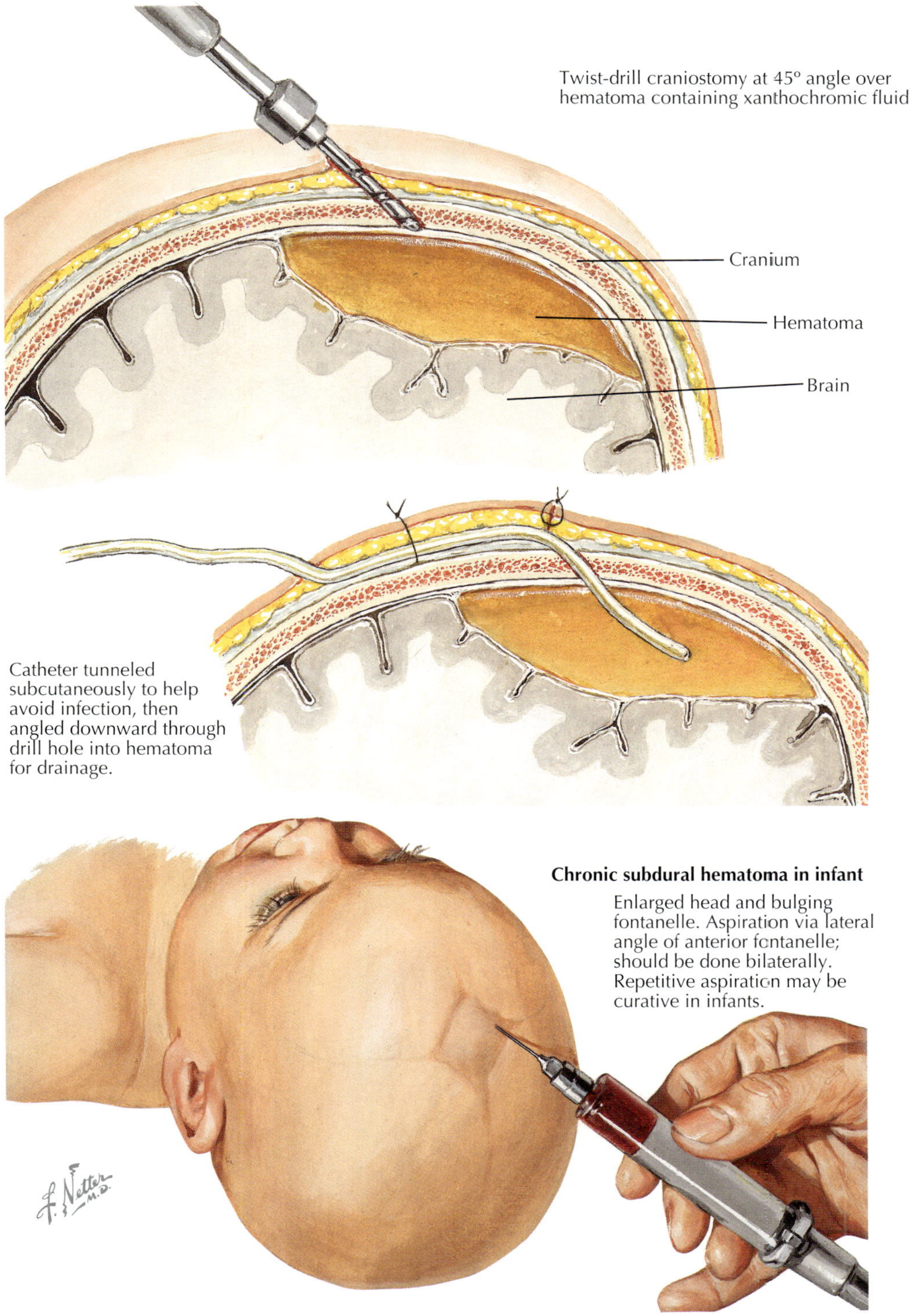

Twist Drill, Burr Hole(s), or Trephine

Coding Atlas

In order to treat the brain, it must first be accessible. Twist drills and burring drills are used to create an opening to the brain. After incising the skin, a small hole can be quickly created in the skull with a twist drill, typically for implanting a thin wire, **catheter**, or needle, without **direct visualization** of the site being treated. A circular **burr hole** is created with a specialized electric drill, allowing for **direct visualization** of the treatment site. A trephine is a generic term for a tool that makes a hole in the skull.

61105 Twist drill hole for **subdural** or ventricular puncture

⃠ **61107** Twist drill hole(s) for subdural, **intracerebral**, or **ventricular** puncture; for implanting ventricular **catheter**, pressure recording device, or other **intracerebral** monitoring device

61108 for evacuation and/or drainage of subdural **hematoma**

61120 **Burr hole**(s) for ventricular puncture (including injection of gas, contrast media, dye, or radioactive material)

61140 Burr hole(s) or trephine; with **biopsy** of brain or **intracranial** lesion

61150 with drainage of brain **abscess** or **cyst**

61151 with subsequent tapping (**aspiration**) of intracranial abscess or cyst

61154 Burr hole(s) with evacuation and/or drainage of hematoma, **extradural** or subdural

61156 Burr hole(s); with aspiration of hematoma or cyst, intracerebral

61210 for implanting ventricular catheter, reservoir, EEG electrode(s), pressure recording device, or other cerebral monitoring device (separate procedure)

61215 Insertion of **subcutaneous** reservoir, pump or continuous infusion system for connection to ventricular catheter

61250 Burr hole(s) or trephine, supratentorial, exploratory, not followed by other surgery

61253 Burr hole(s) or trephine, infratentorial, **unilateral** or **bilateral**

FIGURE 9-6. Burr Hole

A **burr hole** cut into the skull allows the physician to directly access the brain in order to relieve pressure within or to access brain tissue for other **therapeutic** purposes. A drilling burr is an electric saw that creates a hole in the bone (**craniostomy**). For greater access, multiple burr holes may be made and linked using a bone saw. A twist drill is a manually operated drill that creates a smaller hole in the skull. Note: Tools, implants, and/or equipment depicted in the illustration may be outdated but the procedural approach is valid.

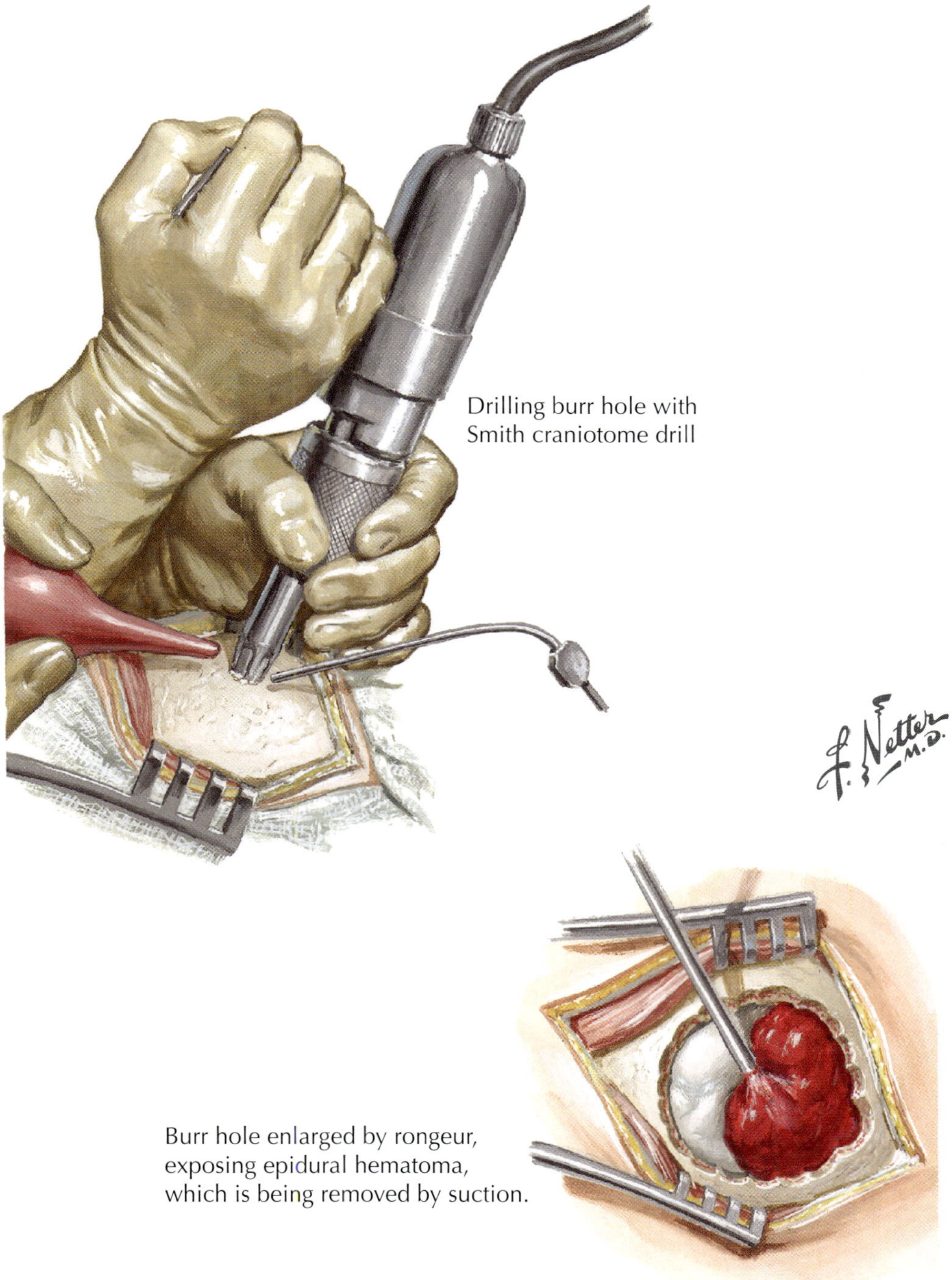

FIGURE 9-7. The Tentorium Cerebelli

The tentorium cerebelli is a dome-shaped fold of dura mater that separates the cerebellum from the cerebrum. The tentorium cerebelli supports the occipital lobes. **Supratentorial** describes a location **superior** to the tentorium, while **infratentorial** describes a location that is **inferior** to the tentorium. Brain surgeries and tumor locations are often described by their location in relation to the tentorium cerebelli.

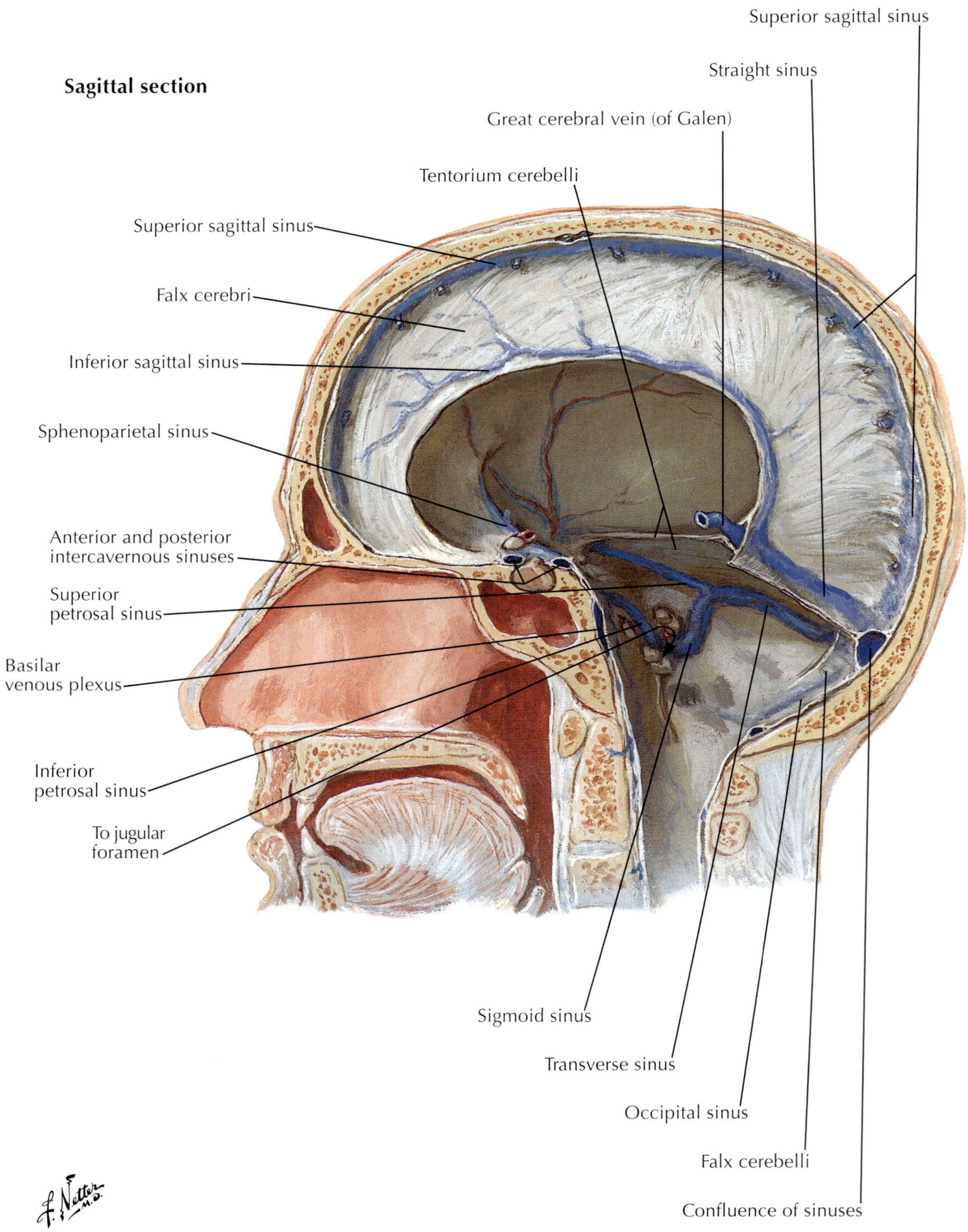

Craniectomy or Craniotomy

Coding Atlas

The procedures reported with codes in this subsection include **burr hole** drilling or **trephination** performed during the same operative session as the **craniectomy/craniotomy**.

61304 Craniectomy or craniotomy, exploratory; supratentorial

61305 infratentorial (posterior fossa)

61312 Craniectomy or craniotomy for evacuation of hematoma, supratentorial; extradural or subdural

61313 intracerebral

61314 Craniectomy or craniotomy for evacuation of hematoma, infratentorial; extradural or subdural

61315 intracerebellar

+ 61316 Incision and subcutaneous placement of cranial bone graft (List separately in addition to code for primary procedure)

61320 Craniectomy or craniotomy, drainage of intracranial abscess; supratentorial

61321 infratentorial

61322 Craniectomy or craniotomy, decompressive, with or without duraplasty, for treatment of intracranial hypertension, without evacuation of associated intraparenchymal hematoma; without lobectomy

61323 with lobectomy

61330 Decompression of orbit only, transcranial approach

61332 Exploration of orbit (transcranial approach); with biopsy

61333 with removal of lesion

61340 Subtemporal cranial decompression (pseudotumor cerebri, slit ventricle syndrome)

61343 Craniectomy, suboccipital with cervical laminectomy for decompression of medulla and spinal cord, with or without dural graft (eg, Arnold-Chiari malformation)

61345 Other cranial decompression, posterior fossa

61450 Craniectomy, subtemporal, for section, compression, or decompression of sensory root of gasserian ganglion

61458 Craniectomy, suboccipital; for exploration or decompression of cranial nerves

61460 for section of 1 or more cranial nerves

61480 for mesencephalic tractotomy or pedunculotomy

61500 Craniectomy; with excision of tumor or other bone lesion of skull

61501 for osteomyelitis

61510 Craniectomy, trephination, bone flap craniotomy; for excision of brain tumor, supratentorial, except meningioma

61512 for excision of meningioma, supratentorial

61514 for excision of brain abscess, supratentorial

61516 for excision or fenestration of cyst, supratentorial

+ 61517 Implantation of brain intracavitary chemotherapy agent (List separately in addition to code for primary procedure)

61518 Craniectomy for excision of brain tumor, infratentorial or posterior fossa; except meningioma, cerebellopontine angle tumor, or midline tumor at base of skull

61519 meningioma

61520 cerebellopontine angle tumor

61521 midline tumor at base of skull

61522 Craniectomy, infratentorial or posterior fossa; for excision of brain abscess

61524 for excision or fenestration of cyst

61526 Craniectomy, bone flap craniotomy, transtemporal (mastoid) for excision of cerebellopontine angle tumor;

61530 combined with middle/posterior fossa craniotomy/craniectomy

61531 Subdural implantation of strip electrodes through 1 or more burr or trephine hole(s) for long-term seizure monitoring

61533 Craniotomy with elevation of bone flap; for subdural implantation of an electrode array, for long-term seizure monitoring

61534 for excision of epileptogenic focus without electrocorticography during surgery

61535 for removal of epidural or subdural electrode array, without excision of cerebral tissue (separate procedure)

61536 for excision of cerebral epileptogenic focus, with electrocorticography during surgery (includes removal of electrode array)

61537 for lobectomy, temporal lobe, without electrocorticography during surgery

61538 for lobectomy, temporal lobe, with electrocorticography during surgery

61539 for lobectomy, other than temporal lobe, partial or total, with electrocorticography during surgery

61540 for lobectomy, other than temporal lobe, partial or total, without electrocorticography during surgery

61541 for transection of corpus callosum

61543 for partial or subtotal (functional) hemispherectomy

61544 for excision or coagulation of choroid plexus

61545 for excision of craniopharyngioma

FIGURE 9-8. The Intracranial Arteries

The **bilateral** internal carotid artery (ICA) enters the brain at the skull base on each side and ascends to split into the **anterior** cerebral artery (ACA) and middle cerebral artery (MCA). This split is shaped like the letter T and may be referred to as the "carotid T" or the "top of the carotid." The bilateral vertebral arteries enter the skull through the foramen magnum at C1 and merge to form the basilar artery.

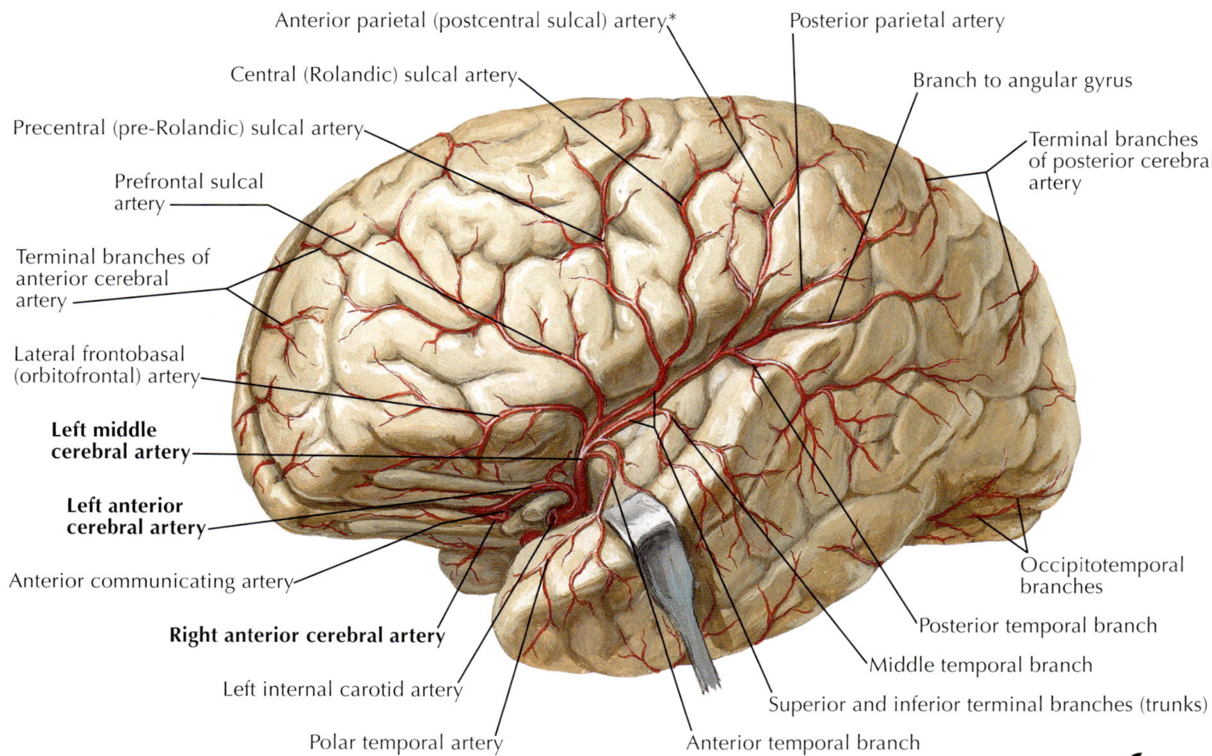

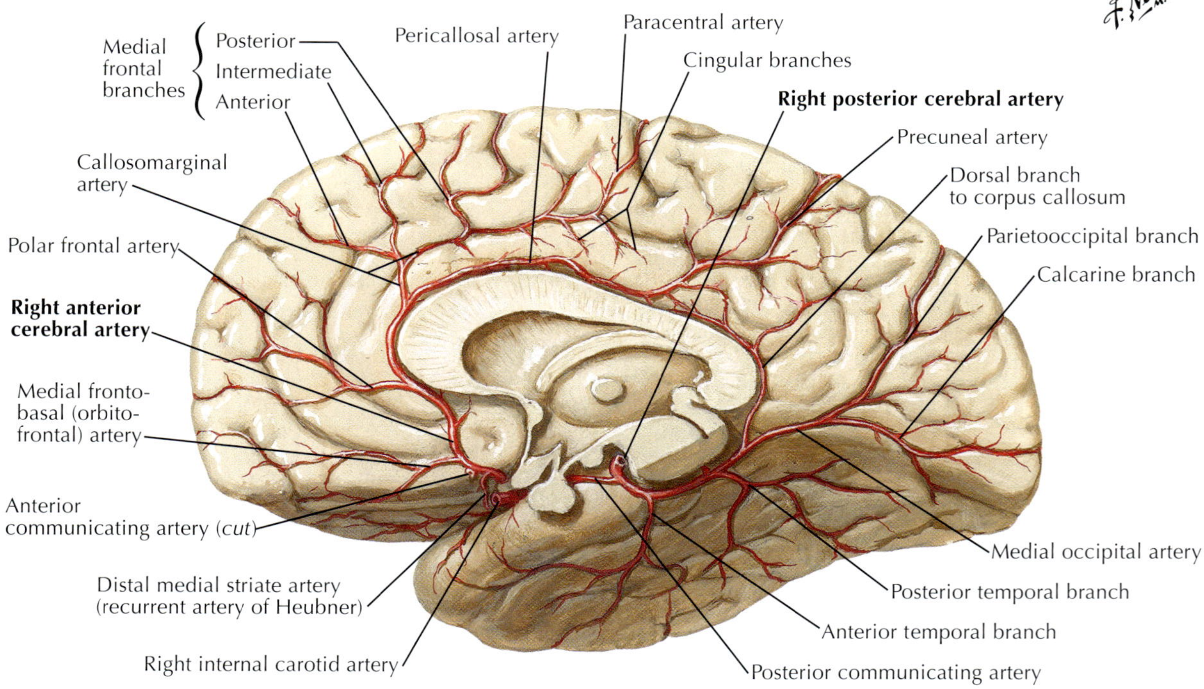

*Note: Anterior parietal (postcentral sulcal) artery also occurs as separate anterior parietal and postcentral sulcal arteries.

FIGURE 9-9. Hematoma

An **epidural** (**extradural**) hemorrhage occurs between the dura mater and the skull. A **subdural** hemorrhage occurs in the space between the dura and arachnoid mater. In **subarachnoid** hemorrhage, bleeding is on the surface of the brain and blood can become trapped in the sulci and fissures. A cerebral (intraparenchymal) hemorrhage occurs within the brain. These hemorrhages lead to the pooling of trapped blood (**hematoma**) that increases **intracranial** pressure, which may damage brain tissue.

Temporal Fossa Hematoma

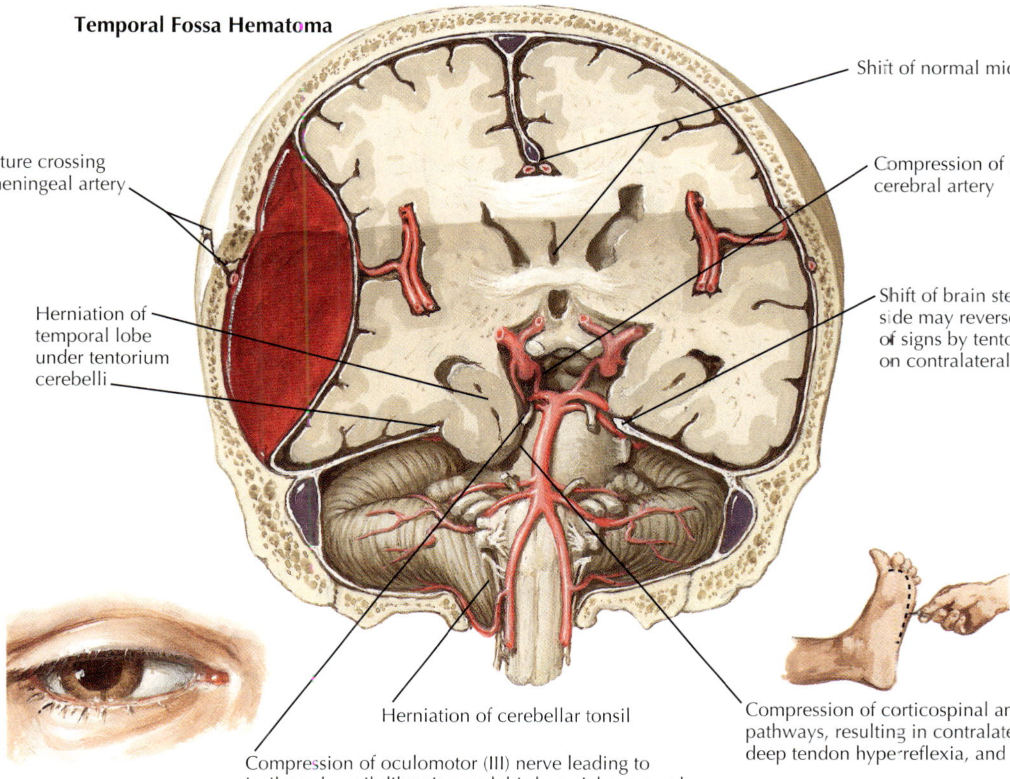

Subfrontal Hematoma

Frontal trauma: headache, poor cerebration, intermittent disorientation, anisocoria

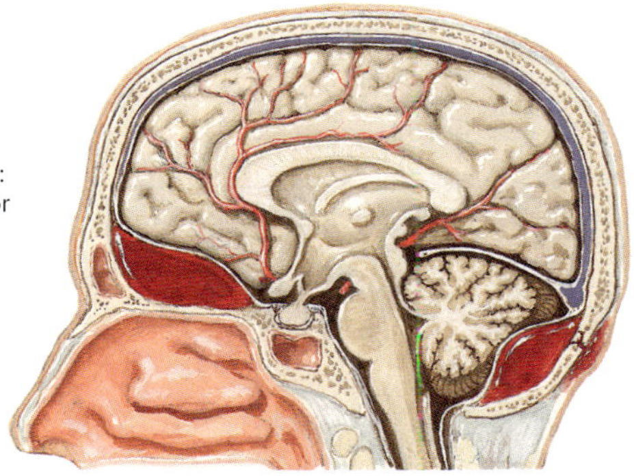

Posterior Fossa Hematoma

Occipital trauma and/or fracture: headache, meningismus, cerebellar and cranial nerve signs, Cushing's triad

Acute Subdural Hematoma

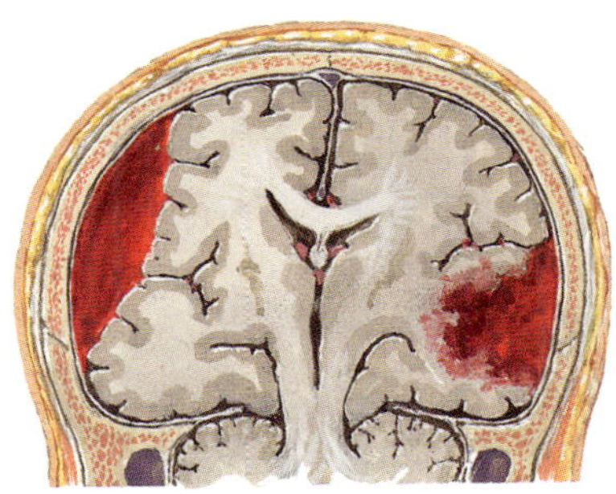

Section showing acute subdural hematoma on right side and subdural hematoma associated with temporal lobe intracerebral hematoma ("burst" temporal lobe) on left

FIGURE 9-10. Transsphenoidal Pituitary Tumor Excision

The pituitary gland is a pea-sized endocrine gland located at the midline of the base of the brain, just posterior to the nasal sinuses. It releases hormones that perform complex functions involving metabolism, growth, and sexual reproduction. Microscopic transsphenoidal surgery is the most common approach for resection of pituitary tumors. Figure 9-10 shows the procedure being performed with direct visualization provided by a nasal speculum. Note: Tools, implants, and/or equipment depicted in the illustration may be outdated but the procedural approach is valid.

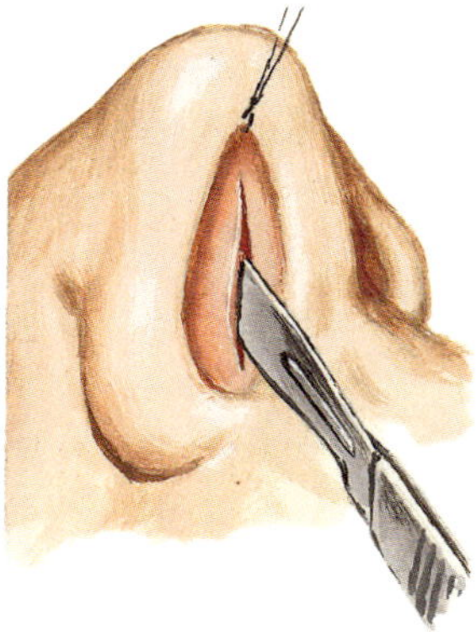

1. Incision in mucosa of nasal septum. Alternate transgingival approach indicated by arrow in figure 2.

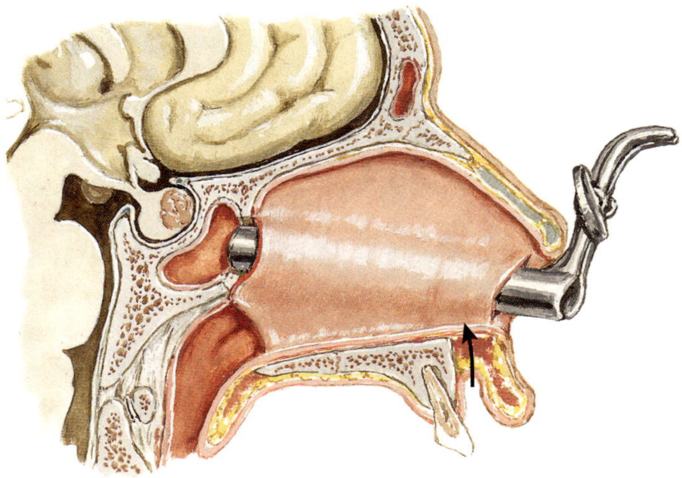

2. Septal mucosa elevated and speculum introduced. Anterior wall of sphenoid sinus removed, exposing its posterior superior wall (roof), which constitutes floor of sella turcica.

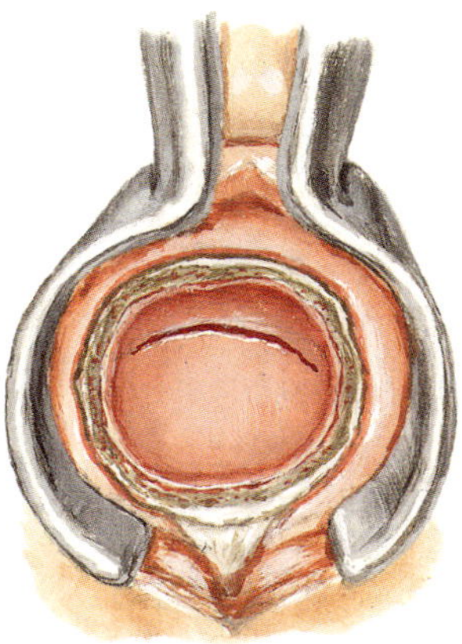

3. View through speculum into sphenoid sinus with incision in roof for opening into sella turcica.

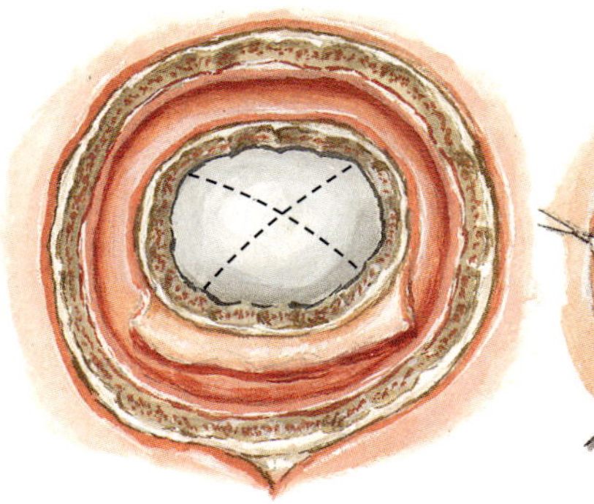

4. Bony floor of sella removed, exposing lining dura. Cruciate incision indicated (view through microscope).

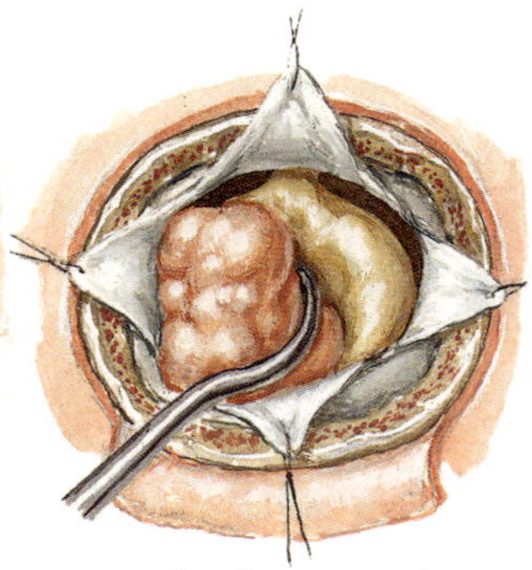

5. Sellar dura opened. Tumor enucleated from remainder of pituitary gland.

Continued on next page

61546 Craniotomy for hypophysectomy or excision of pituitary tumor, intracranial approach

61548 Hypophysectomy or excision of pituitary tumor, transnasal or transseptal approach, nonstereotactic

61550 Craniectomy for craniosynostosis; single cranial suture

61552 multiple cranial sutures

61556 Craniotomy for craniosynostosis; frontal or parietal bone flap

61557 bifrontal bone flap

61558 Extensive craniectomy for multiple cranial suture craniosynostosis (eg, cloverleaf skull); not requiring bone grafts

61559 recontouring with multiple osteotomies and bone autografts (eg, barrel-stave procedure) (includes obtaining grafts)

61563 Excision, intra and extracranial, benign tumor of cranial bone (eg, fibrous dysplasia); without optic nerve decompression

61564 with optic nerve decompression

FIGURE 9-10. Transsphnenoidal Pituitary Tumor Excision ***(continued)***

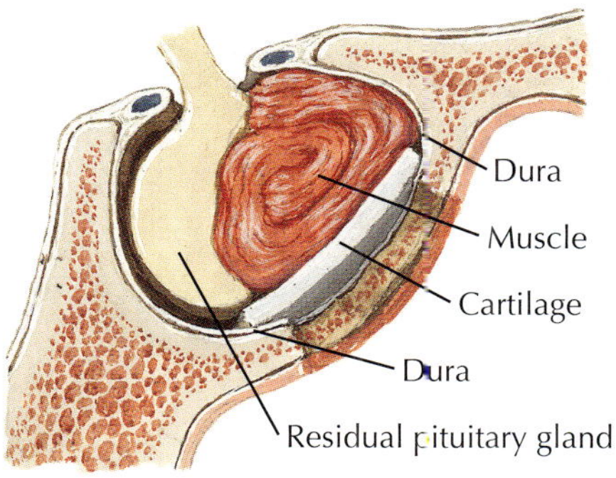

6. After removal of tumor, muscle pack placed in cavity. Piece of cartilage from septum closes opening (enlarged sagittal view).

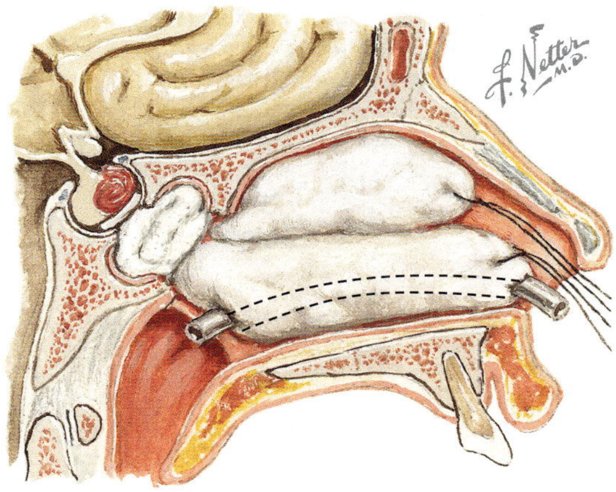

7. Sphenoid sinus packed with Gelfoam; Merocel packs containing airway placed in nose.

61566 Craniotomy with elevation of bone flap; for selective amygdalohippocampectomy

61567 for multiple subpial transections, with electrocorticography during surgery

61570 Craniectomy or craniotomy; with excision of foreign body from brain

61571 with treatment of penetrating wound of brain

61575 Transoral approach to skull base, brain stem or upper spinal cord for biopsy, decompression or excision of lesion;

61576 requiring splitting of tongue and/or mandible (including tracheostomy)

Surgery of Skull Base

Coding Atlas

Because of the complexity of **skull base** surgery, its procedures are reported somewhat differently from other surgical procedures in the CPT code set. In other surgeries, the approach to the surgical site is included in the procedure code. This is not how skull base surgery is coded. Instead, the **approach** is reported, the **therapeutic** or **diagnostic** procedure is reported, and the **repair** or **reconstruction** of the skull entry point is reported. In most cases, a different surgeon will perform each of these tasks. If one surgeon performs multiple components, modifier 51 should be appended to the secondary procedure.

Approach Procedures

Anterior Cranial Fossa

61580 Craniofacial approach to anterior cranial fossa; extradural, including lateral rhinotomy, ethmoidectomy, sphenoidectomy, without maxillectomy or orbital exenteration

61581 extradural, including lateral rhinotomy, orbital exenteration, ethmoidectomy, sphenoidectomy and/or maxillectomy

61582 extradural, including unilateral or bifrontal craniotomy, elevation of frontal lobe(s), osteotomy of base of anterior cranial fossa

61583 intradural, including unilateral or bifrontal craniotomy, elevation or resection of frontal lobe, osteotomy of base of anterior cranial fossa

61584 Orbitocranial approach to anterior cranial fossa, extradural, including supraorbital ridge osteotomy and elevation of frontal and/or temporal lobe(s); without orbital exenteration

61585 with orbital exenteration

61586 Bicoronal, transzygomatic and/or LeFort I osteotomy approach to anterior cranial fossa with or without internal fixation, without bone graft

Middle Cranial Fossa

61590 Infratemporal pre-auricular approach to middle cranial fossa (parapharyngeal space, infratemporal and midline skull base, nasopharynx), with or without disarticulation of the mandible, including parotidectomy, craniotomy, decompression and/or mobilization of the facial nerve and/or petrous carotid artery

FIGURE 9-11. Craniosynostosis and Encephalocele

Primary **craniosynostosis** describes premature **fusion** of cranial sutures in the skull. This fusion usually affects skull shape. In simple craniosynostosis, one suture fuses prematurely. In complex or compound craniosynostosis, multiple sutures are affected. There are specific types of fusion based on the suture affected: scaphocephaly (sagittal); anterior plagiocephaly (coronal); posterior plagiocephaly (lambdoid); brachycephaly (bilateral coronal); and trigonocephaly (metopic). **Encephalocele** is a **neural tube defect** (NTD) that is characterized by a **congenital** sac-like protrusion of brain, cerebrospinal fluid, and meninges.

1

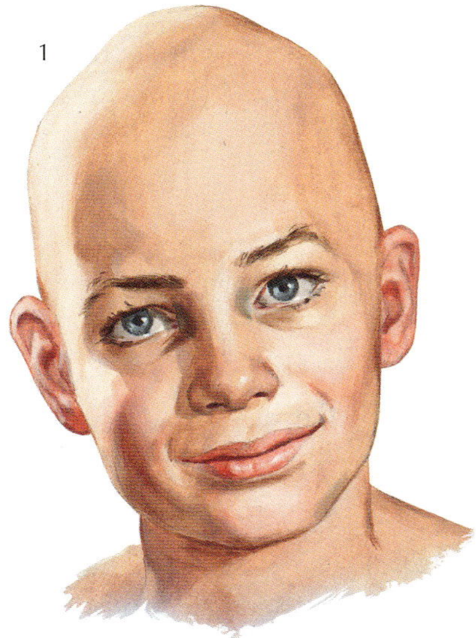

2

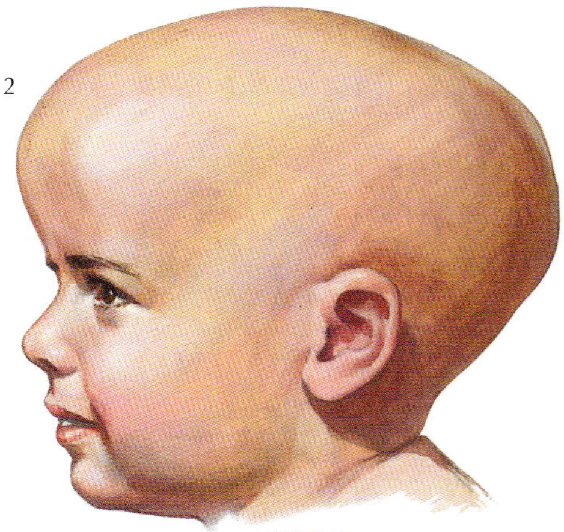

3

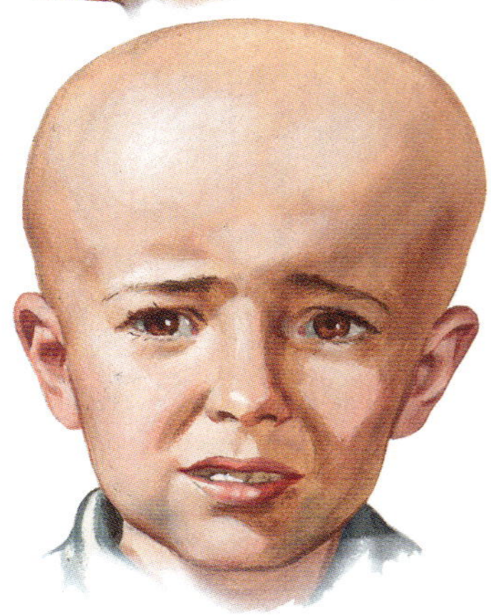

Craniosynostoses
1. Premature closure of coronal and lambdoid sutures (oxycephaly)
2. Premature closure of sagittal suture (scaphocephaly)
3. Premature closure of coronal suture (acrocephaly)

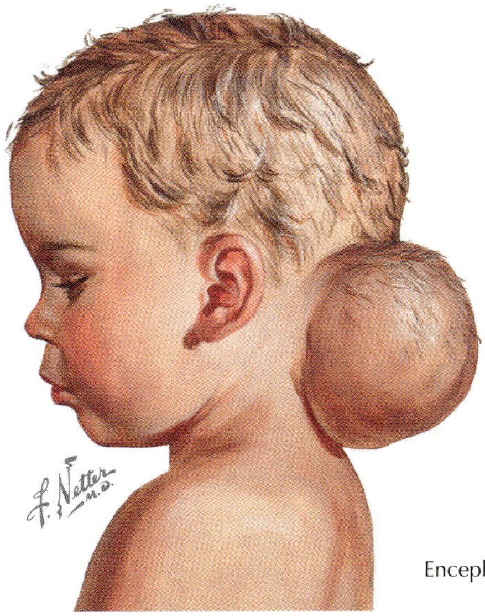

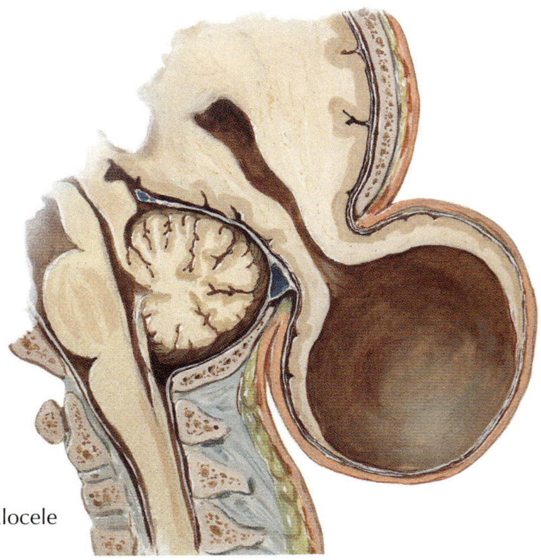

Encephalocele

FIGURE 9-12. Acoustic Neuroma

An acoustic **neuroma** (vestibular **schwannoma**) is a slow-growing **tumor** of the vestibulocochlear nerve (CN VIII) that leads from the inner ear to the brain. It usually develops along the cerebellopontine angle, which is a space filled with CSF, and so may grow quite large before becoming symptomatic. Surgical removal is usually achieved through one of three approaches: **retrosigmoid**, **translabyrinthine**, or **middle cranial fossa**. Most acoustic neuromas are **benign** but can cause significant vestibular symptoms.

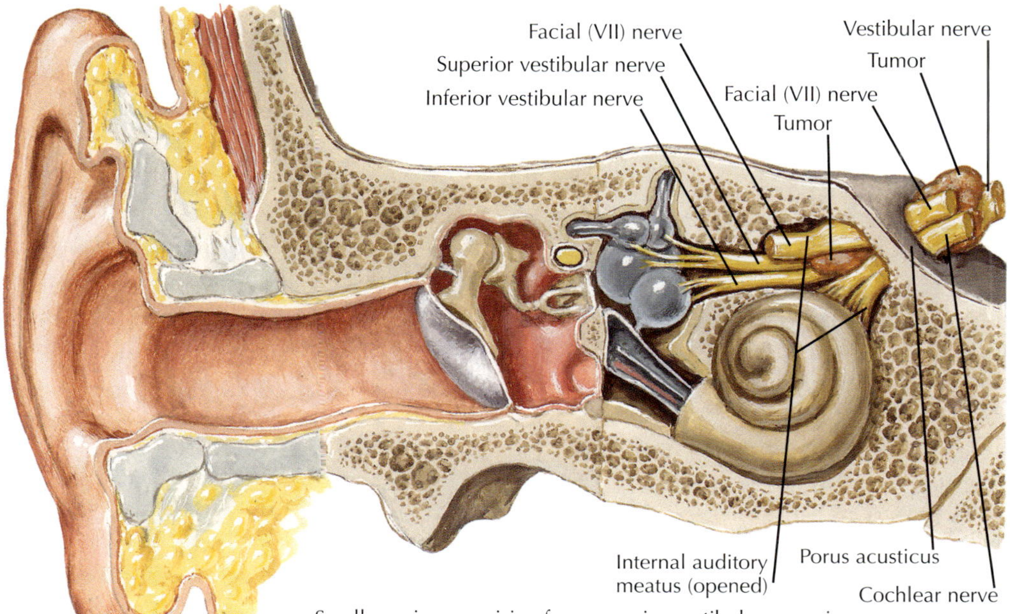

Small neurinoma arising from superior vestibular nerve in internal auditory meatus and protruding into posterior fossa

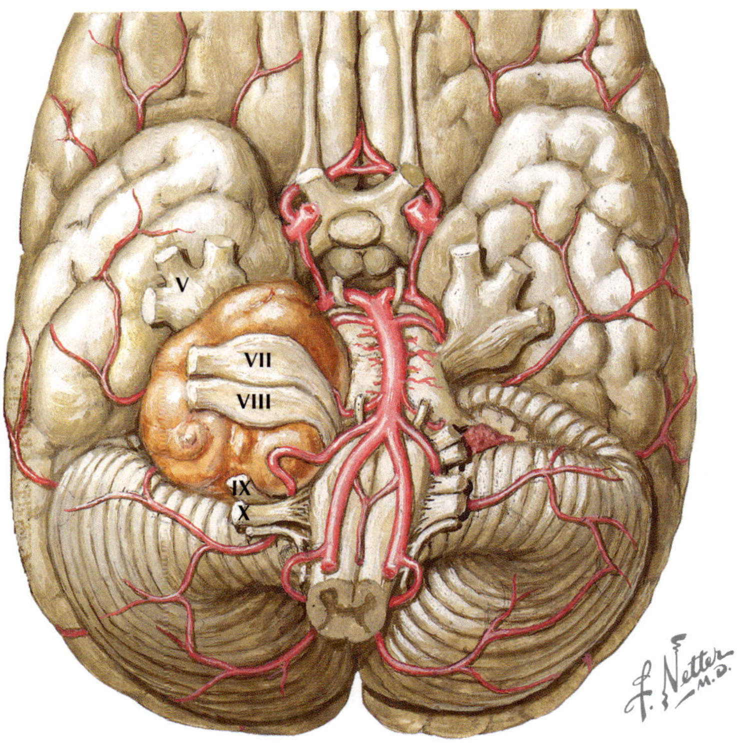

Large acoustic neurinoma filling cerebellopontine angle, distorting brainstem and cranial nerves V, VII, VIII, IX, X

61591 Infratemporal post-auricular approach to middle cranial fossa (internal auditory meatus, petrous apex, tentorium, cavernous sinus, parasellar area, infratemporal fossa) including **mastoidectomy**, resection of sigmoid sinus, with or without decompression and/or **mobilization** of contents of auditory canal or petrous carotid artery

61592 Orbitocranial zygomatic approach to middle cranial fossa (cavernous sinus and carotid artery, clivus, basilar artery or petrous apex) including **osteotomy** of zygoma, craniotomy, extra- or **intradural** elevation of temporal lobe

Posterior Cranial Fossa

61595 **Transtemporal** approach to posterior cranial fossa, jugular foramen or **midline** skull base, including mastoidectomy, decompression of sigmoid sinus and/or facial nerve, with or without mobilization

61596 **Transcochlear** approach to posterior cranial fossa, jugular foramen or midline skull base, including **labyrinthectomy**, decompression, with or without mobilization of facial nerve and/or petrous carotid artery

61597 **Transcondylar** (far lateral) approach to posterior cranial fossa, jugular foramen or midline skull base, including occipital **condylectomy**, mastoidectomy, resection of C1-C3 vertebral body(s), decompression of vertebral artery, with or without mobilization

61598 **Transpetrosal** approach to posterior cranial fossa, clivus or foramen magnum, including **ligation** of superior petrosal sinus and/or sigmoid sinus

Definitive Procedures

Base of Anterior Cranial Fossa

61600 Resection or excision of **neoplastic**, vascular or infectious lesion of base of anterior cranial fossa; extradural

61601 intradural, including **dural** repair, with or without **graft**

Base of Middle Cranial Fossa

61605 Resection or excision of neoplastic, vascular or infectious lesion of infratemporal fossa, **parapharyngeal space**, petrous apex; extradural

61606 intradural, including dural repair, with or without graft

61607 Resection or excision of neoplastic, vascular or infectious lesion of parasellar area, cavernous sinus, clivus or **midline** skull base; extradural

61608 intradural, including dural repair, with or without graft

+ 61610 Transection or ligation, carotid artery in cavernous sinus, with repair by anastomosis or graft (List separately in addition to code for primary procedure)

+ 61611 Transection or ligation, carotid artery in petrous canal; without repair (List separately in addition to code for primary procedure)

+ 61612 with repair by anastomosis or graft (List separately in addition to code for primary procedure)

61613 **Obliteration** of carotid **aneurysm**, arteriovenous malformation, or carotid-cavernous **fistula** by **dissection** within cavernous sinus

Base of Posterior Cranial Fossa

61615 **Resection** or **excision** of **neoplastic**, vascular or infectious lesion of base of **posterior** cranial fossa, jugular foramen, foramen magnum, or C1-C3 vertebral bodies; **extradural**

61616 **intradural**, including dural repair, with or without graft

Repair and/or Reconstruction of Surgical Defects of Skull Base

61618 **Secondary** repair of dura for cerebrospinal fluid leak, **anterior**, middle or **posterior** cranial fossa following surgery of the skull base; by free tissue graft (eg, pericranium, fascia, tensor fascia lata, **adipose** tissue, **homologous** or synthetic grafts)

61619 by local or regionalized vascularized **pedicle flap** or **myocutaneous flap** (including galea, temporalis, frontalis or occipitalis muscle)

Endovascular Therapy

Coding Atlas

Endovascular surgery describes a surgery in which small tools are inserted into the extracranial bloodstream and guided through vessels to the site of a defect, in this case, the brain (intracranial). This allows access to the treatment site without surgical disruption of surrounding brain tissue. Endovascular balloon arterial occlusion codes are based on whether the device is permanent and irreversible (codes 61624, 61626) or temporary and reversible (code 61623). A temporary occlusion is monitored to determine whether the resulting ischemia is detrimental to the patient's cognitive, motor, sensory, visual, memory, or auditory functions before any permanent occlusion is attempted.

61623 Endovascular temporary balloon arterial occlusion, head or neck (extracranial/intracranial) including selective catheterization of vessel to be occluded, positioning and inflation of occlusion balloon, concomitant neurological monitoring, and radiologic supervision and interpretation of all angiography required for balloon occlusion and to exclude vascular injury post occlusion

61624 Transcatheter permanent occlusion or embolization (eg, for tumor destruction, to achieve hemostasis, to occlude a vascular malformation), percutaneous, any method; central nervous system (intracranial, spinal cord)

61626 non-central nervous system, head or neck (extracranial, brachiocephalic branch)

61630 Balloon angioplasty, intracranial (eg, atherosclerotic stenosis), percutaneous

61635 Transcatheter placement of intravascular stent(s), intracranial (eg, atherosclerotic stenosis), including balloon angioplasty, if performed

61640 Balloon dilatation of intracranial vasospasm, percutaneous; initial vessel

✚ 61641 each additional vessel in same vascular family (List separately in addition to code for primary procedure)

✚ 61642 each additional vessel in different vascular family (List separately in addition to code for primary procedure)

Surgery for Aneurysm, Arteriovenous Malformation, or Vascular Disease

Coding Atlas

Codes in this subsection of the CPT code set describe open brain surgery to treat arteriovenous malformation (AVM), aneurysm, or vascular disease. A complex AVM is one that is documented to have a size greater than 3 centimeters and involvement of the eloquent cortex or deep venous drainage.

61680 Surgery of intracranial arteriovenous malformation; supratentorial, simple

61682 supratentorial, complex

61684 infratentorial, simple

61686 infratentorial, complex

61690 dural, simple

61692 dural, complex

61697 Surgery of complex intracranial aneurysm, intracranial approach; carotid circulation

61698 vertebrobasilar circulation

61700 Surgery of simple intracranial aneurysm, intracranial approach; carotid circulation

61702 vertebrobasilar circulation

61703 Surgery of intracranial aneurysm, cervical approach by application of occluding clamp to cervical carotid artery (Selverstone-Crutchfield type)

61705 Surgery of aneurysm, vascular malformation or carotid-cavernous fistula; by intracranial and cervical occlusion of carotid artery

61708 by intracranial electrothrombosis

61710 by intra-arterial embolization, injection procedure, or balloon catheter

61711 Anastomosis, arterial, extracranial-intracranial (eg, middle cerebral/cortical) arteries

FIGURE 9-13. Balloon Embolization

Carotid-cavernous sinus **fistula** is an abnormal communication between a meningeal branch of the internal or external carotid artery and the venous cavernous sinus and can be treated with balloon **embolization** (**occlusion**). The fistula may be treated with **open** surgery, **electrothrombosis**, or balloon embolization. Figure 9-13 shows a **transcatheter** balloon occlusion of the fistula. Note: Tools, implants, and/or equipment depicted in the illustration may be outdated but the procedural approach is valid.

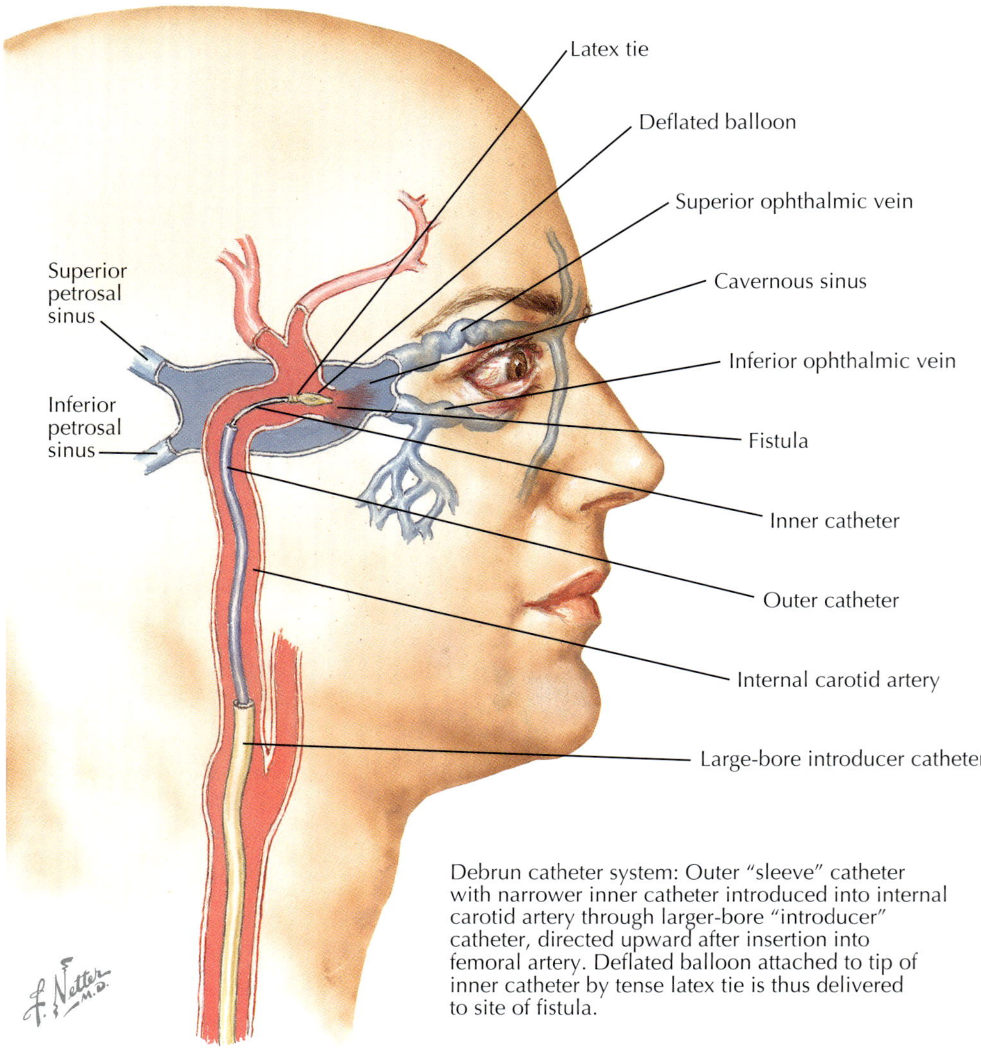

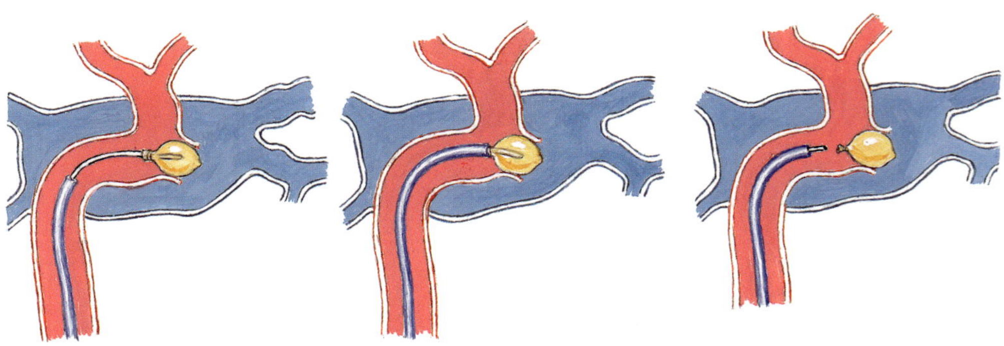

Ballon inflated with radiopaque fluid occluding fistula

Outer catheter advanced over inner catheter to engage balloon cuff

Balloon liberated by slight pull on inner catheter. Balloon neck spontaneously constricted by tense latex tie. All catheters then withdrawn.

Stereotaxis

Coding Atlas

Severe disease, tumor, trauma, or deformity may alter normal anatomic landmarks. Stereotaxis can reduce risk during surgery by precisely mapping individual anatomy for the physician. In stereotactic computer-assisted (navigational) procedures, the surgeon plans the routes and methods for a surgical procedure before the operation begins by creating a three-dimensional image that allows him or her to predict difficulties and assess risks associated with approach and excision or repair.

61720 Creation of lesion by stereotactic method, including burr hole(s) and localizing and recording techniques, single or multiple stages; globus pallidus or thalamus

61735 subcortical structure(s) other than globus pallidus or thalamus

61750 Stereotactic biopsy, aspiration, or excision, including burr hole(s), for intracranial lesion;

61751 with computed tomography and/or magnetic resonance guidance

61760 Stereotactic implantation of depth electrodes into the cerebrum for long-term seizure monitoring

61770 Stereotactic localization, including burr hole(s), with insertion of catheter(s) or probe(s) for placement of radiation source

+ 61781 Stereotactic computer-assisted (navigational) procedure; cranial, intradural (List separately in addition to code for primary procedure)

+ 61782 cranial, extradural (List separately in addition to code for primary procedure)

+ 61783 spinal (List separately in addition to code for primary procedure)

61790 Creation of lesion by stereotactic method, percutaneous, by neurolytic agent (eg, alcohol, thermal, electrical, radiofrequency); gasserian ganglion

61791 trigeminal medullary tract

Stereotactic Radiosurgery (Cranial)

Coding Atlas

Stereotaxis can reduce risk from radiation therapy by precisely mapping individual anatomy for the physician. In stereotactic radiosurgery, radiation treats a defect. The physician maps out a defined target for eradication, and an externally generated ionizing radiation beam is focused on the target. Simple lesions are described as those smaller than 3.5 centimeters in maximum dimension that are not otherwise complex. Complex lesions include those 3.5 centimeters or larger and all schwannomas, AVMs, and tumors in the pituitary, glomus, pineal region, and cavernous sinus/parasellar/petroclival regions. Also, any lesion adjacent to the optic nerve, chasm, or tract or a lesion within the brainstem is considered complex. For stereotactic radiosurgery of the brain, the surgeon uses codes in the range 61796-61800 to report radiosurgery and headframe services. The radiation oncologist would report separately services for clinical treatment planning, dosimetry, physics, treatment delivery, and management.

61796 Stereotactic radiosurgery (particle beam, gamma ray, or linear accelerator); 1 simple cranial lesion

+ 61797 each additional cranial lesion, simple (List separately in addition to code for primary procedure)

61798 1 complex cranial lesion

+ 61799 each additional cranial lesion, complex (List separately in addition to code for primary procedure)

+ 61800 Application of stereotactic headframe for stereotactic radiosurgery (List separately in addition to code for primary procedure)

FIGURE 9-14. Functional Areas for Neurostimulation

Intracranial **neurostimulation** describes surgical placement of an electrical impulse probe for therapeutic reasons. For example, a **deep brain stimulator** (DBS) placed in the globus pallidus interni (GPi) or subthalamic nucleus (STN) may reduce symptoms of Parkinson disease, essential tremor, and multiple sclerosis. Stimulation of the vagal nerve coming from the medulla oblongata may be prescribed for patients with epilepsy who are intolerant of antiepileptic drug therapy or whose seizure activity cannot be adequately controlled.

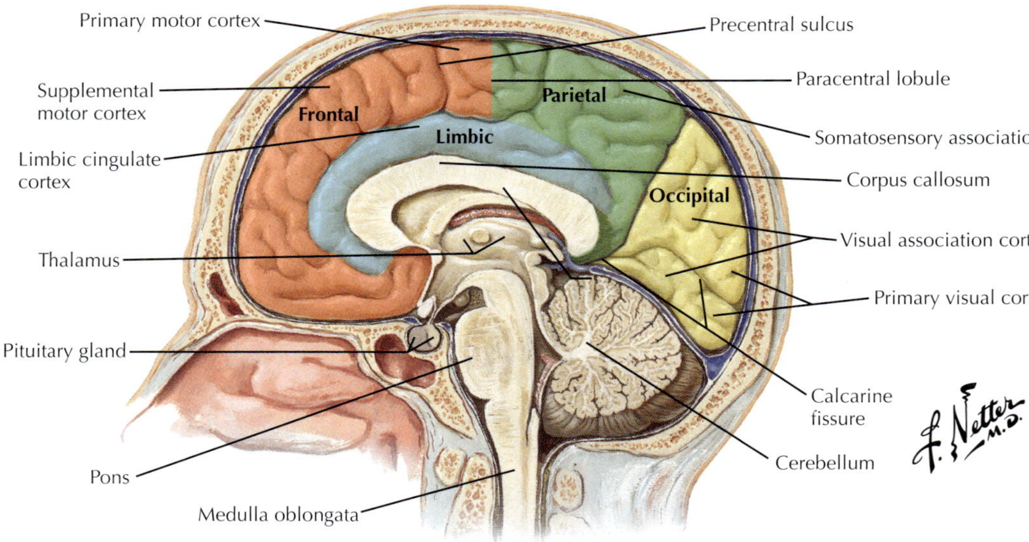

Neurostimulators (Intracranial)

Coding Atlas

An **intracranial** neurostimulator is an electrode array implanted at a predetermined site to suppress tremors, seizures, or other **functional disorders**. **Bilateral** symptoms and findings may require treatment with bilateral electrode arrays. One electrode array may be connected to one pulse generator or receiver, or two electrode arrays (one on each side of the brain) may be required and be connected to one generator or receiver. The **neurostimulator** insertion/removal codes do not include evaluation, testing, programming, or reprogramming. These services are reported with codes from the Medicine section of the CPT code set.

61850 Twist drill or burr hole(s) for implantation of neurostimulator electrodes, cortical

61860 Craniectomy or craniotomy for implantation of neurostimulator electrodes, cerebral, cortical

61863 Twist drill, burr hole, craniotomy, or craniectomy with stereotactic implantation of neurostimulator electrode array in subcortical site (eg, thalamus, globus pallidus, subthalamic nucleus, periventricular, periaqueductal gray), without use of intraoperative microelectrode recording; first array

✚ 61864 each additional array (List separately in addition to primary procedure)

61867 Twist drill, burr hole, craniotomy, or craniectomy with stereotactic implantation of neurostimulator electrode array in subcortical site (eg, thalamus, globus pallidus, subthalamic nucleus, periventricular, periaqueductal gray), with use of intraoperative microelectrode recording; first array

✚ 61868 each additional array (List separately in addition to primary procedure)

61870 Craniectomy for implantation of neurostimulator electrodes, cerebellar, cortical

61880 Revision or removal of intracranial neurostimulator electrodes

61885 Insertion or replacement of cranial neurostimulator pulse generator or receiver, direct or inductive coupling; with connection to a single electrode array

61886 with connection to 2 or more electrode arrays

61888 Revision or removal of cranial neurostimulator pulse generator or receiver

FIGURE 9-15. Depressed Skull Fracture

A depressed skull fracture (DSF) is usually the result of a direct, high-energy blow to the head, eg, a blow from a baseball bat. DSFs create a crater in the skull that translates into an intrusion of the bone into brain tissue. DSFs may be open or closed. In most cases, surgical intervention to elevate the depressed skull bones is performed, with **craniotomy** for removal of any destroyed brain tissue, attention to any **hemorrhage**, and/or repair of any dural tear.

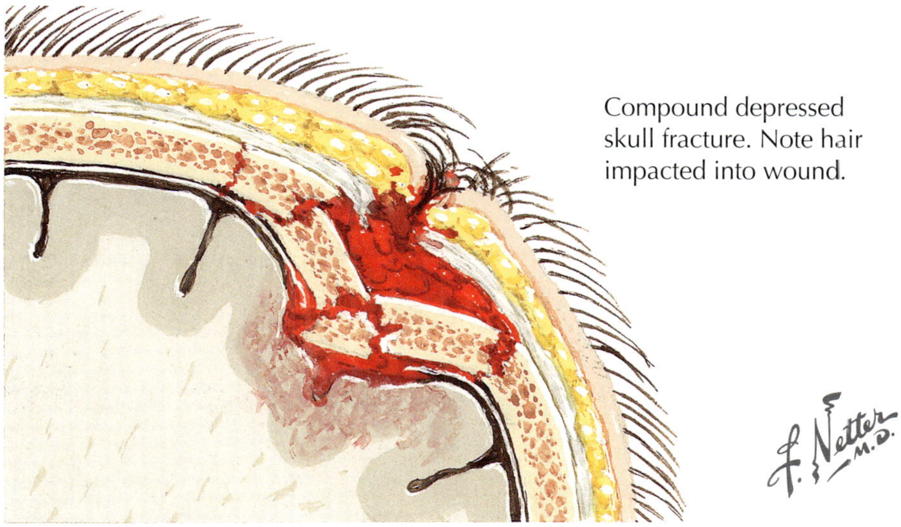

Compound depressed skull fracture. Note hair impacted into wound.

Repair

Coding Atlas

Cerebrospinal fluid (CSF) leaking into the middle ear and Eustachian tube (**otorrhea**) or nasal cavities (**rhinorrhea**) is the hallmark of an abnormal communication between the subarachnoid space and the ear/nose. This puts the patient at risk for meningitis since the sterile subarachnoid space is exposed to the unsterile environment of the ear/nose/throat. The leak may occur following surgery, may be **congenital**, or may be the result of injury or erosive disease.

62000 Elevation of depressed skull fracture; simple, extradural

62005 compound or comminuted, extradural

62010 with repair of dura and/or debridement of brain

62100 Craniotomy for repair of dural/cerebrospinal fluid leak, including surgery for rhinorrhea/otorrhea

62115 Reduction of craniomegalic skull (eg, treated hydrocephalus); not requiring bone grafts or cranioplasty

62117 requiring craniotomy and reconstruction with or without bone graft (includes obtaining grafts)

62120 Repair of encephalocele, skull vault, including cranioplasty

62121 Craniotomy for repair of encephalocele, skull base

62140 Cranioplasty for skull defect; up to 5 cm diameter

62141 larger than 5 cm diameter

62142 Removal of bone flap or prosthetic plate of skull

62143 Replacement of bone flap or prosthetic plate of skull

62145 Cranioplasty for skull defect with reparative brain surgery

62146 Cranioplasty with autograft (includes obtaining bone grafts); up to 5 cm diameter

62147 larger than 5 cm diameter

✚ 62148 Incision and retrieval of subcutaneous cranial bone graft for cranioplasty (List separately in addition to code for primary procedure)

Neuroendoscopy

Coding Atlas

Neuroendoscopy of the brain enables the physician to visually inspect and also treat the brain using a camera that projects an image onto a video display or into an eyepiece. The scope is inserted through a small hole in any portion of the skull and guided to the target site. Tools can be fed through the scoping device to the site of a defect so that the defect can be treated.

✚ **62160** Neuroendoscopy, intracranial, for placement or replacement of ventricular catheter and attachment to shunt system or external drainage (List separately in addition to code for primary procedure)

62161 Neuroendoscopy, intracranial; with dissection of adhesions, fenestration of septum pellucidum or intraventricular cysts (including placement, replacement, or removal of ventricular catheter)

62162 with fenestration or excision of colloid cyst, including placement of external ventricular catheter for drainage

62163 with retrieval of foreign body

62164 with excision of brain tumor, including placement of external ventricular catheter for drainage

62165 with excision of pituitary tumor, transnasal or trans-sphenoidal approach

Cerebrospinal Fluid Shunt

Coding Atlas

A cerebrospinal fluid (CSF) shunt reduces the volume of CSF. Ventriculocisternostomy is the surgical creation of a connection between the ventricle and cisternal space. If a ventriculocisternostomy of the third ventricle is performed using a stereotactic method, endoscopy, or a stereotactic method with endoscopy, code 62201 is reported. A Torkildsen-type operation (code 62180) is normally reserved for acquired obstructive hydrocephalus.

62180 Ventriculocisternostomy (Torkildsen type operation)

62190 Creation of shunt; subarachnoid/subdural-atrial, -jugular, -auricular

62192 subarachnoid/subdural-peritoneal, -pleural, other terminus

62194 Replacement or irrigation, subarachnoid/subdural catheter

62200 Ventriculocisternostomy, third ventricle;

62201 stereotactic, neuroendoscopic method

62220 Creation of shunt; ventriculo-atrial, -jugular, -auricular

62223 ventriculo-peritoneal, -pleural, other terminus

62225 Replacement or irrigation, ventricular catheter

62230 Replacement or revision of cerebrospinal fluid shunt, obstructed valve, or distal catheter in shunt system

62252 Reprogramming of programmable cerebrospinal shunt

62256 Removal of complete cerebrospinal fluid shunt system; without replacement

62258 with replacement by similar or other shunt at same operation

FIGURE 9-16. Cerebrospinal Fluid Circulation

Fresh cerebrospinal fluid (CSF) is produced from blood **plasma** by the choroid plexus in each ventricle. Old CSF is absorbed into the dural venous sinuses via the arachnoid villi. Constantly circulating CSF travels from the **lateral** ventricles to the third ventricle via the aqueduct of Sylvius. From the third ventricle, CSF flows to the fourth ventricle and then out into the subarachnoid space. Some CSF travels into the central canal of the spinal cord via the **median** aperture.

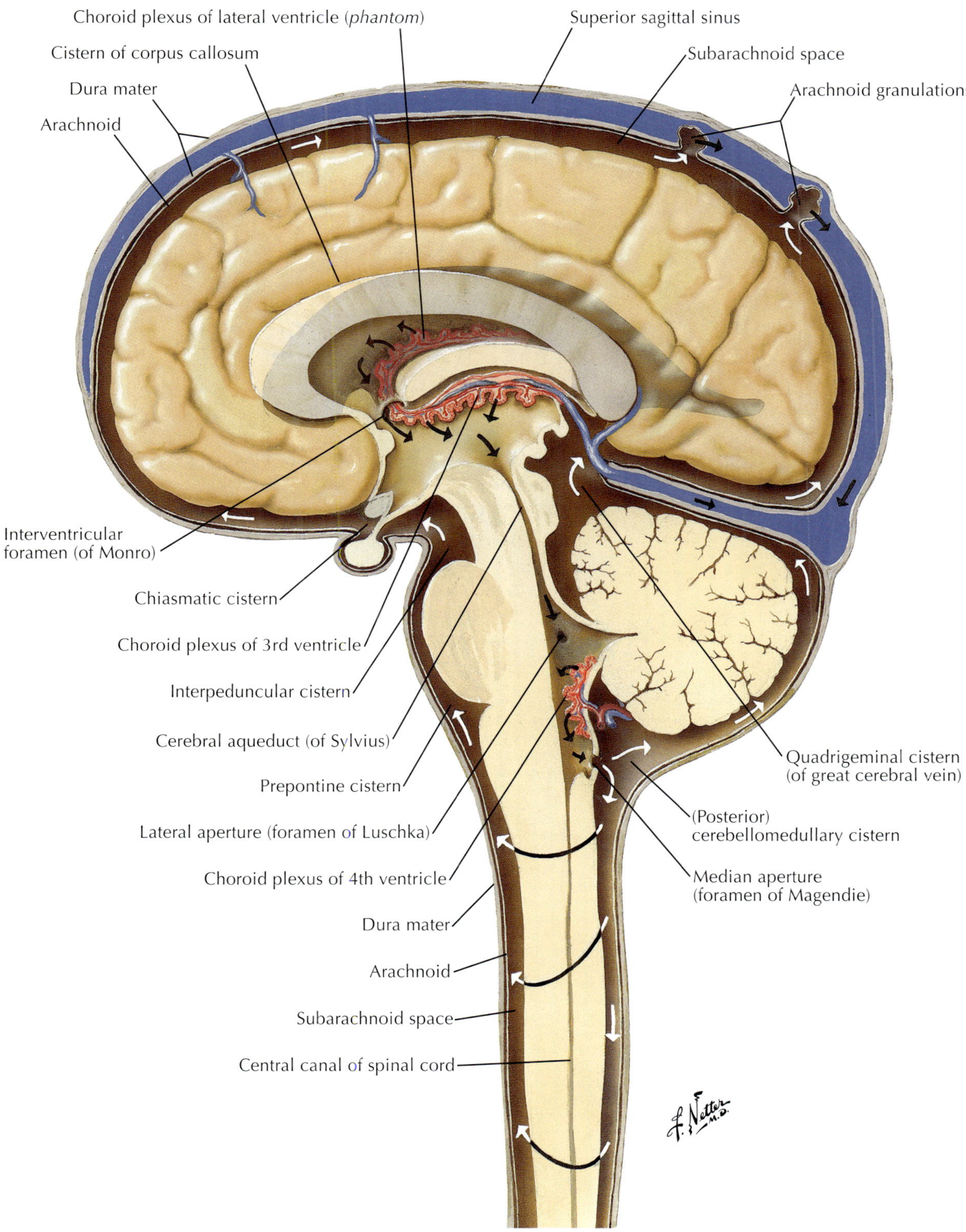

FIGURE 9-17. Hydrocephalus

Hydrocephalus is an abnormal condition in which the cerebrospinal fluid (CSF) balance is disturbed, resulting in a buildup of CSF in the brain. This may lead to increased intracranial pressure (ICP), distortion of the skull bones, and diminished mental capacity. Hydrocephalus may be **congenital** or acquired and can be corrected with surgical placement of a shunt to drain excess CSF. The most common treatment is a ventriculoperitoneal (VP) **shunt**, illustrated in Figure 9-17. Note: Tools, implants, and/or equipment depicted in the illustration may be outdated but the procedural approach is valid.

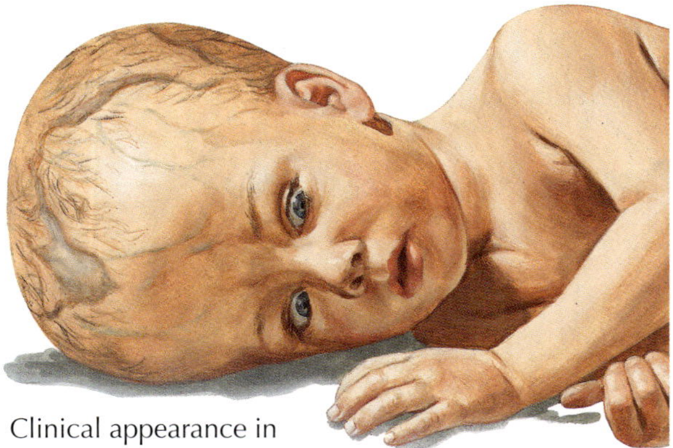

Clinical appearance in advanced hydrocephalus

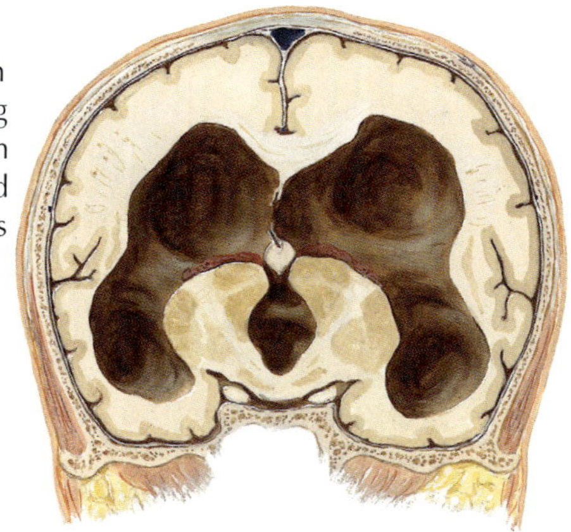

Section through brain showing marked dilatation of lateral and 3rd ventricles

Potential lesion sites in obstructive hydrocephalus

1. Interventricular foramina (of Monro)
2. Cerebral aqueduct (of Sylvius)
3. Lateral apertures (of Luschka)
4. Median aperture (of Magendie)

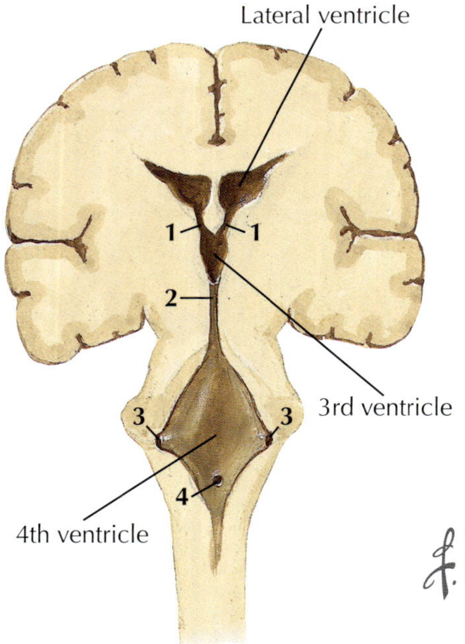

Shunt procedure for hydrocephalus

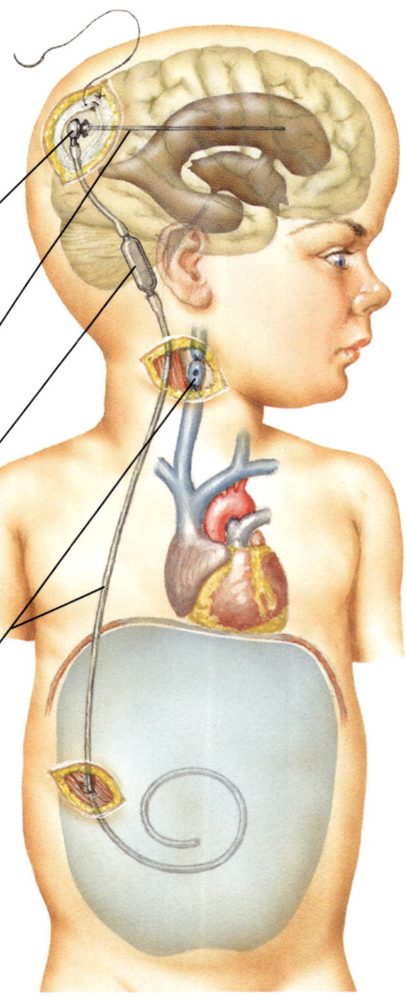

Reservoir at end of cannula implanted beneath galea permits transcutaneous needle puncture for withdrawal of CSF, introduction of antibiotics, or dye to test patency of shunt.

Cannula inserted into lateral ventricle

One-way valve to prevent reflux of blood or peritoneal fluid and control CSF pressure

Drainage tube may be introduced into internal jugular v. and thence into right atrium via neck incision, or may be continued subcutaneously to abdomen.

Spine and Spinal Cord

Injection, Drainage, or Aspiration

Coding Atlas

Scar tissue can be a source of lower back pain (LBP). Epidural **neurolysis** (codes 62263, 62264) breaks up scar tissue and reduces inflammation to treat LBP. **Epidural** neurolysis is also referred to as epidural **neuroplasty** or **lysis** of epidural **adhesions**. Codes 62263 and 62264 should be reported only once during an episode of care, regardless of how many injections/infusions or mechanical lysis procedures are performed.

62263 Percutaneous lysis of epidural adhesions using solution injection (eg, hypertonic saline, enzyme) or mechanical means (eg, catheter) including radiologic localization (includes contrast when administered), multiple adhesiolysis sessions; 2 or more days

62264 1 day

62267 Percutaneous aspiration within the nucleus pulposus, intervertebral disc, or paravertebral tissue for diagnostic purposes

62268 Percutaneous aspiration, spinal cord cyst or syrinx

62269 Biopsy of spinal cord, percutaneous needle

62270 Spinal puncture, lumbar, diagnostic

62272 Spinal puncture, therapeutic, for drainage of cerebrospinal fluid (by needle or catheter)

62273 Injection, epidural, of blood or clot patch

62280 Injection/infusion of neurolytic substance (eg, alcohol, phenol, iced saline solutions), with or without other therapeutic substance; subarachnoid

62281 epidural, cervical or thoracic

62282 epidural, lumbar, sacral (caudal)

62284 Injection procedure for myelography and/or computed tomography, lumbar (other than C1-C2 and posterior fossa)

62287 Decompression procedure, percutaneous, of nucleus pulposus of intervertebral disc, any method utilizing needle based technique to remove disc material under fluoroscopic imaging or other form of indirect visualization, with the use of an endoscope, with discography and/or epidural injection(s) at the treated level(s), when performed, single or multiple levels, lumbar

62290 Injection procedure for discography, each level; lumbar

62291 cervical or thoracic

62292 Injection procedure for chemonucleolysis, including discography, intervertebral disc, single or multiple levels, lumbar

62294 Injection procedure, arterial, for occlusion of arteriovenous malformation, spinal

62302 Myelography via lumbar injection, including radiological supervision and interpretation; cervical

62303 thoracic

62304 lumbosacral

62305 2 or more regions (eg, lumbar/thoracic, cervical/thoracic, lumbar/cervical, lumbar/thoracic/cervical)

62310 Injection(s), of diagnostic or therapeutic substance(s) (including anesthetic, antispasmodic, opioid, steroid, other solution), not including neurolytic substances, including needle or catheter placement, includes contrast for localization when performed, epidural or subarachnoid; cervical or thoracic

62311 lumbar or sacral (caudal)

62318 Injection(s), including indwelling catheter placement, continuous infusion or intermittent bolus, of diagnostic or therapeutic substance(s) (including anesthetic, antispasmodic, opioid, steroid, other solution), not including neurolytic substances, includes contrast for localization when performed, epidural or subarachnoid; cervical or thoracic

62319 lumbar or sacral (caudal)

FIGURE 9-18. The Spinal Cord

Motor nerve roots enter the **anterior** (**ventral**) spinal cord **bilaterally** at each level, sending signals to the brain from the peripheral nervous system (PNS). Sensory nerve roots emerge from the **posterior** (**dorsal**) spinal cord bilaterally at each level, sending signals to the PNS from the brain. Sensory nerves are **afferent** nerves that send signals to the central nervous system (CNS), while motor nerves are **efferent** nerves that send signals from the CNS. There are 8 cervical, 12 thoracic, 5 lumbar, 5 sacral, and 1 coccygeal spinal cord levels.

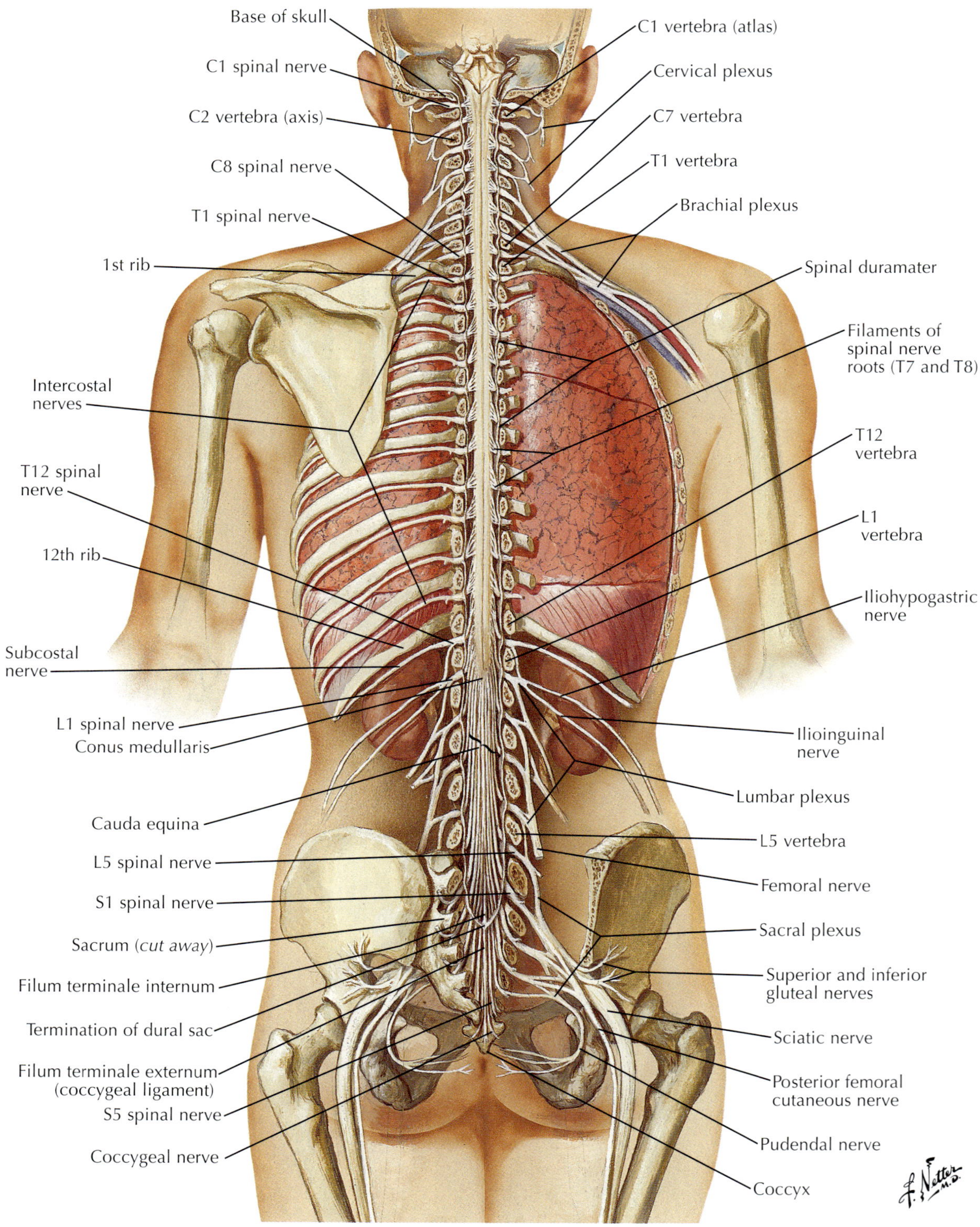

FIGURE 9-19. Dermatomes

Spinal nerve roots are named and numbered according to the site of their insertion or emergence along the vertebral canal. **Dermatomes** have been mapped for each of 31 pairs of spinal nerve roots. A dermatome represents an isolated skin area tied to 1 of the 31 paired spinal nerve roots. Because dermatomes map to only one nerve root level, it may be possible to derive from the site of a skin **neuropathy** the level of a **spinal nerve root** defect.

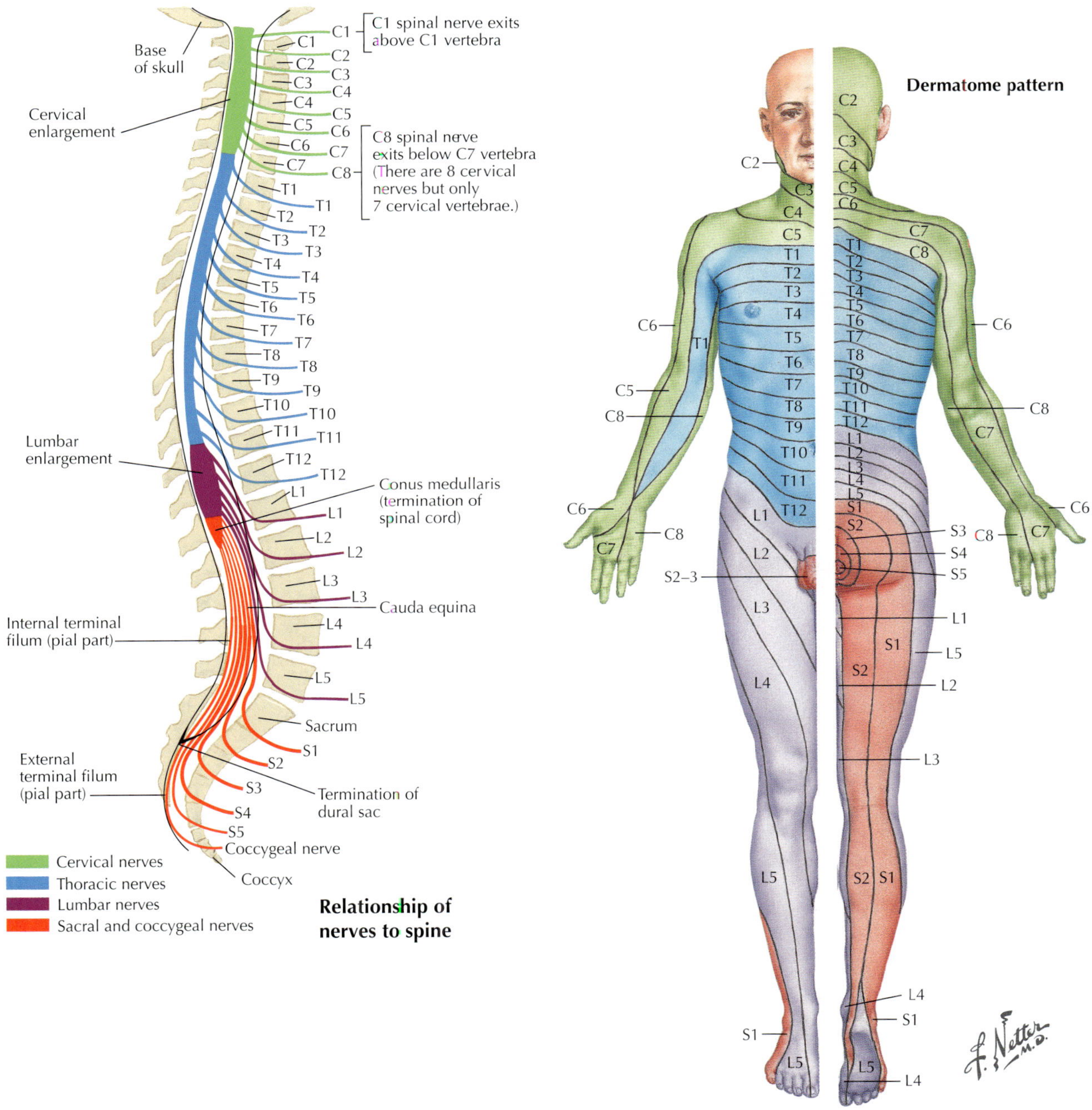

Levels of principal dermatomes

C5	Clavicles
C5, 6, 7	Lateral parts of upper limbs
C8; T1	Medial sides of upper limbs
C6	Thumb
C6, 7, 8	Hand
C8	Ring and little fingers
T4	Level of nipples
T10	Level of umbilicus
T12	Inguinal or groin regions
L1, 2, 3, 4	Anterior and inner surfaces of lower limbs
L4, 5; S1	Foot
L4	Medial side of great toe
L5; S1, 2	Outer and posterior sides of lower limbs
S1	Lateral margin of foot and little toe
S2, 3, 4	Perineum

FIGURE 9-20. Lumbar Puncture and Epidural Injection

Lumbar puncture allows the physician to **aspirate** cerebrospinal fluid (CSF) that is used to obtain information about potentially life-threatening conditions including bacterial meningitis and **subarachnoid** hemorrhage. In some cases, aspiration may also be **therapeutic**. An injection of anesthetic into the **epidural** space of the lumbar spine can provide a regional **pain block** that is common to some surgeries and to labor and delivery. Note: Tools, implants, and/or equipment depicted in the illustration may be outdated but the procedural approach is valid.

Lumbar puncture

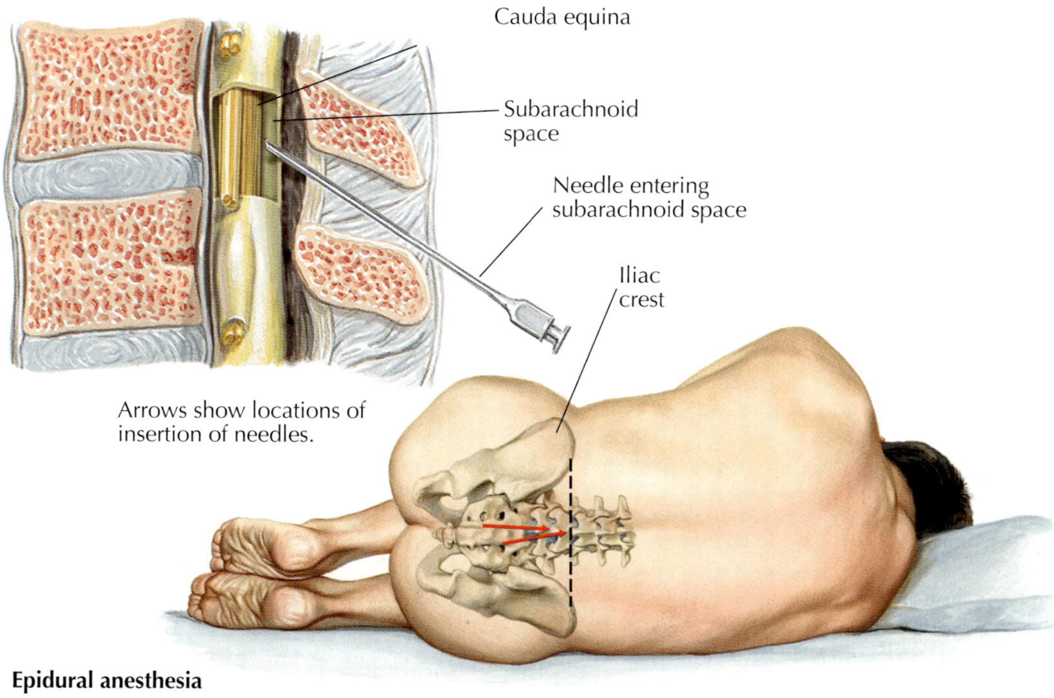

Epidural anesthesia

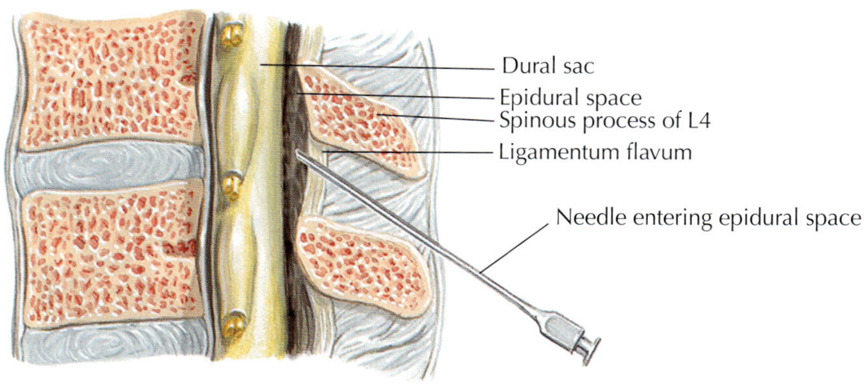

Epidural anesthesia and lumbar puncture are performed by inserting a needle above or below the L4 vertebral spine, which lies at the level of the iliac crest. For epidural anesthesia, the needle passes into the epidural space, and anesthetic agent bathes the nerve roots in proximity. Lumbar puncture, on the other hand, is performed in order to collect a sample of cerebrospinal fluid (CSF) or to introduce an anesthetic agent into the CSF (spinal anesthesia), therefore the needle penetrates the dural sac to enter the subarachnoid space.

Catheter Implantation

Coding Atlas

Codes in the range 62350-62355 are used to report catheter placement/removal for long-term administration of pain medication, chemotherapeutic drugs, antibiotics, and antispasmodic agents via the spine or spinal cord.

62350 Implantation, revision or repositioning of tunneled intrathecal or epidural catheter, for long-term medication administration via an external pump or implantable reservoir/infusion pump; without laminectomy

62351 with laminectomy

62355 Removal of previously implanted intrathecal or epidural catheter

Reservoir/Pump Implantation

Coding Atlas

Epidural or intrathecal implantable infusion delivery pumps deliver drugs to the space just outside the spinal cord in the vertebral canal (epidural) or into the cerebrospinal fluid (CSF) adjacent to the spinal cord (intrathecal). Implantable spinal infusion pumps are intended to delivery therapeutic levels of drugs for a prolonged period. The pump is inserted into a pocket surgically created in the subcutaneous tissue. The reservoir is refilled by inserting a syringe needle through the skin and into the port and injecting a new supply of medication. A catheter from the pump reservoir leads to the epidural or intrathecal infusion site. Typically, this type of system delivers antispasmodics or pain relief.

62360 Implantation or replacement of device for intrathecal or epidural drug infusion; subcutaneous reservoir

62361 nonprogrammable pump

62362 programmable pump, including preparation of pump, with or without programming

62365 Removal of subcutaneous reservoir or pump, previously implanted for intrathecal or epidural infusion

62367 Electronic analysis of programmable, implanted pump for intrathecal or epidural drug infusion (includes evaluation of reservoir status, alarm status, drug prescription status); without reprogramming or refill

62368 with reprogramming

62369 with reprogramming and refill

62370 with reprogramming and refill (requiring skill of a physician or other qualified health care professional)

Posterior Extradural Laminotomy or Laminectomy for Exploration/ Decompression of Neural Elements or Excision of Herniated Intervertebral Discs

Coding Atlas

A spinal interspace is defined as the soft tissue between two vertebrae. Within the interspace is an intravertebral disc, which is encapsulated soft tissue that yields to movement and prevents contact between vertebrae. The interspace also includes the neural foramen through which four spinal nerve roots travel: right and left afferent and right and left efferent nerves. An interspace and the spinal nerves that enter and exit at that level may be identified by the same level as the adjacent and superior vertebra.

63001 Laminectomy with exploration and/or decompression of spinal cord and/or cauda equina, without facetectomy, foraminotomy or discectomy (eg, spinal stenosis), 1 or 2 vertebral segments; cervical

63003 thoracic

63005 lumbar, except for spondylolisthesis

63011 sacral

63012 Laminectomy with removal of abnormal facets and/or pars inter-articularis with decompression of cauda equina and nerve roots for spondylolisthesis, lumbar (Gill type procedure)

63015 Laminectomy with exploration and/or decompression of spinal cord and/or cauda equina, without facetectomy, foraminotomy or discectomy (eg, spinal stenosis), more than 2 vertebral segments; cervical

63016 thoracic

63017 lumbar

63020 Laminotomy (hemilaminectomy), with decompression of nerve root(s), including partial facetectomy, foraminotomy and/or excision of herniated intervertebral disc; 1 interspace, cervical

63030 1 interspace, lumbar

✚ 63035 each additional interspace, cervical or lumbar (List separately in addition to code for primary procedure)

63040 Laminotomy (hemilaminectomy), with decompression of nerve root(s), including partial facetectomy, foraminotomy and/or excision of herniated intervertebral disc, reexploration, single interspace; cervical

63042 lumbar

✚ 63043 each additional cervical interspace (List separately in addition to code for primary procedure)

✚ 63044 each additional lumbar interspace (List separately in addition to code for primary procedure)

FIGURE 9-21. Herniations Affecting the Spinal Cord

A defect in an intervertebral disc may cause it to bulge (**herniate**) against an adjacent nerve root. The herniation compresses the nerve, which may result in weakness if it affects a motor nerve, or numbness if it affects a sensory nerve. In addition, compression of either type of nerve may cause pain. The herniation may be referred to as a slipped or ruptured disc. The most common herniation site is the lumbar spine and the most common symptom is leg pain (sciatica). Cervical herniation is illustrated in Figure 9-21.

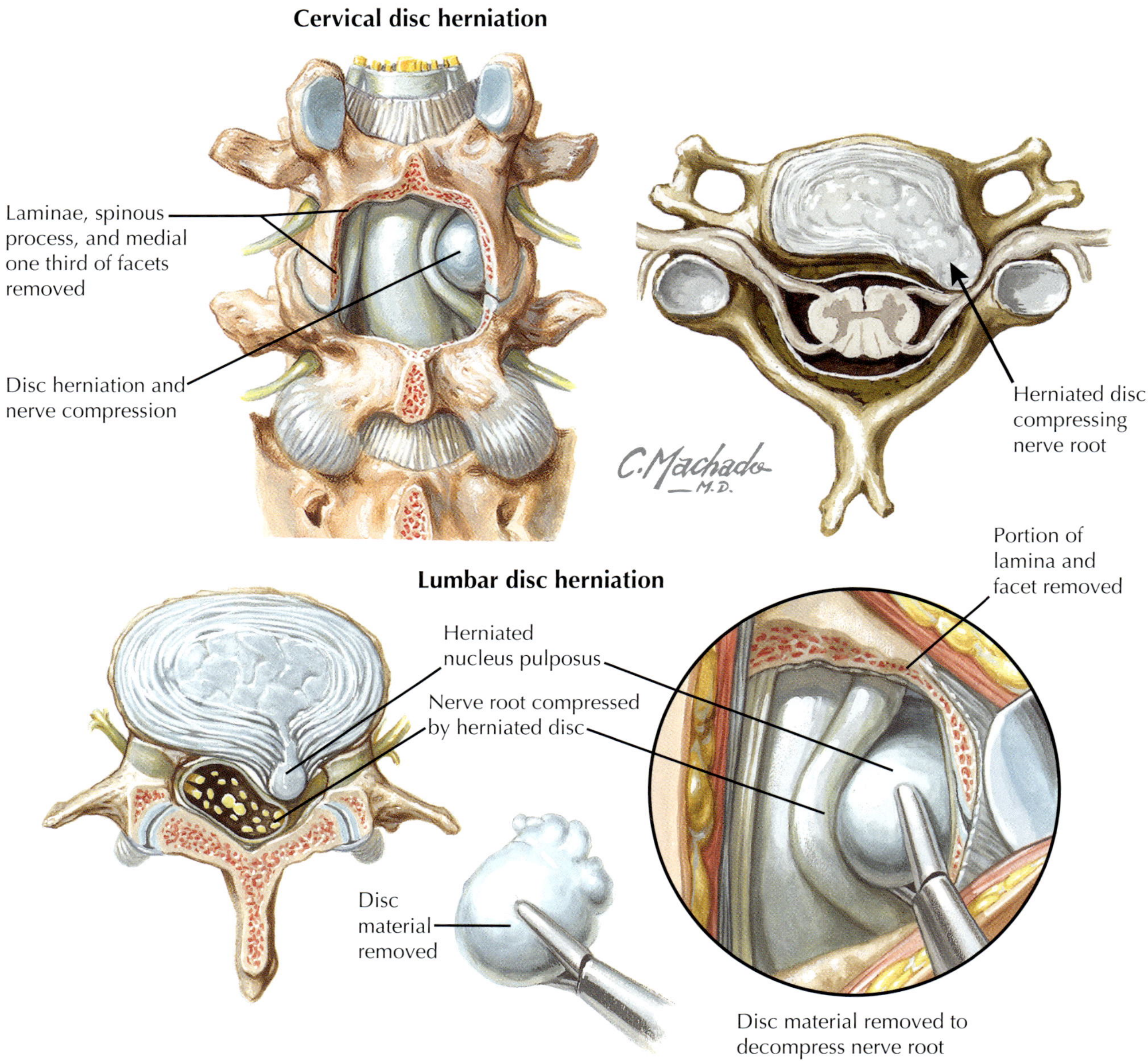

FIGURE 9-22. Spinal Membranes and Nerve Roots

With the exception of the uppermost spinal level, each level of spine has four nerve roots: an **anterior (ventral)** motor nerve and **posterior (dorsal)** sensory nerve on the right side and also on the left side of the spinal column. Each nerve governs sensations and motor signals on the **ipsilateral** side. Within the spinal canal, the ventral and dorsal roots merge to form a mixed spinal nerve that exits through the intervertebral canal. Note: Tools, implants, and/or equipment depicted in the illustration may be outdated but the procedural approach is valid.

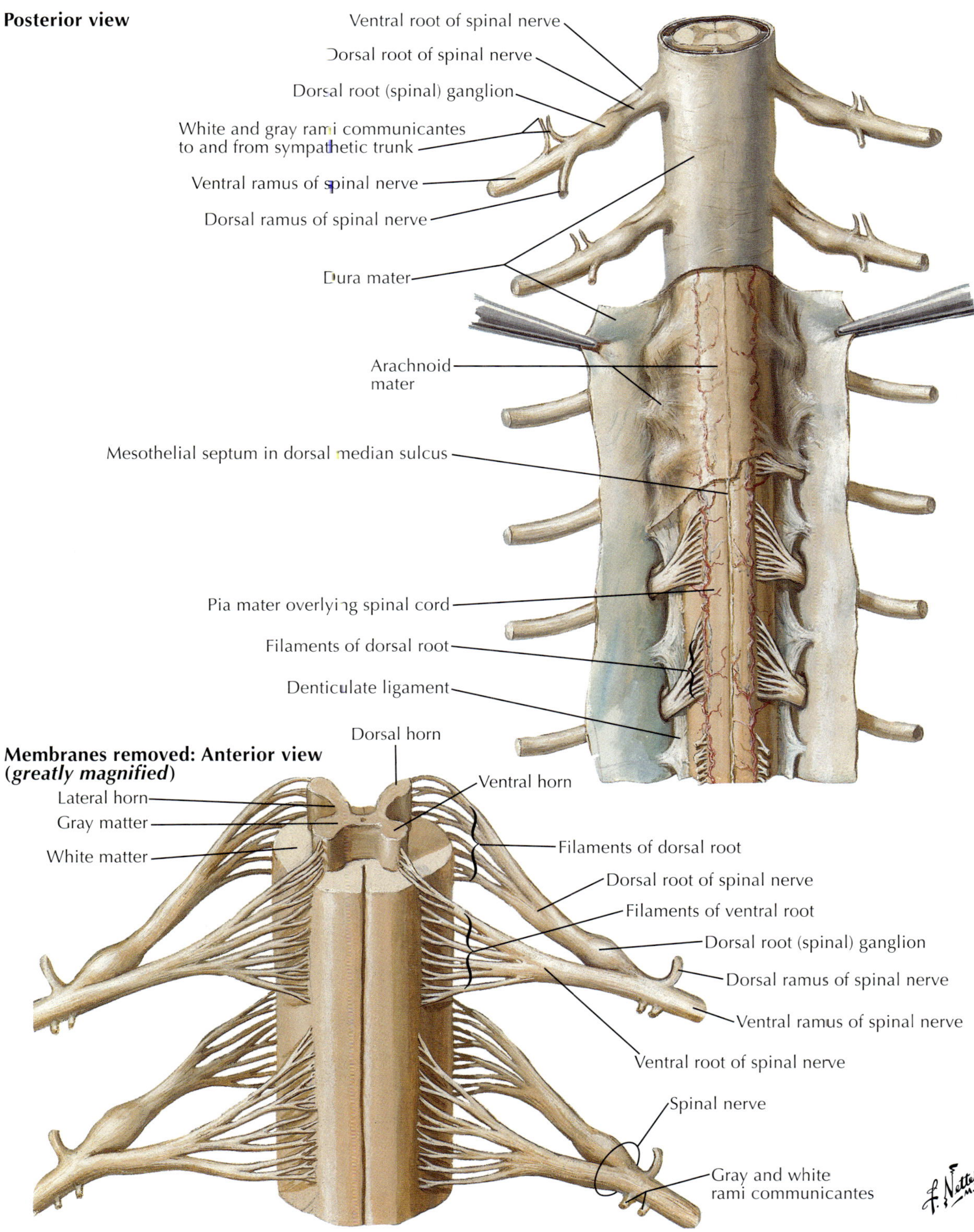

63045 Laminectomy, facetectomy and foraminotomy (unilateral or bilateral with decompression of spinal cord, cauda equina and/or nerve root[s], [eg, spinal or lateral recess stenosis]), single vertebral segment; cervical

63046 thoracic

63047 lumbar

+ 63048 each additional segment, cervical, thoracic, or lumbar (List separately in addition to code for primary procedure)

63050 Laminoplasty, cervical, with decompression of the spinal cord, 2 or more vertebral segments;

63051 with reconstruction of the posterior bony elements (including the application of bridging bone graft and non-segmental fixation devices [eg, wire, suture, mini-plates], when performed)

Transpedicular or Costovertebral Approach for Posterolateral Extradural Exploration/Decompression

Coding Atlas

A **transpedicular** approach describes an approach by way of the narrow portion of the vertebra posterior to the disc (**pedicle**). A **costovertebral** approach is at the site in which the thoracic vertebrae **articulates** with the rib. These approaches are intended to avoid disturbance of local nerve roots and spinal cord.

63055 Transpedicular approach with decompression of spinal cord, equina and/or nerve root(s) (eg, herniated intervertebral disc), single segment; thoracic

63056 lumbar (including transfacet, or lateral extraforaminal approach) (eg, far lateral herniated intervertebral disc)

+ 63057 each additional segment, thoracic or lumbar (List separately in addition to code for primary procedure)

63064 Costovertebral approach with decompression of spinal cord or nerve root(s) (eg, herniated intervertebral disc), thoracic; single segment

+ 63066 each additional segment (List separately in addition to code for primary procedure)

Anterior or Anterolateral Approach for Extradural Exploration/Decompression

Coding Atlas

Anterior and **anterolateral** approaches to the spine involve an incision through the throat or **lateral** neck, **flank** to access the **thorax**, or anterior abdomen. The spinal cord may be explored through this type of incision, and a nerve may be **decompressed** by **resection** of the disc or **vertebral body**.

63075 Discectomy, anterior, with decompression of spinal cord and/or nerve root(s), including osteophytectomy; cervical, single interspace

+ 63076 cervical, each additional interspace (List separately in addition to code for primary procedure)

63077 thoracic, single interspace

+ 63078 thoracic, each additional interspace (List separately in addition to code for primary procedure)

63081 Vertebral corpectomy (vertebral body resection), partial or complete, anterior approach with decompression of spinal cord and/or nerve root(s); cervical, single segment

+ 63082 cervical, each additional segment (List separately in addition to code for primary procedure)

63085 Vertebral corpectomy (vertebral body resection), partial or complete, transthoracic approach with decompression of spinal cord and/or nerve root(s); thoracic, single segment

+ 63086 thoracic, each additional segment (List separately in addition to code for primary procedure)

63087 Vertebral corpectomy (vertebral body resection), partial or complete, combined thoracolumbar approach with decompression of spinal cord, cauda equina or nerve root(s), lower thoracic or lumbar; single segment

+ 63088 each additional segment (List separately in addition to code for primary procedure)

63090 Vertebral corpectomy (vertebral body resection), partial or complete, transperitoneal or retroperitoneal approach with decompression of spinal cord, cauda equina or nerve root(s), lower thoracic, lumbar, or sacral; single segment

+ 63091 each additional segment (List separately in addition to code for primary procedure)

FIGURE 9-23. Thoracic Vertebrae

Each vertebral level is unique. Thoracic vertebrae differ from other sections of the spine in that they contain paired costal **facets** that **articulate** with the **tubercles** of the ribs. Each pair of **pedicles** form that portion of the vertebral arch that connects to the vertebral body. Approaches for **decompression** of the spinal cord may include transpedicular (across the pedicle) or **costovertebral** (at the site of the **costal** facets).

T6 Vertebra: Superior view

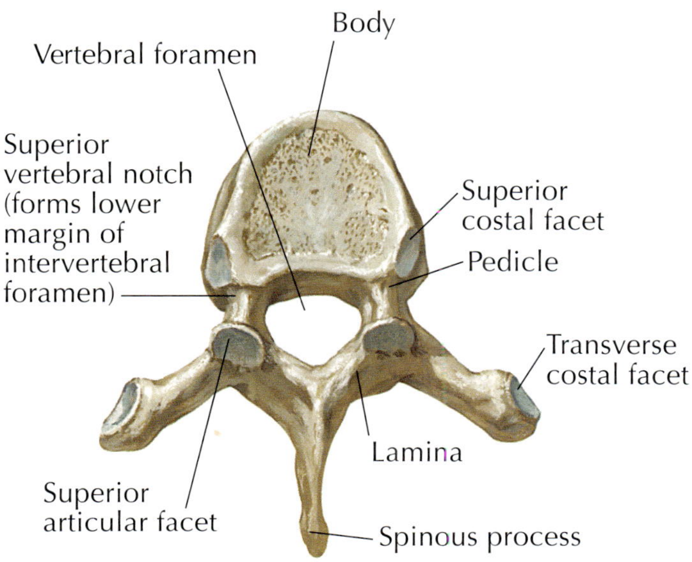

T6 Vertebra: Lateral view

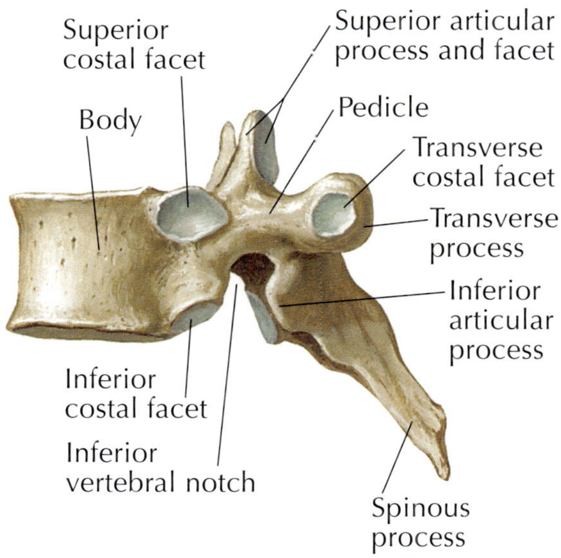

T12 Vertebra: Lateral view

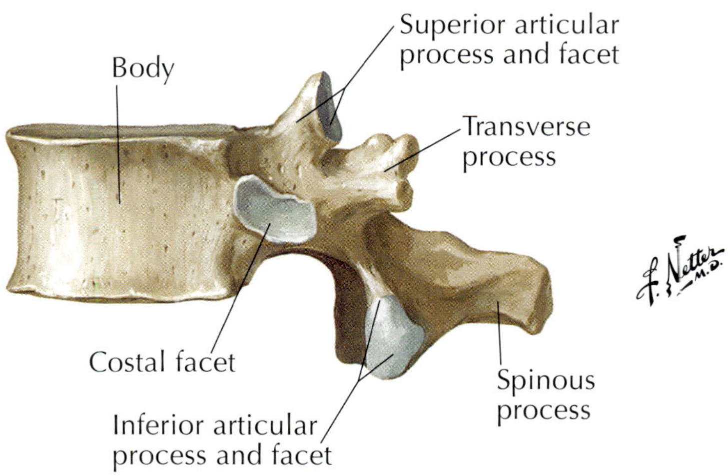

Lateral Extracavitary Approach for Extradural Exploration/Decompression

Coding Atlas

The lateral extracavitary approach includes a posterior incision and resection of the pleura and the peritoneum. A rib and the transverse process of the vertebral body are removed for direct visualization of the vertebral body. This provides better anterior exposure of the vertebral body, allowing limited visualization to the level of the opposite pedicle base.

63101 Vertebral corpectomy (vertebral body resection), partial or complete, lateral extracavitary approach with decompression of spinal cord and/or nerve root(s) (eg, for tumor or retropulsed bone fragments); thoracic, single segment

63102 lumbar, single segment

✚ **63103** thoracic or lumbar, each additional segment (List separately in addition to code for primary procedure)

Incision

Coding Atlas

A segment is defined as two vertebrae attached by ligaments and the intravertebral disc between them. In rhizotomy, nerve roots are severed at the spinal cord, typically for relief of severe pain or spasms. Cordotomy is incision into the spinal cord to disrupt nerve transmissions that are causing pain.

63170 Laminectomy with myelotomy (eg, Bischof or DREZ type), cervical, thoracic, or thoracolumbar

63172 Laminectomy with drainage of intramedullary cyst/syrinx; to subarachnoid space

63173 to peritoneal or pleural space

63180 Laminectomy and section of dentate ligaments, with or without dural graft, cervical; 1 or 2 segments

63182 more than 2 segments

63185 Laminectomy with rhizotomy; 1 or 2 segments

63190 more than 2 segments

63191 Laminectomy with section of spinal accessory nerve

63194 Laminectomy with cordotomy, with section of 1 spinothalamic tract, 1 stage; cervical

63195 thoracic

63196 Laminectomy with cordotomy, with section of both spinothalamic tracts, 1 stage; cervical

63197 thoracic

63198 Laminectomy with cordotomy with section of both spinothalamic tracts, 2 stages within 14 days; cervical

63199 thoracic

63200 Laminectomy, with release of tethered spinal cord, lumbar

Excision by Laminectomy of Lesion Other Than Herniated Disc

Coding Atlas

In a laminectomy, the posterior arch of the vertebra is excised to provide access to the contents of the spinal column or to decompress it. Codes 63250-63290 are used to report laminectomy for reasons other than decompression, including biopsy, excision, evaluation, or therapeutic occlusion of an aberrant vessel.

63250 Laminectomy for excision or occlusion of arteriovenous malformation of spinal cord; cervical

63251 thoracic

63252 thoracolumbar

63265 Laminectomy for excision or evacuation of intraspinal lesion other than neoplasm, extradural; cervical

63266 thoracic

63267 lumbar

63268 sacral

63270 Laminectomy for excision of intraspinal lesion other than neoplasm, intradural; cervical

63271 thoracic

63272 lumbar

63273 sacral

63275 Laminectomy for biopsy/excision of intraspinal neoplasm; extradural, cervical

63276 extradural, thoracic

63277 extradural, lumbar

63278 extradural, sacral

63280 intradural, extramedullary, cervical

63281 intradural, extramedullary, thoracic

63282 intradural, extramedullary, lumbar

FIGURE 9-24. Spinal Cord Tumors

Spinal lesions are classified by their proximity to the spinal cord: within the **dura mater** (**intradural**) or outside of the dura mater (**extradural**). Also noted is whether the spinal cord is involved (**intramedullary**) or not (**extramedullary**) and the location of the lesion along the vertebra (cervical, thoracic, thoracolumbar, lumbar, sacral). CPT code selection is also based on the type of lesion: **neoplasm**, **arteriovenous malformation** (AVM), or other type. Note: Tools, implants, and/or equipment depicted in the illustration may be outdated but the procedural approach is valid.

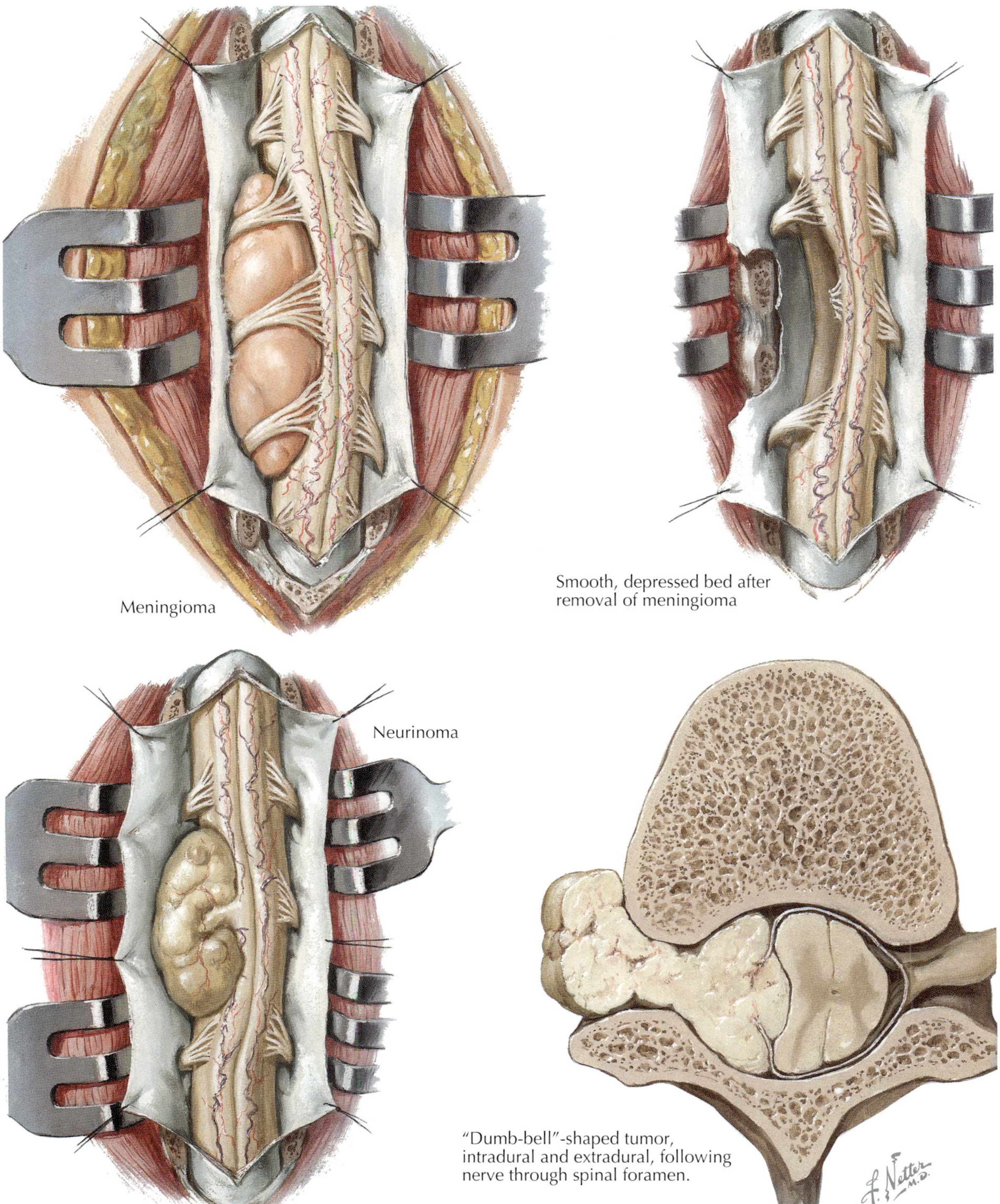

63283 intradural, sacral

63285 intradural, intramedullary, cervical

63286 intradural, intramedullary, thoracic

63287 intradural, intramedullary, thoracolumbar

63290 combined extradural-intradural lesion, any level

+ 63295 Osteoplastic reconstruction of dorsal spinal elements, following primary intraspinal procedure (List separately in addition to code for primary procedure)

Excision, Anterior or Anterolateral Approach, Intraspinal Lesion

Coding Atlas

Anterior and anterolateral approaches to the spine involve an incision through the throat or lateral neck, flank to access the thorax, or anterior abdomen to access the anterior spinal. The spinal cord may be explored through this type of incision, and a lesion may be excised. The procedure may include resection of the vertebral body.

63300 Vertebral corpectomy (vertebral body resection), partial or complete, for excision of intraspinal lesion, single segment; extradural, cervical

63301 extradural, thoracic by transthoracic approach

63302 extradural, thoracic by thoracolumbar approach

63303 extradural, lumbar or sacral by transperitoneal or retroperitoneal approach

63304 intradural, cervical

63305 intradural, thoracic by transthoracic approach

63306 intradural, thoracic by thoracolumbar approach

63307 intradural, lumbar or sacral by transperitoneal or retroperitoneal approach

+ 63308 each additional segment (List separately in addition to codes for single segment)

Stereotaxis

Coding Atlas

Severe disease, tumor, trauma, or deformity may alter normal anatomic landmarks. Stereotaxis can be used to reduce risk during surgery by precisely mapping beforehand individual anatomy for the physician.

63600 Creation of lesion of spinal cord by stereotactic method, percutaneous, any modality (including stimulation and/or recording)

63610 Stereotactic stimulation of spinal cord, percutaneous, separate procedure not followed by other surgery

63615 Stereotactic biopsy, aspiration, or excision of lesion, spinal cord

Stereotactic Radiosurgery (Spinal)

Coding Atlas

Stereotaxis can be used to reduce risk from radiation therapy by precisely mapping individual anatomy for the physician. In stereotactic radiosurgery, radiation therapy treats a defect. The physician maps out a defined target for eradication, and an externally generated beam is focused on the target. For stereotactic radiosurgery of the spine, the surgeon uses codes 63620 and 63621 to report radiosurgery. Any clinical treatment planning, dosimetry, targeting, positioning, or blocking performed by the physician is included in this service.

63620 Stereotactic radiosurgery (particle beam, gamma ray, or linear accelerator); 1 spinal lesion

+ 63621 each additional spinal lesion (List separately in addition to code for primary procedure)

Neurostimulators (Spinal)

Coding Atlas

Spinal nerve stimulation is normally performed to treat and monitor intractable pain. In percutaneous implantation, there is no direct visualization of the lamina or epidural space into which the device is being placed, although an incision may be required to secure the lead to the fascia. A temporary percutaneous trial with electrode array(s) is reported with CPT code 63650 and includes removal of the array during the trial period.

63650 Percutaneous implantation of neurostimulator electrode array, epidural

63655 Laminectomy for implantation of neurostimulator electrodes, plate/paddle, epidural

63661 Removal of spinal neurostimulator electrode percutaneous array(s), including fluoroscopy, when performed

63662 Removal of spinal neurostimulator electrode plate/paddle(s) placed via laminotomy or laminectomy, including fluoroscopy, when performed

63663 Revision including replacement, when performed, of spinal neurostimulator electrode percutaneous array(s), including fluoroscopy, when performed

63664 Revision including replacement, when performed, of spinal neurostimulator electrode plate/paddle(s) placed via laminotomy or laminectomy, including fluoroscopy, when performed

63685 Insertion or replacement of spinal neurostimulator pulse generator or receiver, direct or inductive coupling

63688 Revision or removal of implanted spinal neurostimulator pulse generator or receiver

Repair

Coding Atlas

A meningocele is a congenital defect in the spine or skull with a herniation of the meninges bulging through the gap, creating an externalized sac of cerebrospinal fluid (CSF). A myelomeningocele is a type of spina bifida in which the spinal cord and meninges are exposed along a child's spine. It is also a congenital condition. A pseudomeningocele is an abnormal pocket of CSF that communicates with normal CSF space but is not lined with meninges. Pseudomeningocele is an acquired condition following surgery or injury.

63700 Repair of meningocele; less than 5 cm diameter

63702 larger than 5 cm diameter

63704 Repair of myelomeningocele; less than 5 cm diameter

63706 larger than 5 cm diameter

63707 Repair of dural/cerebrospinal fluid leak, not requiring laminectomy

63709 Repair of dural/cerebrospinal fluid leak or pseudomeningocele, with laminectomy

63710 Dural graft, spinal

Shunt, Spinal CSF

Coding Atlas

Lumbar peritoneal (LP) shunts are, like ventricular peritoneal (VP) shunts, a treatment for hydrocephalus and intracranial hypertension. LP shunts may also be inserted to help manage local spinal pathologies. LP shunts form a communication from the subarachnoid space of the lumbar spine into the peritoneum.

63740 Creation of shunt, lumbar, subarachnoid-peritoneal, -pleural, or other; including laminectomy

63741 percutaneous, not requiring laminectomy

63744 Replacement, irrigation or revision of lumbosubarachnoid shunt

63746 Removal of entire lumbosubarachnoid shunt system without replacement

Extracranial Nerves, Peripheral Nerves, and Autonomic Nervous System

Introduction/Injection of Anesthetic Agent (Nerve Block), Diagnostic or Therapeutic

Coding Atlas

Blocks for treating tarsal nerve syndrome, sural nerve entrapment, or medial calcaneal nerve branch neuritis should be reported with code 64450, which is used to report a block that affects an "other peripheral nerve or branch."

Somatic Nerves

64400 Injection, anesthetic agent; trigeminal nerve, any division or branch

64402 facial nerve

64405 greater occipital nerve

64408 vagus nerve

64410 phrenic nerve

64412 spinal accessory nerve

64413 cervical plexus

64415 brachial plexus, single

64416 brachial plexus, continuous infusion by catheter (including catheter placement)

64417 axillary nerve

64418 suprascapular nerve

64420 intercostal nerve, single

64421 intercostal nerves, multiple, regional block

64425 ilioinguinal, iliohypogastric nerves

64430 pudendal nerve

64435 paracervical (uterine) nerve

64445 sciatic nerve, single

64446 sciatic nerve, continuous infusion by catheter (including catheter placement)

64447 femoral nerve, single

64448 femoral nerve, continuous infusion by catheter (including catheter placement)

64449 lumbar plexus, posterior approach, continuous infusion by catheter (including catheter placement)

64450 other peripheral nerve or branch

64455 Injection(s), anesthetic agent and/or steroid, plantar common digital nerve(s) (eg, Morton's neuroma)

64479 Injection(s), anesthetic agent and/or steroid, transforaminal epidural, with imaging guidance (fluoroscopy or CT); cervical or thoracic, single level

+ 64480 cervical or thoracic, each additional level (List separately in addition to code for primary procedure)

64483 lumbar or sacral, single level

+ 64484 lumbar or sacral, each additional level (List separately in addition to code for primary procedure)

64486 Transversus abdominis plane (TAP) block (abdominal plane block, rectus sheath block) unilateral; by injection(s) (includes imaging guidance, when performed)

64487 by continuous infusion(s) (includes imaging guidance, when performed)

64488 Transversus abdominis plane (TAP) block (abdominal plane block, rectus sheath block) bilateral; by injections (includes imaging guidance, when performed)

64489 by continuous infusions (includes imaging guidance, when performed)

Paravertebral Spinal Nerves and Branches

64490 Injection(s), diagnostic or therapeutic agent, paravertebral facet (zygapophyseal) joint (or nerves innervating that joint) with image guidance (fluoroscopy or CT), cervical or thoracic; single level

+ 64491 second level (List separately in addition to code for primary procedure)

+ 64492 third and any additional level(s) (List separately in addition to code for primary procedure)

64493 Injection(s), diagnostic or therapeutic agent, paravertebral facet (zygapophyseal) joint (or nerves innervating that joint) with image guidance (fluoroscopy or CT), lumbar or sacral; single level

+ 64494 second level (List separately in addition to code for primary procedure)

+ 64495 third and any additional level(s) (List separately in addition to code for primary procedure)

FIGURE 9-25. The Cervical Plexus

The cervical **plexus** is a **bilateral** network of nerves **posterior** to the internal jugular vein and sternocleidomastoid muscles. It is formed by communications between the **anterior** rami of the upper four cervical nerves (C1-C4) and innervates the neck, chest, diaphragm, back of the head, and parts of the face.

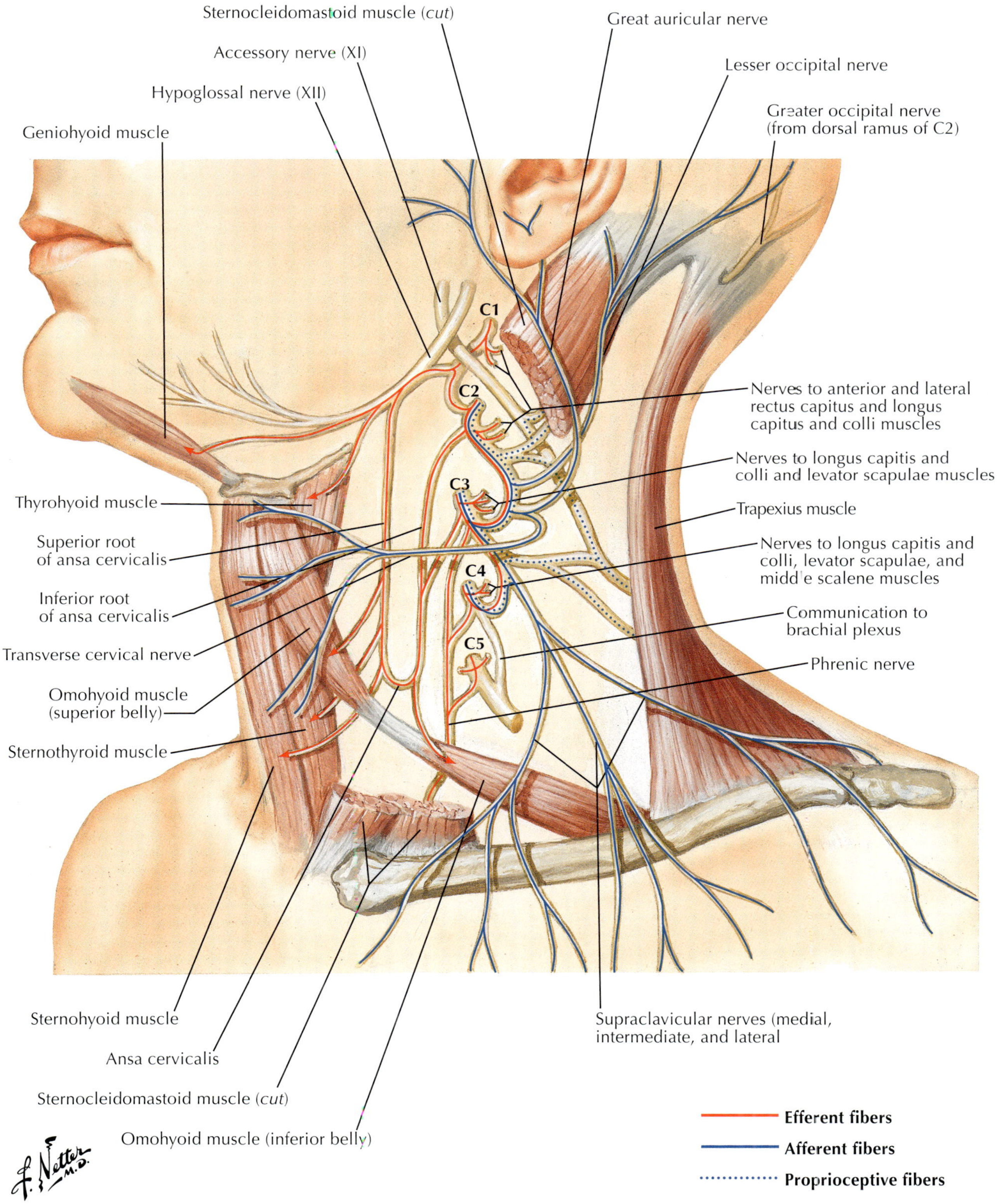

FIGURE 9-26. The Brachial Plexus

The brachial **plexus** is a **bilateral** network of nerves formed by the **ventral** rami of the lower four cervical nerves (C5-C-8) and the first thoracic nerve (T1). It is responsible for motor nerve control of most of the muscles of the upper extremities as well as the **cutaneous** innervation of most of the upper extremities. Brachial plexus injury (BPI) is a common sports injury and also commonly occurs in motorcycle accidents and falls.

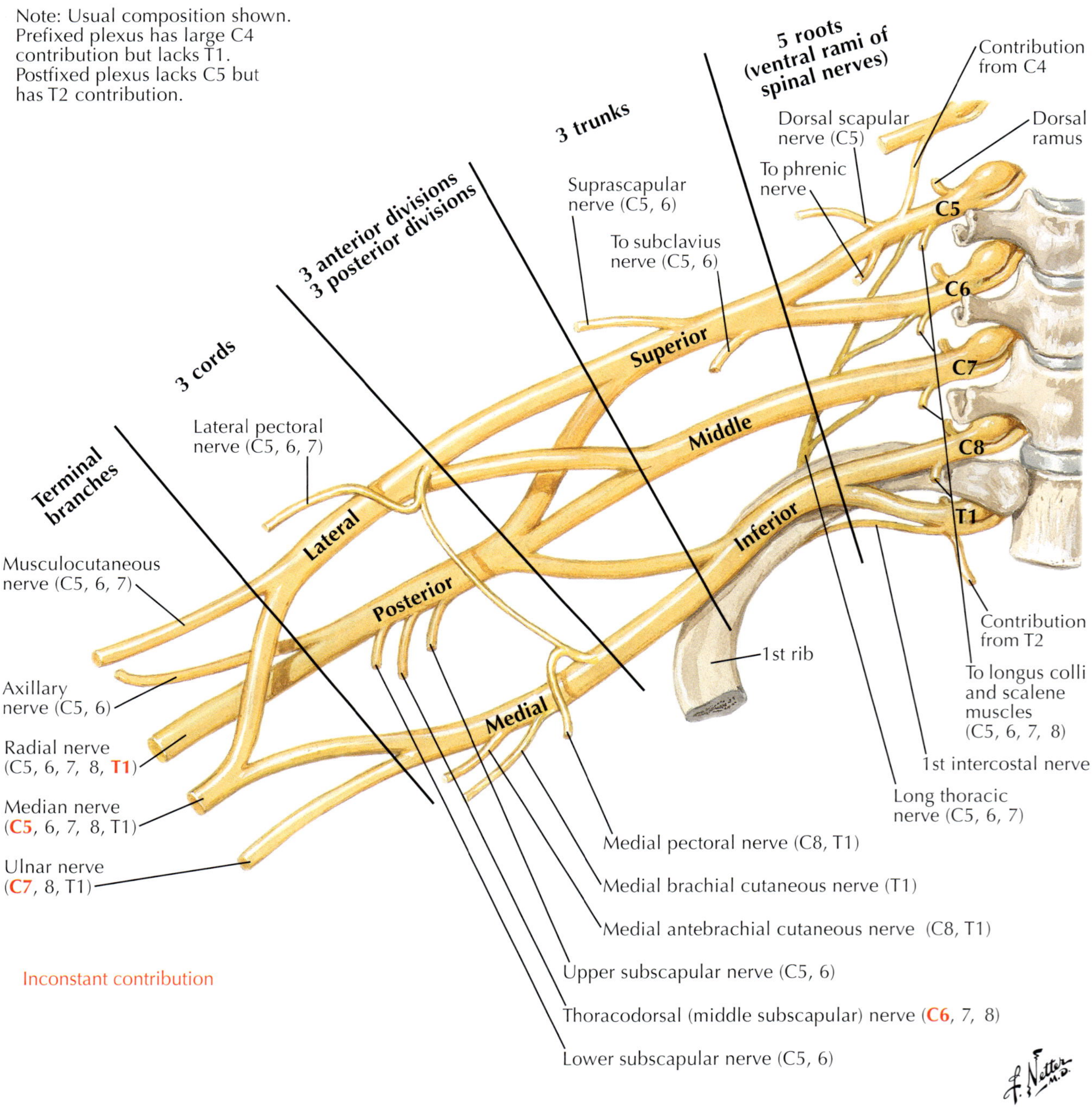

FIGURE 9-27. Lumbosacral and Coccygeal Plexuses

The bilateral lumbosacral plexus is a network of nerves in the lower back that is formed by the divisions of T12 and L1-L4 for lumbar and S1-S3 for sacral. The lumbosacral plexus innervates the pelvic area, buttocks, legs, and feet. The coccygeal plexus arises from the lower part of the ventral branches of S4 and S5 as well as the coccygeal nerves. It supplies the coccygeaus muscle, part of the levator ani, and the sacrococcygeal joint.

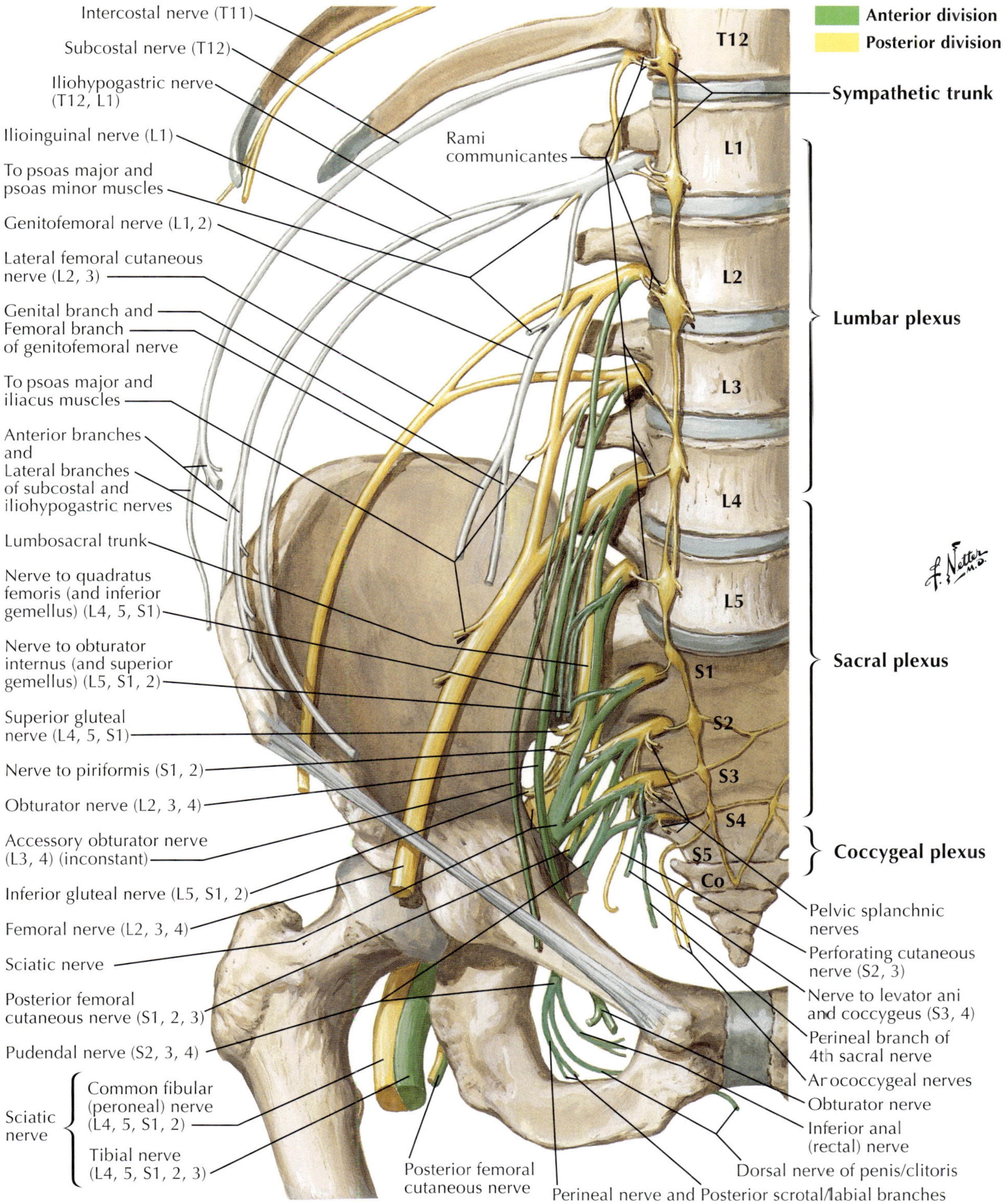

FIGURE 9-28. The Trigeminal Nerve

The **bilateral** trigeminal nerve (cranial nerve V [CNV]) supplies sensations to the face and other structures of the head and motor sensation for **mastication**. It is the largest cranial nerve, exiting the brain at the pons. The trigeminal nerve has three main branches: ophthalmic, maxillary, and mandibular. The ophthalmic and maxillary nerves are entirely sensory; the mandibular nerve has both sensory and motor components. The three branches converge at the trigeminal ganglion, also referred to as the semilunar or gasserian ganglion.

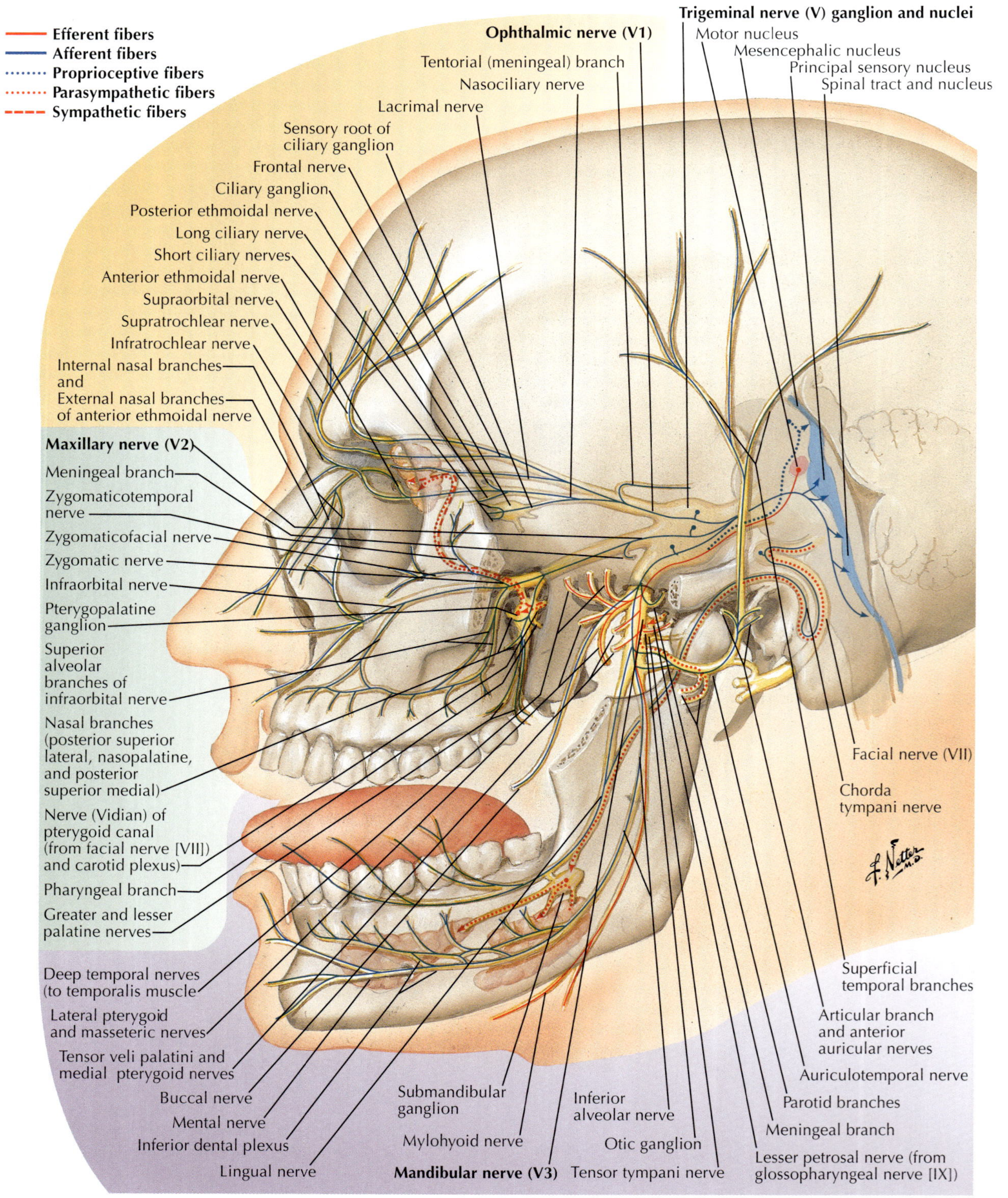

Autonomic Nerves

64505 Injection, anesthetic agent; sphenopalatine ganglion

64508 carotid sinus (separate procedure)

64510 stellate ganglion (cervical sympathetic)

64517 superior hypogastric plexus

64520 lumbar or thoracic (paravertebral sympathetic)

64530 celiac plexus, with or without radiologic monitoring

Neurostimulators (Peripheral Nerve)

Coding Atlas

Urinary symptoms such as urge **incontinence**, urgency, frequency, and nonobstructive retention may be caused by neurological issues and may respond to neurostimulators. Codes 64561 and 64581 are used to report procedures performed on the sacral nerve for treatment of these conditions. Code 64561 is used to report a **percutaneous** approach for lead placement adjacent to the nerve with no direct manipulation of the sacral nerve. An electrically insulated spinal needle is placed percutaneously into the **foramen** and attached to an external stimulation device for testing. Usually, this percutaneous approach is performed to test the efficacy of **neurostimulation**. Following successful testing, the patient may undergo a procedure in which the temporary electrode is replaced with a permanent one, maintaining the ideal location next to the sacral nerve. This more complex and permanent procedure is reported using code 64581. **Tunneling** of the neurostimulator's electrode array through the presacral **fascia** and **subcutaneous** tissues to a separate incision, in which the implantable pulse generator (IPG) will be connected via a lead electrode extension, is reported separately with code 64590.

64550 Application of surface (transcutaneous) neurostimulator

64553 Percutaneous implantation of neurostimulator electrode array; cranial nerve

64555 peripheral nerve (excludes sacral nerve)

64561 sacral nerve (transforaminal placement) including image guidance, if performed

64565 neuromuscular

64566 Posterior tibial neurostimulation, percutaneous needle electrode, single treatment, includes programming

64568 Incision for implantation of cranial nerve (eg, vagus nerve) neurostimulator electrode array and pulse generator

64569 Revision or replacement of cranial nerve (eg, vagus nerve) neurostimulator electrode array, including connection to existing pulse generator

64570 Removal of cranial nerve (eg, vagus nerve) neurostimulator electrode array and pulse generator

64575 Incision for implantation of neurostimulator electrode array; peripheral nerve (excludes sacral nerve)

64580 neuromuscular

64581 sacral nerve (transforaminal placement)

64585 Revision or removal of peripheral neurostimulator electrode array

64590 Insertion or replacement of peripheral or gastric neurostimulator pulse generator or receiver, direct or inductive coupling

64595 Revision or removal of peripheral or gastric neurostimulator pulse generator or receiver

FIGURE 9-29. The Autonomic Nervous System

The autonomic nervous system (ANS) is a network of nerves that manage physiologic balances within the body, contributing to the function of the cardiovascular, gastrointestinal, genitourinary, **thermoregulatory**, and ophthalmological systems. The actions of the ANS are usually characterized as **involuntary**, eg, **peristalsis** and pupillary reaction to light. The system contains both **afferent** (sensory) and **efferent** (motor) pathways. The ANS contains both sympathetic (fight-or-flight) and **parasympathetic** (rest or digest) nerve functions.

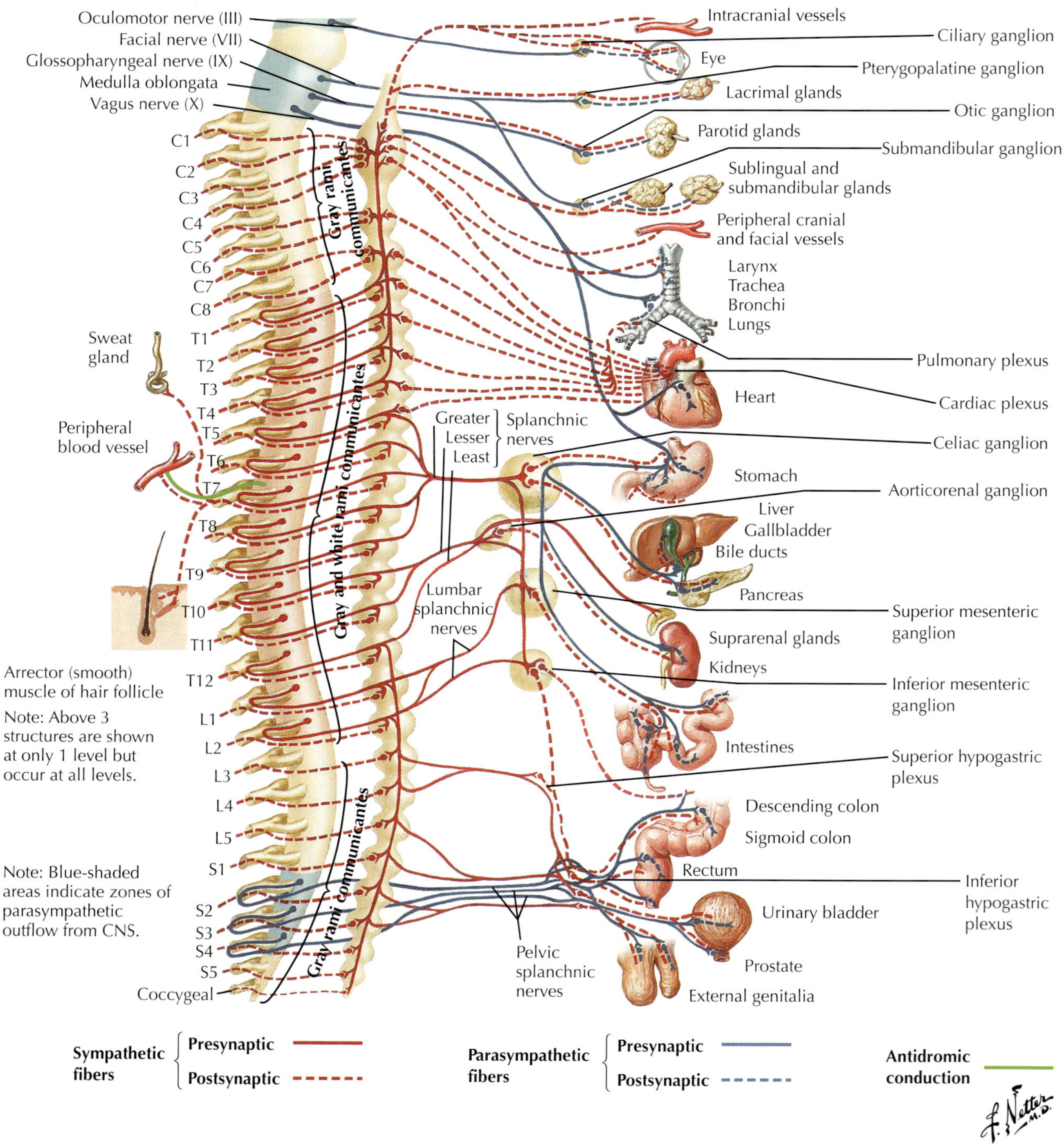

FIGURE 9-30. The Celiac Plexus

The bilateral celiac plexus is sometimes called the solar plexus. It is a dense network of nerve fibers and ganglia surrounding the celiac artery and the root of the superior mesentery artery, posterior to the stomach at the level of L1. The system innervates the abdominal viscera. Celiac blocks may be administered to patients with intractable pain, eg, from pancreatic cancer.

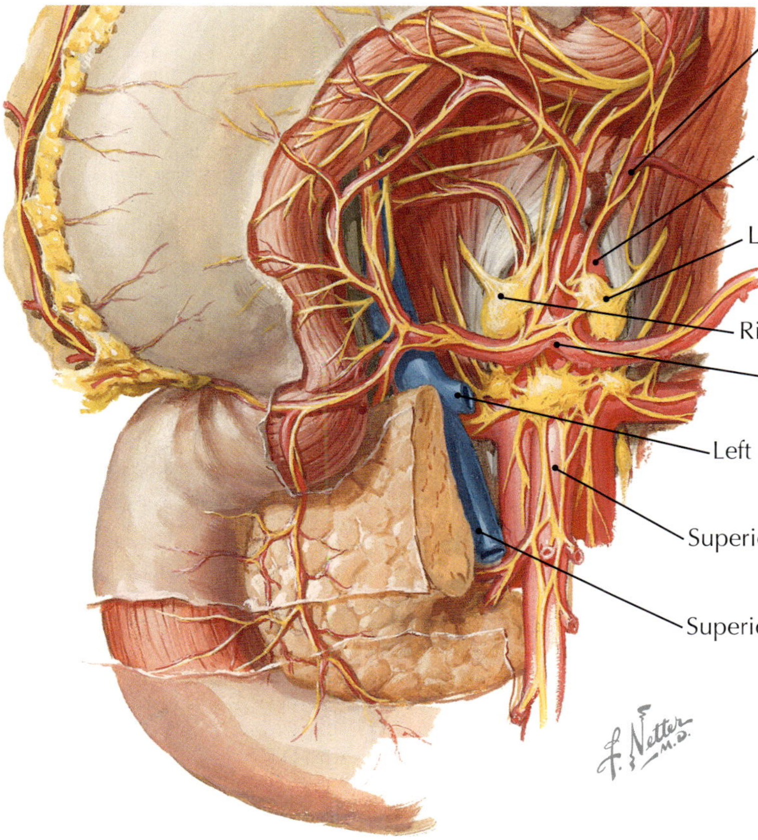

Destruction by Neurolytic Agent (eg, Chemical, Thermal, Electrical or Radiofrequency), Chemodenervation

Coding Atlas

Codes 64600-64681 are used to report injection of other therapeutic agents, eg, cortisone, or for injection of agents for nerve destruction or chemodenervation. Chemodenervation describes the injection of a chemical into the nerve to decrease neural response to stimuli and reduce electrical impulse excitability. The effect may be temporary or permanent, depending on the agent injected. Supply of the chemodenervation agent may be reported separately.

Somatic Nerves

64600 Destruction by neurolytic agent, trigeminal nerve; supraorbital, infraorbital, mental, or inferior alveolar branch

64605 second and third division branches at foramen ovale

64610 second and third division branches at foramen ovale under radiologic monitoring

64611 Chemodenervation of parotid and submandibular salivary glands, bilateral

64612 Chemodenervation of muscle(s); muscle(s) innervated by facial nerve, unilateral (eg, for blepharospasm, hemifacial spasm)

64615 muscle(s) innervated by facial, trigeminal, cervical spinal and accessory nerves, bilateral (eg, for chronic migraine)

FIGURE 9-31. The Sympathetic Nervous System

In addition to regulating the release of **adrenaline** as part of a flight-or-fight response, the **sympathetic** nervous system (SNS) also regulates pupillary diameter in reaction to light, urinary output, regulation of sweat gland secretions, and some heart functions. SNS stimulation also causes **vasoconstriction** of most blood vessels.

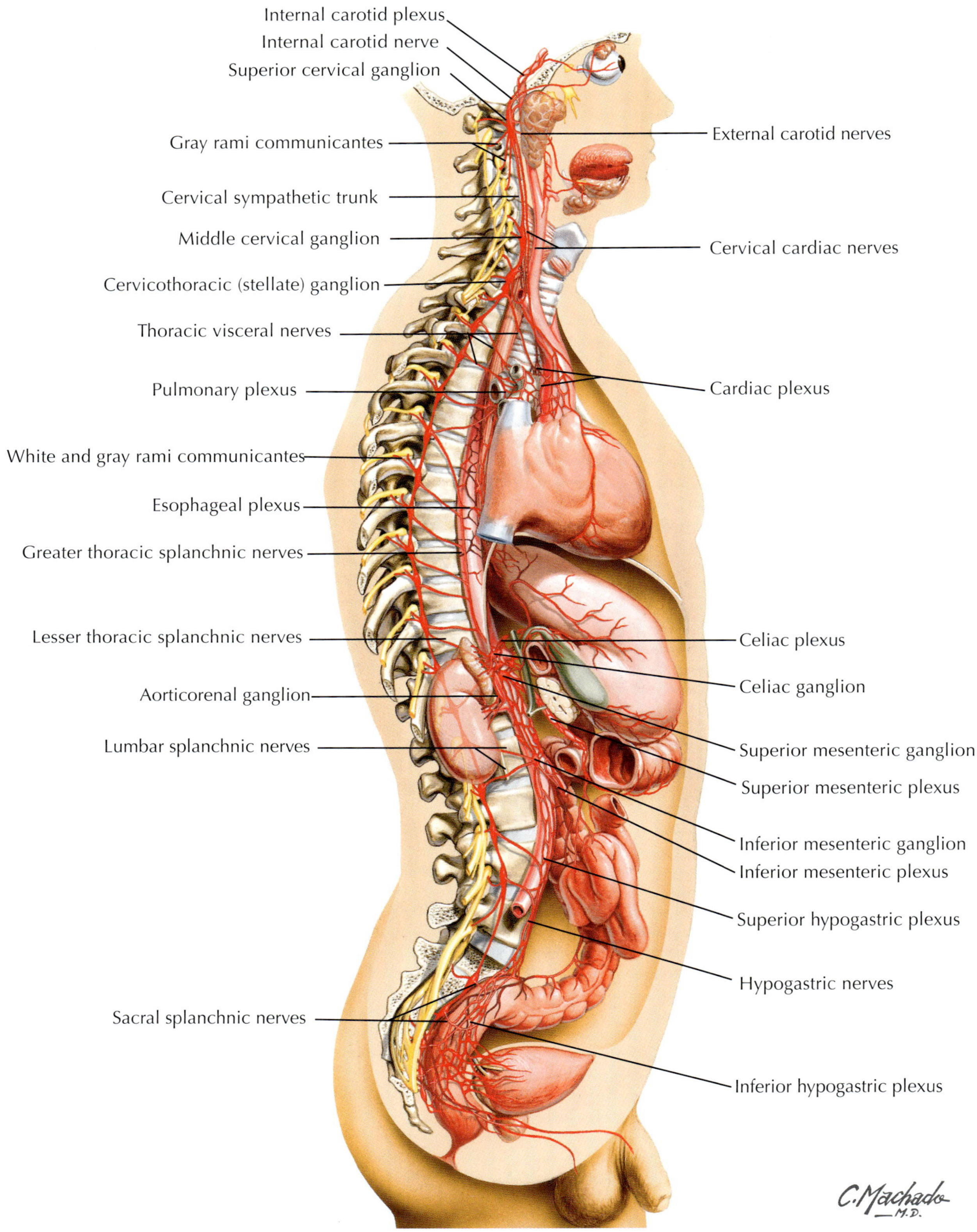

64616 neck muscle(s), excluding muscles of the larynx, unilateral (eg, for cervical dystonia, spasmodic torticollis)

64617 larynx, unilateral, percutaneous (eg, for spasmodic dysphonia), includes guidance by needle electromyography, when performed

64620 Destruction by neurolytic agent, intercostal nerve

64633 Destruction by neurolytic agent, paravertebral facet joint nerve(s), with imaging guidance (fluoroscopy or CT); cervical or thoracic, single facet joint

#✚ **64634** cervical or thoracic, each additional facet joint (List separately in addition to code for primary procedure)

64635 lumbar or sacral, single facet joint

#✚ **64636** lumbar or sacral, each additional facet joint (List separately in addition to code for primary procedure)

64630 Destruction by neurolytic agent; pudendal nerve

64632 plantar common digital nerve

64633 Code is out of numerical sequence. See 64600-64640

64634 Code is out of numerical sequence. See 64600-64640

64635 Code is out of numerical sequence. See 64600-64640

64636 Code is out of numerical sequence. See 64600-64640

64640 other peripheral nerve or branch

64642 Chemodenervation of one extremity; 1-4 muscle(s)

✚ **64643** each additional extremity, 1-4 muscle(s) (List separately in addition to code for primary procedure)

64644 Chemodenervation of one extremity; 5 or more muscles

✚ **64645** each additional extremity, 5 or more muscles (List separately in addition to code for primary procedure)

64646 Chemodenervation of trunk muscle(s); 1-5 muscle(s)

64647 6 or more muscles

Sympathetic Nerves

64650 Chemodenervation of eccrine glands; both axillae

64653 other area(s) (eg, scalp, face, neck), per day

64680 Destruction by neurolytic agent, with or without radiologic monitoring; celiac plexus

64681 superior hypogastric plexus

Neuroplasty (Exploration, Neurolysis or Nerve Decompression)

Coding Atlas

Neuroplasty includes surgical decompression, lysis, and transposition of the nerve to free it from surrounding tissue. CPT codes 64702-64726 are used to report external **neurolysis**, which is performed to release the nerve by dividing perineural **adhesions** and/or perineural scar tissue. Add-on code 64727 is used to report internal neurolysis, which includes microscopic excision of scar tissue from between nerve **fascicles** in order to enhance nerve regeneration after nerve injury or repair.

64702 Neuroplasty; digital, 1 or both, same digit

64704 nerve of hand or foot

64708 Neuroplasty, major peripheral nerve, arm or leg, open; other than specified

64712 sciatic nerve

64713 brachial plexus

64714 lumbar plexus

64716 Neuroplasty and/or transposition; cranial nerve (specify)

64718 ulnar nerve at elbow

64719 ulnar nerve at wrist

64721 median nerve at carpal tunnel

64722 Decompression; unspecified nerve(s) (specify)

64726 plantar digital nerve

✚ **64727** Internal neurolysis, requiring use of operating microscope (List separately in addition to code for neuroplasty) (Neuroplasty includes external neurolysis)

FIGURE 9-32. The Sciatic Nerve

Sciatica is pain that has its origins in a defect in the lumbosacral nerves (L4-S2) with manifestations of leg pain, with or without neurological deficits. The defect is often a compressed nerve. Typically, sciatic nerve pain is worse when standing or during prolonged sitting and improves during walking or by regularly changing positions. Leg pain, disturbances of skin sensation in the leg, and lower extremity muscle wasting are all symptoms of a compromised sciatic nerve.

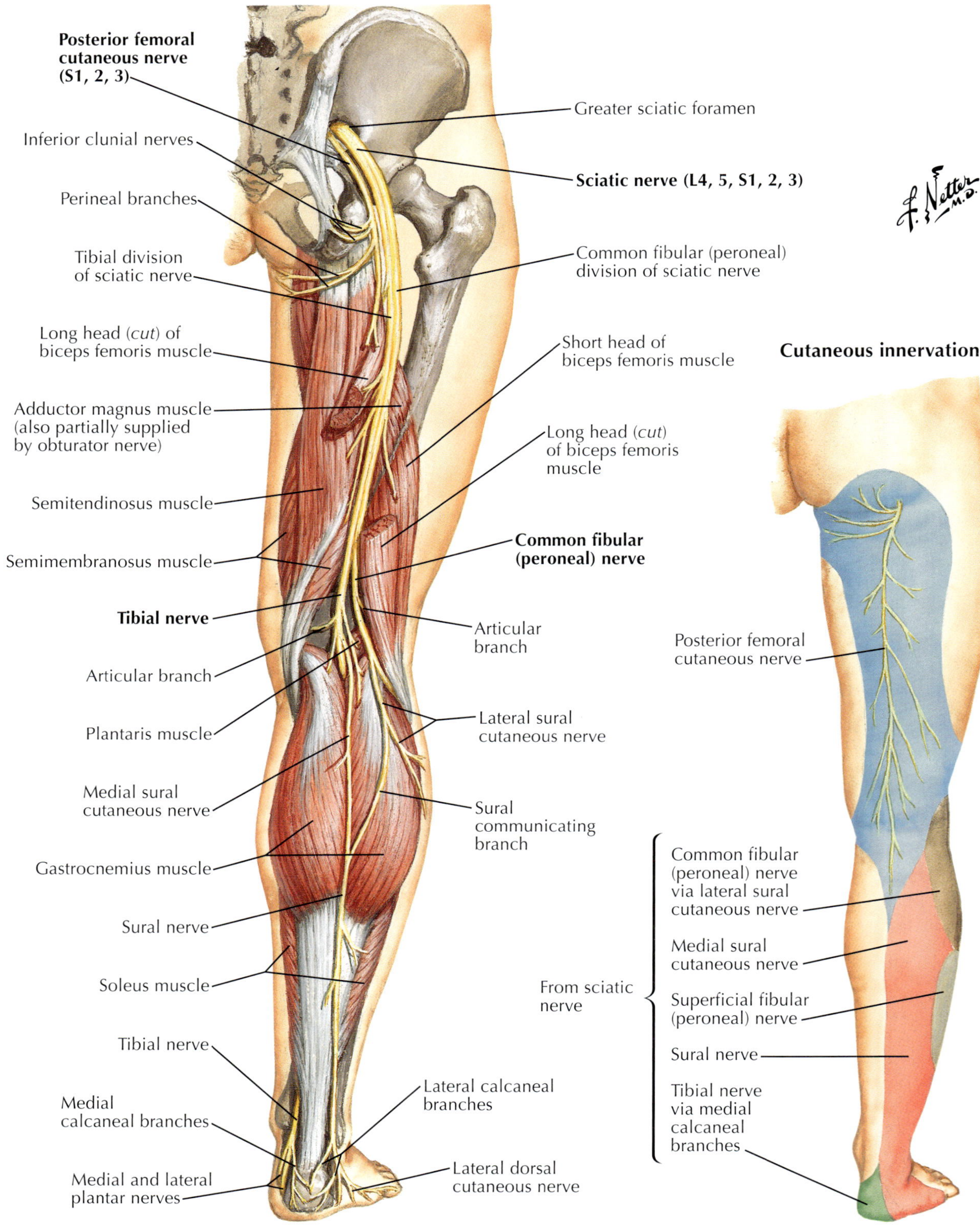

FIGURE 9-33. The Ulnar Nerve

The ulnar nerve is the most **distal** of the medial cord of the brachial **plexus**. Injury or **entrapment** of the ulnar nerve may cause **denervation** or paralysis of the **intrinsic** muscles of the hand. The most common ulnar entrapment site is the cubital tunnel at the elbow. The wrist is the second most common site. The cubital tunnel begins at the medial epicondyle of the humerus and extends across the joint to the ulnar olecranon process. The area also contains the flexor carpi ulnaris (FCU) tendons.

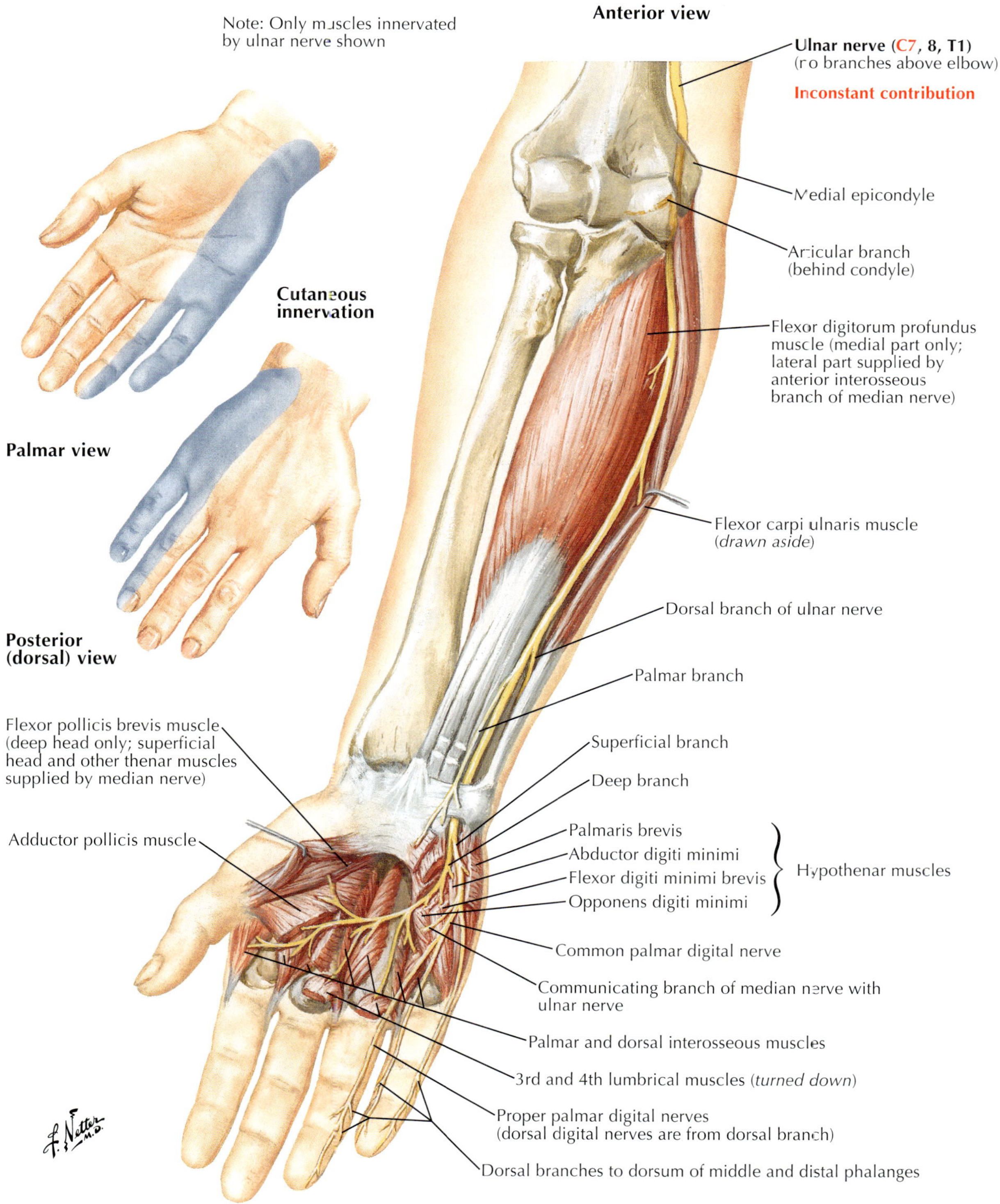

FIGURE 9-34. Digital Nerve Decompression

Nerves in the fingers originate as branches of the median and ulnar nerves that travel down the arm to traverse the wrist into the palm. Digital nerve compression is usually due to occupational repetitive stress that results in nerve **entrapment**, which may be treated surgically by **lysis** or **transposition** of the nerve to a protective location. Note: Tools, implants, and/or equipment depicted in the illustration may be outdated but the procedural approach is valid.

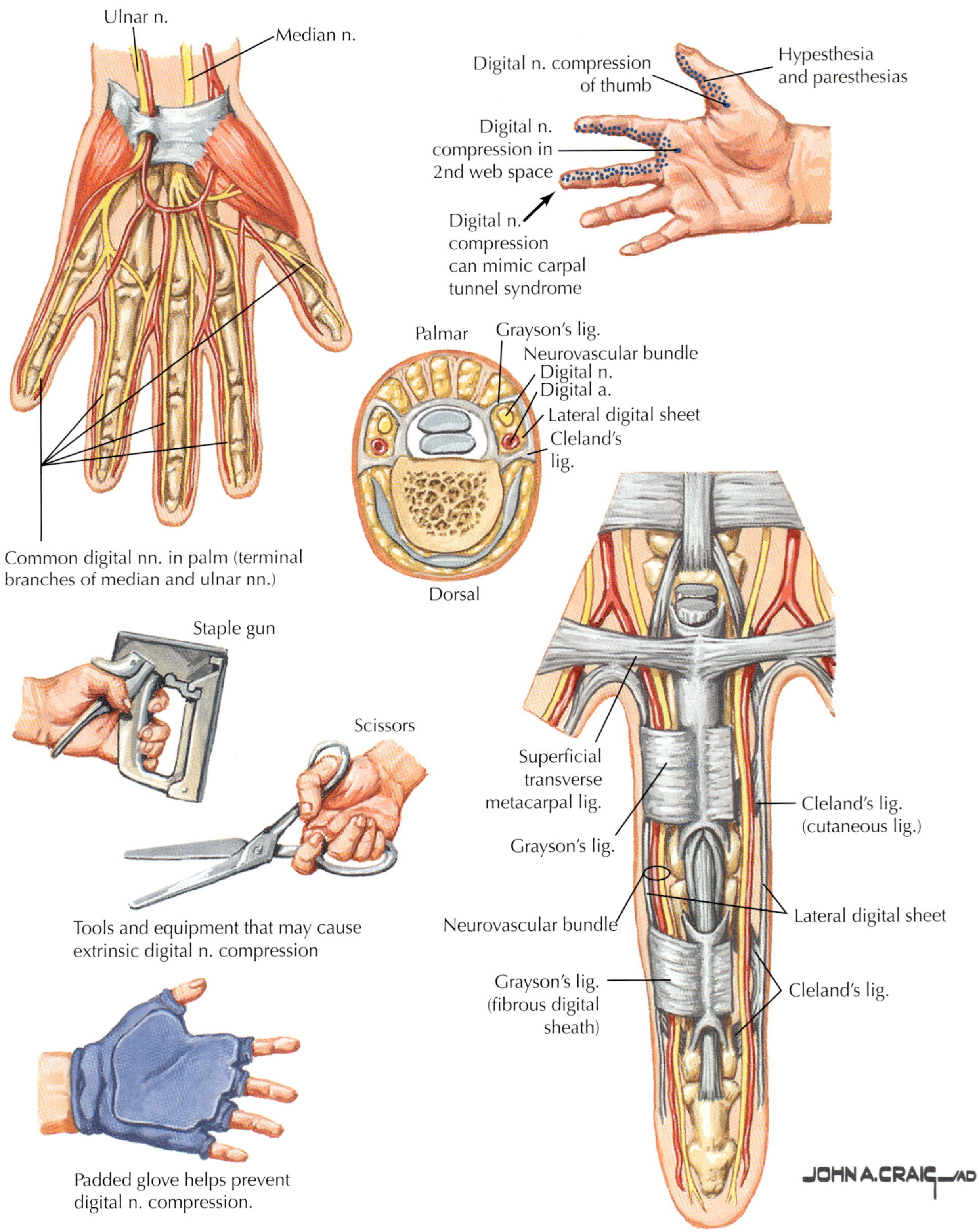

FIGURE 9-35. Median Nerve Neuroplasty

Neuroplasty to **decompress** the medial nerve at the carpal tunnel is commonly called carpal tunnel syndrome (CTS) surgery. Symptoms of CTS include **paresthesias**, pain, and, in some cases, reduction in strength. Surgical release of the **transverse** ligament at the wrist may be performed to decompress the carpal tunnel and its contents. Note: Tools, implants, and/or equipment depicted in the illustration may be outdated but the procedural approach is valid.

Surgical decompression of carpal tunnel

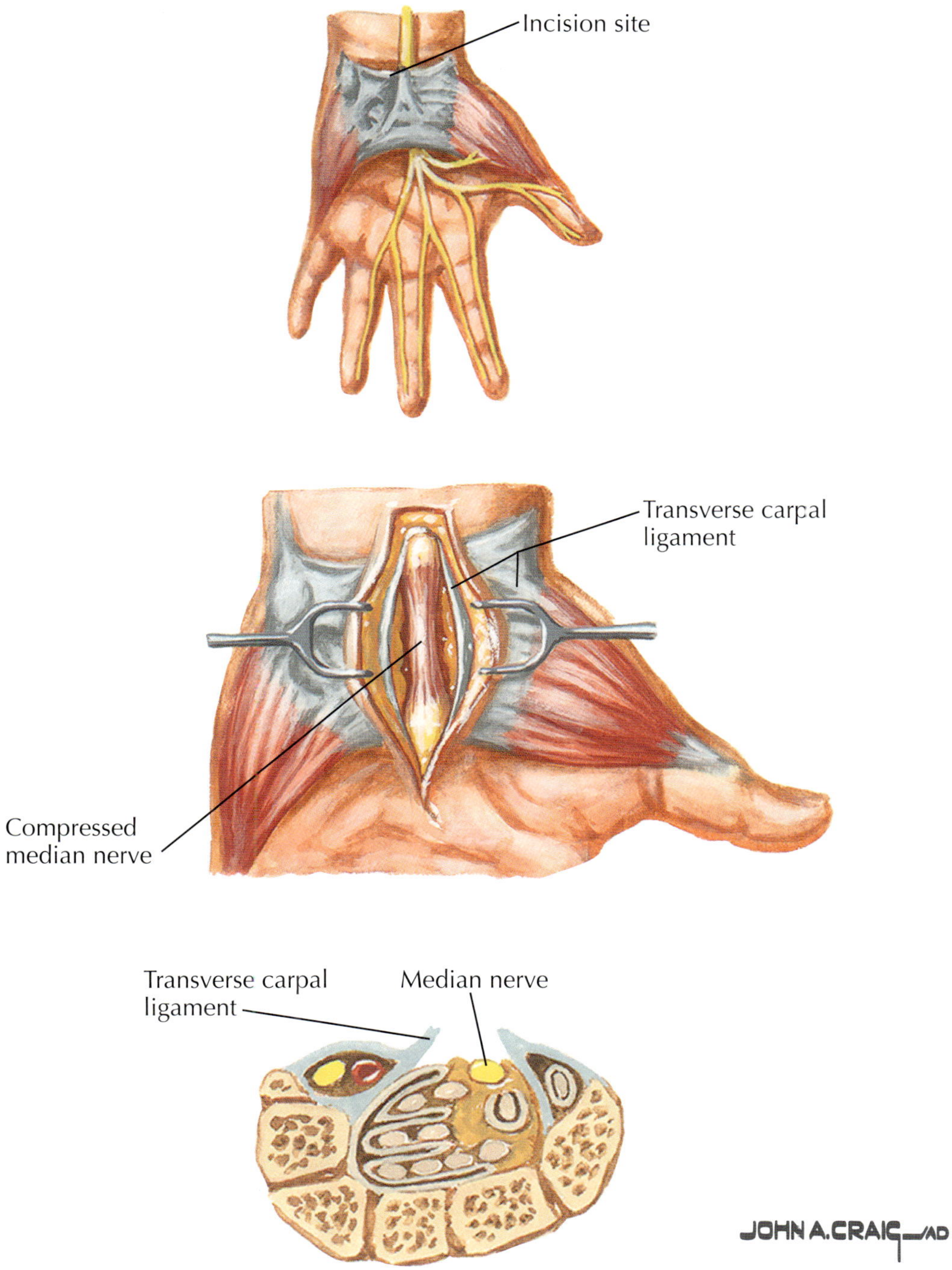

Decompressed carpal tunnel

Transection or Avulsion

Coding Atlas

The vagus nerve may be **resected** in a patient with duodenal or gastric peptic ulcer disease (PUD) if medications are unsuccessful in controlling stomach acid secretions. In highly selective **vagotomy** (HSV), only the **fundus** and body of the stomach are **denervated**. This is sometimes called a parietal cell vagotomy (PCV) or proximal gastric vagotomy (PGV). In HSV, the nerve of Latarjet is spared so that the function of emptying the stomach remains innervated. Less commonly, selective vagotomy (SV) is performed and the nerve of Latarjet is **transected**. In truncal vagotomy, (TV) the main trunk of the vagus nerve is divided, affecting multiple organs.

64732 Transection or avulsion of; supraorbital nerve

64734 infraorbital nerve

64736 mental nerve

64738 inferior alveolar nerve by osteotomy

64740 lingual nerve

64742 facial nerve, differential or complete

64744 greater occipital nerve

64746 phrenic nerve

64755 vagus nerves limited to proximal stomach (selective proximal vagotomy, proximal gastric vagotomy, parietal cell vagotomy, supra- or highly selective vagotomy)

64760 vagus nerve (vagotomy), abdominal

64763 Transection or avulsion of obturator nerve, extrapelvic, with or without adductor tenotomy

64766 Transection or avulsion of obturator nerve, intrapelvic, with or without adductor tenotomy

64771 Transection or avulsion of other cranial nerve, extradural

64772 Transection or avulsion of other spinal nerve, extradural

Excision

Coding Atlas

A **neuroma** is a generic term for a **neoplastic** or **non-neoplastic** source of swelling along a nerve or nerve bundle. A neoplastic neuroma may be called a **schwannoma**, as this type originates from Schwann cells at the nerve. Neuromas are usually **benign**. Non-neoplastic neuromas may occur after trauma or repeated stress, eg, Morton's neuroma, a ball of fibrous tissue in the nerve at the ball of the foot. Neuromas may occur in the CNS (eg, **acoustic neuroma**) or PNS. **Neurofibroma** and **neurolemmoma** (also neurilemmoma) are benign neoplasms of the nerve **sheath** in the PNS only. Neurofibromas are usually seen in patients with **neurofibromatosis**, while neurolemmomas are usually seen in patients with **von Recklinghausen disease**.

Somatic Nerves

64774 Excision of neuroma; cutaneous nerve, surgically identifiable

64776 digital nerve, 1 or both, same digit

+ 64778 digital nerve, each additional digit (List separately in addition to code for primary procedure)

64782 hand or foot, except digital nerve

+ 64783 hand or foot, each additional nerve, except same digit (List separately in addition to code for primary procedure)

64784 major peripheral nerve, except sciatic

64786 sciatic nerve

+ 64787 Implantation of nerve end into bone or muscle (List separately in addition to neuroma excision)

64788 Excision of neurofibroma or neurolemmoma; cutaneous nerve

64790 major peripheral nerve

64792 extensive (including malignant type)

64795 Biopsy of nerve

Sympathetic Nerves

64802 Sympathectomy, cervical

64804 Sympathectomy, cervicothoracic

64809 Sympathectomy, thoracolumbar

64818 Sympathectomy, lumbar

64820 Sympathectomy; digital arteries, each digit

64821 radial artery

64822 ulnar artery

64823 superficial palmar arch

FIGURE 9-36. The Vagus Nerve

The **bilateral** vagus nerve may be documented as the pneumogastric nerve, or cranial nerve X (CNX). It exits the medulla oblongata and, as the longest cranial nerve, travels through the **thorax** to the abdomen. It supplies the **parasympathetic** nerve fibers to all organs except the adrenal glands and has motor and sensory components. Among the critical functions of the vagus nerve is lowering heart rate and blood pressure in response to circulatory changes.

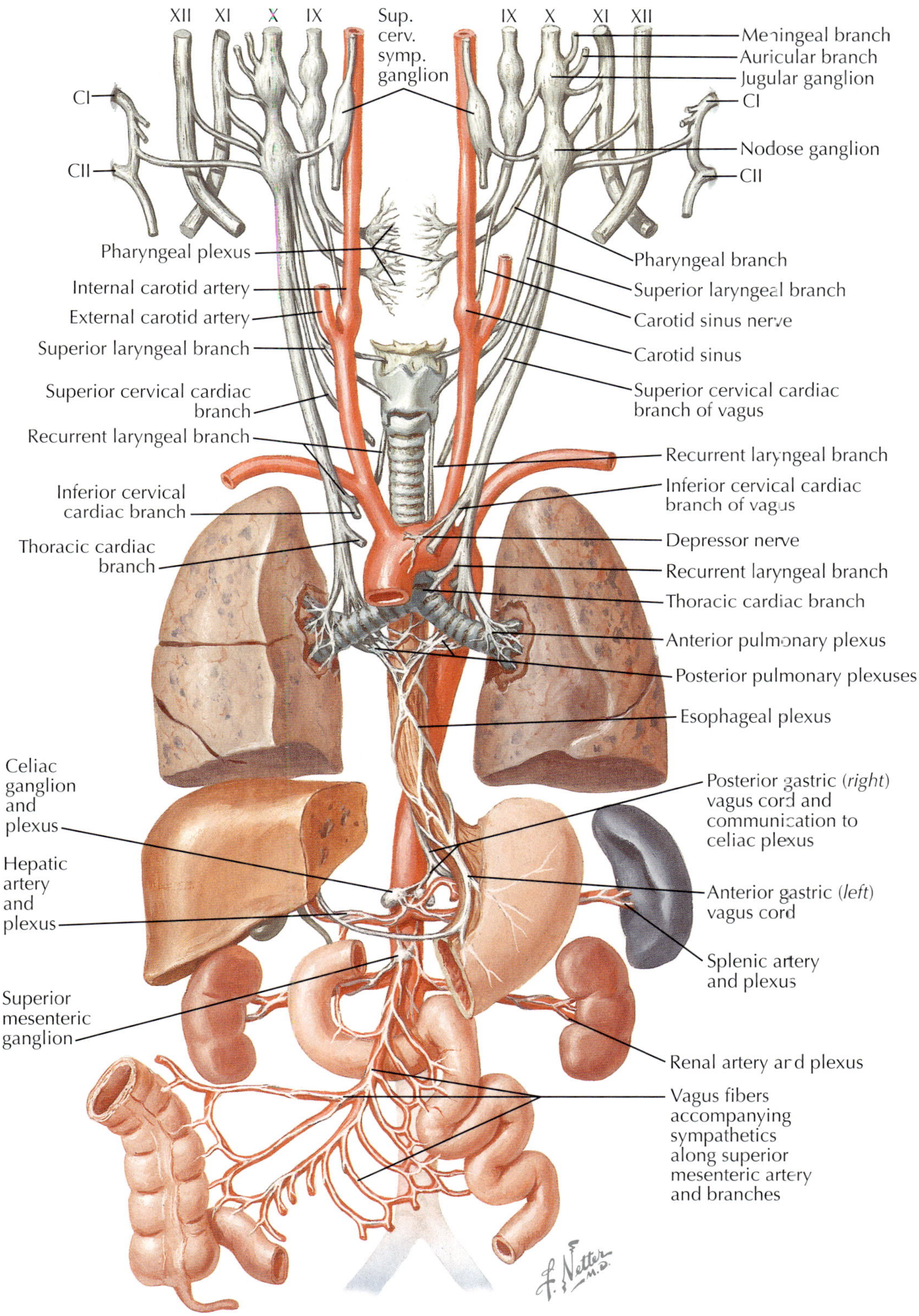

Neurorrhaphy

Coding Atlas

Damage to a nerve can occur at differing scales. Neuropraxia describes inhibited but not destroyed nerve conduction. Axonotmesis describes a more severe disruption, with the disruption of axons and endoneurial sheaths, but with the perineurium and epineurium intact. Neurotmesis may be referred to as Wallerian degeneration and indicates the collapse and sometimes shrinkage of endoneural tubes. The goal of neurorrhaphy is to align the fascicles of the nerve so that, over time, the nerve continuity and electrical impulses are restored.

64831 Suture of digital nerve, hand or foot; 1 nerve

+ 64832 each additional digital nerve (List separately in addition to code for primary procedure)

64834 Suture of 1 nerve; hand or foot, common sensory nerve

64835 median motor thenar

64836 ulnar motor

+ 64837 Suture of each additional nerve, hand or foot (List separately in addition to code for primary procedure)

64840 Suture of posterior tibial nerve

64856 Suture of major peripheral nerve, arm or leg, except sciatic; including transposition

64857 without transposition

64858 Suture of sciatic nerve

+ 64859 Suture of each additional major peripheral nerve (List separately in addition to code for primary procedure)

64861 Suture of; brachial plexus

64862 lumbar plexus

64864 Suture of facial nerve; extracranial

64865 infratemporal, with or without grafting

64866 Anastomosis; facial-spinal accessory

64868 facial-hypoglossal

+ 64872 Suture of nerve; requiring secondary or delayed suture (List separately in addition to code for primary neurorrhaphy)

+ 64874 requiring extensive mobilization, or transposition of nerve (List separately in addition to code for nerve suture)

+ 64876 requiring shortening of bone of extremity (List separately in addition to code for nerve suture)

Neurorrhaphy With Nerve Graft, Vein Graft, or Conduit

Coding Atlas

When a nerve is damaged and the severed ends fall short of the length needed for an anastomosis, an autogenous nerve graft can be sutured in place to bridge the gap. Also, a sleeve can be placed over the severed ends; over time, the gap is filled by regenerated neural tissue composed of axons that bridge the gap so that the electrical impulse circuit is complete. The sleeve may be synthetic (64910) or autogenous vein graft (64911). Use of an operative microscope is included in codes 64910 and 64911.

64885 Nerve graft (includes obtaining graft), head or neck; up to 4 cm in length

64886 more than 4 cm length

64890 Nerve graft (includes obtaining graft), single strand, hand or foot; up to 4 cm length

64891 more than 4 cm length

64892 Nerve graft (includes obtaining graft), single strand, arm or leg; up to 4 cm length

64893 more than 4 cm length

64895 Nerve graft (includes obtaining graft), multiple strands (cable), hand or foot; up to 4 cm length

64896 more than 4 cm length

64897 Nerve graft (includes obtaining graft), multiple strands (cable), arm or leg; up to 4 cm length

64898 more than 4 cm length

+ 64901 Nerve graft, each additional nerve; single strand (List separately in addition to code for primary procedure)

+ 64902 multiple strands (cable) (List separately in addition to code for primary procedure)

64905 Nerve pedicle transfer; first stage

64907 second stage

64910 Nerve repair; with synthetic conduit or vein allograft (eg, nerve tube), each nerve

64911 with autogenous vein graft (includes harvest of vein graft), each nerve

FIGURE 9-37. The Median Nerve

Thenar relates to muscles in the fleshy bulb on the palm at the base of the thumb, and **hypothenar** relates to muscles in the lesser fleshy bulk of the palm at the base of the pinky finger (minimus). The median nerve controls the thenar eminence, while the ulnar nerve controls the hypothenar eminence.

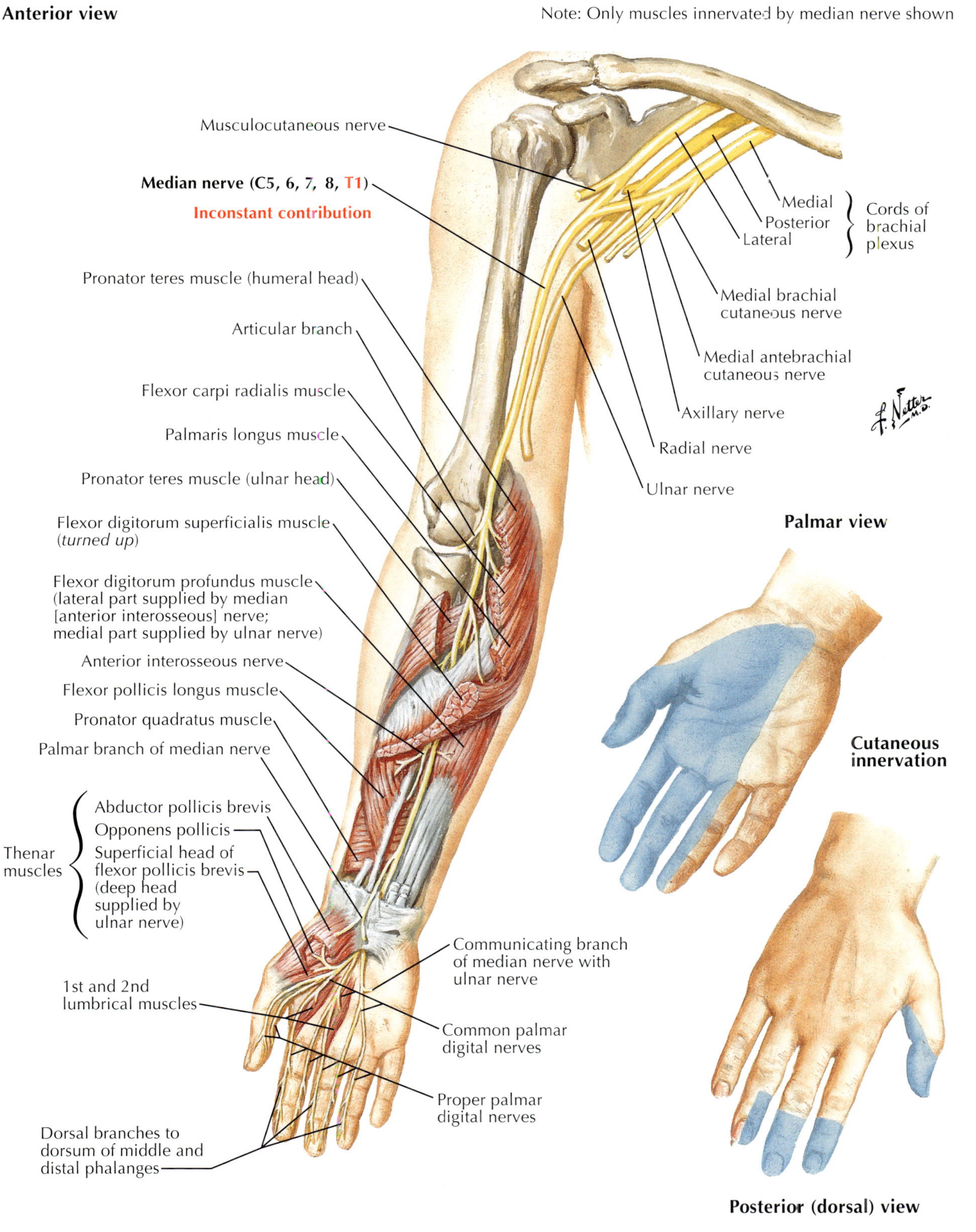

FIGURE 9-38. The Cranial Nerves

Cranial nerve roots emerge from the brain rather than the spinal cord to provide sensory and motor communication to parts of the body. The areas served by cranial nerves are primarily in the head and neck, with the exception of the vagus nerve (cranial nerve X [CNX]), which controls **parasympathetic** responses in the thorax and abdomen.

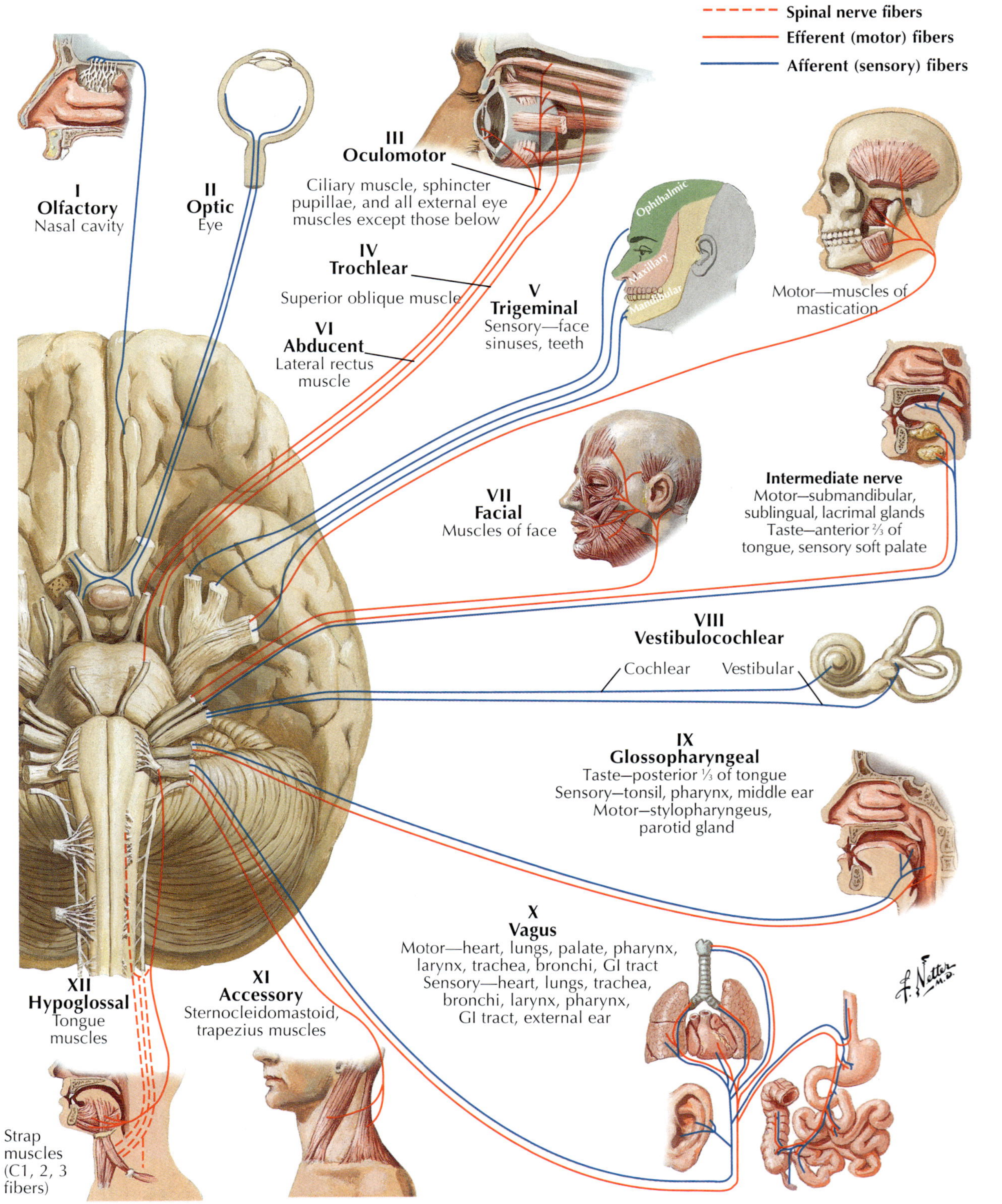

FIGURE 9-39. The Facial Nerve

Facial muscles are thin, **subcutaneous** muscles that control facial expression. They insert into skin of the face, rather than bone, and many have delicate, nuanced movements. Facial muscles are innervated by the **bilateral** facial nerve (cranial nerve VII [CNVII]), which also provides sensory nerves to the anterior two-thirds of the tongue and oral cavity.

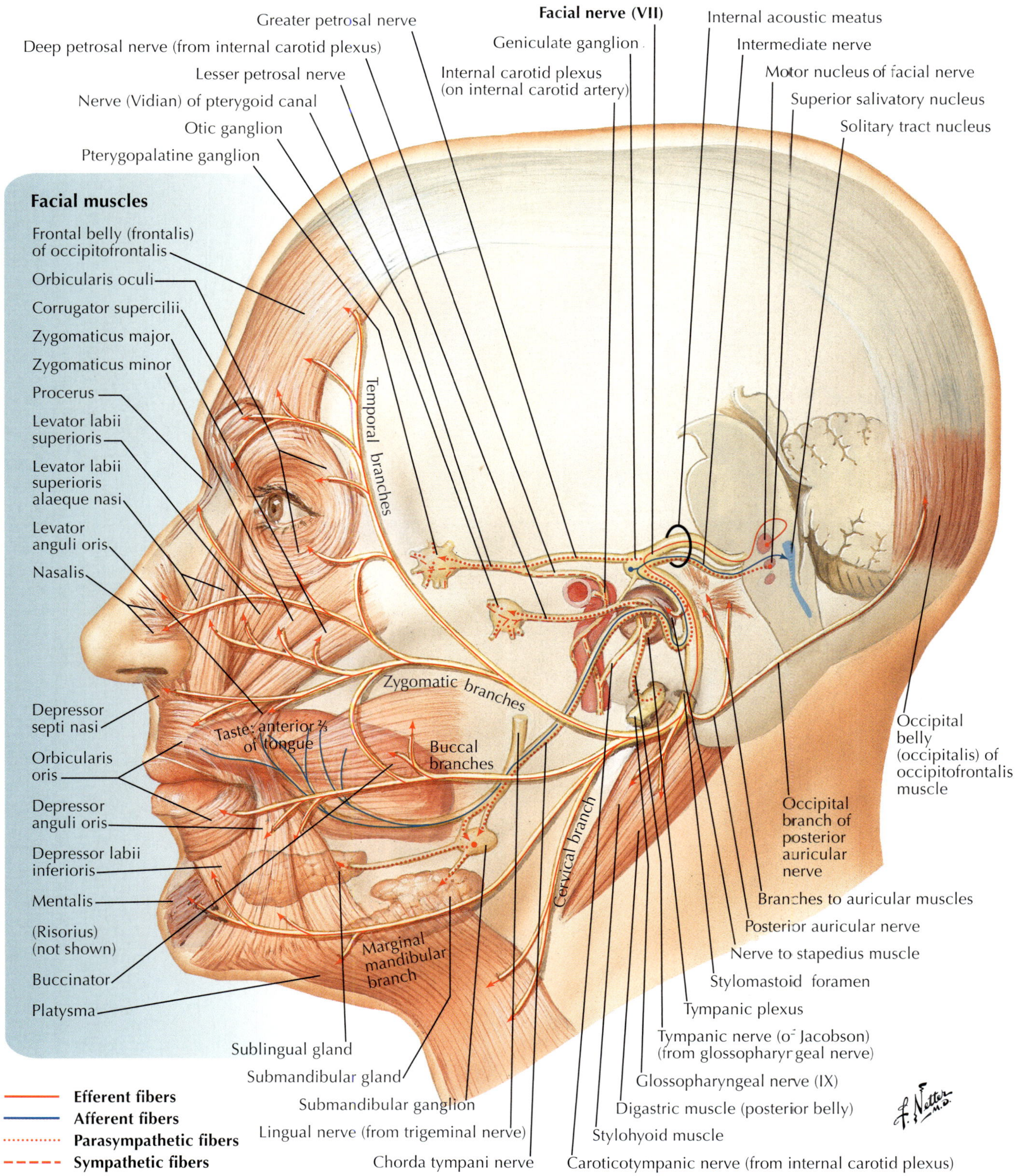

FIGURE 9-40. Peripheral Nerve Anatomy

Nerve fibers are bundled together and surrounded by a **perineurium** layer. Within the perineurium layer, the nerve fibers are protected by layers of connective tissue called **endoneurium**, also referred to as Henle's sheath. Perineurium-bound nerve bundles are further bundled into a larger network by an outer layer called **epineurium**, the outermost layer of the nerve. Blood and lymph vessels also lie within the nerve bundle.

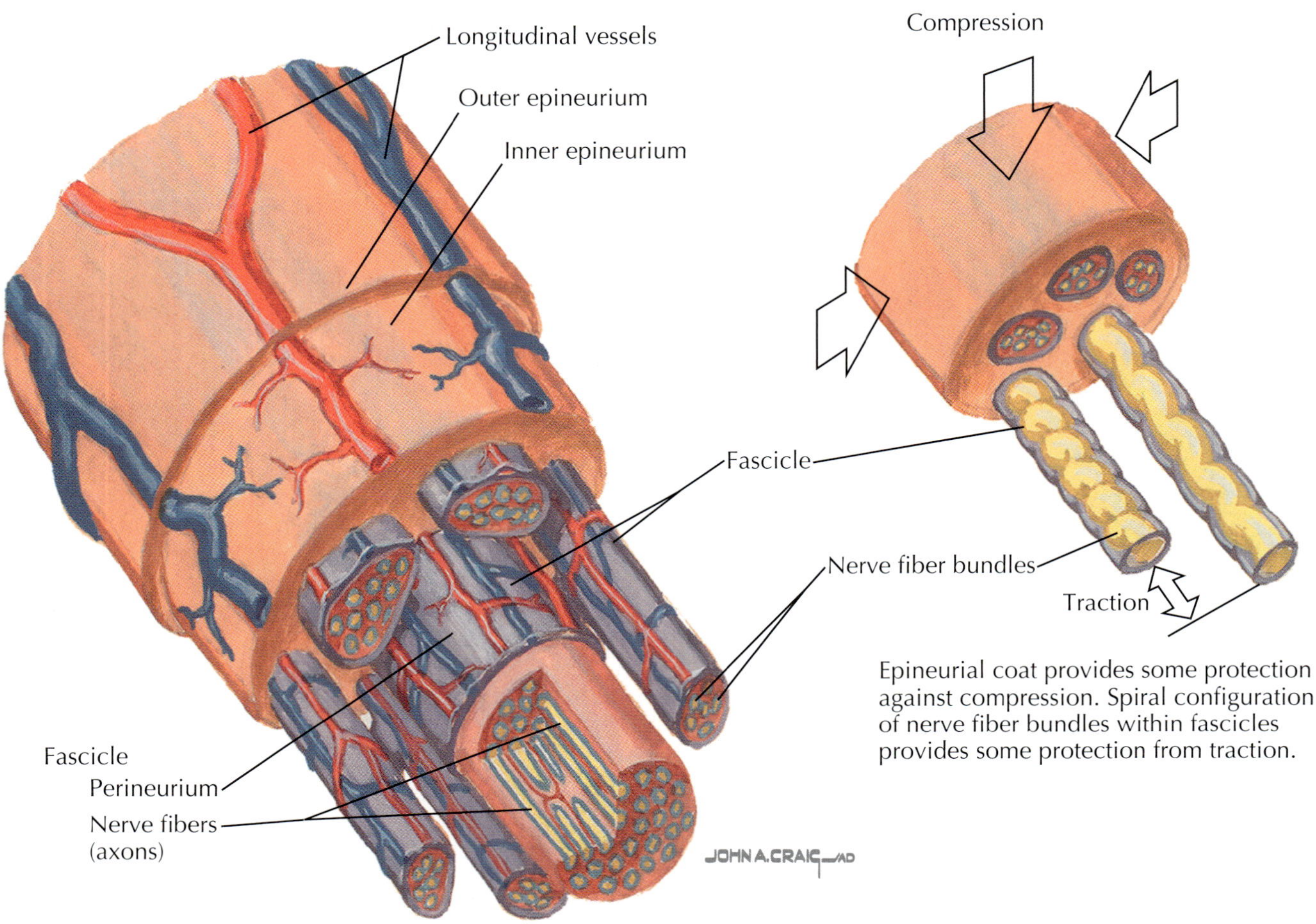

FIGURE 9-41. The Foot and Ankle Nerves

Several nerves serve the foot. The tibial nerve is a branch of the sciatic nerve; when it reaches the sole of the foot, it divides into the **medial** and **lateral** plantar nerves. The dorsal nerves innervate the top of the foot, and the sural nerve runs along the lateral foot to the fifth toe. The saphenous nerve is on the top of the foot but does not penetrate to the toes.

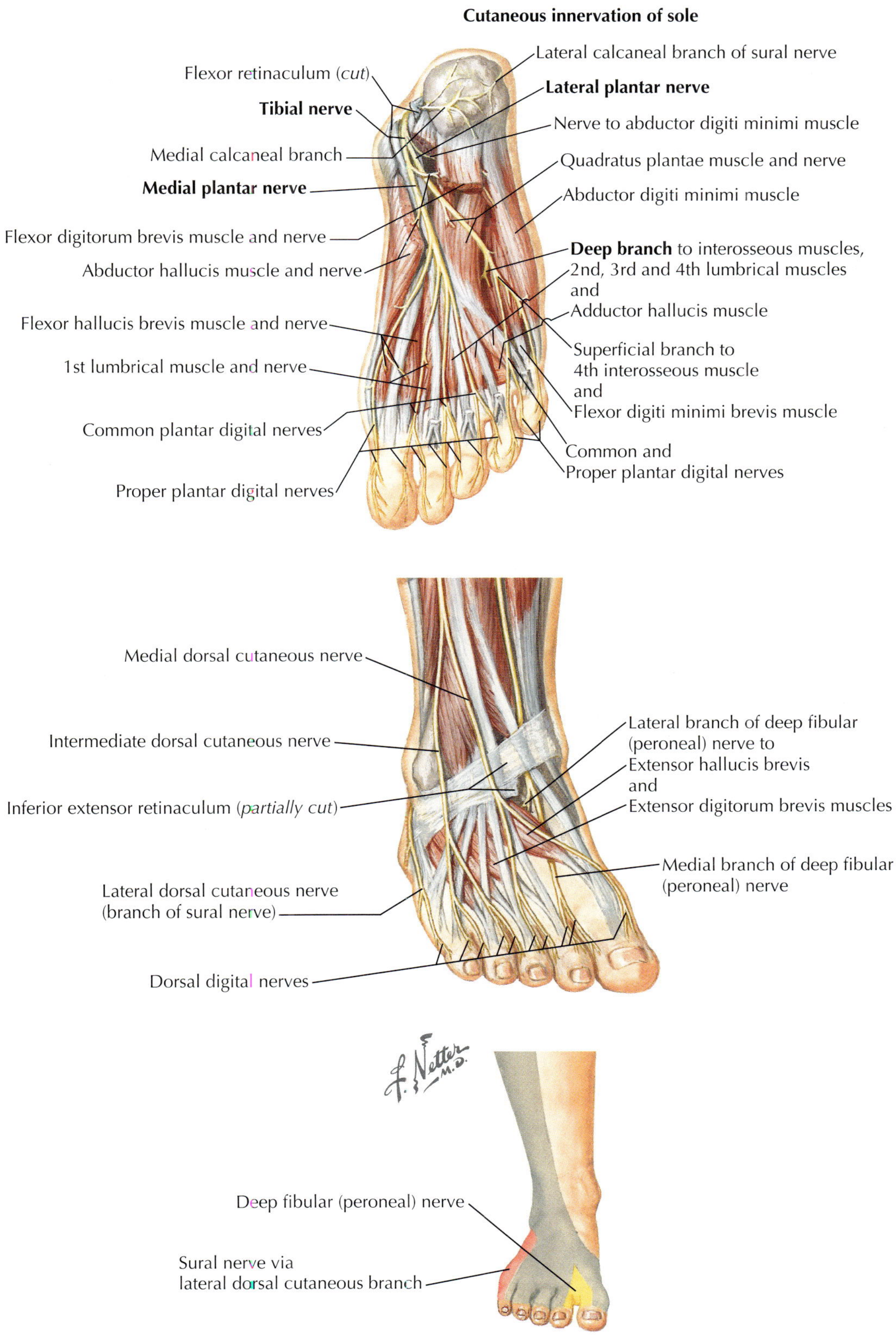

Innervation and action of extrinsic eye muscles: Anterior view of left eye

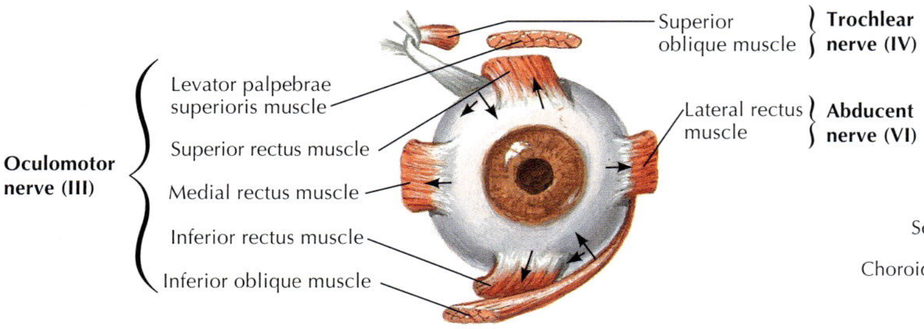

Note: Arrows indicate direction of eye movement produced by each muscle

Ophthalmoscopic view of right retina

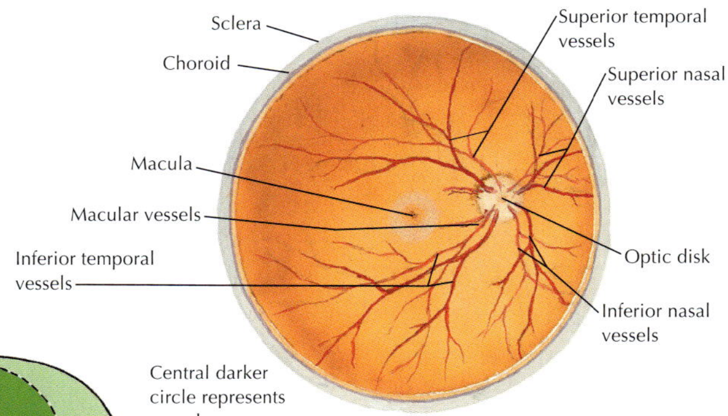

Visual pathway

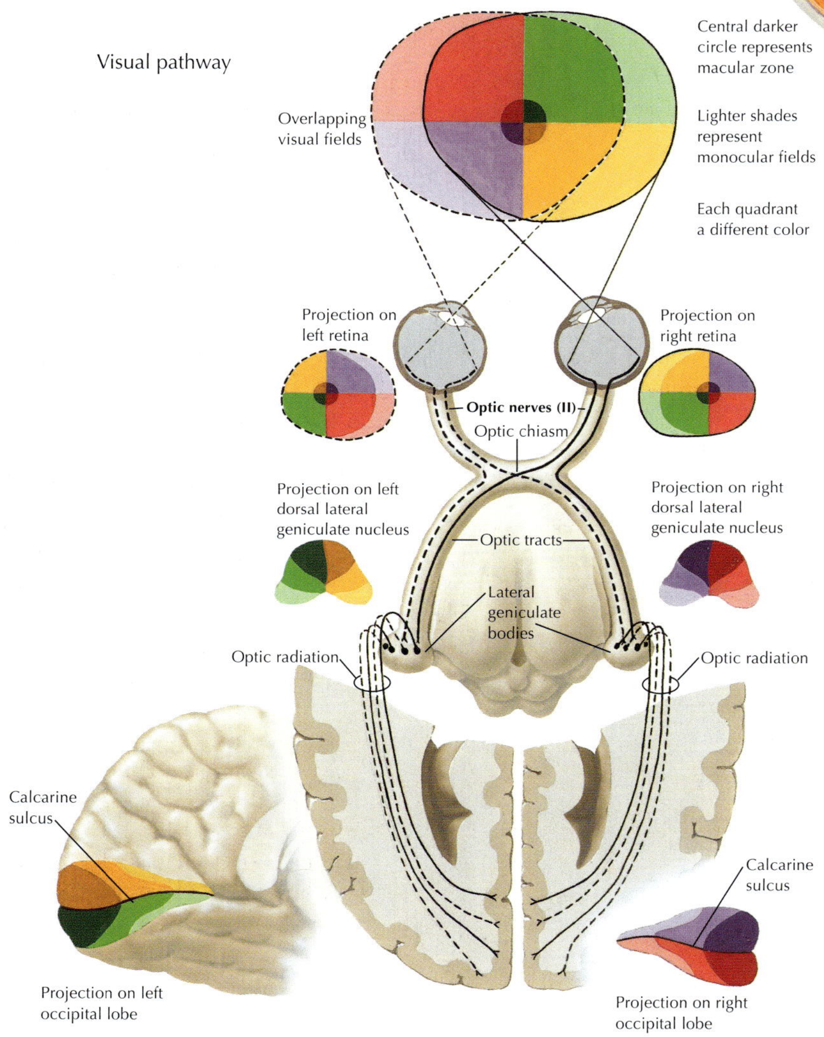

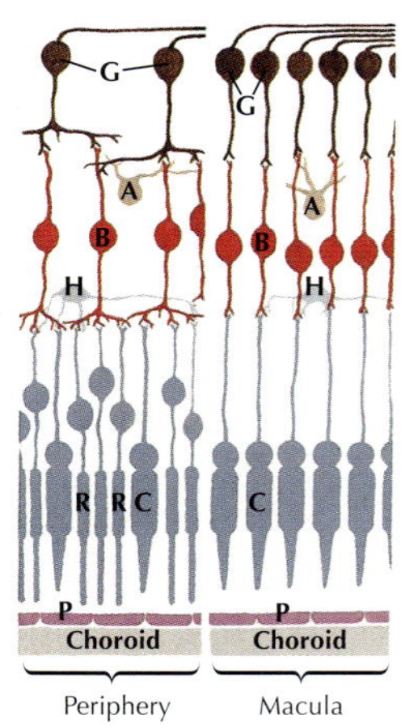

Structure of retina: Schema

- **A** Amacrine cells
- **B** Bipolar cells
- **C** Cones
- **G** Ganglion cells
- **H** Horizontal cells
- **P** Pigment cells
- **R** Rods

CHAPTER 10

Eye and Ocular Adnexa

The eyeball is a complex organ that sits in the eye socket, or **orbit**. The orbit is a deep, bony recess in the skull that protects the eyeball from injury. In addition to the pads of fat that cushion the eye, the orbit houses the optic nerve, **extraocular muscles**, and ocular vasculature. The orbit as well as the lids, extraocular muscles, lacrimal system, and conjunctiva are considered ocular **adnexa**, or an accessory structure to the globe. While some codes within the Eye and Ocular Adnexa section of the CPT code set are used to report **therapeutic** treatment of the orbit, other orbital codes are found in the Musculoskeletal System code set. Similarly, procedures that are performed solely on the skin of the eye may be reported using codes from the Integumentary System code set, and some eye-related surgeries may also be reported using Respiratory System and Nervous System codes.

The eyeball's only function is to facilitate vision. The eyeball's shape is one component of **visual acuity**. If the eyeball is too short, the patient may be nearsighted; if too long, the patient may be farsighted. Also, the fluid within the eye must be kept at a proper pressure and consistent level in order to maintain the shape of the eye for proper **refraction**. The cornea is the clear window at the front one-third of the eye. If the cornea is irregular in shape, the patient's vision is warped by **astigmatism**. In a healthy eye, light travels unobstructed through the transparent structures of the cornea, aqueous humor, pupil, lens, and vitreous humor until it reaches the retina. Each structure contributes to refraction and visual acuity. Light images reach the retina and stimulate it. The stimuli are perceived and transmitted along the optic nerve to the brain (occipital cortex).

The visual pathway has proven to be a key component of modern eye surgery. The advent of lasers revolutionized eye care, as it was discovered that a concentrated beam of light emitted by a laser could be utilized to treat many ocular defects. From its position outside the eye, the beam of a thermal laser can be directed to a target in the eye. The beam travels through the cornea, lens, aqueous humor, and vitreous humor without affecting them. Once the beam reaches the targeted tissue, it may seal blood vessels, destroy **tumors**, reattach retinas, or create new channels for flow of aqueous humor. Another type of laser, the photodisruptive laser, is directed to defects in the clear tissue of the cornea, vitreous humor, or lens.

If the surgeon has a clear visual pathway to the defect, laser surgery is often the approach selected, because it eliminates many risks associated with open surgery on the eye. When laser surgery is not appropriate, the most common approaches for entering the eye are through a **limbal** incision or a **pars plana** approach. A limbal incision is a small cut made by the surgeon into the junction of the cornea and the sclera (limbus). This small cut can be sutured, if needed, once surgery is completed. A limbal incision is commonly used to remove the lens and/or replace it with an intraocular lens (IOL). In a pars plana approach, the posterior segment is entered through a site posterior to the limbus and the ciliary body.

Many ocular surgeries do not require penetration of the globe. These surgeries may be performed to treat **strabismus** (improper alignment of the eyes), commonly seen in children, or eyelid problems such as **ectropion**, **entropion**, or **ptosis**, commonly seen in the elderly population.

Eyeball

Removal of Eye

Coding Atlas

The eyeball is well protected in the bony orbit, where it is surrounded by soft tissue and cushioning fat. In **evisceration**, the cornea is opened and the contents within the sclera are scooped out. The sclera of the eyeball remains attached to eye muscle. In **enucleation**, all connections to the eyeball are severed and the eyeball is removed. **Exenteration** is the resection of all contents of the orbit as well as adjacent eyelids, skin, lacrimal tissue, and sometimes pieces of orbital bone.

65091 Evisceration of ocular contents; without implant

65093 with implant

65101 Enucleation of eye; without implant

65103 with implant, muscles not attached to implant

65105 with implant, muscles attached to implant

65110 Exenteration of orbit (does not include skin graft), removal of orbital contents; only

65112 with therapeutic removal of bone

65114 with muscle or myocutaneous flap

Secondary Implant(s) Procedures

Coding Atlas

A **secondary** implant is indicated when the pathology that led to the removal of the patient's eye is stabilized or when a previous permanent implant needs to be replaced. Any existing permanent or temporary (space-holding) implant is removed and replaced with a new implant. The codes in this subsection are used to report implants within the eye socket. Many implants have multiple parts that are adjusted to fill the patient's ocular void.

65125 Modification of ocular implant with placement or replacement of pegs (eg, drilling receptacle for prosthesis appendage) (separate procedure)

65130 Insertion of ocular implant secondary; after evisceration, in scleral shell

65135 after enucleation, muscles not attached to implant

65140 after enucleation, muscles attached to implant

65150 Reinsertion of ocular implant; with or without conjunctival graft

65155 with use of foreign material for reinforcement and/or attachment of muscles to implant

65175 Removal of ocular implant

Removal of Foreign Body

Coding Atlas

The code range for this subsection does not include removal of **implants**. The codes are used to report embedded **foreign bodies** (FBs) of the eyeball caused by injury and are chosen according to site. The physician mechanically removes FBs; they are not flushed out with fluid. When multiple FBs are in one eye, the appropriate code is used once. If an injury results in FBs in both eyes (**bilateral**), the appropriate codes for each eye are used. Report code 67413 for removal of an orbital FB using a frontal approach or code 67430 for removal using a lateral approach.

65205 Removal of foreign body, external eye; conjunctival superficial

65210 conjunctival embedded (includes concretions), subconjunctival, or scleral nonperforating

65220 corneal, without slit lamp

65222 corneal, with slit lamp

65235 Removal of foreign body, intraocular; from anterior chamber of eye or lens

65260 from posterior segment, magnetic extraction, anterior or posterior route

65265 from posterior segment, nonmagnetic extraction

FIGURE 10-1. The Eyeball

The eye and ocular adnexa can be divided into two parts: **intraocular** and **extraocular**. Intraocular structures are within or comprising the globe. Extraocular structures are beyond the eyeball. The anterior chamber is between the iris and the cornea. Adjacent to the anterior chamber is the posterior chamber, bordered by the iris anteriorly and the lens and zonules posteriorly. The anterior segment includes both the anterior and posterior chambers. The posterior segment is the large area behind the lens.

Horizontal section

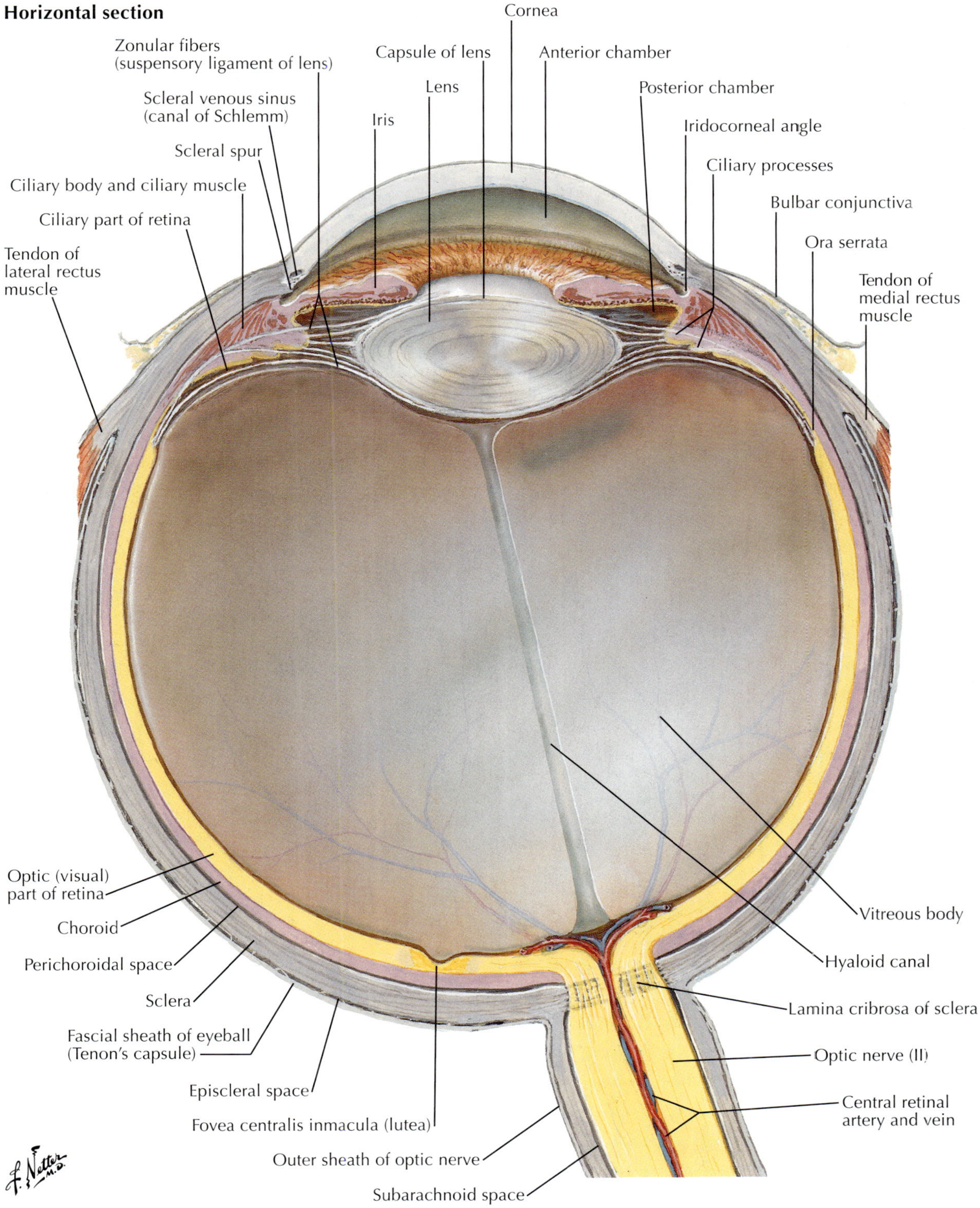

Repair of Laceration

Coding Atlas

The codes in this subsection are used to report injury repairs. The most pertinent information regarding eyeball lacerations is whether the laceration penetrates the globe. Perforation of the sclera may affect the anterior or posterior segments of the eye. Perforation of the cornea leads to leakage of aqueous humor. Repair includes restoration of the anterior chamber by injection as necessary.

65270 Repair of laceration; conjunctiva, with or without nonperforating laceration sclera, direct closure

65272 conjunctiva, by mobilization and rearrangement, without hospitalization

65273 conjunctiva, by mobilization and rearrangement, with hospitalization

65275 cornea, nonperforating, with or without removal foreign body

65280 cornea and/or sclera, perforating, not involving uveal tissue

65285 cornea and/or sclera, perforating, with reposition or resection of uveal tissue

65286 application of tissue glue, wounds of cornea and/or sclera

65290 Repair of wound, extraocular muscle, tendon and/or Tenon's capsule

Anterior Segment

Cornea

Coding Atlas

The cornea is the clear dome that refracts light at the front of the eye. If the dome of the cornea is too flat, too peaked, or irregular in shape, vision is affected. A surgeon may alter the shape of the cornea or remove imperfections from the cornea to improve vision. A diseased corneal layer may be removed or overlaid with a graft. When procedures penetrate the cornea, the pressure of aqueous humor, which is essential to eye shape and **refraction**, must be restored.

Excision

65400 Excision of lesion, cornea (keratectomy, lamellar, partial), except pterygium

65410 Biopsy of cornea

65420 Excision or transposition of pterygium; without graft

65426 with graft

Removal or Destruction

65430 Scraping of cornea, diagnostic, for smear and/or culture

65435 Removal of corneal epithelium; with or without chemocauterization (abrasion, curettage)

65436 with application of chelating agent (eg, EDTA)

65450 Destruction of lesion of cornea by cryotherapy, photocoagulation or thermocauterization

65600 Multiple punctures of anterior cornea (eg, for corneal erosion, tattoo)

Keratoplasty

65710 Keratoplasty (corneal transplant); anterior lamellar

65730 penetrating (except in aphakia or pseudophakia)

65750 penetrating (in aphakia)

65755 penetrating (in pseudophakia)

65756 endothelial

+ 65757 Backbench preparation of corneal endothelial allograft prior to transplantation (List separately in addition to code for primary procedure)

Other Procedures

65760 Keratomileusis

65765 Keratophakia

65767 Epikeratoplasty

65770 Keratoprosthesis

65771 Radial keratotomy

65772 Corneal relaxing incision for correction of surgically induced astigmatism

65775 Corneal wedge resection for correction of surgically induced astigmatism

65778 Placement of amniotic membrane on the ocular surface; without sutures

65779 single layer, sutured

65780 Ocular surface reconstruction; amniotic membrane transplantation, multiple layers

65781 limbal stem cell allograft (eg, cadaveric or living donor)

65782 limbal conjunctival autograft (includes obtaining graft)

FIGURE 10-2. The Anterior Segment

In the presence of bright light, the iris expands and the pupil is reduced. Less light enters the posterior segment. When lighting is dim, the iris contracts and the pupil becomes enlarged, allowing more light to enter the eye. For many laser surgeries, **mydriatic** drops are instilled in the eye to maximize the size of the pupil and improve surgical access. The ciliary process at the base of the iris produces aqueous humor that flows through the anterior segment of the eye.

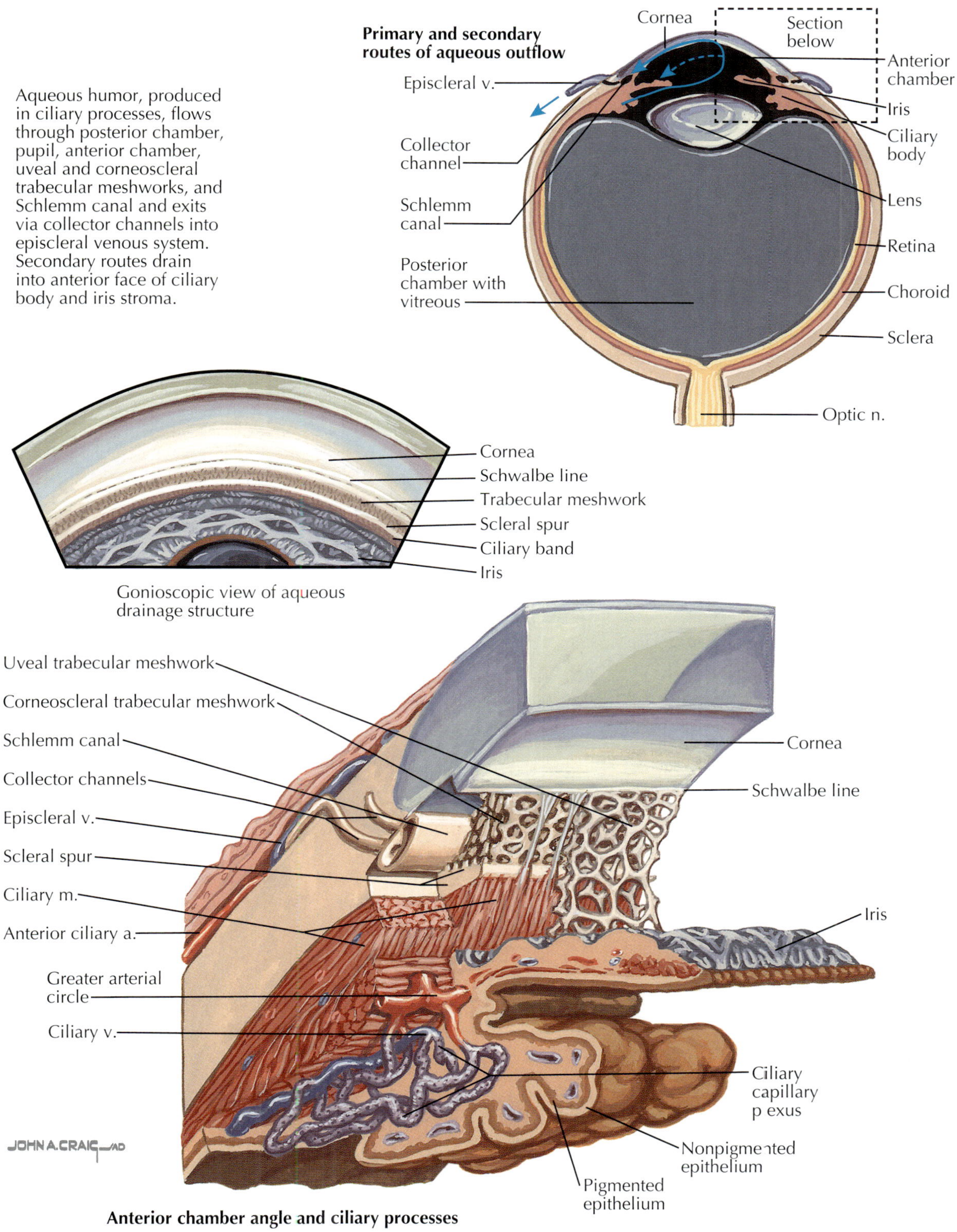

Anterior Chamber

Coding Atlas

Defects anywhere along the visual pathway may affect vision and require intervention. An image is carried through the transparent structures of the eye before stimulating the sensors of the retina. The image is transmitted along the optic nerve to the brain, where it is interpreted. The eye is divided into an anterior segment and a posterior segment, with the anterior segment being the portion anterior to the vitreous humor. The anterior segment is further divided into posterior and anterior chambers. The anterior chamber is the area between the innermost layer of the cornea and the iris and includes the trabecular meshwork. Most anterior chamber procedures are performed to improve the flow of aqueous humor in order to reduce intraocular pressure, to treat glaucoma, or to remove blood from an injury.

Incision

65800 Paracentesis of anterior chamber of eye (separate procedure); with removal of aqueous

65810 with removal of vitreous and/or discission of anterior hyaloid membrane, with or without air injection

65815 with removal of blood, with or without irrigation and/or air injection

65820 Goniotomy

65850 Trabeculotomy ab externo

65855 Trabeculoplasty by laser surgery, 1 or more sessions (defined treatment series)

65860 Severing adhesions of anterior segment, laser technique (separate procedure)

65865 Severing adhesions of anterior segment of eye, incisional technique (with or without injection of air or liquid) (separate procedure); goniosynechiae

65870 anterior synechiae, except goniosynechiae

65875 posterior synechiae

65880 corneovitreal adhesions

Removal

65900 Removal of epithelial downgrowth, anterior chamber of eye

65920 Removal of implanted material, anterior segment of eye

65930 Removal of blood clot, anterior segment of eye

Introduction

66020 Injection, anterior chamber of eye (separate procedure); air or liquid

66030 medication

Anterior Sclera

Coding Atlas

The sclera is the tough, white shell in which the ocular contents reside. It attaches to the cornea at the limbus. The anterior sclera lies between the limbus and the extraocular muscles and is covered in conjunctival tissue. As a treatment for glaucoma, the anterior sclera may be incised to access the anterior chamber and/or to provide a path for aqueous humor release. A shunt, stent, and/or reservoir may be placed.

Excision

66130 Excision of lesion, sclera

66150 Fistulization of sclera for glaucoma; trephination with iridectomy

66155 thermocauterization with iridectomy

66160 sclerectomy with punch or scissors, with iridectomy

66170 trabeculectomy ab externo in absence of previous surgery

66172 trabeculectomy ab externo with scarring from previous ocular surgery or trauma (includes injection of antifibrotic agents)

66174 Transluminal dilation of aqueous outflow canal; without retention of device or stent

66175 with retention of device or stent

Aqueous Shunt

66179 Aqueous shunt to extraocular equatorial plate reservoir, external approach; without graft

66180 with graft

66183 Insertion of anterior segment aqueous drainage device, without extraocular reservoir, external approach

66184 Revision of aqueous shunt to extraocular equatorial plate reservoir; without graft

66185 with graft

FIGURE 10-3. Aqueous Flow and Pressure

Any impediment to the flow of aqueous humor in the trabecular meshwork or **canal of Schlemm** can increase intraocular pressure (IOP). Elevated IOP leads to glaucoma and optic nerve damage if untreated. Surgical intervention may open channels for aqueous flow and reduce risk in patients with angle closure or other flow restrictions. Note: Tools, implants, and/or equipment depicted in the illustration may be outdated but the procedural approach is valid.

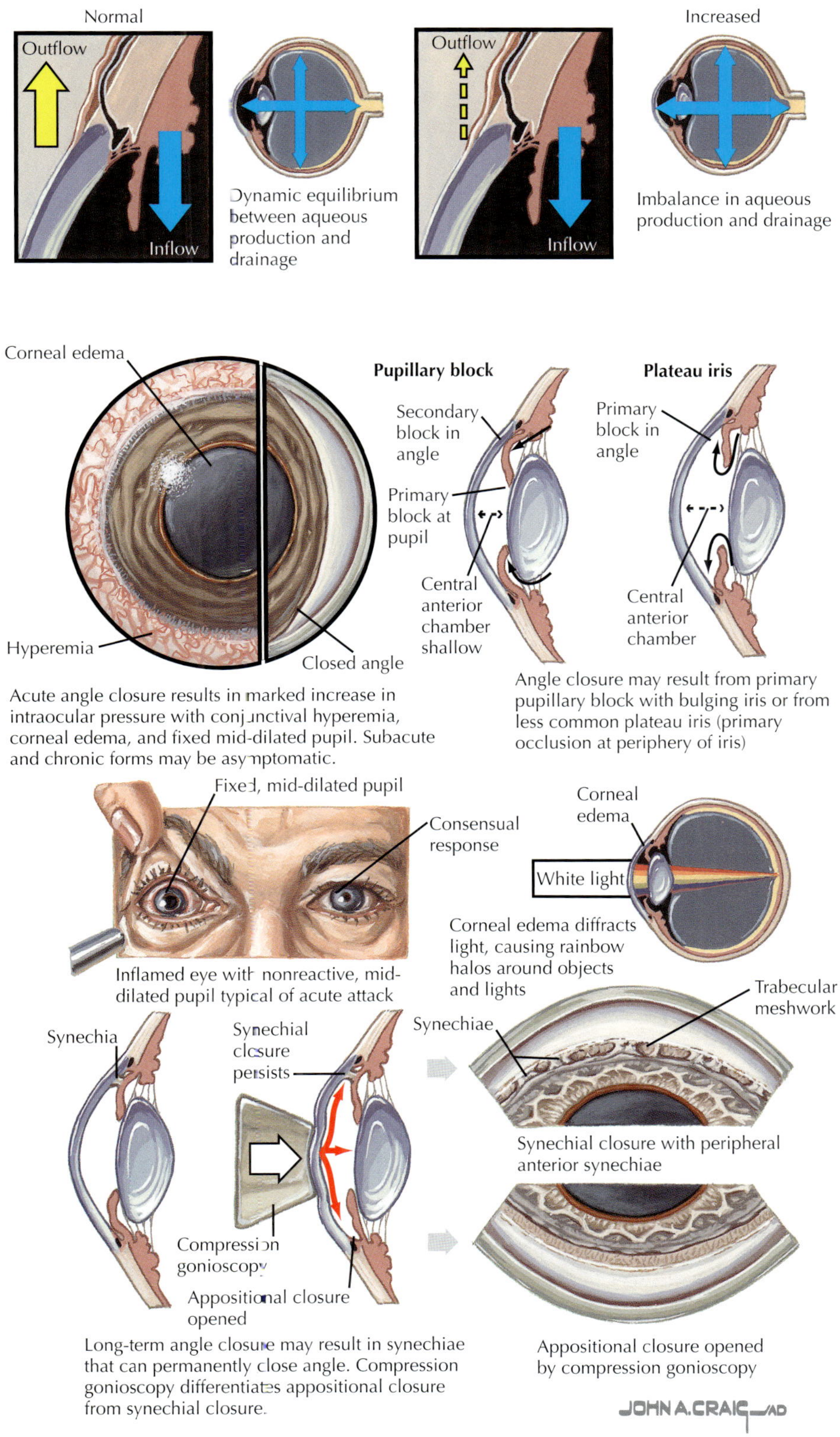

Dynamic equilibrium between aqueous production and drainage

Imbalance in aqueous production and drainage

Acute angle closure results in marked increase in intraocular pressure with conjunctival hyperemia, corneal edema, and fixed mid-dilated pupil. Subacute and chronic forms may be asymptomatic.

Angle closure may result from primary pupillary block with bulging iris or from less common plateau iris (primary occlusion at periphery of iris)

Inflamed eye with nonreactive, mid-dilated pupil typical of acute attack

Corneal edema diffracts light, causing rainbow halos around objects and lights

Synechial closure with peripheral anterior synechiae

Long-term angle closure may result in synechiae that can permanently close angle. Compression gonioscopy differentiates appositional closure from synechial closure.

Appositional closure opened by compression gonioscopy

Repair or Revision

66220 Repair of scleral staphyloma; without graft

66225 with graft

66250 Revision or repair of operative wound of anterior segment, any type, early or late, major or minor procedure

Iris, Ciliary Body

Coding Atlas

The iris is the ring of color in front of the lens. Its purpose is to regulate light entering the eye by contracting and expanding, thus, changing the size of the pupil. The ciliary body is a tissue posterior lateral to the edge of the lens. The ciliary body has two functions: produce aqueous humor and the muscles control the shape of the lens, which contributes to refraction and visual acuity. Some glaucoma patients benefit from procedures that incise or destroy tissue of the iris or ciliary body.

Incision

66500 Iridotomy by stab incision (separate procedure); except transfixion

66505 with transfixion as for iris bombe

Excision

66600 Iridectomy, with corneoscleral or corneal section; for removal of lesion

66605 with cyclectomy

66625 peripheral for glaucoma (separate procedure)

66630 sector for glaucoma (separate procedure)

66635 optical (separate procedure)

Repair

66680 Repair of iris, ciliary body (as for iridodialysis)

66682 Suture of iris, ciliary body (separate procedure) with retrieval of suture through small incision (eg, McCannel suture)

Destruction

66700 Ciliary body destruction; diathermy

66710 cyclophotocoagulation, transscleral

66711 cyclophotocoagulation, endoscopic

⊙ **66720** cryotherapy

66740 cyclodialysis

66761 Iridotomy/iridectomy by laser surgery (eg, for glaucoma) (per session)

66762 Iridoplasty by photocoagulation (1 or more sessions) (eg, for improvement of vision, for widening of anterior chamber angle)

66770 Destruction of cyst or lesion iris or ciliary body (nonexcisional procedure)

Lens

Coding Atlas

The crystalline lens is suspended behind the iris and is crucial to refraction and visual acuity. The convex lens has a capsule and a softer center. Age, injury, or disease may cloud the lens (cataract) or cause the lens to shift from its position in the visual pathway. Vision can be improved if the flawed natural lens is removed and proper refraction restored.

Incision

66820 Discission of secondary membranous cataract (opacified posterior lens capsule and/or anterior hyaloid); stab incision technique (Ziegler or Wheeler knife)

66821 laser surgery (eg, YAG laser) (1 or more stages)

66825 Repositioning of intraocular lens prosthesis, requiring an incision (separate procedure)

Removal

66830 Removal of secondary membranous cataract (opacified posterior lens capsule and/or anterior hyaloid) with corneo-scleral section, with or without iridectomy (iridocapsulotomy, iridocapsulectomy)

66840 Removal of lens material; aspiration technique, 1 or more stages

66850 phacofragmentation technique (mechanical or ultrasonic) (eg, phacoemulsification), with aspiration

66852 pars plana approach, with or without vitrectomy

66920 intracapsular

66930 intracapsular, for dislocated lens

66940 extracapsular (other than 66840, 66850, 66852)

FIGURE 10-4. Lens Removal and Replacement

In **phacoemulsification** or **phacofragmentation**, the lens is fragmented into small pieces and aspirated from the eye. This allows for a smaller surgical incision than would be required if the lens were to be removed in one piece. The new artificial intraocular lens (IOL) is folded and inserted through the same incision, then opened and positioned. **Haptics** secure the new lens. Note: Tools, implants, and/or equipment depicted in the illustration may be outdated but the procedural approach is valid.

Instruments for Cataract Removal

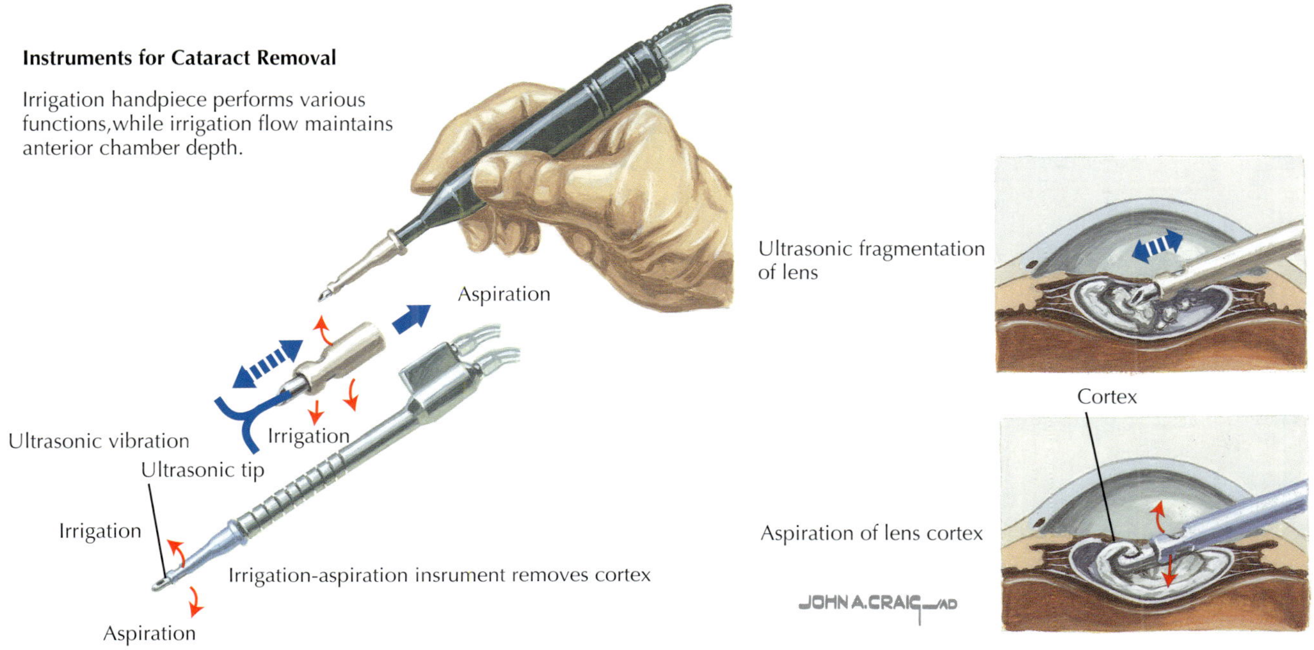

Phacoemulsification and Insertion of Flexible IOL

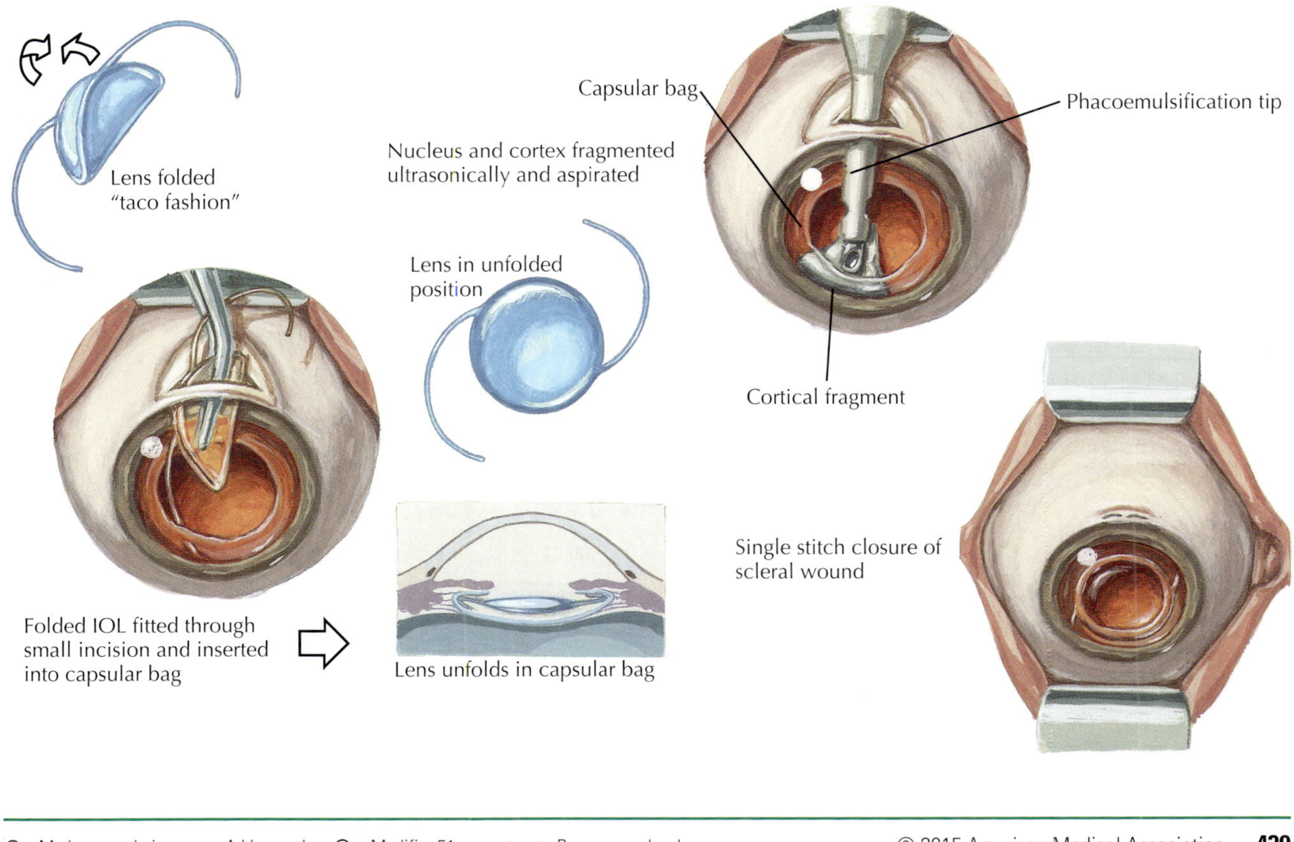

Intraocular Lens Procedures

Coding Atlas

An intraocular lens (IOL) **prosthesis** is often inserted during the same surgical session in which a **cataract** is removed. The surgeon may remove the entire lens either whole or in pieces. This is called **intracapsular cataract extraction (ICCE)**, and an artificial lens may be placed in front of the iris. In **extracapsular intraocular extraction (ECCE)**, the surgeon removes the fragmented lens, leaving in place the posterior capsule of the natural lens. Retention of the posterior shell provides support to the eye. An artificial lens can then be placed behind the iris and in front of the remaining posterior lens.

66982 Extracapsular cataract removal with insertion of intraocular lens prosthesis (1-stage procedure), manual or mechanical technique (eg, irrigation and aspiration or phacoemulsification), complex, requiring devices or techniques not generally used in routine cataract surgery (eg, iris expansion device, suture support for intraocular lens, or primary posterior capsulorrhexis) or performed on patients in the amblyogenic developmental stage

66983 Intracapsular cataract extraction with insertion of intraocular lens prosthesis (1 stage procedure)

66984 Extracapsular cataract removal with insertion of intraocular lens prosthesis (1 stage procedure), manual or mechanical technique (eg, irrigation and aspiration or phacoemulsification)

66985 Insertion of intraocular lens prosthesis (secondary implant), not associated with concurrent cataract removal

66986 Exchange of intraocular lens

Other Procedures

Coding Atlas

An ophthalmic **endoscope** provides the ophthalmologist with real-time magnified video of the surgical field through a scope that may also contain surgical tools. Code 66990 can be used to report endoscopic procedures only with the following codes: 65820, 65875, 65920, 65985, 65986, 67039, 67040, 67041, 67042, 67043, 67112, and 67113.

+ 66990 Use of ophthalmic endoscope (List separately in addition to code for primary procedure)

Posterior Segment

Vitreous

Coding Atlas

Vitreous is the clear gel that fills the chamber of the eye behind the lens, helping the globe retain its shape and pressing the retina firmly against the vascular choroid. Light travels through vitreous to reach the retina. Flaws in vitreous may cause flaws in vision. Vitreous may be removed if it is flawed, diseased, or interfering with the function of the retina, as in **proliferative vitreoretinopathy**. Vitreous may be replaced with vitreous substitute in order to maintain the shape of the eye or to anchor the retina.

67005 Removal of vitreous, anterior approach (open sky technique or limbal incision); partial removal

67010 subtotal removal with mechanical vitrectomy

67015 Aspiration or release of vitreous, subretinal or choroidal fluid, pars plana approach (posterior sclerotomy)

67025 Injection of vitreous substitute, pars plana or limbal approach (fluid-gas exchange), with or without aspiration (separate procedure)

67027 Implantation of intravitreal drug delivery system (eg, ganciclovir implant), includes concomitant removal of vitreous

67028 Intravitreal injection of a pharmacologic agent (separate procedure)

67030 Discission of vitreous strands (without removal), pars plana approach

67031 Severing of vitreous strands, vitreous face adhesions, sheets, membranes or opacities, laser surgery (1 or more stages)

67036 Vitrectomy, mechanical, pars plana approach;

67039 with focal endolaser photocoagulation

67040 with endolaser panretinal photocoagulation

67041 with removal of preretinal cellular membrane (eg, macular pucker)

67042 with removal of internal limiting membrane of retina (eg, for repair of macular hole, diabetic macular edema), includes, if performed, intraocular tamponade (ie, air, gas or silicone oil)

67043 with removal of subretinal membrane (eg, choroidal neovascularization), includes, if performed, intraocular tamponade (ie, air, gas or silicone oil) and laser photocoagulation

Retina or Choroid

Coding Atlas

When the retina detaches, it loses its normal blood supply. The retina may be reattached surgically by sealing it back into place, by using a scleral band to create pressure inside the posterior segment, or by injecting a vitreous substitute to force the retinal tissue back into place. In **retinopathy**, new vessels (**neovascularization**) threaten vision. Retinopathy is commonly treated using a laser. Retinal detachment and retinopathy treatments may require multiple sessions. Codes that specify "1 or more sessions" are used once to report multiple treatments occurring over time as part of a treatment plan.

Repair

67101 Repair of retinal detachment, 1 or more sessions; cryotherapy or diathermy, with or without drainage of subretinal fluid

67105 photocoagulation, with or without drainage of subretinal fluid

67107 Repair of retinal detachment; scleral buckling (such as lamellar scleral dissection, imbrication or encircling procedure), with or without implant, with or without cryotherapy, photocoagulation, and drainage of subretinal fluid

67108 with vitrectomy, any method, with or without air or gas tamponade, focal endolaser photocoagulation, cryotherapy, drainage of subretinal fluid, scleral buckling, and/or removal of lens by same technique

67110 by injection of air or other gas (eg, pneumatic retinopexy)

67112 by scleral buckling or vitrectomy, on patient having previous ipsilateral retinal detachment repair(s) using scleral buckling or vitrectomy techniques

67113 Repair of complex retinal detachment (eg, proliferative vitreoretinopathy, stage C-1 or greater, diabetic traction retinal detachment, retinopathy of prematurity, retinal tear of greater than 90 degrees), with vitrectomy and membrane peeling, may include air, gas, or silicone oil tamponade, cryotherapy, endolaser photocoagulation, drainage of subretinal fluid, scleral buckling, and/or removal of lens

67115 Release of encircling material (posterior segment)

67120 Removal of implanted material, posterior segment; extraocular

67121 intraocular

Prophylaxis

67141 Prophylaxis of retinal detachment (eg, retinal break, lattice degeneration) without drainage, 1 or more sessions; cryotherapy, diathermy

67145 photocoagulation (laser or xenon arc)

Destruction

67208 Destruction of localized lesion of retina (eg, macular edema, tumors), 1 or more sessions; cryotherapy, diathermy

67210 photocoagulation

67218 radiation by implantation of source (includes removal of source)

67220 Destruction of localized lesion of choroid (eg, choroidal neovascularization); photocoagulation (eg, laser), 1 or more sessions

67221 photodynamic therapy (includes intravenous infusion)

+ 67225 photodynamic therapy, second eye, at single session (List separately in addition to code for primary eye treatment)

67227 Destruction of extensive or progressive retinopathy (eg, diabetic retinopathy), 1 or more sessions, cryotherapy, diathermy

67228 Treatment of extensive or progressive retinopathy, 1 or more sessions; (eg, diabetic retinopathy), photocoagulation

67229 preterm infant (less than 37 weeks gestation at birth), performed from birth up to 1 year of age (eg, retinopathy of prematurity), photocoagulation or cryotherapy

Posterior Sclera

Coding Atlas

The sclera is the tough, white shell in which the ocular contents reside. The posterior sclera covers that portion of the globe located behind the site at which the **extraocular** muscles are attached to the globe.

Repair

67250 Scleral reinforcement (separate procedure); without graft

67255 with graft

Ocular Adnexa

Extraocular Muscles

Coding Atlas

In **strabismus**, the eyes do not line up properly or do not work in unison. A surgeon may be able to correct strabismus by treating one or more of the six intraocular muscles in each eye. These muscles work in pairs: **lateral** with **medial** rectus (horizontal muscles), **superior** with **inferior** rectus (vertical muscles), and superior with inferior oblique (vertical muscles). The muscles may be shortened (**resection**) or lengthened (**recession**). Previous surgeries may make these corrections more complex.

67311 Strabismus surgery, recession or resection procedure; 1 horizontal muscle

67312 2 horizontal muscles

67314 1 vertical muscle (excluding superior oblique)

67316 2 or more vertical muscles (excluding superior oblique)

67318 Strabismus surgery, any procedure, superior oblique muscle

+ 67320 Transposition procedure (eg, for paretic extraocular muscle), any extraocular muscle (specify) (List separately in addition to code for primary procedure)

+ 67331 Strabismus surgery on patient with previous eye surgery or injury that did not involve the extraocular muscles (List separately in addition to code for primary procedure)

+ 67332 Strabismus surgery on patient with scarring of extraocular muscles (eg, prior ocular injury, strabismus or retinal detachment surgery) or restrictive myopathy (eg, dysthyroid ophthalmopathy) (List separately in addition to code for primary procedure)

+ 67334 Strabismus surgery by posterior fixation suture technique, with or without muscle recession (List separately in addition to code for primary procedure)

+ 67335 Placement of adjustable suture(s) during strabismus surgery, including postoperative adjustment(s) of suture(s) (List separately in addition to code for specific strabismus surgery)

+ 67340 Strabismus surgery involving exploration and/or repair of detached extraocular muscle(s) (List separately in addition to code for primary procedure)

67343 Release of extensive scar tissue without detaching extraocular muscle (separate procedure)

67345 Chemodenervation of extraocular muscle

67346 Biopsy of extraocular muscle

Orbit

Coding Atlas

The orbit is the bony cradle that houses and cushions the eyeball, the extraocular muscle, and all soft tissue within the orbit except the eyeball. A **retrobulbar** injection is an injection from a syringe into the space in the orbit behind the eyeball. An injection into the **Tenon's capsule** is from a syringe into a sheath that surrounds most of the eye and ocular muscles. Fractures and bone grafts of the orbit are reported using codes from the Musculoskeletal System code set.

Exploration, Excision, Decompression

67400 Orbitotomy without bone flap (frontal or transconjunctival approach); for exploration, with or without biopsy

67405 with drainage only

67412 with removal of lesion

67413 with removal of foreign body

67414 with removal of bone for decompression

67415 Fine needle aspiration of orbital contents

67420 Orbitotomy with bone flap or window, lateral approach (eg, Kroenlein); with removal of lesion

67430 with removal of foreign body

67440 with drainage

67445 with removal of bone for decompression

67450 for exploration, with or without biopsy

Other Procedures

67500 Retrobulbar injection; medication (separate procedure, does not include supply of medication)

67505 alcohol

67515 Injection of medication or other substance into Tenon's capsule

67550 Orbital implant (implant outside muscle cone); insertion

67560 removal or revision

67570 Optic nerve decompression (eg, incision or fenestration of optic nerve sheath)

FIGURE 10-5. The Extraocular Muscles

Binocular vision depends on a balanced push-and-pull action between paired muscles. When there is an imbalance between paired muscles, the patient has symptoms such as double vision and flawed depth perception. The patient also may have cosmetic symptoms such as crossed eyes (esotropia), walleye (exotropia), or uncoordinated eye movements. Surgery may restore balance and eliminate these symptoms.

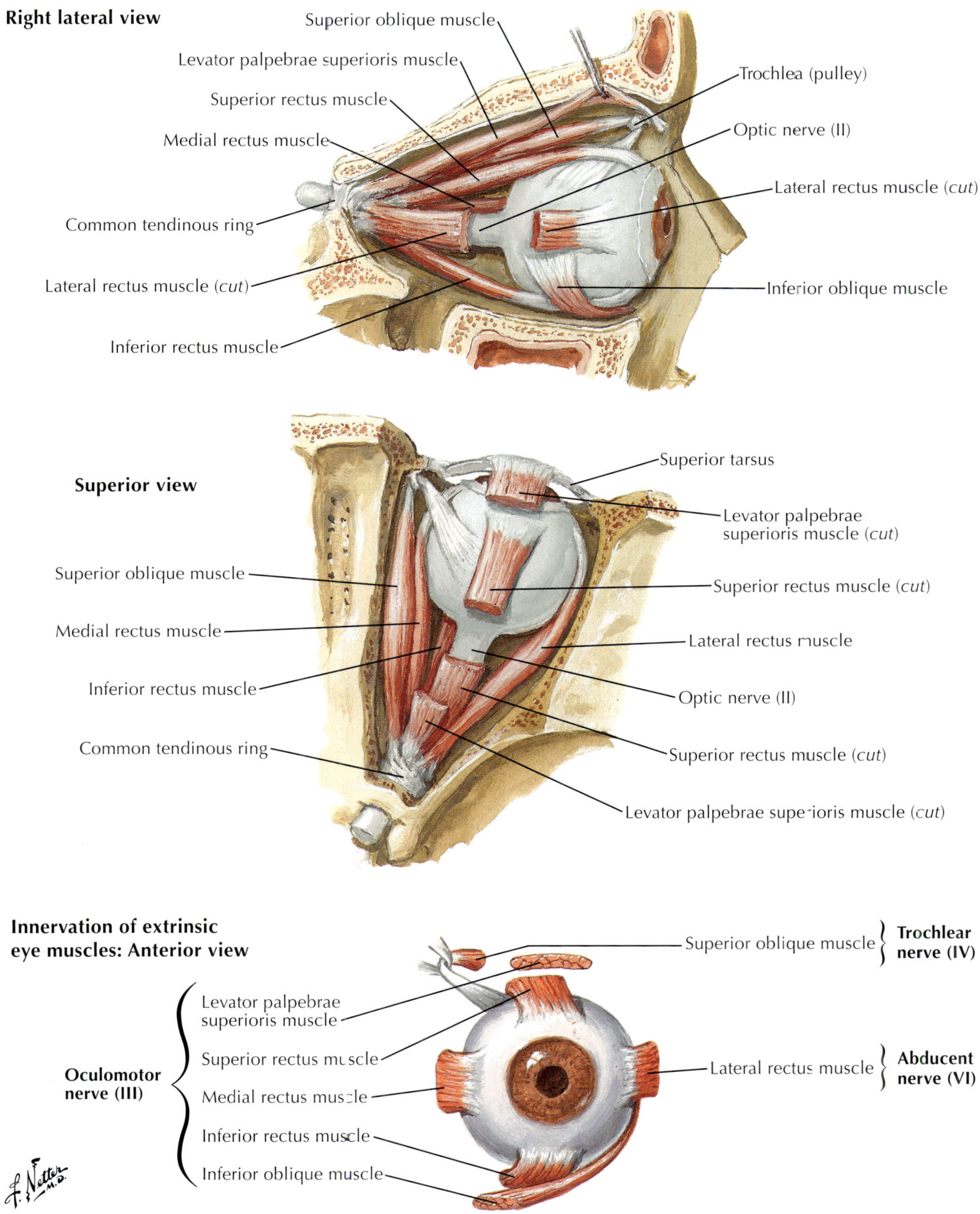

Eyelids

Coding Atlas

Eyelids protect the eye and distribute moisture during blinking. Many disorders of the eyelids may be the result of aging as skin or muscle loses its elasticity. Other disorders are due to disease, injury, or nerve damage. Conjunctival tissue lines the inside of the eyelids, which are edged in eyelashes and glands. The meibomian glands secrete a protective film to prevent evaporation of tears. Some eyelid procedures involve only skin. These are reported using codes from the Integumentary System code set.

Incision

67700 Blepharotomy, drainage of abscess, eyelid

67710 Severing of tarsorrhaphy

67715 Canthotomy (separate procedure)

\# **67810** Incisional biopsy of eyelid skin including lid margin

Excision, Destruction

67800 Excision of chalazion; single

67801 multiple, same lid

67805 multiple, different lids

67808 under general anesthesia and/or requiring hospitalization, single or multiple

67810 Code is out of numerical sequence. See 67700-67810

67820 Correction of trichiasis; epilation, by forceps only

67825 epilation by other than forceps (eg, by electrosurgery, cryotherapy, laser surgery)

67830 incision of lid margin

67835 incision of lid margin, with free mucous membrane graft

67840 Excision of lesion of eyelid (except chalazion) without closure or with simple direct closure

67850 Destruction of lesion of lid margin (up to 1 cm)

Tarsorrhaphy

67875 Temporary closure of eyelids by suture (eg, Frost suture)

67880 Construction of intermarginal adhesions, median tarsorrhaphy, or canthorrhaphy;

67882 with transposition of tarsal plate

Repair (Brow Ptosis, Blepharoptosis, Lid Retraction, Ectropion, Entropion)

67900 Repair of brow ptosis (supraciliary, mid-forehead or coronal approach)

67901 Repair of blepharoptosis; frontalis muscle technique with suture or other material (eg, banked fascia)

67902 frontalis muscle technique with autologous fascial sling (includes obtaining fascia)

67903 (tarso) levator resection or advancement, internal approach

67904 (tarso) levator resection or advancement, external approach

67906 superior rectus technique with fascial sling (includes obtaining fascia)

67908 conjunctivo-tarso-Muller's muscle-levator resection (eg, Fasanella-Servat type)

67909 Reduction of overcorrection of ptosis

67911 Correction of lid retraction

67912 Correction of lagophthalmos, with implantation of upper eyelid lid load (eg, gold weight)

67914 Repair of ectropion; suture

67915 thermocauterization

67916 excision tarsal wedge

67917 extensive (eg, tarsal strip operations)

67921 Repair of entropion; suture

67922 thermocauterization

67923 excision tarsal wedge

67924 extensive (eg, tarsal strip or capsulopalpebral fascia repairs operation)

FIGURE 10-6. Eyelid Anatomy

The upper eyelid extends to the eyebrow and the lower eyelid extends to the orbital bone rim. In **blepharoptosis**, the visual field is reduced due to upper eyelid drooping. This can be eliminated by resecting or advancing the muscles of the eyelid. **Ectropion** refers to a laxity of the eyelid that causes the lower eyelid to pull away from the globe. This can be repaired by tightening the tissue with a suture, by application of heat to shrink tissue, or by excising a wedge of eyelid tissue. Note: Tools, implants, and/or equipment depicted in the illustration may be outdated but the procedural approach is valid.

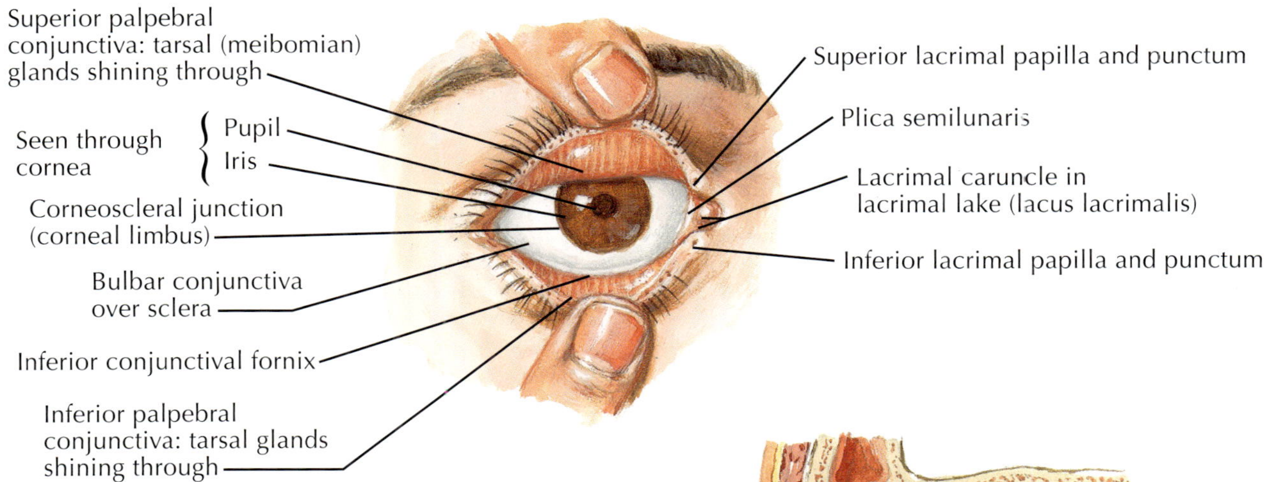

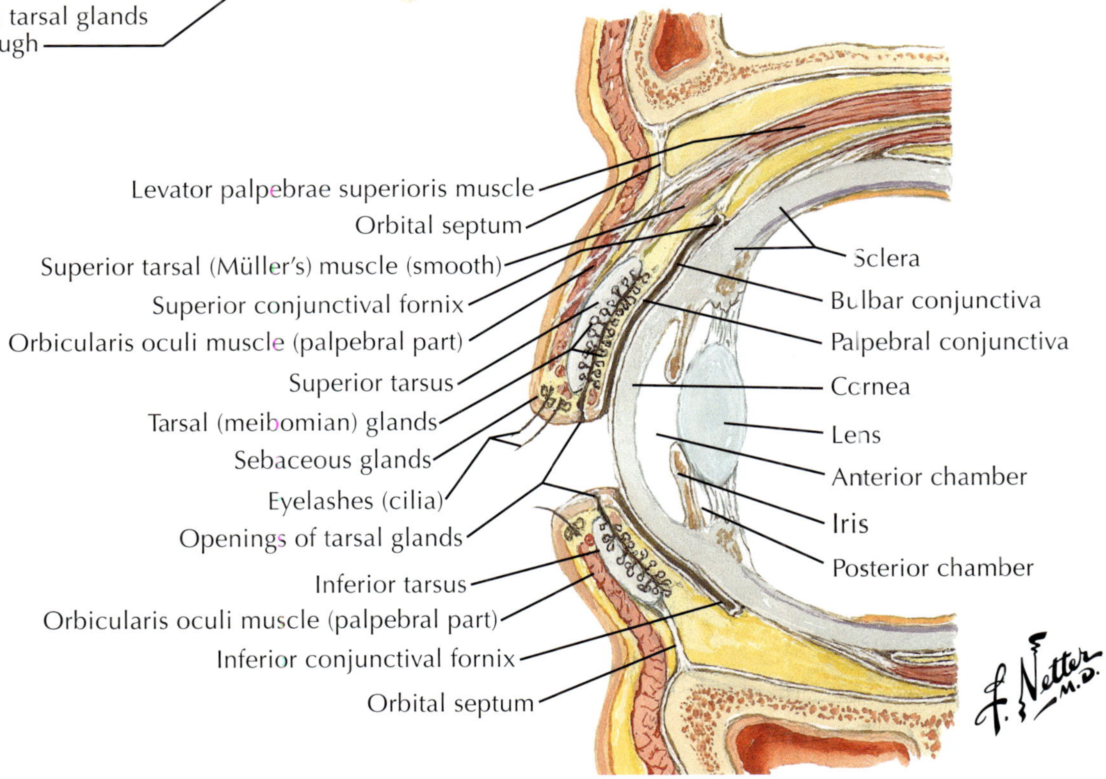

Reconstruction

67930 Suture of recent wound, eyelid, involving lid margin, tarsus, and/or palpebral conjunctiva direct closure; partial thickness

67935 full thickness

67938 Removal of embedded foreign body, eyelid

67950 Canthoplasty (reconstruction of canthus)

67961 Excision and repair of eyelid, involving lid margin, tarsus, conjunctiva, canthus, or full thickness, may include preparation for skin graft or pedicle flap with adjacent tissue transfer or rearrangement; up to one-fourth of lid margin

67966 over one-fourth of lid margin

67971 Reconstruction of eyelid, full thickness by transfer of tarsoconjunctival flap from opposing eyelid; up to two-thirds of eyelid, 1 stage or first stage

67973 total eyelid, lower, 1 stage or first stage

67974 total eyelid, upper, 1 stage or first stage

67975 second stage

Conjunctiva

Incision and Drainage

Coding Atlas

The conjunctiva is the thin mucous membrane covering the eyelids and anterior sclera. A cul-de-sac of conjunctival tissue prevents foreign bodies such as contact lenses from becoming lost in the orbit. The cul-de-sac is formed from conjunctiva that lines the eyelids and continues until it is reflected back toward the front of the eye along the sclera, terminating at the limbus.

68020 Incision of conjunctiva, drainage of cyst

68040 Expression of conjunctival follicles (eg, for trachoma)

Excision and/or Destruction

Coding Atlas

No distinction is made in coding excisions of the conjunctiva based on the type of lesion excised. Code selection is based on the purpose of the procedure (biopsy, excision, or destruction), size of the lesion, and whether adjacent sclera is removed.

68100 Biopsy of conjunctiva

68110 Excision of lesion, conjunctiva; up to 1 cm

68115 over 1 cm

68130 with adjacent sclera

68135 Destruction of lesion, conjunctiva

Injection

Coding Atlas

A subconjunctival injection delivers medication into the space between the conjunctiva and the sclera.

68200 Subconjunctival injection

Conjunctivoplasty

Coding Atlas

In conjunctivoplasty, conjunctival tissue is excised, rearranged, or grafted to improve coverage of the anterior sclera. Conjunctivoplasty may be performed adjunct to other procedures, eg, pyterygium excision or evisceration. If additional tissue is required for conjunctivoplasty, mucosa from inside the patient's cheek (buccal mucosa) may be excised and grafted into the eye. A symblepharon is an adhesion between conjunctiva lining the eyelid (palpebral) and conjunctiva lining the sclera (bulbar).

68320 Conjunctivoplasty; with conjunctival graft or extensive rearrangement

68325 with buccal mucous membrane graft (includes obtaining graft)

68326 Conjunctivoplasty, reconstruction cul-de-sac; with conjunctival graft or extensive rearrangement

68328 with buccal mucous membrane graft (includes obtaining graft)

68330 Repair of symblepharon; conjunctivoplasty, without graft

68335 with free graft conjunctiva or buccal mucous membrane (includes obtaining graft)

68340 division of symblepharon, with or without insertion of conformer or contact lens

Other Procedures

68360 Conjunctival flap; bridge or partial (separate procedure)

68362 total (such as Gunderson thin flap or purse string flap)

68371 Harvesting conjunctival allograft, living donor

Lacrimal System

Coding Atlas

The lacrimal system manufactures and distributes tears. The majority of fluid is manufactured in the bilateral **lacrimal gland**, but also in lacrimal glands deep in the conjunctiva and mucous cells from the conjunctiva above the eye. The fluid drains into the eyes through lacrimal puncta. Tears can drain from the eye through the nasolacrimal **duct**; these tears exit from the nose. Inadequate tear production or a blockage in any of the ducts can create complications to the other structures of the eye.

Incision

68400 Incision, drainage of lacrimal gland

68420 Incision, drainage of lacrimal sac (dacryocystotomy or dacryocystostomy)

68440 Snip incision of lacrimal punctum

Excision

68500 Excision of lacrimal gland (dacryoadenectomy), except for tumor; total

68505 partial

68510 Biopsy of lacrimal gland

68520 Excision of lacrimal sac (dacryocystectomy)

68525 Biopsy of lacrimal sac

68530 Removal of foreign body or dacryolith, lacrimal passages

68540 Excision of lacrimal gland tumor; frontal approach

68550 involving osteotomy

Repair

68700 Plastic repair of canaliculi

68705 Correction of everted punctum, cautery

68720 Dacryocystorhinostomy (fistulization of lacrimal sac to nasal cavity)

68745 Conjunctivorhinostomy (fistulization of conjunctiva to nasal cavity); without tube

68750 with insertion of tube or stent

68760 Closure of the lacrimal punctum; by thermocauterization, ligation, or laser surgery

68761 by plug, each

68770 Closure of lacrimal fistula (separate procedure)

Probing and/or Related Procedures

68801 Dilation of lacrimal punctum, with or without irrigation

68810 Probing of nasolacrimal duct, with or without irrigation;

68811 requiring general anesthesia

68815 with insertion of tube or stent

68816 with transluminal balloon catheter dilation

68840 Probing of lacrimal canaliculi, with or without irrigation

68850 Injection of contrast medium for dacryocystography

FIGURE 10-7. The Lacrimal System

A fine network of canals and ducts is required for the lacrimal system to effectively flush the eyes with tears. At times, patients will undergo surgery to widen or clear lacrimal passages that may be obstructed due to **calculi**, neoplasms, **foreign bodies**, or **stenosis**.

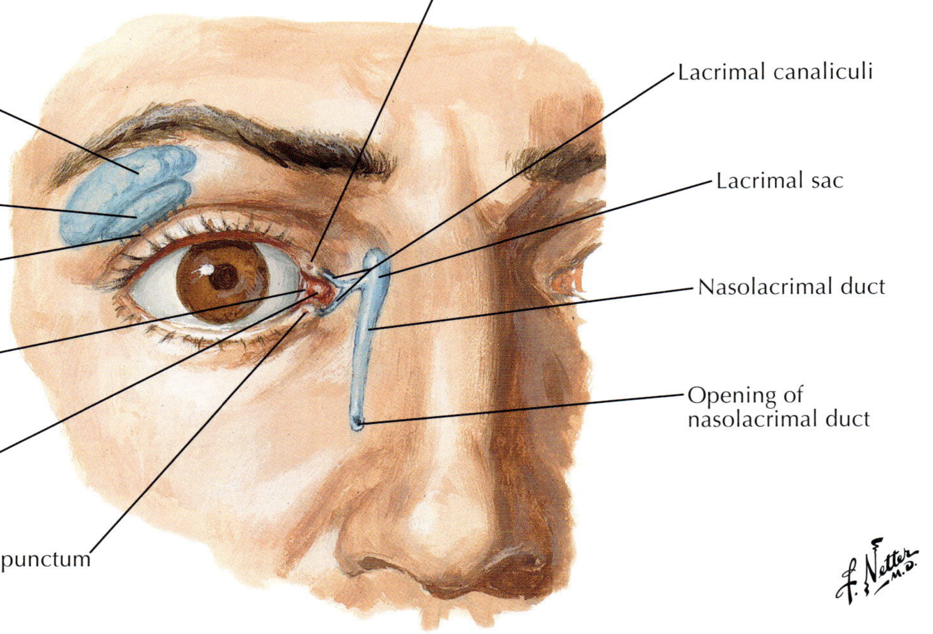

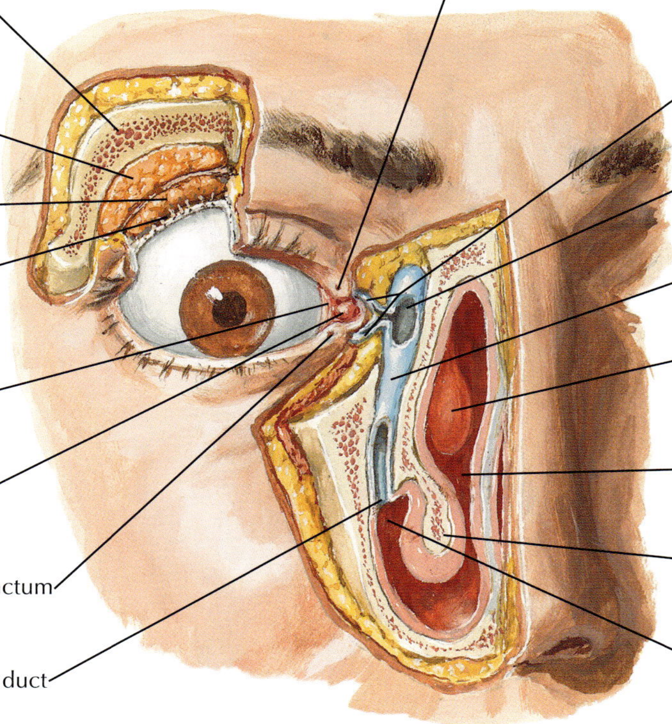

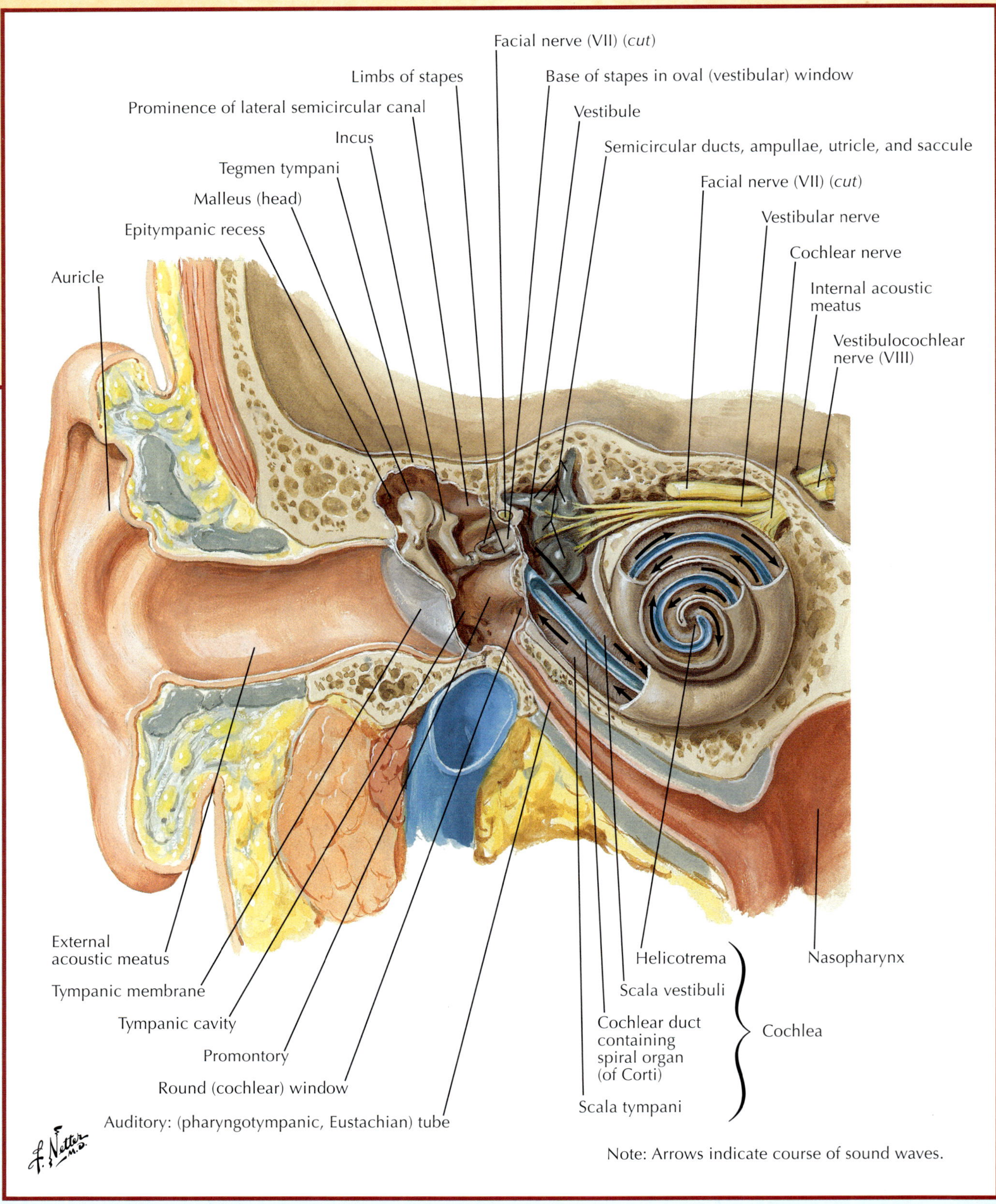

Facial nerve (VII) (cut)
Limbs of stapes
Base of stapes in oval (vestibular) window
Prominence of lateral semicircular canal
Vestibule
Incus
Semicircular ducts, ampullae, utricle, and saccule
Tegmen tympani
Facial nerve (VII) (cut)
Malleus (head)
Vestibular nerve
Epitympanic recess
Cochlear nerve
Auricle
Internal acoustic meatus
Vestibulocochlear nerve (VIII)
External acoustic meatus
Tympanic membrane
Tympanic cavity
Promontory
Round (cochlear) window
Auditory: (pharyngotympanic, Eustachian) tube
Helicotrema
Scala vestibuli
Cochlear duct containing spiral organ (of Corti)
Scala tympani
Cochlea
Nasopharynx
Note: Arrows indicate course of sound waves.
F. Netter M.D.

◈ CHAPTER 11 ◈

Auditory System

The auditory system is divided into three segments: external, middle, and inner ear. Hearing loss can occur if any of these segments is defective or no longer able to conduct sound or if the nerve carrying sensory information to the brain is damaged. There are two types of hearing loss: conductive and sensorineural. In **conductive hearing loss**, sound vibrations are impeded en route to the inner ear or acoustic nerve. In **sensorineural hearing loss**, the ability of the inner ear or acoustic nerve to sense and transmit sound is affected.

The external ear includes the fleshy concha and external auditory **meatus**. This segment is designed to collect sound and funnel it toward the tympanic membrane (eardrum). The external auditory meatus is a canal composed of cartilage and bone and lined in skin, **cilia** (small hairs), and glands that secrete **cerumen** (earwax). Cerumen traps foreign matter and inhibits bacterial growth. Cilia are activated by jaw movement, causing foreign bodies to migrate toward the outer ear. Any significant buildup of cerumen may affect auditory acuity.

The middle ear is composed of the tympanic membrane, Eustachian tube, and ossicles. When sound waves reach the tympanic membrane, they set off vibrations that are passed through the eardrum and bony ossicles (malleus, incus, stapes) to the oval window leading to the inner ear. The Eustachian tube connects the middle ear to the nasopharynx and functions to equalize pressure between the middle ear and the external atmosphere. Pressure differences can be painful and can lead to conductive hearing loss. Otitis media is middle ear inflammation. Some children have chronic otitis media; small ventilation tubes may be placed in their eardrums to aid in pressure equalization (PE) until they outgrow the condition.

The inner ear includes the oval window, round window, semicircular canals, vestibule, and cochlea, which transmit the sound waves to the auditory nerve. In this way, sensations are carried to the brain for interpretation. When the stapes vibrates against the oval window, a vibratory reaction in the fluid within the cochlea is generated. The round window vibrates in tandem with the oval window, equalizing the pressure caused by oval window vibrations. When the cochlea is damaged and no longer able to transmit sensory information to the auditory nerve, a **cochlear implant** may be considered. The cochlear implant does not replace a normal functioning cochlea but does provide the patient with sound sensations.

In addition to its function of capturing and transmitting sound waves, the ear also plays an important role in balance. The inner ear's semicircular canals and vestibule sense **equilibrium**. Each of the three fluid-filled semicircular canals is oriented to a different plane. Motion sensors within the fluid detect change in physical orientation. The sensors, which are cilia embedded in canal walls, transmit information regarding head rotation and speed of movement to the brain.

The mastoid process is the portion of temporal bone behind the ear. The mastoid process contains air cells that act to enhance vibration and sound. Occasionally, middle ear infections can extend into the mastoid cells, causing **mastoiditis**. Codes for procedures involving the mastoid process can be found in the External, Middle, and Inner Ear subsections of the Auditory System code set. In some cases, the middle or inner ear may be accessed through the middle fossa of the temporal bone to decompress or resect a nerve or to remove a tumor. These procedures are reported using codes in the range 69950-69970; these are found at the end of the Auditory System section.

External Ear

Incision

Coding Atlas

The ear has two functions: to perceive and transmit sound sensations to the auditory nerve and to sense **equilibrium** via the semicircular canals. Any disruption in the pathway of sound reception can cause hearing loss. Procedures described in the Auditory System code set are aimed at preserving or improving hearing or equilibrium or treating disease or cosmetic defects. Codes in the External Ear subsection are used to report procedures that extend beyond superficial skin into the deeper tissues and structures of the **pinna** and external auditory **meatus**. For procedures limited to the integument, see the Integumentary System code set.

69000 Drainage external ear, abscess or hematoma; simple

69005 complicated

69020 Drainage external auditory canal, abscess

69090 Ear piercing

Excision

Coding Atlas

Lesions within the external auditory **meatus** may be soft or bony. **Exotoses** are formations of new bone in the ear canal; these formations can narrow the canal and lead to hearing loss. Any skin **graft** required following an excision of the ear or auditory canal would be reported separately.

69100 Biopsy external ear

69105 Biopsy external auditory canal

69110 Excision external ear; partial, simple repair

69120 complete amputation

69140 Excision exostosis(es), external auditory canal

69145 Excision soft tissue lesion, external auditory canal

69150 Radical excision external auditory canal lesion; without neck dissection

69155 with neck dissection

Removal

Coding Atlas

Occasionally, a physician or other qualified health care professional must remove **foreign bodies** or dense and impacted **cerumen**. In patients who have undergone previous **mastoidectomy**, the ear canal may communicate with an exposed mastoid cavity. The mastoidectomy cavity collects debris and usually requires regular **debridement**.

69200 Removal foreign body from external auditory canal; without general anesthesia

69205 with general anesthesia

69210 Removal impacted cerumen requiring instrumentation, unilateral

69220 Debridement, mastoidectomy cavity, simple (eg, routine cleaning)

69222 Debridement, mastoidectomy cavity, complex (eg, with anesthesia or more than routine cleaning)

Repair

Coding Atlas

Otoplasty refers to the cosmetic correction of a protruding ear. In **meatoplasty**, the ear canal, also called the external auditory **meatus**, is reconstructed due to injury, infection, or congenital **atresia**. Reconstruction may include removing soft tissue as well as shaving or drilling the underlying bony canal. Any graft is reported separately using codes from the Integumentary System code set.

⊙ **69300** Otoplasty, protruding ear, with or without size reduction

69310 Reconstruction of external auditory canal (meatoplasty) (eg, for stenosis due to injury, infection) (separate procedure)

69320 Reconstruction external auditory canal for congenital atresia, single stage

FIGURE 11-1. The External Ear

The external ear may be referred to as the auricle or **pinna**. It is formed primarily of skin and **cartilage**. The helix is the outermost cartilaginous curve of the ear. The external auditory **meatus** is a canal of bone and cartilage that is lined with **cilia** and skin. The external auditory meatus terminates at the tympanic membrane (eardrum).

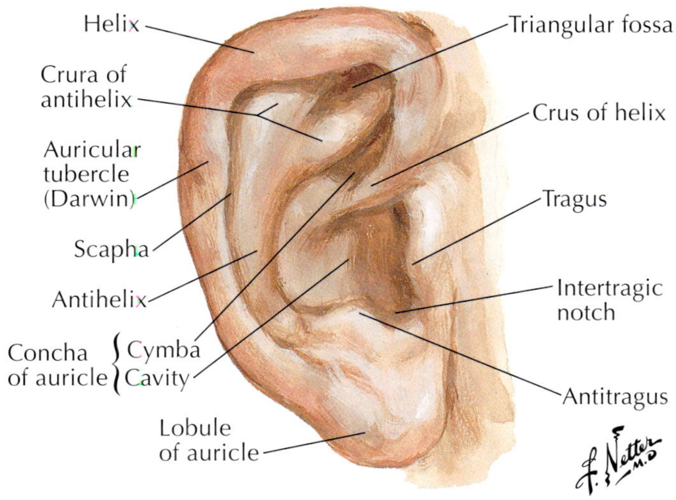

Middle Ear

Incision

Coding Atlas

Myringotomy or **tympanotomy** refers to an incision into the tympanic membrane. In **tympanostomy**, a small tube is inserted into the tympanic membrane to create a communication between the external auditory canal and the middle ear. Tympanostomy is a common therapy for children with immature Eustachian tubes that prevent air from reaching the middle ear, leading to chronic otitis media. The tubes are a temporary solution until the Eustachian tubes mature. Eustachian tubes may be referred to as auditory or pharyngotympanic tubes.

69420 Myringotomy including aspiration and/or eustachian tube inflation

69421 Myringotomy including aspiration and/or eustachian tube inflation requiring general anesthesia

69424 Ventilating tube removal requiring general anesthesia

69433 Tympanostomy (requiring insertion of ventilating tube), local or topical anesthesia

69436 Tympanostomy (requiring insertion of ventilating tube), general anesthesia

69440 Middle ear exploration through postauricular or ear canal incision

69450 Tympanolysis, transcanal

Excision

Coding Atlas

A **mastoidectomy** is performed to remove infection or growths. The **mastoid bone** is approached through an incision behind the ear. Typically, a high-speed drill and suction irrigation are used to remove mastoid bone.

69501 Transmastoid antrotomy (simple mastoidectomy)

69502 Mastoidectomy; complete

69505 modified radical

69511 radical

69530 Petrous apicectomy including radical mastoidectomy

69535 Resection temporal bone, external approach

69540 Excision aural polyp

69550 Excision aural glomus tumor; transcanal

69552 transmastoid

69554 extended (extratemporal)

FIGURE 11-2. The Middle Ear

The air-filled middle ear begins with the tympanic membrane and continues to the fenestra vestibule (oval window) of the inner ear. The malleus connects the tympanic membrane to the incus, which is attached to the stapes. The stapes terminates at the oval window. Because there is interaction between these tiny bones and their muscle attachments, they are able to enhance small sounds or suppress loud ones.

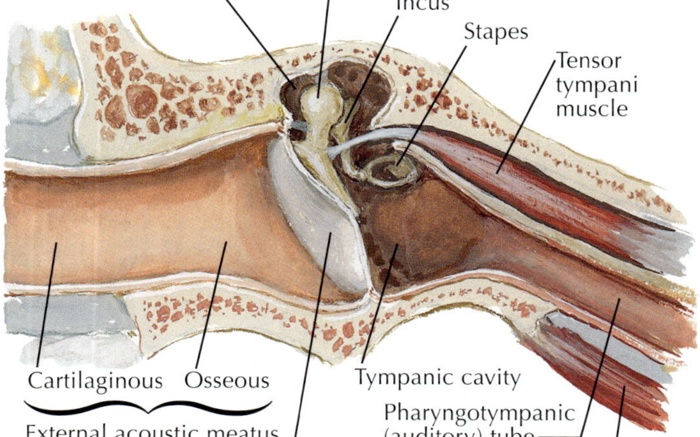

Coronal oblique section of external acoustic meatus and middle ear

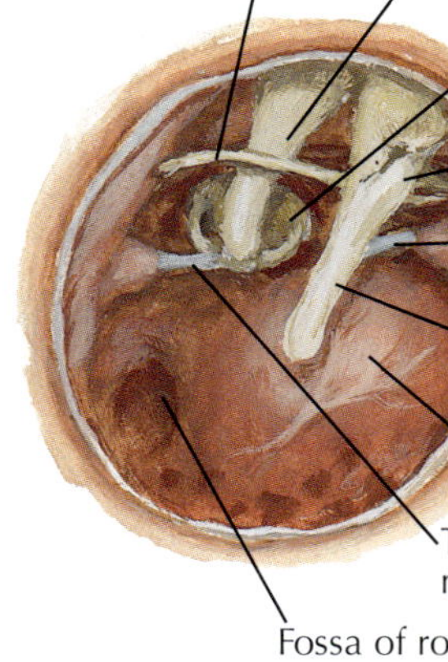

View into tympanic cavity after removal of tympanic membrane

Auditory Ossicles

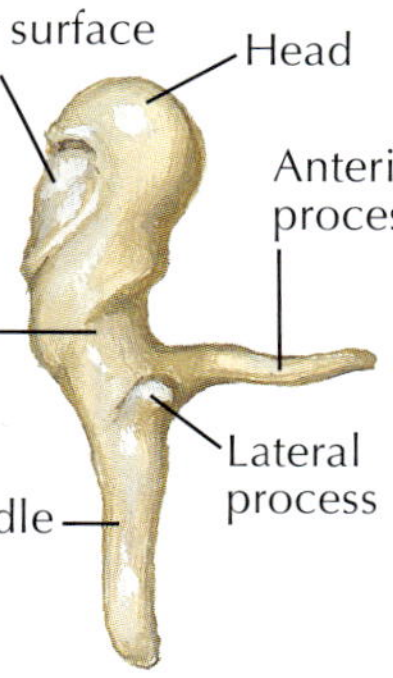

Malleus: Lateral View

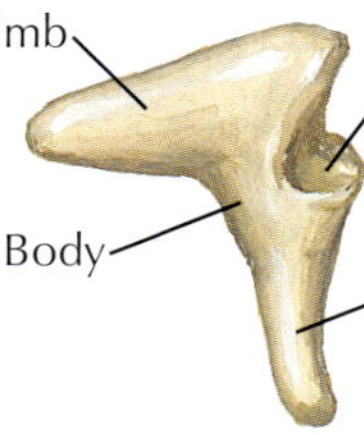

Incus: Lateral View

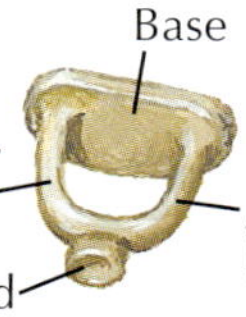

Stapes: Superolateral View

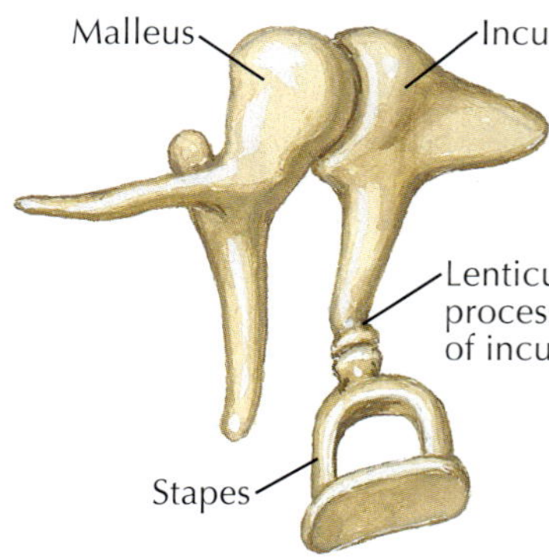

Ossicles Articulated: Medial View

Repair

Coding Atlas

Ossicular chain reconstruction (OCR), or **ossiculoplasty**, is the surgical alteration of the ossicular chain in an attempt to mitigate **conductive hearing loss**. The ossicles may have become disconnected or their movement impeded. Reconstruction may be partial (partial ossicular replacement prosthesis [PORP]) or complete (total ossicular replacement prosthesis [TORP]) and may include **autograft**, **homograft**, or, most commonly, **prosthetic** implant.

69601 Revision mastoidectomy; resulting in complete mastoidectomy

69602 resulting in modified radical mastoidectomy

69603 resulting in radical mastoidectomy

69604 resulting in tympanoplasty

69605 with apicectomy

69610 Tympanic membrane repair, with or without site preparation of perforation for closure, with or without patch

69620 Myringoplasty (surgery confined to drumhead and donor area)

69631 Tympanoplasty without mastoidectomy (including canalplasty, atticotomy and/or middle ear surgery), initial or revision; without ossicular chain reconstruction

69632 with ossicular chain reconstruction (eg, postfenestration)

69633 with ossicular chain reconstruction and synthetic prosthesis (eg, partial ossicular replacement prosthesis [PORP], total ossicular replacement prosthesis [TORP])

69635 Tympanoplasty with antrotomy or mastoidotomy (including canalplasty, atticotomy, middle ear surgery, and/or tympanic membrane repair); without ossicular chain reconstruction

69636 with ossicular chain reconstruction

69637 with ossicular chain reconstruction and synthetic prosthesis (eg, partial ossicular replacement prosthesis [PORP], total ossicular replacement prosthesis [TORP])

69641 Tympanoplasty with mastoidectomy (including canalplasty, middle ear surgery, tympanic membrane repair); without ossicular chain reconstruction

69642 with ossicular chain reconstruction

69643 with intact or reconstructed wall, without ossicular chain reconstruction

69644 with intact or reconstructed canal wall, with ossicular chain reconstruction

69645 radical or complete, without ossicular chain reconstruction

69646 radical or complete, with ossicular chain reconstruction

69650 Stapes mobilization

69660 Stapedectomy or stapedotomy with reestablishment of ossicular continuity, with or without use of foreign material;

69661 with footplate drill out

69662 Revision of stapedectomy or stapedotomy

69666 Repair oval window fistula

69667 Repair round window fistula

69670 Mastoid obliteration (separate procedure)

69676 Tympanic neurectomy

Other Procedures

Coding Atlas

Bone-anchored hearing aids (BAHAs) transmit sound waves into an external sound processor secured on the patient's scalp. The processor sends the sound through a tube implanted in bone, usually the mastoid process. The tube terminates in the inner ear. This system allows conduction to bypass the middle ear. In patients with chronic middle ear disease, a concurrent **mastoidectomy** may be performed as **prophylaxis**.

69700 Closure postauricular fistula, mastoid (separate procedure)

69710 Implantation or replacement of electromagnetic bone conduction hearing device in temporal bone

69711 Removal or repair of electromagnetic bone conduction hearing device in temporal bone

69714 Implantation, osseointegrated implant, temporal bone, with percutaneous attachment to external speech processor/cochlear stimulator; without mastoidectomy

69715 with mastoidectomy

69717 Replacement (including removal of existing device), osseointegrated implant, temporal bone, with percutaneous attachment to external speech processor/cochlear stimulator; without mastoidectomy

69718 with mastoidectomy

69720 Decompression facial nerve, intratemporal; lateral to geniculate ganglion

69725 including medial to geniculate ganglion

69740 Suture facial nerve, intratemporal, with or without graft or decompression; lateral to geniculate ganglion

69745 including medial to geniculate ganglion

FIGURE 11-3. The Labyrinth and the Auditory Nerve

The vestibulocochlear nerve may be documented as the auditory vestibular nerve, or the cranial nerve VIII (CNVIII). It has dual functions of sensory transmission of sound from the cochlea and equilibrium from the labyrinth. Cilia lining the cochlea are activated by sound, and this vibration is sensed by the nerve. Fluid within each duct of the labyrinth shifts when the head moves, and this movement is also transmitted to the nerve for interpretation by the brain.

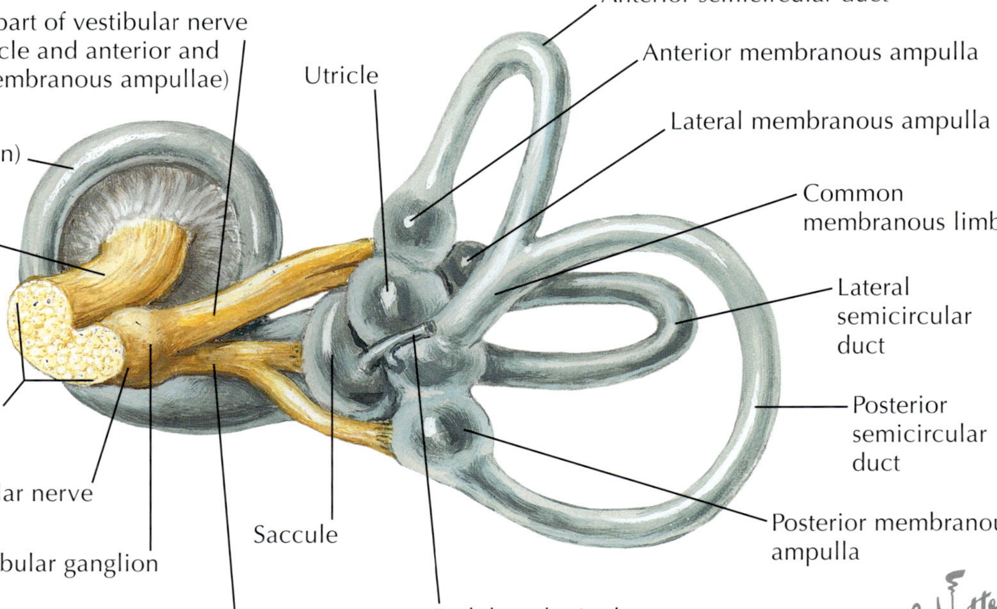

Inner Ear

Incision and/or Destruction

Coding Atlas

The inner ear, or labyrinth, is composed of the cochlea, utricle, saccule, and semicircular canals. The labyrinth may be treated with drugs that are infused via a transtympanic injection or catheter into the middle ear. The medication reaches the inner ear as the patient is placed in a position during which the affected ear is facing up for a brief period. Gentamicin infusion by this method may be referred to as chemical labyrinthectomy.

69801 Labyrinthotomy, with perfusion of vestibuloactive drug(s); transcanal

69805 Endolymphatic sac operation; without shunt

69806 with shunt

69820 Fenestration semicircular canal

69840 Revision fenestration operation

Excision

Coding Atlas

Labyrinthectomy is a destructive procedure that is performed in order to eliminate equilibrium symptoms in a patient with vestibular dysfunction. The sensitive epithelium of the inner ear is stripped via a transcanal or mastoid approach. Any hearing is sacrificed. Another destructive approach to vestibular dysfunction is sectioning of the vestibular nerve.

69905 Labyrinthectomy; transcanal

69910 with mastoidectomy

69915 Vestibular nerve section, translabyrinthine approach

FIGURE 11-4. Inner Ear Fluid

The interior of the cochlea and semicircular canals has two fluid layers. A bony outer shell is filled with **perilymph**, which is similar to cerebrospinal fluid. The perilymph layer is continuous through both structures and the vestibule that connects them. A membranous inner series of tubes is filled with electrolyte-rich **endolymph** that also continues through both structures. The two fluids do not normally mix.

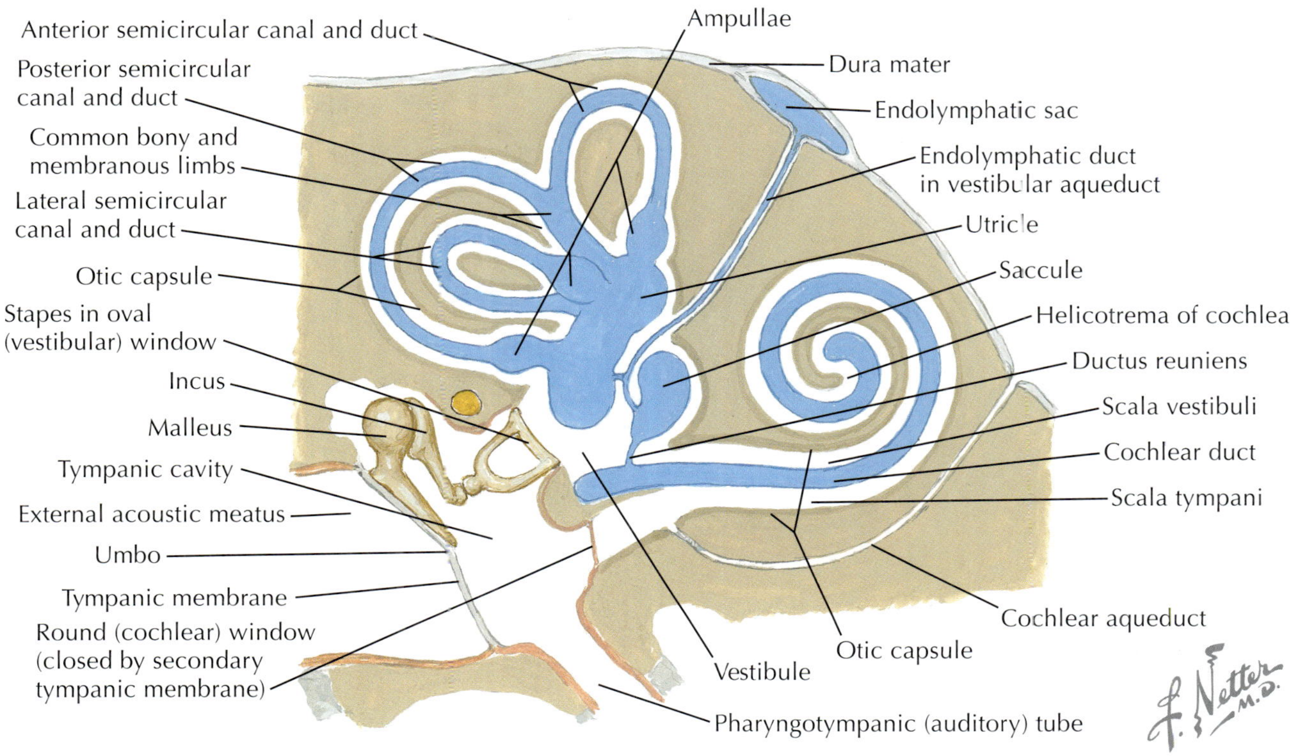

Introduction

Coding Atlas

A **cochlear implant** replaces the functions of the external, middle, and inner ear. The implant includes a microphone, speech processor, translator, and electrode relay. The relay communicates sensory information directly to the auditory nerve. This is similar to a bone-anchored hearing aid (BAHA), with the exception that the BAHA transmits the message to the cochlea, while the cochlear implant transmits directly to the auditory nerve.

69930 Cochlear device implantation, with or without mastoidectomy

Temporal Bone, Middle Fossa Approach

69950 Vestibular nerve section, transcranial approach

69955 Total facial nerve decompression and/or repair (may include graft)

69960 Decompression internal auditory canal

69970 Removal of tumor, temporal bone

Operating Microscope

+ 69990 Microsurgical techniques, requiring use of operating microscope (List separately in addition to code for primary procedure)

◆ APPENDIX A ◆

Glossary

abdominal cavity. Anatomic site bounded by the diaphragm, abdominal walls, and pelvis.

abduction. Movement of a limb away from the body; opposite of adduction.

aberrant. Abnormal, or varying from standard.

ablation. Surgical removal or destruction of the function of a body part.

abscess. Localized inflammation within a tissue or organ that forms a cavity containing pus.

acetabuloplasty. Surgical reconstruction of the cup-shaped socket of the hip joint.

achalasia. Disorder of esophageal muscle movement; an impediment to swallowing.

acid reflux. Backflow of stomach acid into the esophagus.

acoustic nerve. Division of the eighth cranial nerve (CNVIII, vestibulocochlear nerve) that transmits sound sensations to the brain.

acoustic neuroma. Tumor, usually benign, arising from the eighth cranial nerve (CNVIII).

acquired. Occurring after birth.

acrochordon. Cutaneous skin tag, usually benign.

acromionectomy. Surgical excision of all or part of the bony process of the shoulder blade (scapula).

acromioplasty. Surgical reconstruction of the bony process of the shoulder blade (scapula).

acute. Of sudden onset and usually of brief course.

adduction. Movement of a limb toward the body; opposite of abduction.

adenoma. Benign epithelial tumor that resembles or arises in glandular tissue.

adenopathy. Swelling or enlargement of lymph nodes.

adhesiolysis. Surgical cutting or stripping out of band(s) of scar tissue between organs or body surfaces.

adhesions. Bands or scars between organs or body surfaces that cause tension and obstruct normal movement.

adipose. Anatomical fat.

adjacent tissue transfer. Surgical rearrangement of nearby healthy tissue around a wound, sometimes called a local flap.

adjuvant. Supplemental, eg, a therapy in addition to a primary therapy.

adnexa, adnexal. Anatomical structures that are in close proximity to another structure.

adrenalectomy. Surgical excision of all or part of the adrenal gland, also called suprarenal gland.

adrenaline. Neurohormone produced in high-stress situations, also called epinephrine.

advancement. Surgical repositioning to a more distal point.

afferent. Flowing toward the center, eg, the brain or lymph node; opposite of efferent.

afterloading. Practice of filling after surgical insertion, eg, with brachytherapy devices that can be surgically placed, then injected with a radioactive substance afterward.

albumin. Simple protein found throughout biological tissues and fluids.

alimentary duct. Main duct of the lymphatic system found in the chest anterior to the spine and discharging lymph and chyle into the bloodstream.

alimentary tract. Mucosa-lined passageway from the mouth to the anus, through which food is ingested, digested, absorbed, and eliminated; also called digestive tract.

allogeneic. From the same species.

allograft. Tissue for grafting from a donor of the same species.

alloimmunization. Immune response to foreign antigens from the same species, eg, transplanted tissue or maternal response to a fetus.

alloplastic. Adapting to the environment.

allotransplantation. Tissue from one member of a species grafted into another member of the same species.

alveolar. Relating to a small cavity or sac, usually referencing the sacs where the exchange of oxygen and carbon dioxide occurs in the lung, or the bony socket in the mandible or maxilla into which a tooth root inserts.

alveolectomy. Surgical removal of tooth-supporting bone along the mandible or maxilla, usually performed to facilitate a dental prosthesis.

alveolus. Small cavity or sac, usually referencing the sacs where the exchange of oxygen and carbon dioxide occurs in the lung, or the bony socket in the mandible or maxilla into which a tooth root inserts.

alveoloplasty. Surgical reconstruction and shaping of the bone into which the tooth inserts along the mandible or maxilla, usually in preparation for dental prosthesis.

amblyogenic. Causing a lack of development of vision in one eye.

amniocentesis. Aspiration of fluid from the fluid-filled sac that contains a fetus, performed by inserting a needle through the abdomen and into the uterus and amniotic sac.

amnioinfusion. Therapeutic instillation of fluid through a catheter into the amniotic cavity, typically after labor has begun to augment amniotic fluid volume.

amniotic membrane. Composition of the fetal sac, sometimes repurposed for eye wound healing.

amputation. Surgical removal of all or part of an extremity by surgery, trauma, or prolonged constriction; surgical amputation is performed when an organ is no longer viable, is painful, or contains a disease process that compromises health.

amygdalohippocampectomy. Treatment for epilepsy resistant to treatment in which the amygdala, parahippocampal gyrus, and hippocanthus are resected.

anal speculum. Instrument inserted into the anus for viewing anal and rectal tissue.

anal verge. Junction where mucosa ends and perianal skin begins in the distal anus.

anastomosis, anastomosed. Surgical connection or surgically connected, usually two anatomical lumens of similar size.

anatomic nervous system. Network of nerves that control involuntary actions such as heartbeat and respiration.

anatrophic pyelolithotomy. Open surgery on the renal pelvis to remove calculus or calculi, especially staghorn stones, through an incision in the plane of the kidney that is relatively avascular.

anesthetic. Medication causing loss of sensation.

aneurysm. Arterial ballooning caused by a weakened arterial wall.

angioplasty. Surgical reconstruction or widening of a blood vessel.

angioscopy. Visualization of blood vessels, either from the inside using a fiberoptic endoscope or using microscopy following the injection of radiopaque agents.

annuloplasty. Surgical reconstruction of the annulus, or ring, of a cardiac valve.

anomaly, anomalous. Feature that is unusual, abnormal, or nonconforming.

anoscope, anoscopy. Device inserted into the anus for inspection of anal mucosa and structures; may contain a light source; may be called an anal speculum.

antagonist muscle. Muscle that opposes the action of another muscle and so provides stability and control; antagonist muscle pairs work in tandem, with one muscle relaxing while the other contracts.

antegrade. Extending or moving forward; flowing with the current.

antepartum. During pregnancy and before delivery.

anterior. Situated in front of.

anterolateral. Situated in front and to one side of.

antero-latero-vertical. Situated above, in front, to the side of.

anterovertical. Situated above and in front of.

antibiotic. Therapeutic agent that inhibits the growth of a microorganism.

antibody. Protein that attacks foreign bodies in the blood stream as part of the immune system; also called immunoglobulin.

anticarcinogenic. Therapeutic agent that inhibits or prevents the growth of cancer.

antispasmodic. Therapeutic agent that inhibits or prevents muscle spasms; also called spasmolytic.

antrotomy. Incision into the paranasal sinus under the eye.

antrum. Paranasal sinus located under the eye in a space in the maxillary bone lined by mucous membrane; synonymous with maxillary sinus; plural of antrum is antra.

aortic arch. Curving portion of aorta between ascending and descending aorta and giving rise to the brachiocephalic trunk, left common carotid, and left subclavian arteries.

aortic valve. Semilunar valve that lies between the left ventricle of the heart and the aorta; oxygenated blood is pumped through the aortic valve to be disseminated throughout the body.

aortopexy. Surgical fixation of the aortic arch, usually to the sternum.

aphakia. Without the natural lens in the eye.

apheresis. Removal of plasma from the blood; whole blood is withdrawn from the body, plasma is separated from the whole blood, and the blood is returned to the patient.

apicectomy. Surgical excision of that portion of the temporal bone called the petrous apex.

aponeurosis. Broad glistening sheet of tendon-like tissue that serves mainly to connect a muscle with the parts that it moves.

approach. In surgery, the method chosen for accessing the targeted site.

arrest. Stoppage.

arterial blood gasses. Measurement of the pressures exerted by the dissolved oxygen and carbon dioxide in the arterial blood and a measurement of the free hydrogen ion concentration (pH) that reflects the acid–base balance of the blood.

arterioles. Small vascular branches that connect arteries to capillaries.

arteriotomy. Surgical incision into an artery wall.

arteriovenous. Including both vein and artery.

arteriovenous fistula. Acquired abnormal direct connection between an artery and a vein; it may be surgically created or formed following injury or due to disease.

arteriovenous malformation. Congenital abnormal connection between an artery and vein.

arthrocentesis. Diagnostic or therapeutic aspiration of fluid from a joint.

arthrodesis. Fixation or stiffening of a joint by surgical means; also called artificial ankylosis; joint stiffness or immobility due to disease or injury.

arthrography. Radiographic image of a joint after it has been infused with contrast media.

arthroplasty. Reconstructive surgery of a joint or joints to restore motion because of ankyloses or trauma or to prevent excessive motion; this repair and reconstruction may use silicone, metallic, or other implants.

arthroscopy. Endoscopic examination of the interior of a joint.

arthrotomy. Surgical incision into a joint capsule.

articulate, articulation. Movement at a joint.

artificial insemination. Introduction of semen into the vagina or uterus by any means other than coitus.

arytenoidectomy. Surgical excision of arytenoid cartilage to widen the laryngeal inlet as a treatment for vocal cord disorders.

arytenoidopexy. Surgical fixation of arytenoid cartilage or muscle.

ascites. Abnormal accumulation of fluid in the peritoneal cavity.

aspirate, aspiration. Withdrawing or the withdrawal of fluid by suction or negative pressure.

assisted reproductive technology. Fertility treatments in which the egg and sperm are handled outside the body.

astigmatism. Condition in which the cornea has an irregular shape, affecting visual acuity.

astragalectomy. Surgical excision of all or part of the talus bone of the ankle joint; also called talectomy.

asymptomatic. Clinically nonapparent condition.

atelectasis. Collapse of a lung or part of a lung, resulting in a partial or complete airless state of a lung.

atherectomy. Surgical excision of plaque from the interior wall of a blood vessel.

atherosclerosis. Deposits of hardened fat and cholesterol built up on the walls of an artery or arteries.

atherosclerotic. Having deposits of hardened fat and cholesterol built up on the walls of an artery or arteries.

atresia. Congenital absence.

atrial fibrillation. Heartbeat in which the normal rhythmical contractions of the atria are replaced by rapid irregular twitchings of the muscular wall; the ventricles respond irregularly to the dysrhythmic bombardment from the atria.

atrium. Chamber or cavity connected to another chamber or cavity, eg, right and left atria of the heart, which are connected to the right and left ventricles; plural of atrium is atria.

atticotomy. Surgical incision and opening of the superior tympanic cavity (attic), which contains the upper half of the malleus and most of the incus.

auditory nerve. Eighth cranial nerve (CNVIII, vestibulocochlear nerve) that transmits sound sensations and balance information to the brain.

augmentation. Process of making greater, more numerous, larger, or more intense.

aural glomus tumor. Vascular tumor of the middle ear arising from glomus bodies.

aural polyp. Benign, fleshy growth in the external ear canal or tympanic membrane.

auricle. Exterior protrusion of the ear (pinna); also the upper part of each coronary atria.

autogenous. Originating within the body and not acquired from any outside source.

autograft. Tissue taken from one part of the body and transplanted to another part of the same body.

autoimmunity. Immune response in which the immune system mistakenly attacks its own cells.

autologous. From the same person, eg, blood withdrawn from a patient and later transfused into the same patient.

autotransplantation. Graft of tissue from one person onto another site of the same person.

AV fistula. Abnormal connection between an artery and a vein that may be congenital or acquired, or may be surgically created for hemodialysis cannula access.

AV graft. Abnormal connection between an artery and a vein made of artificial tubing and used for hemodialysis cannula access.

avascular. Without blood supply.

avulsion. Tearing away of a body part.

axial pattern flap. Oblong autograft that remains attached to a longitudinal blood supply while being transferred to its new location.

axilla. Armpit or underarm region.

axon. Nerve fiber that conducts electrical impulses along a nerve.

axonotmesis. Nerve injury that includes disruption of the axon and myelin sheath, but with the epineurium and perineurium preserved so that the injury site can regenerate.

backbench preparation. Work by a surgeon to prepare a graft for implantation.

backflow. Abnormal regurgitation or backward flow of fluids.

balance. Equilibrium; for fluid within the body, the stability of water and electrolytes in relation to ingestion and secretion.

balloon dilation. Enlargement of a lumen by placing an uninflated balloon into it then inflating the balloon multiple times until the lumen is stretched.

balloon embolization. Surgical occlusion of a vessel by placing a balloon and then inflating it; may also be called balloon occlusion.

balloon occlusion. Surgical occlusion of a vessel by placing a balloon then inflating it; may also be called balloon embolization.

band ligation. Use of elastic bands to treat hemorrhoids or other varices to stop bleeding or to destroy the abnormal tissue.

bariatrics. Branch of medicine concerned with the management, prevention, and control of obesity and allied diseases.

barrel-stave procedure. Bone grafting or osteotomies to create expansion bands in the skull, like barrel staves, that can accommodate the capacity of the cranium in infants with skull deformity.

basal cell. Normal cell found at the base of the epidermis; source of basal cell carcinoma, a slow-growing skin cancer.

benign. Not harmful; in neoplasms, describing a neoplasm that does not metastasize.

benign prostatic hyperplasia. Nonmalignant proliferation of the epithelial and stromal cells of the prostate gland, causing overall enlargement.

bifrontal. Bilateral, frontal incisions adjacent to coronal sutures or craniotomies.

bifurcation. Division or forking into two branches, or the site where such a division occurs.

bilateral. Occurring on both sides of the body, eg, kidneys, nostrils, and thumbs.

bilateral pelvic lymphadenectomy. Surgical excision of lymph nodes on both sides of the pelvis, including internal, external, and common iliac nodes.

bile. Fluid manufactured in the liver and stored in the gallbladder that aids in digestion.

biliary atresia. Congenital blockage of the ducts that carry bile from the liver to the gallbladder.

biliary tract. Organs and ducts that store bile and release it into the small intestine, including the gallbladder and bile ducts.

binocular. With both eyes working in unison.

biopsy. Removal and examination (usually microscopic) of tissue from the living body performed to establish a precise diagnosis.

biotransformation. Process by which a substance is changed from one chemical to another by chemical reaction within the body.

bipolar. Having two poles.

bipolar cautery. Hemostasis achieved by using an electrocautery tool that releases electrical current into tissue from an active electrode; from there, the electricity is transferred to a passive electrode.

bisection. Surgical division into two parts.

blastocyst. Cluster of cells in early embryonic development.

blepharoplasty. Surgical repair of the eyelid to remove excess fat or skin.

blepharoptosis. Abnormal drooping of the upper or lower eyelid.

blepharospasm. Uncontrolled contraction, twitch, or closing of the eyelid.

blepharotomy. Surgical incision into the eyelid.

block. In Mohs micrographic surgery, a piece or pieces of tissue flattened, embedded in mounting medium placed on a single disk, and frozen in a cryostat for frozen sectioning and slide preparation.

blood clot. Coagulated blood forming a solid or semisolid mass.

blood-borne. Carried throughout the body through the bloodstream.

blowout. Fracture of one or more of the walls of the orbit.

blunt trauma. Forceful physical injury that is nonpenetrating and may include contusion, fracture, abrasion, and laceration.

bolus. One-time rapid infusion or intake of a substance or agent.

bone-anchored hearing aid. Surgically implanted sensor that uses the conduction of sound through bone to improve the hearing of patients.

bone flap. Portion of bone temporarily removed from the skull but left attached to overlying muscle and blood supply; its removal provides access to the brain.

bone graft. Piece(s) of bone either harvested from the patient or supplied by a bone bank and used to support surrounding bone during bone surgery.

bone marrow. Highly vascular, soft, pulpy network of reticular tissue that fills the cavities of most bones.

bone marrow transplant. Replacement of damaged or diseased bone marrow with healthy bone marrow stem cells; the transplant may involve cells previously harvested from the patient, cells from another person, or umbilical cord stem cells.

botulinum toxin. Pharmacological toxin administered therapeutically for chemodenervation in cases of dystonia, spasticity, other involuntary muscle activity, chronic pain, smooth muscle hyperactive disorders, cosmesis, sweating disorders, and salivary disorders.

boutonniere deformity. Tendon defect that prevents the middle joint of the finger from being straightened.

brachytherapy. Use of radioactive sources placed directly into a tumor-bearing area to generate local regions of high-intensity radiation.

breech. In childbirth, a presentation in which the baby is positioned to exit the pelvic outlet buttocks first or feet first.

bronchial thermoplasty. Application of heat, delivered through a bronchoscope, to the surface of the bronchial tubes to reduce the volume of smooth muscle and improve breathing in a patient with asthma.

bronchoplasty. Surgical reconstruction or repair of the bronchus to restore the patency and integrity of the lumen.

bronchoscopy. Endoscopic examination of the bronchus.

broncho-tracheal. Relating to the bronchi and trachea.

brush biopsy, brushings. Sample tissue obtained by sweeping a small brush across the targeted surface for pathological examination; commonly performed using an endoscopic approach.

buccal. Of the cheek, as in buccal mucosa, a graft tissue harvested from inside the patient's cheek.

Buck's fascia. Strong layer of penile fascia immediately superficial to the tunica albuginea.

bulbocavernosus. Muscle that in the male compresses the bulb of the penis and the bulbar urethra; in the female, the muscle serves to compress the vagina.

bulbourethral gland. Bilateral gland at the base of the prostate that contributes fluid to semen; also called Cowper's gland.

burr. Rotary drill used in surgery involving bone, especially cranial surgery.

burr hole. Opening in the skull made by a burr drill; may be a therapeutic hole for releasing pressure or may be for access to the skull's interior.

bursa. Friction-reducing, fluid-filled sac or cavity within a joint capsule.

bypass. To go around, eg, a lumen anastamosed above and below a blockage so that flow is not interrupted.

cadaver. Corpse or dead body.

calculus. Abnormal concretion or stone formed within an organ from mineral salts, cholesterol, calcium, or other deposits; also called a stone.

calices. Cup-shaped subdivisions within the renal pelvis; singular is calyx.

calycoplasty. Surgical reconstruction of the cup-shaped subdivisions within the renal pelvis.

canalplasty. Surgical reconstruction of the external auditory canal; also called canaloplasty.

cannula, cannulation. Small hollow tube that is inserted into the body, or the insertion of the tube.

canthopexy. Suture stabilization of the eyelid tendon.

canthoplasty. Plastic repair or reconstruction of the juncture of the upper and lower eyelids.

canthorrhaphy. Suture of the upper eyelid to the lower eyelid.

canthotomy. Incision of the juncture of the upper and lower eyelids.

capillary. Tiny vessel that connects artery to vein.

capsulectomy. Excision of all or part of a capsule.

capsulodesis. Suturing of a joint capsule to bone to increase its stability.

capsulopalpebral. Referring to fascia lying near the surface of the interior lower eyelid.

capsulorrhaphy. Suture repair of a capsule, especially a joint capsule.

capsulorrhexis. Continuous surgical tear of the lens capsule.

capsulotomy. Incision into the capsule, usually referring to the crystalline lens of the eye.

cardiac event. Occurrence of a serious cardiovascular defect, eg, myocardial infarct, ventricular fibrillation, or unstable angina.

cardiac filling. Ventricles filling to capacity with blood in preparation for the next impulse, which will cause the ventricles to contract and squeeze their contents into the lungs or into circulation; any abnormal pressure against the heart, eg, cardiac tamponade, may impede the ability of the ventricles to fill completely.

cardiac massage. Rhythmic compression of the chest in a patient with no heartbeat in an attempt to restore cardiac function; may also be performed by directly compressing an exposed heart.

cardiac output. Volume of blood that is pumped by the heart in a 60-second period, reflecting the strength and frequency of cardiac contractions.

cardiac tamponade. Pressure against the heart muscle due to fluid buildup between the heart and parietal pericardium.

cardiopulmonary bypass. During heart or lung surgery, diversion of blood to oxygenator pumps outside the body with the return of oxygenated blood into circulation.

cardiopulmonary insufficiency. Inadequate performance of the heart and/or lung.

cardiotomy. Incision into the heart.

cardiovascular system. System of heart, great vessels, veins, and arteries that circulates blood throughout the body.

cardioversion. Therapeutic electrical shock of a dysrhythmic heart in an attempt to restore a normal heart rhythm.

carpectomy. Surgical excision of all or part of a bone of the carpus, or wrist joint; bones include hamate, capitate, trapezoid, trapezium, triquetral, lunate, scaphoid.

cartilage. Rubbery connective tissue associated with joints and also found in soft tissues elsewhere in the body.

caruncle. Fleshy benign mass.

casting. Stiff dressing used to immobilize a body part.

cataract. Opacity of the lens of the eye, the lens capsule, or both.

catheter, catheterization. Tubular instrument that allows passage of fluid from or into a body cavity, or the placement of the tubular instrument.

cauda equina. Bundle of spinal nerves and nerve roots innervating the hips, knees, ankles, feet, and anal sphincter.

caudal. Anatomically posterior or inferior.

cauterization, cautery. To destroy tissue with heat.

cecostomy. Surgical creation of a communication between the large intestine and the skin of the abdomen; the cecum is secured to the skin so that feces can be excreted through the surgically created stoma; the large intestine distal to the stoma site is bypassed entirely.

celiotomy. Incision into the abdomen; also called laparotomy.

cell harvesting. In stem cell services, the collection of cells from blood using an apheresis machine.

cell washing. In sample cell collection, flushing an area, eg, the bronchus, with saline using bronchoscopy and then aspirating the saline to retrieve cells from the site.

central nervous system. Portion of the nervous system that interprets signals and controls actions; includes the brain and spinal cord.

central venous catheter. Tubular instrument passed through a peripheral or central vein, ending in the thoracic vena cava or right atrium, for measurement of venous pressure or for infusion of concentrated solutions.

cerclage. Technique in which a wire or other nonabsorbable material is placed around a body part to hold it in place or, in the case of the cervix uteri, to keep its os closed.

cerebrospinal fluid leak. Seepage of cerebrospinal fluid surrounding the brain or spinal cord into neighboring tissues, caused by a tear in the arachnoid and dura mater; may be iatrogenic, traumatic, or idiopathic.

cerumen. Ear wax.

cervical approach. Surgical access through the neck.

cervical cap. Pliable cup-shaped disc inserted into the vagina to fit over the cervix uteri for the prevention of pregnancy.

cervical stump. Distal portion of uterus (cervix uteri) attached to proximal vagina and retained in a subtotal hysterectomy.

cervicothoracic. Of the neck and chest.

cesarean. Childbirth accomplished through an incision in the abdomen and through the uterine wall.

chalazion. Cyst of the eyelid's meibomian gland.

cheilectomy. Surgical excision of bone spurs from a joint cavity, eg, the base of the big toe.

chelating agent. Chemical that bonds to deposits, eg, ethylenediaminetetraacetic acid (EDTA) for calcium deposits on the cornea.

chemical peel. Use of caustic agents to accelerate exfoliation or resurface skin so that the skin increases in volume.

chemocauterization. Destruction by chemical.

chemodenervation. Weakening of a muscle by damaging its nerve with a toxic agent.

chemonucleolysis. Injection of a nucleus-dissolving enzyme into a bulging vertebral disc.

chemoreceptor. Sensory nerve cell responsive to chemical stimulation.

chemosurgery. Therapeutic destruction of tissue by chemicals.

chemotherapy. Use of drugs or medications to directly attack a cancer at the cellular level by disrupting the cell metabolic cycle.

choanal atresia. Congenital stenosis of the nasal airway.

cholangiography. Radiographic imagery of the biliary ducts with injection of contrast media.

cholangiopancreatography. Radiological examination of the biliary and pancreatic ductal systems with the infusion of contrast.

cholecystectomy. Surgical excision of all or part of the gallbladder.

cholecystitis. Inflammation of the gallbladder.

cholecystoenterostomy. Surgically created communication between the gallbladder and the small intestine.

cholecystostomy. Surgical creation or presence of a communication from the gallbladder to the external skin surface for drainage of the gallbladder.

cholecystotomy. Surgical incision into the gallbladder.

choledochal cyst. Congenital bile duct anomaly with dilatation of bile ducts.

choledochoenterostomy. Surgical creation or presence of a communication from the common bile duct to the small intestine.

choledocholithiasis. Stone or calculus in the common bile duct.

choledochoscopy. Endoscopic examination of the common bile duct.

choledochostomy. Surgical creation or presence of a communication from the common bile duct to the external skin surface for drainage.

choledochotomy. Surgical incision into the common bile duct.

cholelithiasis. Stone or calculus in the gall bladder.

chondroplasty. Reconstructive surgery of torn or damaged cartilage.

chordee. Malformation in which the penis bends downward.

chorioamnionitis. Inflammation of the fluid-filled membrane sac that encloses the fetus.

chorionic villus sampling. Excision of fetal placental tissue for chromosome analysis; the sampling is performed through a catheter passed through the maternal cervix and into the pregnant uterus.

chromotubation. Injection of a radiopaque dye into the uterus and fallopian tubes for radiographic evaluation of patency.

chronic. Continuing over time with persistence.

chronic venous insufficiency. Vascular disorder of leg extremities in which the venous valves or walls are ineffective, causing venous stasis.

chyle, chyliferous. Product of digestion consisting of fluid fat and lymph; containing chyle.

cilia. Hair-like projections that often have a sweeping motion or function.

cineplasty. Surgical reconstruction of muscle at the site of an amputation to facilitate operation of a prosthesis, eg, to enable muscle contractions to trigger movements in the mechanical limb.

circulation. Movement of fluid through a body system.

circulatory system. Organ structures that distribute fluids throughout the body, including the cardiovascular and lymphatic systems.

cirrhosis. Scarring and fibrotic disease of the liver.

claviculectomy. Surgical excision of all or part of the shoulder bone that articulates with the sternum and the scapula.

cleft palate. Congenital defect in which the two sides of the bony or soft roof of the mouth do not fuse, usually causing an opening from the mouth into the nasal sinuses; also called cheiloschisis.

clitoroplasty. Surgical construction, reconstruction, or reduction of the clitoris.

cloacal anomaly. Congenital malformation of the female digestive and genitourinary tracts in which the rectum, vagina, and urethra develop as one merged lumen, a cloaca, that opens onto the perineum.

closed fracture. Broken bone that does not break through the skin; the opposite of a compound fracture.

closed reduction, closed treatment. Nonsurgical treatment in which manual maneuvering returns a bone or other body part to its proper location.

closure. Suture or stapling of a wound or operative site.

coagulation. Thickening of blood to turn from a liquid to a gel; also called clotting.

coagulum pyelolithotomy. Technique for removing multiple small calculi from the renal pelvis by injecting a substance that forms clots around the stones.

coarctation. Congenital narrowing of the aorta.

coccygectomy. Surgical excision of all or part of the coccyx, or tailbone.

cochlea. Circumvoluted inner ear structure that converts sound from vibrations to nerve impulses.

cochlear implant. Electronic device that improves the hearing of a profoundly deaf or hard-of-hearing patient; consists of an external sound receptor and speech processor and an implanted transmitter and electrode array that send messages to the auditory nerve.

coitus. Sexual intercourse with a person of the opposite sex.

cold preservation. Process to keep donor organs viable; may include continuous pumping of a chilled and nourishing oxygen-rich solution through the organ.

colectomy. Excision of part or all of the colon.

collagen. Insoluble protein that is the chief component of connective tissue.

colonoscopy. Endoscopic examination of the large intestine from the anus to the ileocecal junction; may include examination of the terminal ileum ileocecal junction.

coloproctostomy. Anastomosis of a proximal segment of colon to the rectum after resection of a distal segment of colon.

colorrhaphy. Suture repair of the colon.

colostomy. Surgical creation of a communication between the large intestine and the skin of the abdomen; a portion of large intestine is secured to the skin so that feces can be excreted through the surgically created stoma; the large intestine distal to the stoma site is bypassed entirely.

colpocentesis. Aspiration of fluid through a needle inserted through the posterior wall of the vagina into the pouch of Douglas; also called culpocentesis or culdocentesis.

colpocleisis. Surgical closure of the vagina following the removal of vaginal epithelium and plication of vaginal tissues to strengthen the septum.

colpoperineorrhaphy. Suture repair of the vagina and perineum.

colpopexy. Surgical suspension of a relaxed and prolapsed vagina; vaginofixation.

colporrhaphy. Suture repair of the vagina.

colposcopy. Examination of the vagina using an illuminating magnifying device (colposcope).

colpotomy. Incision into the vaginal wall.

colpo-urethrocystopexy. Suture and lift of the urethra and bladder using a vaginal approach.

comminuted. Broken, crushed, or shattered into a number of small or large pieces, eg, multiple fragmented pieces in a bone fracture.

commissurotomy. Surgical incision or digital break-up of adherent or thickened leaflets in a valve of the heart.

compartment syndrome. High pressure from swelling or bleeding within a fascia-bound muscle compartment, compromising blood flow; may be acute or chronic.

composite graft. Graft composed of more than one type of tissue, eg, cartilage and fat, or more than one vessel segment, eg, two lengths of harvested vein

compound. In fracture care, a fracture that pierces the skin, exposing the broken bone; the opposite of a closed fracture.

compression. Force that tends to push two objects together.

computed tomography. Series of X rays processed through a computer to produce three-dimensional images.

concha. Shell-shaped object; commonly the hollow of the external ear or the nasal turbinates.

concha bullosa. Extension of the ethmoid sinus located in the middle turbinate.

concomitant. Occurring at the same time or together.

concretion. Small, hard deposit in tissue.

concurrent. Occurring at the same time.

conduction. Transfer.

conductive hearing loss. Hearing loss caused by an interruption or distortion in the vibrations that travel through the external and middle ear and into the cochlea, where the vibrations are converted to neural impulses.

condylectomy. Excision of all or part of a rounded projection of a bone.

condyloma. Sexually transmitted wart-like growth around the anus or genitalia.

conformer. Device placed over a portion of the globe of the eye to help the globe maintain its spherical shape.

congenital. Existing before birth.

conization. Surgical excision of a central, cone-shaped plug of tissue from the cervix.

conjunctivoplasty. Plastic repair of the conjunctiva.

continent. Having voluntary control of the bladder and/or bowel.

contracture. Deformity caused by a tightening of muscle, skin, ligament, or tendon.

contralateral. Relating to, located on, or occurring on the opposite side.

contrast. Substance applied to enhance imaging of a body structure; may be swallowed, injected, or inserted into the structure being examined.

cor triatriatum. Congenital presence of three atrial chambers in the heart.

cordectomy. Surgical excision of all or part of a vocal cord.

cordocentesis. Aspiration of fetal blood for analysis; this is done by inserting a needle through the maternal abdomen and into the umbilical cord.

cordotomy. Severing of select nerve fibers in the spinal cord.

core samples. Tissue obtained through a hollow core needle biopsy.

corn. Benign and thickened cone of skin, usually over a bony prominence or in an area of friction on the foot.

coronal. Describing a surgical approach, essentially an incision from ear to ear, over the top of the head; this approach prevents facial scarring.

coronary artery disease. Narrowing of the arteries that supply blood to the muscles of the heart.

coronoidectomy. Surgical excision of all or part of the coronoid process, eg, the mandible.

corpectomy. Removal of the body of a vertebrae (the portion anterior to the spinal canal).

corpora cavernosography. X-ray examination of the structures of the corpus cavernosa following administration of contrast media.

cortex. Outer layer of an organ or other body structure, as distinguished from the internal substance.

cosmesis. Physical beauty.

cosmetic. Of aesthetic value.

costal. Relating to the ribs or rib cage.

costotransversectomy. Surgical excision of the joint connecting a rib to a transverse process of a vertebra.

costovertebral. Relating to the junction of a rib and the transverse process of a vertebra.

cranial nerve. Afferent or efferent nerve of the brain, of which there are 12: olfactory (I), optic (II), oculomotor (III), trochlear (IV), trigeminal (V), abducent (VI), facial (VII), vestibulocochlear (VIII), glossopharyngeal (IX), vagus (X), accessory (XI), and hypoglossal (VII).

cranial tongs. Traction or immobility device that attaches through pins in the skull, usually bilaterally at the temples.

craniectomy. Surgical excision of all or a part of the cranium.

craniomegalic skull. Misshapen skull with enlarged skullcap.

craniopharyngioma. Benign pituitary tumor.

cranioplasty. Surgical reconstruction or repair of a defect of the skull.

craniosynostosis. Congenital defect in which the cranial suture(s) fuses prematurely, preventing normal brain growth.

craniotomy. Surgical incision into the cranium.

craterization. Surgical excision of a bowl-shaped piece of bone.

cryocautery. Surgical destruction of tissue by freezing, usually with a freezing probe.

cryopreservation. Frozen storage.

cryosurgery. Surgical destruction of tissue by freezing, usually with a freezing probe.

cryotherapy. Surgical destruction of tissue by freezing, usually with a freezing probe.

crystalline lens. Transparent, convex contributor to refraction located behind the iris and anterior to the vitreous.

C-tube. Cecostomy tube; communication between the abdominal skin and the cecum through which water is infused to flush the bowel.

cul-de-sac. Anatomical cavity through which there is no passage, commonly referencing the pouch of Douglas between the rectum and the uterus, and the conjunctival cul-de-sac, where the eyelid (palpebral) conjunctiva connects to the scleral (bulbar) conjunctiva.

curettage. Surgical removal of tissue using a scraping instrument (curette).

curettement. Act of scraping to achieve surgical removal of tissue.

cutaneous. Of the skin.

cutdown. Dissection of a vein for insertion of a cannula or needle for administration of intravenous fluids or medications or for insertion of an intraluminal device.

cyanosis. Low oxygen levels in the blood that lead to low oxygen in tissues, which take on a bluish hue.

cyclectomy. Ciliary body excision.

cyclodialysis. Creation of a path for aqueous flow between the anterior chamber and suprachoroidal space.

cyclophotocoagulation. Destruction of ciliary body tissue using a laser.

cyst. Encapsulated lesion filled with fluid or semi-fluid material.

cystectomy. Surgical excision of a cyst, or surgical removal of all or a part of the urinary bladder.

cystocele. Herniation of the posterior bladder and trigone at the anterior vaginal wall.

cystography. Radiologic examination of the urinary bladder after infusion of contrast media.

cystometrogram, cystometrography. Testing device and procedure for measuring pressures intermittently as the urinary bladder is instilled with fluid infused through a urethral catheter.

cystoplasty. Surgical reconstruction of the urinary bladder, eg, to increase its capacity.

cystorrhaphy. Suture repair of the urinary bladder.

cystoscopy, cystoscopic. Endoscopic examination of the urinary bladder and urethra.

cystostomy. Surgical creation or presence of a communication between the bladder and the skin of the abdomen; urine may be eliminated through this communication.

cystotomy. Incision into the urinary bladder.

cystourethrogram. Radiologic examination of the urinary bladder and urethra after infusion of contrast media.

cystourethroplasty. Surgical reconstruction of the urinary bladder and urethra.

cystourethroscopy. Endoscopic examination of the urinary bladder and urethra.

D&C. Dilation and curettage, usually referencing the scraping of the endometrium of the uterus requiring dilation of the cervix for cervical approach.

dacryocystorhinostomy. Surgical creation of communication between the lacrimal sac and the nasal cavity.

dacryolith. Concretion or calculus found in the lacrimal sac or lacrimal duct.

debridement, debride. Removal, usually by sharp separation, of foreign material and devitalized or contaminated tissue until surrounding healthy tissue is exposed.

debulking. Removal of the majority of the targeted tissue.

decompress, decompression. To release pressure within or against a structure; the act of releasing pressure.

decompression fasciotomy. Incision through the skin and into muscle fascia to release pressure on muscle within the fascial compartment.

decortication. Surgical removal of the outer covering or shell of an organ or body part.

decubitus. Relating to a supine position or other position while lying down, usually referencing pressure ulcers seen in bedridden patients.

deep brain stimulator. System that triggers electrical impulses to the thalamus or other deep brain tissue; consists of an electrode lead surgically implanted in the brain and attached by wire to a subcutaneous neurostimulator.

defibrillator. Device that provides an electric shock to the heart in order to return the heart to a normal rhythm.

dehiscence. Bursting open, splitting, or gaping along natural or sutured lines.

deligation. Removal of a ligature or wire.

denervate. To interrupt a nerve supply to a specific body site.

dentition. Upper and lower dental arches and teeth.

dentoalveolar. Referring to the hard and soft tissues of teeth and their support structures.

depressed skull fracture. Fracture of a skull bone in which the bone is displaced into the cranial cavity.

dermabrasion. Use of a mechanical device to accelerate exfoliation of or damage to skin so that the skin increases in volume.

dermatome. Anatomic skin site supplied by an individual spinal nerve.

dermatoplasty. Surgical reconstruction of skin with the use of grafts.

dermoid cyst. Solitary thick-walled tumor of the skin containing fatty or horny masses and sometimes hair.

destruction. Eradication of tissue.

diagnostic. Describing a procedure that will provide information regarding the patient's condition.

dialysis. Removal of waste products and excess fluid from the blood for patients whose kidneys can no longer perform that function.

diaphragm. Muscular wall that separates the abdomen from the thoracic cavity.

diaphragmatic hernia. Displacement of abdominal contents into the chest cavity through a hole in the diaphragm.

diaphysectomy. Surgical excision of all or part of the shaft of a long bone.

diathermy. Altering of tissue by use of heat generated by electricity.

digital. With a finger or hand.

dilatation. Act of increasing the circumference of a lumen.

dilation. Act of increasing the circumference of a lumen or other body part, eg, pupil.

dilation and curettage. D&C, usually referencing the scraping of the endometrium of the uterus requiring dilation of the cervix for cervical approach.

dilation and evacuation. D&E, usually referencing the evacuation of the contents of the uterus requiring dilation of the cervix for cervical approach; a common abortion method.

dilator. Surgical instrument applied to a lumen to increase its circumference.

direct laryngoscopy. Direct visualization of the larynx using a scope.

direct repair. Surgical suture or repair in which the physician has direct visualization of the operative field, eg, laparotomy vs laparoscopy or open biopsy vs endoscopic biopsy.

direct visualization. Situation in which the physician can examine directly the operative site.

disarticulation. Amputation of a limb by separation of the joint without cutting of bone.

discectomy. Surgical excision of all or part of a vertebral disc.

discission. Incision or a cutting, as into a soft cataract.

discography. Radiologic examination of a vertebral disc after infusion of contrast media.

dislocation. Abnormal displacement of a body part, usually a bone.

displaced. Malpositioned.

dissection. Blunt dissection involves the separation of tissue along natural lines using a finger or blunt instrument instead of cutting; sharp dissection involves the separation of tissue by cutting with a scalpel, scissors, or other sharp instrument.

distal. Farther from any point of reference, or farthest from the center of the body.

diversion. To cause a change in flow, usually around a defect.

diverticulectomy. Surgical excision of diverticulum or diverticula.

diverticulum. Circumscribed pouch of variable size protruding from the wall of a tube or hollow organ; plural of diverticulum is diverticula.

division. To cut apart or separate.

donor. One who gives, eg, tissue or an organ, to another.

dorsal. Relating to the back or the posterior part of an organ.

dosimeter. Device for measuring exposure to or dose of radiation.

drainage. Fluid or other discharge from an organ, body part, or wound.

duct. Small lumen for distribution of fluid, eg, bile, tears, lymph, or saliva.

ductogram. Radiologic image of a duct after infusion of contrast media, eg, lactiferous duct in the breast.

ductus arteriosus. Normal connection between the aorta and pulmonary artery in fetal circulation that should close following birth; in some cases, the ductus arteriosus remains open and must be closed surgically.

duodenoileostomy. Surgical connection between the duodenum and the ileum, or the creation of this surgical connection.

duodenostomy. Surgical incision into the duodenum.

dura mater. Outer layer of the spinal cord.

dural. Relating to the outer layer of the spinal cord or brain, the dura mater.

duraplasty. Reconstruction or repair of the outer layer of the spinal cord, the dura mater.

dysphagia. Difficulty swallowing.

dysplasia. Abnormal growth and development of an anatomical structure or of cells within that structure.

dysthyroid ophthalmopathy. Disease of the eye and eye muscles associated with defective functioning of the thyroid gland.

dystocia. Difficulty(ies) during labor.

dystonia. State of abnormal (hypo- or hyper-) tonicity in any tissue.

dystrophic. With degeneration of tissue.

Ebstein anomaly. Congenital tricuspid valve displacement.

eccrine glands. Sweat-producing glands on the forehead, neck, back, palms, and soles for thermoregulation; eccrine glands differ from apocrine sweat glands, which occur in axillae, pubic, and periumbilical tissues.

extracorporeal membrane oxygenation (ECMO). Heart–lung bypass support in which the blood is oxygenated outside the body.

ectopic. Congenital malposition; in pregnancy, implantation of an embryo outside the uterus.

ectropion. Turning out of the margin of the eyelid.

eczema. Inflammatory skin disease with crusting, scaling, and itching.

edema. Presence of abnormally large amounts of fluid in the intercellular tissue spaces of the body.

efferent. Flowing away from the center, eg, the brain or lymph node; opposite of afferent.

effusion. Collection of fluid leached from local tissues.

electrocautery. Tissue destruction using direct or alternating current to produce heat.

electrocorticography. Electroencephalogram performed with the electrodes placed directly on the brain.

electrodesiccation. Tissue destruction using direct or alternating electrical current to produce heat.

electroejaculation. Electrical stimulation that generates ejaculation, usually performed to collect the semen of a patient otherwise incapable of ejaculation who desires procreation through artificial means.

electrofulguration. Tissue destruction using electrical current to produce heat.

electromyography. Measuring and recording electrical nerve activity produced by skeletal muscle.

electrosurgery. Cutting or destroying tissue using electrical current.

electrothrombosis. Application of direct electrical current through a needle into a targeted site for thrombus production to block a vessel.

embolectomy. Surgical excision of a blood clot that has traveled through the vascular system and become lodged in a vessel, blocking blood flow.

embolic. Relating to an embolus (blood clot) in a blood vessel.

embolization. Occlusion of a vascular site.

embolus. Thrombus that breaks free and is carried antegrade from the site at which it formed.

embryo. Human oocyte that has been fertilized and has undergone mitotic division but has not yet been classified as a fetus.

emergent. Unplanned and changing.

emphysematous. With permanent damage to lung alveoli.

empyema. Pocket of pus in the pleural space.

empyemectomy. Surgical excision of a pocket of pus in the pleural space.

emulsify. Breakdown of fat into smaller particles.

en bloc. In one piece or segment; as a whole.

encephalocele. Congenital neural tube defect with a herniation of brain tissue through an opening in the skull.

end-stage heart failure. When the heart is unable to sustain circulation of blood throughout the body.

end-stage renal disease. When the kidneys are unable to remove waste and excess water from the body.

endarterectomy. Surgical excision of the plaque and underlying lining from an artery.

endobronchial ultrasound (EBUS). Use of sound waves delivered through an endoscopic probe to view the bronchial airway anatomy, eg, for diagnostics and for staging cancer.

endocervical sampling. Obtaining scrapings or brushings from the epithelium of the canal of the cervix uteri for diagnostic purposes.

endocrine. Relating to glands that secrete hormones into the blood stream, eg, the pancreas, pituitary, hypothalamus, thymus, gonads and pituitary, pineal, thyroid, parathyroid, and adrenal gonads.

endolymph. Potassium-rich fluid of the membranous labyrinth.

endometrial sampling. Obtaining scrapings or brushings from the lining of the uterus for diagnostic purposes.

endometrioma. Ectopic endometrial tissue that forms a cyst on the ovary.

endoneural tube. Endoneurium.

endoneurium. Connective tissue surrounding each neuron in a bundle of neurons.

endoprosthesis. Prosthetic lumen that is surgically implanted in a duct or vessel of the body.

endopyelotomy. Surgical incision of the renal pelvis using an endoscopic approach.

endoscope. Narrow tube with a light source and camera that can be fed into a lumen of the body for inspection; the scope may also carry tools for therapeutic intervention.

endoscopic ultrasound. Use of sound waves delivered through an endoscopic probe to view the targeted anatomy, eg, for diagnostics.

endoscopy. Examination of a body tube or cavity using a lighted instrument specifically designed for that purpose; the instrument may be a rigid metal tube or a flexible fiberoptic endoscope and has a fiberoptic light source attached to it for illuminating the tissues during examination.

endothelial, endothelium. Thin layer of cells lining the interior surface of a body part, eg, blood vessel, heart, lymphatic vessel.

endovascular. Describing access through blood vessel lumens to reach a surgery or examination site.

endovenous. Within or through a vein.

enteral. Passing through or into the small intestine, eg, enteral feeding is through a stoma from the skin surface directly into the small intestine, bypassing the esophagus and stomach.

enterectomy. Surgical excision of all or part of the small intestine.

enteric. Of or through the small intestine.

enterocele. Protrusion of peritoneum containing small intestine into the area between the rectum and vagina.

enterocystoplasty. Surgical reconstruction to enlarge the bladder using a piece of bowel tissue.

enteroenterostomy. Anastomosis of two segments of intestine.

enterolysis. Surgical incision or excision of intestinal adhesions.

enterorrhaphy. Suture repair of the intestine.

enteroscopy. Endoscopic examination of the small intestine; the scope is inserted through the mouth and into the upper gastrointestinal tract to access the small intestine.

enterostomy. Surgical creation of a communication between the small intestine and the skin of the abdomen; a segment of the small intestine is secured to the skin so that feces can be excreted through the surgically created stoma; bowel distal to the stoma site is bypassed entirely.

enterotomy. Surgical incision into the small intestine.

entrapment. Symptomatic, chronic pinching of a body part, eg, a nerve.

entropion. Abnormal inward turning of the edge of the eyelid.

enucleation. Surgical removal en masse, as in the removal of an eyeball from the orbit after severing the optic nerve and intraocular muscles.

environmental. Relating to outside factors rather than genetic or acquired internal physiologic disorders.

enzyme. Protein that causes a reaction, eg, breaks down food particles in the alimentary canal or breaks down heart tissue during a myocardial infarct.

epicardial. Referring to the outer layer of tissue of the heart.

epicondylitis. Inflammation of the tendons surrounding a projection at the end of a long bone at a joint (epicondyle).

epididymectomy. Surgical excision of all or part of the bony projection at the end of a long bone at the joint (epicondyle).

epididymovasostomy. Surgical cutting of the vas deferens with anastomosis to the epididymis, usually as a method of surgical vasectomy reversal.

epidural. Relating to the dura mater; sometimes a shortened term for epidural anesthetic.

epigastric hernia. Bulging of the peritoneum through the abdominal wall.

epiglottidectomy. Surgical excision of all or part of the cartilage plate that opens and closes the windpipe during alimentation.

epikeratoplasty. Creating a refractive change in the cornea by shaping donated corneal tissue and securing it to the patient's corneal epithelium.

epilation. Removal of hair, as in eyelashes.

epileptogenic. Inciting seizure in a patient with epilepsy.

epineurium. Connective tissue surrounding bundled groups of neurons.

epiphyseal. Relating to the bone that forms the rounded end of long bones, where growth occurs in long bones before adulthood.

epiphyseal arrest. Defect in the growth of a long bone that stops the lengthening of an immature bone.

epiphyseal separation. Damage to the epiphyseal growth plate, usually occurs when a bone is fractured.

epiphysiodesis. Fusion of the pediatric epiphyseal growth plate in a patient with legs of differing lengths; the fusion may be temporary or permanent and allows the shorter leg to become as long as the other leg.

episiotomy. Surgical incision into the perineum to facilitate delivery during childbirth.

epispadias. Congenital malformation of the urethra in which the lumen is not closed but is exposed and open along the dorsum of the penis.

epithelial downgrowth. Growth of aberrant epithelial tissue following eye surgery or injury.

epithelium. Outermost layer of cells.

eschar. Dry, crusty, and contracted skin caused by a serious burn.

escharotomy. Surgical incision into dry, crusty, and contracted skin caused by a serious burn in order to release pressure in the viable tissues beneath.

esophagectomy. Surgical excision of all or part of the esophagus.

esophagoenterostomy. Anastomosis of the distal esophagus to the proximal small intestine, usually performed in patients who have undergone complete gastrectomy.

esophagogastroduodenoscopy (EGD). Endoscopic examination of the esophagus, stomach, duodenum, and sometimes the jejunum; therapeutic procedures may be performed during EGD.

esophagojejunostomy. Surgical suture (anastomosis) of the esophagus to the jejunum.

esophagomyotomy. Incision into the sphincter muscle of the esophagus.

esophagoplasty. Surgical reconstruction of the esophagus.

esophagoscopy. Endoscopic examination of the esophagus; therapeutic procedures may be performed during esophagoscopy.

esophagotomy. Surgical incision into the esophagus.

esophagus. Lumen that carries food and liquids from the mouth to the stomach via peristalsis.

estradiol. Female estrogen hormone released by ovaries and adrenal glands; helps regulate the reproductive cycle.

ethmoidectomy. Surgical excision of bone or cells in the ethmoid sinus.

etiology. Origination or cause of a condition.

Eustachian tube. Lumen connecting the middle ear to the nasopharynx to equalize pressure in and to drain mucus from the middle ear.

eventration. Congenital anomaly of the diaphragm in which the dome of the diaphragm is abnormally high and the diaphragm is abnormally thin and sometimes lacking in muscle.

evisceration. Removal of the contents of an organ, eg, incision into the eyeball and removal of the contents while retaining the sclera and its attachments to the optic nerve and extraocular muscles; may also describe postoperative protrusion of viscera through a ruptured abdominal incision.

exchange transfusion. Blood transfusion in which all of an infant's blood is replaced using one or two catheters; in neonates, an umbilical vessel may be used as one of the catheter sites.

excision. Act of removing a portion or all of an organ or body part by cutting it out or off.

exclusion. Surgical separation of a body part without excision.

exenteration. Surgical resection of a body organ, eg, removal of the eyeball, eyelids, and contents of the orbit.

exfoliation. Procedure to remove the top layers of epidermis.

exocrine. Relating to glands that secrete fluids into ducts, eg, sweat, salivary, mammary glands, and organs of the digestive system.

exostectomy. Surgical excision of all or part of a bony overgrowth.

exotosis. Bony overgrowth.

expiration. Exhaled breath that removes waste and carbon dioxide from the body.

exploration. Diagnostic examination of a body part or system.

exstrophy. Congenital defect in which a malformed bladder is herniated through the abdominal wall.

extensor. Muscle that extends the bone away from the body's center; the opposite of flexor.

external. On the outside of the body or organ.

external auditory canal/meatus. Bilateral lumen from the external ear to the tympanic membrane lined with skin and hair; transmits sound.

external cephalic version. Manual repositioning of a fetus to a head-down position by applying pressure to the pregnant abdomen.

external fixation. Stabilization and alignment of a fracture achieved by the percutaneous placement of pins or wires through the skin and into bone; attached externally to bars or other devices.

extra-abdominal. Outside or beyond the walls of the abdomen.

extra-articular. Outside or beyond the capsule of a joint.

extracapsular intraocular extraction (ECCE). Removal of most of the eye's natural lens, except the posterior shell, and replacement with an artificial intraocular lens placed between the iris and the remaining shell.

extracapsular. An artificial intraocular lens placed behind the iris.

extracavitary. Lateral approach for spinal surgery in which muscle is retracted and the vertebra is approached from the side.

extracorporeal. Outside or beyond the body.

extracorporeal shock wave. Treatment for a urinary calculus in which ultrasonic vibrations are administered from outside the body and focused on the site of the calculus; the vibrations break the calculus into smaller pieces.

extracranial. Outside or beyond the cranium.

extradural. Outside or beyond the dura mater.

extraforaminal. Outside or adjacent to the neural foramen of the spine.

extrahepatic. Outside or beyond the liver.

extramedullary. Outside or beyond the medulla.

extranasal. Outside or beyond the nose.

extraocular. Outside or beyond the globe of the eye.

extraoral approach. Surgical approach that does not go through the mouth.

extraparenchymal. Outside or beyond the parenchyma or fundamental part of an organ.

extrapelvic. Outside or beyond the pelvis.

extraperitoneal. Outside or beyond the peritoneum.

extrapleural. Outside or beyond the pleural cavity.

extratemporal. Outside or beyond the temporal bone; as an approach, usually in front of the ear.

extravasation. Abnormal seepage of fluid into nearby tissues.

extrinsic. In muscles, being distant from the body part the muscle moves, eg, a muscle in the forearm activating a finger.

facet. Bilateral projection in the posterior vertebra that forms a facet joint and provides spinal articulation.

facet joint. Joint located on the back of the spine on each side where one vertebra slightly overlaps the adjacent vertebrae; these joints, which are smooth like the facets of a diamond, guide and allow the complicated movements of the spine.

facetectomy. Excision of part or all of a vertebral facet.

facial nerve. Cranial nerve VII, the nerve of facial expression; also transmits sensations from the tongue and mouth.

false aneurysm. Ruptured aneurysm in which the blood is contained by the surrounding tissue; also called a pseudoaneurysm or aneurysmal hematoma.

fascia, fascial. Connective sheath consisting of fibrous tissue and fat that unites the skin and underlying tissues or contains muscle groupings.

fascia lata. Strong and tough fascia that envelops the muscles of the thigh.

fascicle. Bundle of muscle, nerve, or tendon fibers.

fasciectomy. Surgical incision into fascia.

fasciocutaneous flap. Skin flap that includes subcutaneous tissue and underlying deep fascia.

fasciotomy. Surgical incision into fascia of a muscle compartment.

fecal. Relating to waste from the bowel.

fecal microbiota. Flora within feces that promote intestinal health and are transplanted via colonoscopy in patients with refractory *Clostridium difficile* colitis.

feces. Waste from the bowel.

femoral hernia. Bulging loop of intestinal tissue at the groin at the femoral canal.

femoroplasty. Surgical reconstruction or recontouring of the femoral head.

fenestra vestibule. Opening in the medial wall of the middle ear; also called the oval window.

fenestrated. Containing a window or windows.

fenestration. Surgical opening of a window in a structure.

fertility. Ability of a man to impregnate a woman or of a woman to conceive and give birth to a live infant.

fetal. Until birth, a developing unborn offspring that has advanced from the embryo stage.

fetal biophysical profile. Analysis of the health of an unborn infant based on fetal heart rate, movement, breathing, amniotic fluid, and muscle tone; performed in the third trimester.

fiberoptic. Optical system consisting of thin transparent fibers of glass or plastic that transmits light and is used to visualize images.

fibrin glue. Absorbable blood-derived tissue glue.

fibrinolysis. Breaking down of blood clots.

fibroadenoma. Benign tumor containing fibrous and glandular tissue.

fibrocutaneous. Benign skin tissue containing tough fibers.

fibroid. Benign fibrous tumor of muscle and fibrous tissue, eg, uterine fibroid tumor.

fibroma. Benign fibrous tumor of connective tissue, eg, oral fibroma.

fiducial marker. Surgically implanted localization device for targeting tissue to be treated or excised during a separate encounter.

filiform and follower. Urethral dilation system that consists of a thin, thread-like guide passed through the urethra over which catheters or other instruments may be introduced into the urethra.

fimbria. Fringe or finger-like tissue; plural of fimbria is fimbriae.

fimbrioplasty. Surgical reconstruction of fringe or finger-like tissue, eg, fallopian tube fimbriae reconstruction.

fine needle aspiration. Biopsy procedure in which cells are aspirated for pathological examination; to remove a larger sample containing tissue, a core needle biopsy is performed.

first-order branch. Initial branch off of the aorta or the initial access vessel, as described in vascular catheter placement.

fissure. Tear or narrow opening in tissue, eg, within the anal mucosa.

fissurectomy. Surgical excision of a tear or narrow opening in tissue.

fistula, fistula tract. Abnormal tube-like communication between two body surfaces or cavities or between an internal organ and the body surface, usually the result of injury or disease but may be surgically created for therapeutic reasons.

fistulectomy. Surgical excision of an abnormal communication between two structures or one structure and the skin surface.

fistulization. Surgical creation of a tube-like communication between two body parts.

fistulotomy. Surgical incision into a fistula.

fixation. Act or operation of holding, suturing, pinning, or fastening in a stable position.

fixation device. Apparatus used to obtain bony fixation.

flank. Anatomical location on the lateral back, below the ribs and above the buttocks.

flap. Grafting tissue that remains attached to its vascular supply as it is repositioned to compensate for a defect.

flexible fiberoptic. Describing an endoscope that has a small circumference and is equipped with light and a camera; can be inserted into the nose, mouth, anus, or stoma and advanced along the lumen for diagnostic or therapeutic reasons.

flexor. Muscle that draws the bone toward the body's center; the opposite of extensor.

fluoroscopic, fluoroscopy. X-ray technique for study of movement within an anatomical site; images are displayed on a video monitor.

fluorouracil. Topical cream used in the treatment of actinic keratoses and Bowen's disease; it is administered systemically to treat some cancers.

flutter. Rapid and pulsing beat, eg, atrial flutter.

fontanelle. Any of several spaces between skull bones in an infant, providing potential access sites to the infant brain; cranial sutures seal the bones as the fontanelles close.

footplate drill-out. Removal of a diseased crura of the stapes; the drill-out is usually followed by placement of a prosthesis to replace the crura, restoring hearing.

foramen. Natural anatomic opening that allows passage of vessels, nerves, or other structures, eg, through bone or the walls of an organ.

foramen ovale. In fetal circulation, an opening between the right atrium and left atrium; this opening closes shortly after birth.

foraminotomy. Incision into a foramen to enlarge its circumference and decompress nerves or vessels within.

forceps. Hinged instrument for grasping objects during medical procedures; in childbirth, a large instrument that cups the infant head on both sides to facilitate birth.

foreign body. Something that has become lodged in the body during trauma.

fragmentation. Break-up of bone or hard tissue.

free flap. Dissected skin excised from one location and secured elsewhere within the same body, with anastomosis of vessels at the new site.

free graft. Transplanted tissue that has had all connections severed before it is placed in its new location.

frenectomy. Excision of a small attachment of skin that restricts movement of a body part, eg, on the tongue, lip, or inferior penis.

frenoplasty. Surgical reconstruction of the small attachment of skin that restricts movement of a body part.

frenotomy. Incision into the small attachment of skin that restricts movement of a body part, eg, on the tongue, lip, or inferior penis.

frenulotomy. Incision into the small attachment of skin that restricts movement of a body part, eg, on the tongue, lip, or inferior penis.

frenulum, frenum. Small attachment of skin that restricts movement of a body part, eg, on the tongue, lip, or inferior penis; plural of frenulum is frenula.

frenumectomy. Excision of a small attachment of skin that restricts movement of a body part, eg, on the tongue, lip, or inferior penis.

fulguration. Use of electric energy produced by a high-frequency current to cut through tissue or destroy lesions that are pathologic.

functional disorder. Medical condition that restricts an unrelated body process, eg, dementia causing incontinence or generalized weakness causing gait disturbances.

functional endoscopic sinus surgery. Endoscopic opening of stenosed sinus passages.

fundic patch. Widening of a stenosed esophagus using a patch of tissue from the fundus of the stomach.

fundoplasty. Surgical repositioning of the upper portion of the stomach around the lower end of the esophagus.

fundoplication. Surgical folding and suturing of the fundus of the stomach around the lower end of the esophagus.

fundus. Upper dome-like portion of an organ, eg, the stomach, bladder, or uterus.

furuncle. Painful, pus-filled nodule on the skin caused by Staphylococcus; a boil.

fused. Joined together.

fusiform. Oblong and tapered at both ends.

fusion. Uniting of two bony segments, whether a fracture or a vertebral joint.

galactogram. Radiographic image of a mammary duct after it has been infused with contrast media.

gamete. Male or female component of fertilization, eg, sperm or oocyte.

ganglion. Nerve cluster.

ganglion cyst. Benign growth arising from an aponeurosis or tendon of the foot or hand; cyst is filled with fluid.

gas tamponade. Use of gas, eg, C3F8 or SF6, as a vitreous substitute to pressurize the posterior segment and provide pressure to hold the retina against the choroid.

gastrectomy. Surgical excision of all or part of the stomach.

gastric bypass. High division of the stomach, anastomosis of the small upper pouch of the stomach to the jejunum, and closure of the distal part of the stomach that is retained; a bariatric surgery for treatment of morbid obesity.

gastric reflux. Backward flow of stomach acid into the esophagus.

gastroduodenostomy. Surgical creation of a connection between the stomach and a remote segment of duodenum.

gastroesophageal reflux disease. Chronic backward flow of stomach acid into the esophagus, causing pain and, in some cases, damaging the esophagus.

gastrojejunostomy. Surgical creation of a connection between the stomach and a segment of jejunum.

gastroplasty. Surgical reconstruction of the stomach.

gastrorrhaphy. Suture repair of the stomach.

gastroschisis. Congenital defect in the abdominal wall with evisceration of abdominal contents, uncovered by peritoneum.

gastrostomy. Creation of a communication between the stomach interior and the skin surface, through which a feeding tube may be placed or the stomach may be decompressed of gasses.

gastrostomy tube. Feeding tube that is inserted through a small incision in the skin, abdominal wall, and stomach so that the patient may be fed directly into the stomach, bypassing the mouth and esophagus.

gastrotomy. Incision into the stomach.

geniculate ganglion. Bundle of sensory nerves of the facial nerve.

genioplasty. Surgical reconstruction of the chin.

Gerota's fascia. Tough fascia forming the exterior of the kidney.

gestation. Duration of pregnancy.

GFR. Glomerular filtration rate; the efficiency of the kidney in filtering blood of impurities.

gingiva. Mucosal tissue lining the mandible and maxilla and surrounding the teeth.

gingivectomy. Excision of gingival tissue from around the teeth.

glans penis. Bulb at the distal end of the penis that is covered in foreskin.

glaucoma. Blockage of the Schlemm's canal that prevents the normal outflow of aqueous humor, resulting in accumulation of fluid, increased intraocular pressure, and, eventually, blindness.

glossectomy. Surgical excision of all or a part of the tongue.

glucagon. Pancreatic hormone that raises blood glucose levels by triggering the release of glycogen in the liver.

glucose. Simple sugar that is readily absorbed into the bloodstream during digestion.

glycogen. Sugar stored in the liver; its release is triggered by glucagon.

goniosynechiae. Adhesion of the iris to the cornea, occurring at the angle of the anterior chamber.

goniotomy. Incision into the trabecular meshwork and Schlemm's canal.

graft, grafting. Transfer of tissue from one location to another location.

granulomatous. Having abnormal local inflammatory nodular response in tissue.

greater curvature. Large, inferior curve of the stomach.

G-tube. Feeding tube that is inserted through a small incision in the skin, abdominal wall, and stomach so that the patient may be fed directly into the stomach, bypassing the mouth and esophagus; also referred to as a gastrostomy tube.

guided saturation sampling. Technique of obtaining multiple samples in order to increase the odds that any abnormality will be sampled; in prostate sampling, 20 to 40 samples are included in the saturation sample.

halo. Medical device to keep head immobile following cervical injury.

haptics. Appendages on an artificial intraocular lens that secure the lens to the eye.

hard palate. Bony inferior plate of the skull that comprises the roof of the mouth.

harvest. To collect tissue from a donor.

heart–lung machine. Equipment attached to a patient's vascular system that takes over the function of the heart and lungs temporarily, eg, during surgery.

heater probe. Endoscopic hemostatic device that uses electrical current to generate heat.

helix. Skin-covered cartilage that forms the outer rim of the external ear.

hemangioma. Benign tumor composed of an abnormal cluster of blood vessels.

hematoma. Localized mass of blood, usually clotted, within a tissue or body part.

hematopoietic progenitor cell. Bone marrow cells critical to the formation of blood.

hematuria. Blood in the urine.

hemiarthroplasty. Joint reconstruction in which only one of the two surfaces of the joint is replaced with a prosthesis.

hemiepiphyseal arrest. Surgical insertion of a device to stop growth on one side of a bone, usually to correct an angular deformity; the arrest may be temporary.

hemifacial. Involving half of the face.

hemiglossectomy. Surgical excision of one half of the tongue, usually of one side.

hemilaminectomy. Exposure of the foramen of the spinal cord by excision of a small piece of the lamina to access the foramen where an incision is made to decompress the nerve; also called laminoforaminotomy.

hemipatellectomy. Surgical excision of part of the knee cap (patella).

hemiphalangectomy. Surgical excision of a part of a toe.

hemispherectomy. Surgical excision of a cerebral hemisphere.

hemodialysis. Process of removing metabolic waste products, other toxins, and excess fluids from the blood and replacing essential blood constituents by a process of diffusion through a semi-permeable membrane.

hemodynamic. Relating to the functional properties of blood circulation.

hemorrhage. Excessive or abnormal bleeding.

hemorrhoidectomy. Surgical excision of a hemorrhoid.

hemorrhoidopexy. Repositioning of hemorrhoidal tissue after treatment of a hemorrhoid.

hemorrhoid. Dilation of a vein in the rectum or anus that causes a varicosity.

hemostasis. Natural or medical cessation of blood flow.

hemothorax. Blood accumulation in the pleural cavity.

hepatectomy. Surgical excision of all or part of the liver.

hepaticoenterostomy. Surgical creation of a communication between the hepatic duct and the small intestine.

hepaticostomy. Surgical incision into the hepatic duct with placement of a drainage tube that is secured to the skin.

hepaticotomy. Surgical incision into the hepatic duct.

hepatotomy. Surgical incision into the liver.

hernia. Bulging of tissue from its normal location through a weakened anatomical site.

herpetic vesicle. Skin or mucosal blistering eruption caused by the herpes virus.

Heyman capsule. Irradiated ovoid secured in an intracavitary site for radiation treatment of cancer.

hidradenitis. Inflammation of sweat glands; may lead to development of pus-filled lesions at the site of apocrine glands or excessive sweating at the site of eccrine glands.

histopathologic. Relating to the study of microscopically visible changes in diseased cells or tissue.

Hodgkin's disease. Cancer of the lymphatic system.

homograft. Tissue for grafting from the same species, eg, human tissue for grafting.

homologous. From the same species, eg, human.

horizontal. On the transverse plane.

hormone. Chemical substance formed in one organ or part of the body and carried in the blood to another organ or part of the body.

horseshoe kidney. Congenital anomaly in which the kidneys are joined inferiorly.

hot biopsy forceps. Tool used to obtain endoscopic biopsies and provide electrocoagulation for hemostasis at the biopsy site.

hyaloid. Transparent membrane that separates the retina from the vitreous.

hydatidiform mole. Form of gestational trophoblastic disease that may be benign or malignant; a mass that is part of a nonviable pregnancy.

hydrocele. Swelling due to accumulation of serous fluid.

hydrocelectomy. Surgical excision of a hydrocele.

hydrocephalus. Congenital or acquired abnormal collection of cerebrospinal fluid within the skull; may lead to elevated intracranial pressure.

hymenectomy. Surgical excision of a thin membrane at the introitus.

hymenotomy. Surgical incision to the thin membrane at the introitus.

hyoid myotomy and suspension. Surgical incision into the muscle of the hyoid and fixation of the hyoid to thyroid cartilage with suture or by wrapping it with fascia lata; treatment for obstructive sleep apnea.

hyperkeratotic. Exhibiting a thickening of the skin.

hyperplasia, hyperplastic. Numerical or quantitative increase in the cells of a tissue or organ wherein the bulk of the organ is increased.

hypertension. Chronic elevated blood pressure.

hyperthermia. Therapeutic application of excessive heat.

hypertrophic, hypertrophy. Abnormal increase in size or volume of an organ or tissue.

hyphema. Condition in which blood fills the anterior chamber of the eye.

hypodermis. Subcutaneous skin; the deepest layer of the integument.

hyponychium. Nail bed underlying the nail at the tip of the finger or toe.

hypopharyngeal. Relating to the inferior portion of the pharynx or the portion that terminates at the esophagus.

hypophysectomy. Surgical excision of all or part of the pituitary gland.

hypoplasia, hypoplastic. Having less growth or development than is normal.

hypospadias. Congenital defect in which the urethra does not fully extend to the tip of the glans penis but rather opens into the perineum or some site along the inferior shaft of the penis.

hypothalamus. Segment of the brain that controls fluid balance and hormone production; organ linking the functions of the endocrine glands with the nervous system.

hypothenar. Referring to the fleshy bulb of skin at the edge of the palm proximal to the pinky finger.

hypoxia. Low oxygen in body tissue.

hysterectomy. Surgical excision of the uterus.

hysteroplasty. Surgical reconstruction or repair of the uterus.

hysterorrhaphy. Suture repair of the uterus.

hysterosalpingography. Radiographic image of the uterus and fallopian tubes after they have been infused with contrast media.

hysteroscopic, hysteroscopy. Endoscopic examination of the endometrium of the uterus; a scope is inserted into the vagina and cervical os to access the uterus.

hysterotomy. Surgical incision into the uterus.

ileal conduit. Urinary diversion in which the distal ends of the ureters are anastamosed to an excised segment of ileum that is brought out to the skin surface as a stoma.

ileocolostomy. Surgical connection between the ileum and the large intestine.

ileoileostomy. Surgical connection between two segments of ileum.

ileoproctostomy. Surgical connection between the ileum and the rectum.

ileoscopy. Endoscopic examination of the ileum, usually occurring during colonoscopy and from an anal approach.

ileostomy. Surgical creation of a communication between the small intestine and the skin of the abdomen; the terminal end of the ileum is secured to the skin so that feces can be excreted through the surgically created stoma; bowel distal to the stoma site is bypassed entirely.

iliac fossa. Broad, flat bilateral bone of the pelvis superior to the arcuate line.

ileum. Lower three-fifths of the small intestine lying between the jejunum and the cecum; it is about 12 feet long.

imbrication. Surgical overlapping of tissue layers in wound closure or repair.

immunity. Ability to ward off infection, either generally or to a specific organism.

immunodeficiency. Flaw in the immune system that increases risk of infection.

impairment. Functioning at less than the norm.

in situ. In the natural or normal place; confined to the site of origin without invasion of neighboring tissues.

in vitro fertilization. Union of sperm and egg in a laboratory.

incarcerated. Abnormally imprisoned part, such as a hernia, that is irreducible.

incision. To cut into, or the cut itself.

incision and drainage (I&D). To cut into and actively drain and explore a cavity.

incompetent. Not able to perform its normal function, eg, a valve or cervix uteri.

incomplete abortion. Therapeutic or spontaneous termination of a pregnancy that is ≤22 weeks gestation, with retention of some products of conception.

incontinence, incontinent. Inability to control the flow of urine or the movement of bowels.

incus. Ossicle of the middle ear located between the malleus and the stapes; transmits vibrations from the outer ear to the inner ear.

indirect laryngoscopy. Visual examination of the vocal cords and surrounding tissue using a light source and a mirror.

induced abortion. Medical or surgical intervention to stop a pregnancy that is ≤22 weeks gestation.

inelastic. Not stretchable.

infarction. Localized area of ischemic necrosis produced by occlusion of the arterial blood supply.

inferior. Anatomically below or beneath a point of reference; lower.

infracardiac. Under or below the heart.

infrared coagulation. Methodology in which bursts of infrared light from a rectal probe are administered to coagulate hemorrhoidal tissue.

infratemporal. Surgical approach anterior to the ear and inferior to the temporal bone.

infratentorial. Inferior to the tentorium, usually referencing a portion of the brain inferior to the cerebrum.

infraumbilical. Inferior to the umbilicus, usually referencing a surgical approach.

infusion. Introduction of a fluid through a route other than oral, eg, intravenous, intrathecal, or epidural.

inguinal canal. Pathway in the abdomen through which the ilioinguinal nerve travels as well as the spermatic cord in males and the round ligament in females.

inguinal hernia. Bulging of abdominal contents, usually small intestine, through the inguinal canal.

inguinal ring. Anterior (superficial) or posterior (deep) entrance to the inguinal canal.

injection. Use of a syringe to introduce liquid into the body for diagnostic or therapeutic purposes.

innervate. To provide neural sensation to.

inorganic. Substance not having its origins as a life form.

insertion of bronchial valve. Surgical procedure to place valves in the bronchial tubes to control air leaks in the lung.

inspiration. Breathing in; taking oxygen into the lungs.

instillation. Placing liquid into a body part.

insufficiency. Inadequacy.

insulin. Hormone produced in the pancreas that regulates the metabolism of sugars and fats.

interdental. Between teeth.

intermaxillary. In fixation, wires, ie, binds the maxilla to the mandible.

intermittent claudication. Disorder that presents as pain when exercising; due to ischemia of the extremities.

internal. On the inside; within.

internal fixation. Firmly attaching bony parts internally with surgical wires, screws, pins, rods, or plates.

interpolation flap. Skin flap that retains its vascular connection and is moved to a new location.

intersex state or surgery. Congenital condition in which the sexual organs are ambiguous or surgery to correct this ambiguity.

interspace. Space between two structures, eg, ribs or, more commonly, vertebrae.

intersphincteric. Contained within the sphincter tissue of the anus.

interstitial. Referring to the space between tissue or body parts.

interstitial cystitis. Chronic inflammatory condition of the bladder with urinary frequency, urgency, and pain; also referred to as bladder pain syndrome.

interstitial fluid pressure. Measurement of tissue within a swollen muscle compartment; data for assessment of compartment syndrome.

interstitial radioelement. Irradiated device secured between body parts for radiation treatment of cancer.

intra-abdominal. Within the abdomen.

intra-aortic balloon assist device. Intraluminal mechanical pump that supports cardiac function by inflating and deflating a balloon.

intra-arterial. Within the artery.

intra-articular. Within the joint.

intracapsular cataract extraction (ICCE). Removal of an entire natural lens and replacement with an artificial intraocular lens placed in front of the iris.

intracapsular. Referring to an artificial intraocular lens placed in front of the iris.

intracardiac. Within the heart.

intracatheter. Within the catheter.

intracavitary. Directly into a body cavity, as in placement of an intracavitary chemotherapy agent.

intracerebellar. Within the cerebellum.

intracerebral. Within the cerebrum.

intracervical. Within or through the cervical os.

intracranial. Within the cranium.

intradiscal. Within the disc.

intradural. Within the dura mater.

intrahepatic. Within the liver.

intraluminal. Within a lumen or through a lumen.

intramedullary. Within the bone.

intramural. Inside the walls of an organ or structure.

intranasal. Within the nose or through the nose.

intraocular lens prosthesis. Artificial refractive device inserted into the eye to replace an absent natural lens.

intraocular pressure. Force exerted by the fluid inside the eye that presses out against the eyeball; if intraocular pressure is abnormally high, it can result in a higher risk for developing glaucoma.

intraocular. Within the globe of the eye.

intraoperative. Occurring during a surgical procedure.

intraoperative microelectrode recording. Adjunct procedure performed prior to deep brain stimulation (DBS); electrode placement to validate the site of DBS electrode placement.

intraoral. Within the mouth or through the mouth.

intraosseous. Within the bone or through the bone.

intrapelvic. Within the pelvis or through the pelvis.

intrapleural. Within the pleural cavity or through the pleural cavity.

intrapulmonary. Within the lung.

intraspinal. Within the spine.

intratemporal. Approaching through the temporal bone.

intrathecal. Within or going under or between the meninges of the brain or spinal cord, such as an intrathecal injection.

intrathoracic. Within the chest cavity or through the chest cavity.

intrauterine. Within the uterus.

intrauterine device (IUD). Method of birth control that consists of a small, free-floating implant within the uterine cavity.

intravascular. Within the blood vessel or through the blood vessel.

intravenous. Within the vein or through the vein.

intravesical. Within the bladder.

intrinsic. In muscles, being adjacent to the body part the muscle moves, eg, deltoideus of the shoulder joint.

intubation. Placement of a tube into a lumen in the body for breathing or insertion or removal of fluids.

intussusception. Disorder in which a section of intestine slips back on itself, forming a double-walled length, much like a collapsed telescope; this can cause bowel blockage.

inverted. In an opposite position compared to the norm.

involuntary. Without the ability to consciously control, eg, involuntary muscle movements that perform peristalsis of the bowel or cause the heart to beat.

ipsilateral. Situated or appearing on the same side; affecting the same side.

iridectomy. Surgical removal of iris tissue.

iridencleisis. Surgical implantation of a portion of the iris into the corneoscleral junction to increase aqueous circulation and drainage.

iridocapsulectomy. Surgical excision of tissue from the capsule of the lens with approach through the iris.

iridocapsulotomy. Surgical incision through the iris and into the capsule of the lens.

iridodialysis. Injury in which the iris is separated from the sclera.

iridoplasty. Plastic surgery of the iris.

iridotasis. Surgical stretching of the iris.

iridotomy. Small hole-like incision into the iris.

iris bombe. Defect in which the iris bulges forward due to aqueous pressure in the posterior chamber.

irradiation. Process of exposing an object or body part to radiation; a treatment for cancer.

irrigation. Flushing of a surgical or wound site with fluid.

ischemia. Reduction or cessation of blood flow to an anatomical site due to the blockage of blood vessels to the site.

island flap. Skin for grafting that is cut free of all surrounding skin but retains its vascular supply as it is relocated; also called island pedicle flap.

islets of Langerhans. Clusters of insulin-producing cells found in the pancreas.

isthmus. Band of tissue connecting two larger anatomical bodies.

isthmusectomy. Excision of all or part of a band of tissue connecting two larger anatomical bodies.

J-tube. Feeding or venting tube placed into the part of the small intestine between the duodenum and the ileum; also called a jejunostomy tube.

jejunostomy. Surgical creation of a communication between the small intestine and the skin of the abdomen; the terminal end of the jejunum is secured to the skin so that feces can be excreted through the surgically created stoma; bowel distal to the stoma site is bypassed entirely.

jejunostomy tube. Feeding or venting tube placed into the part of the small intestine between the duodenum and the ileum; also called a J-tube.

Kaposi sarcoma. Malignant neoplasm of the connective tissues often associated with AIDS.

keel. Device used as a brace to maintain laryngeal structure during reconstructive surgery of the larynx.

keloid. Hypertrophic scar tissue.

keratectomy. Removal of corneal tissue.

keratomileusis. Surgery in which a middle layer of corneal tissue is removed, sculpted, and reinserted to improve visual acuity.

keratophakia. Surgery in which a layer of donor corneal tissue is sculpted and inserted in between layers of the patient's cornea to improve visual acuity.

keratoplasty. Plastic surgery on the cornea.

keratoprosthesis. Surgery in which a defective cornea is replaced with an artificial cornea.

keratosis. Localized growth on the skin or mucosa, eg, actinic keratosis or keratoses linguae.

keratotomy. Incision into the cornea.

kyphectomy. Surgical excision of all or part of a deformity of the lumbar spine.

kyphoplasty. Surgical reconstruction of a deformity of the lumbar spine.

labyrinth. Canals of the inner ear responsible for sound perception and balance.

labyrinthectomy. Surgical excision of all or part of the inner ear.

laceration. Injury of soft tissue caused by accidental cutting or tearing.

lacrimal gland. Organ that secretes tears.

lactiferous. Relating to milk, eg, lactiferous ducts.

lagophthalmos. Defect that prevents full closure of the eyelid.

lamellar. Of a layer; eg, in keratoplasty, replacement of a layer of corneal tissue without penetrating the cornea.

lamina. Thin, flat plate or arch of a vertebra comprising the posterior roof of the spinal canal; laminae, plural of lamina.

laminaria. Small, water-absorbent rod inserted into the cervical os to induce dilation of the cervix; may be used to induce abortion.

laminectomy. Surgical excision of the posterior portion of the vertebra (lamina); may be performed to decompress the spinal cord adjacent to it.

laminotomy. Surgical incision into the posterior portion of the vertebra (lamina) as an approach to the intervertebral disc.

laparoscope. Lighted instrument inserted through a small incision for viewing the interior of the abdomen for diagnostic or therapeutic purposes.

laparoscopic, laparoscopy. Visual examination of the contents of the abdominal cavity with an instrument attached to a light source (laparoscope); the laparoscope is a rigid or flexible tube lined with glass fibers that transmit light and images; a video camera, which is attached to the external end of the laparoscope, transmits the images to a video monitor or eyepiece.

laparotomy. Surgical opening into the abdomen that allows for direct visualization of the operative site.

laryngeal web. Congenital anomaly of the voice box characterized by a mucous membrane web across the larynx.

laryngocele. Congenital, anomalous, air-filled sacs within the larynx.

laryngofissure. Incision into the larynx through the thyroid cartilage.

laryngoplasty. Surgical reconstruction of the larynx.

laryngotomy. Incision into the larynx.

laser. Light amplified by stimulated emission of radiation; a focused beam of light that can be used therapeutically in a surgical setting.

laser vaporization. Destruction of tissue using a focused beam of light.

lateral. Away from the middle; to the side or the outside or periphery.

laterovertical. In a manner that is oriented up-and-down and to the side.

latissimus dorsi flap. Transference of back muscle and skin to the chest for breast reconstruction; the flap retains its vascularity.

lavage. Wash and irrigate.

lead. Insulated conduit of electricity or signal.

left lymphatic duct. Central trunk of the lymphatic system located along the thoracic spine in the chest cavity; also called thoracic duct.

leiomyomata. Tumor of the smooth muscle, usually benign and commonly found in the uterus and small intestine.

lesion. Any pathological change in the continuity or structure of a bodily tissue; may be caused by trauma or disease.

lid retraction. Abnormal eyelid position in which the sclera is exposed at the top or bottom of the open eye.

ligament. Tough connective joint fiber that joins bone and/or cartilage.

ligate, ligation. To tie off, ie, occlude a lumen or the act of doing so; eg, ligation of a hemorrhaging vessel, a fallopian tube, or a hemorrhoid.

lingual. Relating to the tongue or to speech.

lipectomy. Surgical removal of fat or fatty tissue.

lipoma. Benign, fatty tumor that is usually found in subcutaneous tissue or muscle.

litholapaxy. Surgical crushing of a calculus or calculi in the urinary system (usually the bladder) followed by flushing of the fragments out through the urethra.

lithotripsy. Crushing of a calculus or calculi in the urinary system using shock waves administered outside the body and targeted to the stones; the stones naturally pass through the urethra during urination.

lobe. Anatomically differentiated portion of an organ, eg, liver or lung.

lobectomy. Removal of a single lobe.

local skin flap. Adjacent skin stretched or rotated to cover a defect; the skin is not entirely severed from the donor site.

loop electrode biopsy. Diagnostic removal of tissue from the cervix uteri for pathological examination; a cone of tissue is excised using electrosurgical technique, providing tissue from high in the lining of the cervical canal.

loop electrode conization. Removal of abnormal tissue from the cervix uteri for therapeutic reasons; a cone of tissue is excised using electrosurgical technique, removing abnormal tissue from high in the lining of the cervical canal.

loop ileostomy. Construction of stoma for elimination of feces; constructed from anastomosis of a loop of ileum rather than anastomosis of a severed end of ileum; stoma has a communication to both the proximal and distal portions of the bowel.

lumen. Channel of a tubular structure.

lung volume reduction. Surgical excision of wedges of diseased pulmonary tissue to optimize function of remaining lung tissue as a treatment for emphysema.

lymph. Interstitial fluid and chyle collected and then circulated through the lymphatic system and into the bloodstream.

lymph node sampling. Surgical excision and biopsy of multiple lymph nodes to determine if they have metastatic disease.

lymphadenectomy. Surgical excision of lymph nodes for diagnostic or therapeutic reasons.

lymphadenitis. Inflammation and enlargement of the lymph node(s).

lymphangiography. Radiographic image of a lymphatic vessel and nodes after they have been infused with contrast media.

lymphangiotomy. Surgical incision into a lymphatic vessel.

lymphatic. Relating to the vessels, nodes, and fluid that make up the system that filters and cleans pathogens and debris from the body and transports fatty acids (chyle) from the intestines to the bloodstream.

lymphocele. Abnormal collection of lymphatic fluid within the body, usually a complication of surgery.

lymphocyte. B cells and T cells that respond to infection in the body as part of an immune response.

lymphoma. Cancer of the lymphatic and immune system.

lysis. Surgical destruction or severing, especially of scar tissue between organs.

macrodactyly. Abnormally enlarged finger or toe.

macular edema. Fluid collection in the central area of the retina.

macular hole. Full-thickness defect in the central area of the retina.

macular pucker. Scar tissue in the central area of the retina; also called epiretinal membrane.

magnetic resonance guidance. Imaging technique in which strong magnetic fields are used to create electronic mapping of the body; the maps are used to perform surgery with greater precision.

malignancy, malignant. Progressive and worsening of a condition, especially describing invasive neoplastic behavior.

malleus. Small bone in the ossicular chain of the middle ear that transmits sound vibrations from the tympanic membrane (eardrum) to the incus; also called the hammer.

malocclusion. Improper contact between the upper and lower teeth; sometimes due to deviations in tooth development and sometimes due to deviations in jaw development.

malrotation. Congenital anomaly that involves twisting of the small bowel around its malpositioned mesenteric attachments; the risks are obstruction and ischemia.

malunion. Bone healing into a position that is not its normal position.

mammaplasty. Surgical reconstruction of the breast to change its shape or size.

mandibulectomy. Surgical excision of a piece of lower jaw bone.

manipulation. Skillful use of the hands to return a body part to its natural position, eg, fractured bones or hernias.

manometer, manometric. Instrument for measuring the pressure of a gas or liquid.

margin. In surgical excision, the amount of normal tissue between the edge of the abnormal tissue and the edge of the excision site, eg, a rim of normal tissue around an excised tumor.

marsupialization. Surgical incision of a cyst or abscess with suture fixation of the skin to permanently open the site; performed to prevent recurrence.

mass. Abnormal lump or bump of undetermined etiology.

mastication, masticator. Act of chewing food; a muscle or other body part that contributes to chewing.

mastoid process. Bony prominence posterior to the ear that contains sound-conducting air cells.

mastoidectomy. Excision of all or part of the mastoid bone.

mastoidectomy cavity. Communication between the external auditory canal and an area posterior to the ear where mastoid cells have been obliterated.

mastopexy. Surgical procedure to lift sagging breast for cosmesis.

mastotomy. Surgical incision into the breast.

maxillectomy. Surgical removal of all or part of the maxillary bone.

maze procedure. Cardiac surgery with ablation of atrial nodes to treat atrial fibrillation; approach varies from mini-thoracotomy to open surgery with cardiopulmonary bypass.

meatal. Relating to a lumen or canal.

meatoplasty. Surgical reconstruction of a lumen or canal

meatotomy. Surgical incision into a lumen or canal.

meatus. Lumen or canal, eg, urinary or external auditory meatus.

Meckel's diverticulum. Congenital anomaly consisting of a pouch in the distal ileum.

media. Relating to the middle; plural of medium.

medial. Relating to or near the middle.

median. Middle or midline.

median tarsorrhaphy. Suturing closed eyelids together.

mediastinoscopy. Endoscopic examination of the space posterior to the sternum and between the heart and lungs.

mediastinotomy. Incision into the space between the lungs that is bounded by the lungs on either side, the sternum in front, the vertebrae in back, and the diaphragm on the bottom.

mediastinum. Space between the lungs that is bounded by the lungs on either side, the sternum in front, the vertebrae in back, and the diaphragm on the bottom.

medium. Substance used for diagnostic tests, eg, a contrast media; plural of medium is media.

medulla. Inner part of an organ, eg, medulla renalis or medulla oblongata.

megacolon. Abnormal dilation of the colon that affects peristalsis; may be congenital or acquired and may be acute or chronic.

melanoma. Malignant tumor derived from cells that are capable of forming melanin; it often metastasizes to the liver.

membranous urethra. Portion of the male urethra at the perineum surrounded by the external urinary sphincter muscle; lies adjacent and distal to the prostatic urethra and proximal to the bulb of the penis.

meninges. Layer surrounding the brain and spinal cord; between the pia mater and arachnoid membrane.

meningioma. Tumor that develops from the lining of the brain or spinal cord.

meningocele. Congenital neural tube defect with a herniation of the membranes that line the spine and brain, forming a cyst filled with cerebrospinal fluid.

meniscectomy. Surgical excision of all or part of the meniscus, usually the excision of a torn portion of cartilage.

menses. Menstrual flow.

Merkel cell. Specialized epithelial skin cells that give rise to a very metastatic form of carcinoma with a high rate of mortality.

mesentery. Large fold of peritoneum that is the conduit for blood vessels, nerves, and lymphatics to the intestine, forming an attachment between the intestine and posterior abdominal wall.

mesh. Woven implantable sheet that provides support to organs following surgery, especially hernia or prolapse repair; may be synthetic or organic and temporary or permanent.

metabolism. Chemical or physical process by which the body converts or uses energy.

metastasis, metastasize. Transference of bacteria or body cells, especially cancer cells, from the original site to another part of the body, usually via blood or lymph, and resulting in development of a similar lesion at the new site.

metastatic. Having transferred to another site from the primary site and resulting in development of a similar lesion at the new site.

metatarsectomy. Surgical excision of a metatarsal bone in the foot.

methylmethacrylate. Acrylic resin used as prosthetic bone in arthroplastic surgery.

micrognathia. Congenital undersized jaw.

microsurgical. Technique in which small vessels and/or nerves are anastamosed using an operating microscope.

microvascular anastomosis. Technique in which small vessels that may have been severed or may be part of a new graft are attached end-to-end with the use of an operating microscope to form patent lumens.

microwave thermotherapy. Use of an instrument that emits microwaves to heat tissue, eg, in transurethral prostate surgery.

middle cranial fossa. Area of the brain that houses the temporal lobes laterally and the hypothalamus medially.

midline. Along the middle plane of the body or of a body part.

missed abortion. Death of a fetus at ≤22 weeks gestation without subsequent natural expulsion of the fetus from the uterus.

mitral valve. Bicuspid valve that controls the flow of blood from the left atrium to the left ventricle.

modality. Method of applying or using a therapeutic agent or procedure.

modified radical neck dissection. Preservation of one or more structures, excluding lymph nodes, that are usually excised in a radical neck dissection.

Mohs micrographic surgery. Excision of a skin lesion during which the physician prepares and views slices of excised tissue under the microscope and maps the boundaries of the lesion in order to ensure all margins are clear after completion of the procedure.

molluscum contagiosum. Virus that causes benign, painless skin lesions; lesions resolve spontaneously over time.

morbid obesity. Clinically severe obesity defined as being 100 pounds over ideal weight or having a body mass index of greater than 35-40.

morcellated, morcellation, morcellized. Cut into small pieces, or the process of cutting into small pieces.

morphology. Science that deals with the form and structure of living things as a whole and apart from their function.

mosaicplasty. Transplant of autologous chondrocyte to repair and reconstruct joint cartilage.

motor. Causing or transmitting information about movement, eg, motor nerves produce impulses that cause muscles to contract or relax.

moulage. Prosthetic device created using a mold or model.

mucocele. Abnormal cyst along a salivary duct that is filled with mucous, often found in the mouth.

mucofistula. Stoma created to release mucous or gas from the bowel; the stoma is in a portion of the bowel that is interrupted and does not contain feces.

mucosa, mucous membrane. Epithelial lining of the entire digestive tract and some of the respiratory and genitourinary tracts; tissue has heightened absorption and secretion capabilities.

Mullerian duct. Embryonic structure that becomes the fallopian tube in females, and disappears in males during normal fetal development.

multiplane. Referring to a fixation device that is applied in more than one direction or along multiple planes, as seen in fractures fitted with ring fixation or with multiple bars screwed into bone at different angles.

muscle transfer. Grafting muscle so that it performs a new function.

muscularis propria. Layer of smooth muscle responsible for peristalsis.

mycotic. Fungal; infected with fungus.

myelography. Radiographic image of the spinal cord after the injection of a contrast medium into the subarachnoid space.

myelomeningocele. Congenital neural tube defect with a herniation of the membranes that line the spine and brain, forming a cyst filled with cerebrospinal fluid and the spinal cord.

myelotomy. Surgical incision into a nerve to interrupt sensory signals.

myocardial infarction. Death of heart tissue; a heart attack.

myocutaneous flap. Skin and muscle for grafting that are separated from their current positions without severing all of their vascular and/or nerve connections.

myomectomy. Surgical excisions of fibroid tumors from the uterus; also called fibroidectomy or leiomyomectomy.

myotomy. Surgical incision into a muscle.

myringoplasty. Surgical reconstruction of a perforated eardrum.

myringotomy. Surgical incision into the eardrum.

nasolabial. Relating to the nasal cavity and the space posterior to the upper lip.

nasolacrimal ducts. Bilateral lumen connecting the lacrimal sac to the nasal cavity; carries tears, the product of the lacrimal gland.

nasopharynx. Throat above the soft palate.

nasotracheal. Related to intubation of the trachea by advancing a tube into the nose and down the throat.

native. Original; natural to the patient.

navicular fossa. Spongy portion of the male urethra located within the glans penis.

navigational bronchoscopy. Electromagnetic navigation and imaging used to find, sample, or treat neoplasms within the lungs; also used to perform suction, control bleeding, and place stents and catheters.

necrosis, necrotizing. Death of tissue or undergoing death of tissue.

needle. Slender, hollow instrument used to puncture tissue in order to deliver medication or retrieve core samples.

needle core biopsy. Diagnostic procedure involving the insertion of a large, hollow needle into a lesion; the needle is equipped with a cutter that cuts the tissue trapped inside; the tissue is retrieved for separate analysis.

neobladder. Creation of a urinary bladder from other tissue, eg, from a segment of ileum.

neonatal, neonate. Person from birth through the 28th day following birth.

neoplasm, neoplastic. Abnormal, progressive, uncontrolled growth of cells that serve no useful purpose; a tumor.

neovascularization. Development of new blood vessels in tissue.

nephrectomy. Surgical removal of a kidney or part of a kidney.

nephrocutaneous. Relating to the kidney and skin.

nephrolithotomy. Incision into the kidney for the removal of a kidney stone.

nephropexy. Surgical fixation, usually with sutures, of the kidney.

nephrorrhaphy. Suture repair of the kidney.

nephrostomy. Surgically created passageway between the kidney and the skin.

nephrostomy tube. Temporary pathway for urine to be drained from the kidney; an incision is made through the skin and into the kidney, and a tube is inserted into the kidney and secured to the skin with sutures; urine drains into a collection bag.

nerve root. First nerve branch immediately off the central nervous system.

nerve sparing. In surgery, avoidance of severing or damaging nerves to preserve function, eg, in prostatectomy.

neural tube defect. Congenital defect of the brain, spine, or spinal cord.

neurectomy. Surgical excision of all or part of a nerve.

neurolemmoma. Benign nerve sheath tumor; also called a schwannoma.

neuritis. Inflammation of a nerve.

neuroendoscopy. Endoscopic cranial or spinal surgery; in cranial surgery, the endoscope is inserted through a small hole in the skull.

neurofibroma. Benign tumor of the nerve sheath.

neurofibromatosis. Genetic disorder that causes tumors to form on neural tissue, usually near the skin's surface.

neurolysis, neurolytic. Administration of an agent that interferes with nerve fibers so that signals are disrupted, usually for pain relief.

neuroma. Benign growth on a nerve, eg, Morton's neuroma.

neuromuscular pedicle. Tissue for grafting that includes nerves for anastomosis to nerves at the new site.

neuropathy. Disease or disorder of a nerve or nerves.

neuroplasty. Surgical reconstruction.

neuropraxia. Nerve injury with physiologic block of nerve conduction without any anatomical interruption; a minor injury.

neurorrhaphy. Suture repair of a nerve.

neurostimulation, neurostimulator. Electrical excitation of the central or peripheral nervous system, or the device that creates the electrical excitation.

neurotmesis. Nerve injury with complete anatomical disruption or rupture; the most severe type of nerve injury.

neurovascular. Relating to both nerves and blood vessels.

nevus. Congenital cutaneous patch of skin caused by overgrowth of skin cells and usually benign; plural of nevus is nevi.

newborn. Person from birth through the 28th day following birth.

no man's land. Area in the hand from the distal palmar crease to the proximal interphalangeal joint; considered to be more difficult to repair than other sites in the hand.

nocturnal penile tumescence. Erection that occurs during normal sleep; is measured to evaluate the cause of impotence as organic or inorganic.

nonautogenous. Graft tissue from a human other than the patient.

nondystrophic. Normal, eg, normal toenails.

noninvasive. Performed without introduction of instrumentation into the body.

nonneoplastic. Not related to new growth.

nonobstetrical. Not involving pregnancy, eg, describing a procedure on a nonpregnant patient.

nonselective. Catheter placement in the aorta or vena cava, or remaining in the punctured vessel and not entering any branches beyond.

nonstereotactic. Not involving three-dimensional computerized location of a defect that is the target of surgery.

nonunion. Failure of progression of healing with expectation of no further healing.

nonviable. Not compatible with life.

nutrient. Substance that provides biological energy and fuel for growth.

obese. Having a body mass index of 30 or greater; being significantly overweight.

obliteration. Destruction or removal of tissue.

obstruction. Blockage, partial or complete.

obstructive sleep apnea. Condition in which the flow of air is disrupted during sleep to the extent there are long breaks between breaths; due to anatomic anomalies.

obturator. Any natural or artificial thing that closes an opening.

occiput. Back of the head.

occluded, occlusion, occlusive. Completely or partially blocked; the blockage.

ocular implant. Temporary or permanent prosthesis to replace the eye; its purpose may be to fill the ocular void or to cosmetically replace the natural eye.

omentectomy. Removal of all or part of the double layer of peritoneum that covers the stomach and hangs down like an apron, covering the anterior surface of the abdominal organs.

omentopexy. Suture fixation of the greater omentus to a nearby organ.

omentum. Double layer of peritoneum that covers the stomach and hangs down like an apron, covering the anterior surface of the abdominal organs.

omphalectomy. Excision of all or part of the navel.

omphalocele. Herniation of abdominal contents into the base of the umbilical cord, covered by peritoneum.

onychocryptosis. Ingrowing toenail in which the nail grows into the skin of the toe.

oophorectomy. Surgical removal of all or part of an ovary, or both ovaries.

open. Through a direct incision overlying the site.

open sky technique. Approach through the anterior segment of the eye.

operating microscope. Binocular surgical microscope used to visualize small objects for anastomosis or other diagnosis or treatment.

operculectomy. Excision of a flap of gum that forms around the site of a newly erupted tooth.

opponensplasty. Surgical reconstruction to restore function of the opposable grasping movements of the thumb, usually dysfunctional due to nerve damage; the procedure involves transfer of a finger tendon to an insertion site in the thumb.

optical endomicroscopy. Microscopic examination of tissue in situ during an endoscopic procedure; a miniature microscope captures and transmits microscopic images for histologic evaluation.

orbital implant. Prosthesis that resides outside the globe and its attached muscles.

orbitotomy. Incision into orbit.

orchiectomy. Surgical removal of all or part of a testis, or both testes.

orchiopexy. Surgical fixation of a testicle in the scrotum.

organic. Biological, eg, from a plant or animal.

orifice. Natural opening in the body, eg, mouth, ear, urethra, anus.

oromaxillary. Relating to the mouth and jaw.

oronasal. Relating to the mouth and nose.

oropharynx. Relating to the mouth and pharynx.

orthotopic. Occurring in the normal position.

osseous. Relating to bone.

ossicles. Malleus, incus, and stapes of the middle ear; bones that transmit sound vibrations to the inner ear.

ossicular chain reconstruction. Surgical repair of the continuity of the malleus, incus, and stapes in the middle ear to reestablish sound conduction to the inner ear; also called ossiculoplasty.

ossiculoplasty. Surgical repair of the continuity of the malleus, incus, and stapes in the middle ear to reestablish sound conduction to the inner ear; also called ossicular chain reconstruction.

ostectomy. Surgical excision of all or part of a bone.

osteitis. Inflammation of the bone.

osteoma. Benign tumor of the bone.

osteomyelitis. Inflammation of bone caused by infection with a pyogenic (pus-forming) organism.

osteophytectomy. Surgical excision of anomalous bony spur(s) along the superior and inferior edges of a vertebral body; these outgrowths may compress the spinal cord.

osteoplastic, osteoplasty. Surgical reconstruction or replacement of bone.

osteoporosis. Condition of reduced quality of bone; atrophy of the skeletal system.

osteotomy. Incision into the bone, usually for drainage.

ostiomeatal complex. Nasal sinus channel that links the middle meatus to the frontal, anterior, and middle ethmoid and maxillary sinuses.

ostium, ostia. Door or opening; ostia is plural of ostium.

ostomy. Creation of an external stoma through which waste may be removed from the bowel or kidney; also called a stoma.

otoplasty. Surgical reconstruction of the external ear.

otorrhea. Drainage or discharge from the ear.

oval window. Membrane that connects the middle and inner ear; also called the fenestra ovalis.

ovarian vein syndrome. Disorder in which the vein to the ovary compresses the ureter, leading to symptoms that may include pain and urinary tract infection.

ovariolysis. Surgical freeing of the ovary from adhesions.

oviducts. Bilateral duct between the uterus and ovary that provides a pathway for the ovum during ovulation; also called the fallopian tube.

ovum. Female reproductive cell that, after fertilization, develops into a new member of the same species; plural of ovum is ova.

oxytocin. Hormone that is key to sexual reproduction; it is produced by the hypothalamus and stored in the pituitary gland; may be administered to a pregnant patient to induce labor or to strengthen contractions during labor.

pacemaker. Device implanted either temporarily or permanently that electrically stimulates the myocardium of one or more chambers of the heart to contract when the heart fails to do so on its own (eg, myocardial infarction, drug toxicity); placed in order to restore or maintain hemodynamic stability.

pain block. Injection of anesthetic into a nerve in order to block regional pain signals to the brain; may be performed for surgical or post-surgical pain relief or as a therapy for chronic neuropathic pain.

palate. Roof of the mouth; it separates the mouth from the nasal cavities; contains bony hard palate anteriorly and soft palate posteriorly.

palatopharyngoplasty. Surgical reconstruction of the soft palate and pharynx to remove excess tissue that may contribute to obstructive sleep apnea and to reposition other tissues in the oropharynx; the goal is to enlarge the airway; also called uvulopalatopharyngoplasty or uvulopharyngoplasty.

palatoplasty. Surgical reconstruction of the palate with suture repair and tissue repositioning, usually performed to repair a congenital cleft palate and/or create an anatomy compatible with speech and unobstructed dento-alveolar growth in children.

palliation. Treatment, such as an operation, that does not cure a problem but makes adjustments to improve the situation.

palmar. Relating to the palm of the hand.

palpebral. Relating to the eyelids.

Pancoast tumor. Pulmonary malignancy on the surface area of the superior sulcus of the lung; its location raises the likelihood that any metastasis will be extrapulmonary (into lymphatics, intercostal nerves, chest wall, or vertebrae) rather than intrapulmonary (deeper into lung).

pancreatectomy. Surgical excision of all or part of the pancreas.

pancreaticojejunostomy. Surgical creation of a connection between the pancreatic duct or a transected portion of pancreas and the jejunum, usually as a treatment for chronic pancreatitis.

pancreatitis. Inflammation of the pancreas; may be chronic or acute.

pancreatography. Radiographic imaging of the pancreas and/or its ducts after they have been infused with contrast media.

panniculectomy. Surgical excision of excess skin and fat, eg, excision of a redundant apron of skin and fat hanging from the abdomen.

papilla. Small anatomical projection; may be a normal structure, eg, papillae on the tongue or duodenum, or a defect, eg, anal papillae (skin tags).

papillary. Referring to a papilla or papillae.

papilloma. Small, warty, nipple-shaped skin growth.

papillotomy. Incision into the opening of the pancreatic duct and into the duodenum (duodenal papilla), usually for the removal of calculi.

paracentesis. Removal of fluid through a syringe or catheter.

paramedian forehead flap. Reconstructive procedure in which full-thickness skin containing the supratrochlear artery is mobilized from the forehead to a pedicle flap in order to repair a major nose defect.

parapharyngeal space. Area in the neck that contains the maxillary artery and ascending pharyngeal artery, lateral to the upper pharynx; a common route for infection from the tongue, salivary glands, or tonsils.

parasympathetic. Part of the involuntary nervous system that activates functions associated with feeding and reproduction, eg, saliva production and digestion while eating, sexual activity, urination, and defecation.

paratendon. Tissue between a tendon and a tendon sheath; may be fatty or synovial.

parathyroidectomy. Surgical excision of all or part of a parathyroid gland.

paravaginal. Tissue adjacent to the vagina.

paravertebral. Tissue adjacent to the vertebra.

parenchyma. Portion of an organ that performs the function of the organ, as compared to supporting structures, encasing capsules, or connective tissues.

paresthesia. Abnormal sensation caused by damage to peripheral nerve, eg, tingling, prickling, or phantom sensations.

parietal. Relating to the walls of a cavity.

paronychia. Inflammation of the skin tissue surrounding a fingernail or toenail.

paroxysmal. Sudden, short, frequent spasm or intensification of symptoms.

pars plana approach. Surgical access through an incision posterior to the limbus and through the sclera into the posterior segment.

partial ossicular reconstruction prosthesis (PORP). Artificial replacement for some of the structures (malleus, incus, or stapes) in the middle ear.

patch graft. Small amount of tissue that is secured at the site of a defect, eg, at the site of a vessel graft.

patellectomy. Surgical excision of the kneecap (patella).

patency. Having an open state.

patent ductus arteriosus. Transient fetal circulatory shunt that fails to close at birth; the ductus arteriosus allows fetal blood to bypass the lungs and if it remains open (patent) after birth, blood flowing out of the aorta to the body is directed back to the lungs via the pulmonary artery, causing excessive blood flow in the lungs.

pedicle. Narrow stalk of tissue.

pedicle flap. Graft that is separated from its current position without severing all of its vascular and/or nerve connections.

pedunculotomy. Surgical incision into all or part of the cerebral peduncle, a bilateral motor nerve tract; performed to mitigate involuntary movement.

pelvic floor. Muscles and fascia that form the structure from the anus to the genitals.

pelvic ring. Continuity of bone formed by the bilateral ilium, ischium and pubis, and sacrum.

pendulous urethra. Portion of the male urethra that runs from the bulbous urethra at the penile base to the glans penis at its distal end.

penile urethra. Portion of the male urethra that runs the length of the penis.

percutaneous. Approaching through the skin, often using a needle puncture.

percutaneous endoscopic gastrostomy (PEG) tube. Communication from the stomach to the skin surface in the form of a tube that is used to feed the patient; it bypasses the mouth and esophagus.

perfusion. Flow of blood or other perfusate per unit volume of tissue, as in ventilation/perfusion ratio.

periarticular. Adjacent to or near a joint.

pericardial window. Creation of a portal in the pericardium for the release of fluid that has built up between the pericardium and the heart.

pericardiectomy. Excision of all or part of the pericardial sac surrounding the heart.

pericardioscopy. Endoscopic examination of the pericardium, usually through a subxiphoid approach.

pericardiotomy. Surgical incision into the pericardial sac surrounding the heart.

pericardium. Double fibroserous membranous sac that envelops the heart.

pericoronal. Adjacent to or near the crown of a tooth.

perilymph. Fluid with a composition similar to that of cerebrospinal fluid; contained in the bony labyrinth.

perineal urethra. That portion of the urethra that traverses the perineum.

perineorrhaphy. Suture repair of the perineum.

perinephric. Near or associated with the kidney.

perineum. Structured muscle, fascia, and skin between the genitalia and the anus.

perineurium. Connective tissue that surrounds each bundle of neurons.

periodontal. Tissue (gums) that holds the teeth in place.

perionychium. Soft tissue and skin that surround the base and sides of a toenail or fingernail.

periorbital. Within or surrounding the orbit.

peripancreatic. Adjacent to or near the pancreas.

peripheral. On the outer edges or situated away from the center of a structure; opposite of central.

peripheral artery disease. Atherosclerosis, ie, narrowed arteries that reduce blood flow to limbs, usually the lower extremity.

peripheral nervous system. Sensory, motor, and autonomic nerves that are outside of the brain and spinal cord.

peripheral vascular disease. Diseased vessels that reduce blood flow to or from limbs, usually the lower extremity; also called venous disease.

peripherally inserted central catheter (PICC). Intravenous access port at a peripheral site, eg, the arm, which delivers medication through a thin tube that continues from the intravenous site to a large vessel near the heart.

periprostatic. Adjacent to or near the prostate.

periprosthetic capsulotomy. Incision into fibrous scar tissue that surrounds a breast implant; the operative goal is to enlarge the implant pocket.

perirectal. Relating to tissues near the rectum.

perirenal. Relating to tissues near the kidney.

peristalsis. Smooth muscle contractions that advance the contents of a lumen antegrade along its route; involuntary muscle action.

peritoneal. Relating to abdominal organs, space between abdominal organs, or the serous membrane that lines the abdomen.

peritoneum. Smooth, delicate, transparent, serous membrane that lines the abdominal and pelvic cavities and forms a sac over these organs.

peritonitis. Inflammation of the peritoneum.

peritonsillar. Adjacent to or near the tonsil.

periurethral. Relating to tissues near the urethra.

perivesical. Relating to tissues near the bladder.

pessary. Device inserted into the vagina to provide support to the uterus, bladder, vagina, or rectum, or to deliver medication.

pH. Measurement of the acidity or alkalinity of a solution, as defined by power of hydrogen.

phacoemulsification. Surgical disintegration of a cataract, followed by aspiration and removal.

phacofragmentation. Surgical procedure to break up a cataract and remove it in multiple pieces.

phagocyte. Cell in the immune system that eats detritus and bacteria.

phalangectomy. Surgical excision of all or part of a segment of a finger or toe.

pharyngectomy. Surgical excision of all or part of the pharynx.

pharyngoplasty. Surgical reconstruction of the pharynx.

pharyngostomy. Incision and creation of an artificial communication in the pharynx; may be followed by placement of a feeding tube.

photocoagulation. Use of controlled light energy (eg, laser beam) to alter and ablate tissue.

photodynamic therapy. Administration of photoactive drugs that destroy cancer cells by making them sensitive to light.

photopheresis. Extracorporeal (outside the body) treatment of blood followed by reinfusion.

physiologic. Normal; not pathological; characteristic of or conforming to the normal functioning or state of the body.

pilonidal. Hair trapped within a cyst; common location for a pilonidal cyst is superior to the gluteal cleft.

pinna. External ear.

placenta. Organ of pregnancy that transfers oxygen and nutrients from the mother to the fetus; it adheres to the wall of the uterus and is attached to the fetus via the umbilical cord.

plane. Flat smooth surface; there are three directions of planes, all in reference to a standing person facing the examiner: vertical anterior to posterior (sagittal), vertical side to side (coronal or longitudinal), and horizontal (transverse).

plaque. Small differentiated area of abnormal skin or mucosa; also, deposits in tissue that build up over time, eg, dental or arterial plaque.

plasma. Component of whole blood that transports waste and also serves as a protein reserve; plasma volume can be changed by depositing or withdrawing fluids from extravascular tissue.

plasma coagulator. Endoscopic laser device that provides hemostasis.

plastic. Related to the appearance, rather than the function, of a body part.

plastic operation/repair. Reconstructive surgery to restore or enhance the normal appearance of a body part.

platelet. Blood component that functions to stop bleeding; also called thrombocyte.

plethysmography. Image from a device that measures the change in volume within an organ, eg, lung or penis, during a test.

pleural effusion. Abnormal collection of fluid between the layers that line the lungs.

pleural scarification. Procedure in which intentional scarification of the pleura, eg with electrocautery or other modality, is a therapy for a malignant pleural effusion.

pleurectomy. Surgical excision of all or part of the pleura.

pleurodesis. Production of adhesions between the parietal and visceral pleura.

plexus. Convergence of multiple vessels or nerves; a network.

plication. Taking of tucks in tissue to make it smaller or stronger; a folding.

pneumatic retinopexy. Injection of gas into the posterior segment of the eye to treat retinal detachment.

pneumonectomy. Surgical excision of a lung, usually referencing removal of an entire lung.

pneumonolysis. Surgical separation of the two pleural layers or of the outer pleural layer from the chest wall to collapse the lung.

pneumonostomy. Surgical incision into the lung.

pneumoperitoneum. Air in the peritoneum; often referencing air released into the peritoneum to enhance visualization during laparoscopic surgery.

pneumothorax. Collapsed lung; air has leaked into the pleural cavity, putting pressure on the lung.

pollicization. Reconstructive surgery in which a finger is revised so that it can be used as a thumb.

polydactyl. Congenital condition in which the patient has more toes and/or fingers than is normal.

polyhydramnios. Excess amniotic fluid in the amniotic sac.

polyp. Abnormal growth in mucous membrane, usually considered benign.

polypectomy. Surgical excision of all or part of a polyp.

PORP. Partial ossicular reconstruction prosthesis; artificial replacement for some of the structures (malleus, incus, or stapes) in the middle ear.

portal hypertension. High pressure in the venous system that leads to the liver.

port, portal. Small medical implant through which infusions can be performed.

portoenterostomy. Creation of a communication between the jejunum and duodenum and the liver to allow for bile drainage into the intestine; a treatment for biliary atresia.

portography. X-ray visualization of the hepatic portal system after the infusion of contrast media.

postauricular. Behind the ear.

posterior. Situated toward the rear or behind a structure.

postfenestration. Condition in which the patient has previously undergone fenestration, ie, creation of a mastoid cavity and a window in the lateral semicircular canal; a fascial graft is placed over the window, and sound is transmitted through the graft into the inner ear.

postpartum. Related to childbirth, specifically the six weeks following childbirth.

pouch of Douglas. Anatomical cavity between the rectum and the uterus.

pre-auricular. In front of the ear.

premalignant. Tissue that histologically is not malignant but has characteristics that indicate it could become malignant.

preservation. During surgical excision or resection, sparing of targeted tissue.

preterm infant. Neonate who is <37 weeks gestation at the time of birth.

prevesical. In front of the bladder.

priapism. Persistent and painful penile erection; may be due to medication overdose or caused by dysfunction in the veins or arteries of the corpora caveronosa.

primary. First or most important in order of time or development.

procidentia. Prolapse, eg, of the uterus or rectum.

procreation. Sexual intercourse and reproduction.

proctectomy. Surgical excision of all or part of the rectum.

proctopexy. Surgical fixation of the rectum, usually with sutures, to adjacent structures, eg, the sacrum.

proctoplasty. Surgical reconstruction of the rectum.

proctosigmoidoscopy. Endoscopic examination of the rectum and, possibly, a portion of the sigmoid colon.

prolapse. Downward displacement of an organ.

proliferative vitreoretinopathy (PVR). Complication of retinal detachment in which scar tissue complicates successful reattachment.

pronator. Muscle that has the function of turning toward or turning down an extremity, eg, a muscle at the radius that moves the hand to a palm-down position.

prophylactic treatment. Preventive care.

prophylaxis. Preventive measure.

prostaglandin. Hormone that contributes to function of smooth muscle, control of blood pressure, induction of labor, and reaction to infection and injury.

prostatectomy. Excision of all or part of the prostate.

prostatic urethra. That portion of the male urethra that begins at the bladder neck and continues through the prostate gland.

prostatotomy. Incision into the prostate.

prosthesis, prosthetic. Artificial substitute for a body part.

proximal. Closer to any point of reference, or closest to the center of the body.

pseudoaneurysm. Ruptured aneurysm in which the blood is contained by the surrounding tissue; also called a false aneurysm or aneurysmal hematoma.

pseudocyst. Abnormal expansion of a cavity that is cystic in appearance but is not a true cyst.

pseudomeningocele. Pocket of cerebrospinal fluid in extradural soft tissue.

pseudophakia. Artificial intraocular lens.

pterygium. Benign overgrowth of conjunctival tissue onto the cornea.

pterygomaxillary. Relating to the bony palate and the upper jaw.

ptosis. Drooping or casting downward from normal anatomical position.

ptyalism. Drooling or excessive salivary gland secretions.

pulmonary valve. Cardiac valve between the right ventricle and the pulmonary artery.

pulse generator. Equipment that houses the battery and circuitry used to deliver an electrical charge; permanent devices are placed surgically; temporary devices are located outside the patient's body.

punch. Removal of cylindrical or disc-shaped tissue using a tool equipped with a circular blade; punch technique may be used for biopsy or for excision; the depth of the tissue removed may be full-thickness or partial-thickness skin or other tissue, eg, sclera.

Purkinje fibers. System of specialized conducting fibers that allow rapid transmission of a cardiac impulse from the atrioventricular node to the ventricles.

purulent. With pus.

push transfusion. Manual injection of blood during a transfusion; the blood is injected slowly using a needle or catheter.

pyelocutaneous. Refers to the pelvis of the kidney and skin, usually as a description of the path of a fistula or stoma.

pyelolithotomy. Surgical excision of the kidney through the skin and into the pelvis, with removal of a calculus from the kidney; also called pelviolithotomy.

pyeloplasty. Surgical reconstruction of the renal pelvis.

pyeloscopy. Endoscopic examination of the renal pelvis.

pyelostomy. Formation of an opening into the pelvis of the kidney to establish urinary drainage.

pyelotomy. Incision into the pelvis of the kidney.

pyloromyotomy. Surgical incision into the sphincter muscle of the pylorus to widen its aperture.

pyloroplasty. Surgical reconstruction of the pylorus of the stomach, usually performed to increase the width of the pylorus.

quadrant. One part of an organ or body part divided into four segments, eg, upper right, upper left, lower right, and lower left.

quadricepsplasty. Surgical reconstruction of the quadriceps femoris, a group of large extensor muscles on the anterior thigh.

quinsy. Peritonsillar abscess; a complication of tonsillitis.

radiation therapy. Targeted treatment of disease, principally malignant neoplasms, using high-energy ionizing radiation beams to kill tissue by damaging its DNA; the radiation may come from an external source, from a source implanted in the body, or from an intraoperative source.

radical neck dissection. Unilateral treatment for metastatic neck disease in which lymph nodes, muscles, veins, salivary glands, and nerves are removed from the neck.

radical resection. Surgical excision of an organ or body part including local connective tissue, blood vessels, lymphatic supply, and other neighboring tissues, usually associated with a malignancy.

radioactive. Emitting high-energy ionizing radiation beams.

radiofrequency ablation. Destruction of tissue through the use of a specific form of energy (radiofrequency).

radiofrequency microremodeling. Urethroscopic application of a radiofrequency heat probe to scar and thereby strengthen urethral tissue in order to reduce female stress urinary incontinence.

radiofrequency thermotherapy. Urethroscopic application of a radiofrequency heat probe to destroy prostate tissue in order to reduce male urethral stenosis.

ranula. Acquired and benign pseudocyst on the floor of the mouth, usually caused by mucous extravasation and/or a sublinqual salivary gland obstruction.

raphe. Delineating line or ridge along the midline of the scrotum and continuing along the underside of the penis.

re-amputation. Second amputation occurring as an extension of a previous amputation at the same site or limb.

reanastomosis. Surgical reconnection of two lumens; often a reversal of an earlier procedure that severed a connection.

recession. Displacement of a muscle or tendon to a position posterior to its anatomic insertion site; this makes the muscle more taut than it was before surgery.

recipient cardiectomy–pneumonectomy. Removal of the heart and lungs from a patient who is to receive donor heart and lungs.

reconstruction. Surgical repair and/or restoration of an organ or body part.

rectocele. Bulging of the rectum into the posterior vaginal wall.

recurrent. Happening again.

reducible. With the ability to restore to its normal place or position, either manually or surgically.

reduction. Restoration to its original position, eg, restoring a bone in a fracture or returning a herniated organ to its proper location.

redundant. Characterized by containing duplicate or excess amounts.

reflux. Condition in which acid from the stomach flows retrograde into the esophagus.

refraction. Sharpening of a perceived image by bending of light waves; refraction naturally occurs in the eyes and can be measured during a refraction process to provide a patient with lenses that correct any naturally occurring refraction errors.

reinnervation. Restoration of nerve and nerve continuity, either surgically or through natural healing.

renal pelvis. Funnel-shaped urine collection site within the kidney that is connected to the proximal ureter.

repair. Restoration of a diseased or damaged tissue naturally, by healing processes, or artificially with therapeutic intervention.

resection. Surgical removal of a section or segment of an organ or structure; in the case of muscle or tendon, this will result in the muscle being more lax than it was before surgery.

restrictive myopathy. In Grave's disease, impaired movement of extraocular muscles.

retention suture. Stitch placed in muscle or fascia to reduce tension on skin sutures.

retinal detachment. Separation of the light-sensitive membrane at the back of the eye from the vascular choroid.

retinopathy. Abnormal blood vessel development in the retina.

retrobulbar. Behind the globe of the eye.

retrocaval ureter. Congenital displacement of the inferior vena cava that may cause compression and nephrohydroureter; also called circumcaval ureter.

retrograde. Extending or going backward; flowing against the current.

retrolingual. Occurring posterior to the tongue or near its base.

retroperitoneal, retroperitoneum. From behind the peritoneum.

retropubic. Occurring behind the pubic bone(s) of the pelvis.

retrosigmoid. Surgical approach to the brain through the occipital bone posterior to the sigmoid sinus posterior to the ear.

rhinectomy. Surgical excision of all or a part of the nose.

rhinophyma. Disfiguring granulomatous growth of the nose.

rhinoplasty. Reconstruction of the nose.

rhinorrhea. Free discharge of nasal secretions, eg, mucous, cerebrospinal fluid, blood, and pus.

rhinotomy. Incision into the nose.

rhizotomy. Selective surgical severing of nerve roots of the spine, usually performed for pain relief.

rhytidectomy. Surgical excision of skin of the face to reduce laxity of tissue and wrinkles; a facelift.

rhytid. Wrinkle in the skin associated with age or sun exposure.

robotic assistance. Surgical instruments implemented through the use of computer and software technology.

rotation. To pivot on an axis.

round window. Complementary membrane between the middle ear and the cochlea that provides pressure relief so that vibrations received at the oval window can be easily transmitted in the fluid-filled cochlea.

Roux-en-Y. Y-shaped pattern of the bowel formed by the anastomosis of the distal end of the divided jejunum to the stomach, bile duct, or another structure, with implantation of the proximal end into the side of the jejunum at a suitable distance below the first anastomosis.

rubber band ligation. Nonsurgical treatment of an internal hemorrhoid through placement of a rubber band around the base of the hemorrhoid, cutting off its blood supply; the physician performs ligation using an anoscope or proctoscope for direct visualization of the hemorrhoid and rubber band device.

rugae. Accordion-like folds on the inside of an organ that allow it to expand, eg, inside the stomach, bladder, and vagina.

sac. Pouch-like structure.

saccular. Pouch-like.

saccule. Small pouch-like structure.

sacroperineal. Of the sacrum and perineum, usually referencing an approach for cloacal anomaly repair in which an attempt is made to spare the anal sphincter muscle.

saline infusion sonohysterography (SIS). Salt solution infused into the uterus to improve imaging during an ultrasound scan.

salpingectomy. Surgical excision of all or part of the fallopian tube(s).

salpingolysis. Severing of scar tissue or adhesions from the fallopian tube.

salpingo-oophorectomy. Surgical excision of all or part of the fallopian tube(s) and ovary(ies).

salpingostomy. Surgical incision into a fallopian tube, eg, to remove an ectopic pregnancy; also called salpingotomy.

salpingotomy. Surgical incision into the fallopian tube, eg, to remove an ectopic pregnancy; also called salpingostomy.

sampling. Removal of tissue or fluid from body from multiple sites or at multiple times for biopsy or other evaluation.

sarcoma. Malignant neoplasm of connective tissue.

saucerization. Surgical excision of integument or bone to form a scooped out depression.

scapulopexy. Surgical fixation of the scapula, usually to the chest wall or vertebra.

schwannoma. Benign nerve sheath tumor; also called a neurolemmoma.

sciatica. Pain that originates in the sciatic nerve, causing pain in the leg.

scleral buckling. Surgical treatment of retinal detachment; it is done by applying pressure outside the globe to seal the retina to the choroid within the globe.

sclerectomy. Removal of the tough white outer shell of the globe of the eye (sclera).

sclerosing. Hardening or to cause to harden or stiffen, eg, injection of varicose veins with an agent that renders them too scarred for circulating blood to pass through them.

sclerosis. Stiffening or hardening of tissue.

scrotoplasty. Surgical reconstruction of the scrotum.

second order. Branch coming off the initial branch of the aorta or the initial access vessel, as described in vascular catheter placement; branch vessel emanating from a first-order vessel.

secondary. Caused by another condition or happening after another event.

secondary closure. Suture repair of a surgical wound in a setting that is different from that of the original operation.

secondary fibrosis. Formation of excessive fibrous tissue as the result of something else; eg, after injection of a sclerosing agent, a secondary fibrosis occurs in veins.

secondary revision. Surgical revision of an operative site that occurs in a setting that is different from that of the original operation.

secundines. Afterbirth; placenta.

segmentectomy. Removal of a discrete bronchopulmonary segment from either the left or right lung.

selective catheter placement. Placement of a working catheter into a branch off the aorta or the access vessel; the catheter is established for another procedure, eg, angioplasty, atherectomy, or stent placement.

semicircular canal. One of a trio of tubes in the inner ear; these tubes sense body planes and motion and are important to balance.

semilunar valve. Valve located at the opening of the aorta or pulmonary artery of the heart; structure that prevents backflow of blood into the ventricle of the heart.

sensorineural hearing loss. Defect in the inner ear, vestibulocochlear nerve, or brain that affects the transmission or interpretation of sound signals.

sensory. Relating to the neural reception and transmission of sensation-related information to the brain.

sentinel lymph node. First lymph node distal to the site of a malignancy; biopsy of the sentinel node is performed to evaluate potential metastasis.

septal. Relating to a natural partition that divides two anatomical sites.

septal defect. Hole in the natural partition that divides two anatomical sites.

septectomy. Surgical excision of all or part of a natural partition that divides two anatomical sites.

septic abortion. Spontaneous or planned termination of pregnancy that results in sepsis to the patient.

septoplasty. Surgical reconstruction of a natural partition that divides two anatomical sites.

septostomy. Surgical incision of the natural partition that divides two anatomical sites.

septum. Natural partition that divides two anatomical sites, eg, nasal septum and atrial septum.

sequestrectomy. Surgical removal of necrotic bone (sequestrum) that has separated from nearby bone; healthy bone is not incised or excised.

seroma. Tumor-like collection of serum in tissue.

serous membrane. Moisture-producing outer lining of membranes that enclose bodily cavities, eg, pleura and peritoneum; also called the serosa.

sesamoidectomy. Surgical excision of the small bone embedded in a tendon (sesamoid), usually referencing sesamoid bone of the hand or foot.

seton. Material threaded through tissue to facilitate drainage or to mark the route of a fistula.

sheath. Covering or lining on the exterior of a body part.

shunt. Abnormal flow between two body parts; may be congenital or acquired; if acquired, may be a natural anomaly or surgically created to correct an anatomical problem.

sialodochoplasty. Surgical reconstruction of a salivary duct.

sialography. Radiographic imagery of a salivary duct with injection of contrast media.

sialolithotomy. Surgical incision into a salivary gland, usually for the extraction of a stone.

sialorrhea. Excessive drooling or uncontrollable salivation.

sigmoidoscopy. Endoscopic examination of the entire rectum, sigmoid colon, and, possibly, part of the descending colon.

sinus tract. Hollow path through which fluid can travel, usually a defect, eg, a fistula.

sinusoscopy. Endoscopic examination of the nose and nasal sinuses.

sinusotomy. Surgical incision into a sinus.

skeletal fixation. Securing fractured bone in place using screws, plates, wires, or nails.

skeletal traction. Applying tension to bone in order to realign it or to relieve pressure on neighboring structures, eg, nerves.

Skene's gland. Bilateral female gland that drains through the Skeen's duct to the vulva; also called the paraurethral gland.

skin flap. Integumentary tissue that remains connected to its own blood supply as it is repositioned locally to cover a defect.

skin graft tube. Use of skin to create a lumen, eg, a urethral lumen created from foreskin in hypospadias repair.

skin tag. Benign cutaneous growth on a narrow stalk, commonly seen in the groin and armpit; also called acrochordon.

skull base. Inferior portion of the skull composed of ethmoid, sphenoid, occipital, and bilateral frontal and temporal bones; also describes surgery performed on the contents of the skull base, which is a portion of the brain with complex and crowded anatomical structures.

SLAP lesion. Superior labral tear from the anterior to the posterior; injury to the cartilage surrounding the shoulder socket (glenoid).

sleeve gastrectomy. Bariatric procedure in which the greater curvature of the stomach is excised, reducing the stomach capacity by approximately 75%.

slit lamp. Diagnostic device that shines a thin beam of light into the eye.

smooth muscle. Muscle within a hollow organ that performs involuntary actions as directed by the autonomic nervous system, eg, muscles that perform peristalsis in the gastrointestinal and urinary tracts and blood vessels.

snare. Endoscopic excision and retrieval device that consists of a loop that is secured around tissue to be excised, eg, a polyp.

soft palate. Muscle and connective tissue that extends from the hard palate to block the nasopharynx during sucking and swallowing.

somatic nervous system. Network of nerves responsible for voluntary movements and feedback in the peripheral nervous system, eg, body movement and sensory perception.

somatostatin. Hormone that affects the release of other hormones; it is released by the stomach, intestine, and pancreas.

sonogram. Recorded image from an ultrasound.

sound. Instrument for the dilation of a lumen or inserted into a lumen during examination.

space of Retzius. Retropubic, prevesical area.

spasmodic dysphonia. Chronic muscle spasms within the vocal cords that interfere with speech.

spasmodic torticollis. Chronic muscle spasms within the neck muscles causing involuntary neck movement and pain.

spasmolytic. Drug that acts to relax muscle and reduce or eliminate muscle spasms.

speculum. Instrument inserted into an orifice, eg, vagina or anus, to facilitate visual inspection or treatment within the orifice.

sperm washing. Laboratory process by which spermatozoa are separated from the fluid in semen.

spermatocele. Benign cyst on the epididymis that is filled with spermatozoa.

sphenoidectomy. Surgical excision of all or part of the sphenoid sinus.

sphenoidotomy. Incision or creation of a surgical opening in the sphenoid sinus, located posterior to the ethmoid sinus bilaterally.

sphincter. Circular muscle surrounding a lumen that is contracted to control flow through the lumen.

sphincteroplasty. Surgical reconstruction of the sphincter, usually referencing a sphincter within the digestive system, eg, anal or transduodenal sphincter.

sphincterotomy. Surgical incision into sphincter tissue.

Spigelian hernia. Spontaneous protrusion of preperitoneal fat, a peritoneal sac, or a sac containing a viscous material that occurs through the Spigelian zone (fascia).

spina bifida. Congenital spinal defect that is the result of incomplete closure of the neural tube, causing incomplete closure of the vertebra around the spinal cord; condition may be mild or very severe.

spinal nerve root. Motor and sensory nerves that connect directly at the spinal cord.

spinal puncture. Insertion of a needle into the spinal canal, usually into the space between two vertebrae, with aspiration of cerebrospinal fluid for diagnostic or therapeutic reasons.

spinothalamic tract. Pathway of electrical signals from the peripheral nervous system to the brain; it is involved with perceptions of touch, itch, temperature, and pain.

spleen. Highly vascularized, lymphocyte-producing organ in the upper left abdomen.

splenectomy. Surgical removal of all or part of the spleen.

splenic flexure. Angle of colon at which the transverse colon transitions into the descending colon.

splenoportography. Radiographic imagery of the portal system with injection of contrast media into the spleen.

splenorrhaphy. Suture repair of the spleen.

splint. Rigid device for immobilizing a broken bone.

spondylolisthesis. Anterior displacement of a vertebra so that it rests on the vertebra inferior to it.

squamous cell. In carcinoma, an epithelial cancer.

stab phlebectomy. Surgical excision of segments of varicose veins through small incisions overlying the excision sites.

staging. Diagnostic evaluation of the course of a disease, eg, to determine the extent of a malignancy based on evaluation of regional lymph nodes, size of original tumor, and distant metastatic activity.

stapedectomy. Surgical excision of the stapes, a bone in the ossicular chain; may be followed by placement of a prosthesis for continuity of the ossicular chain.

stapedotomy. Surgical incision into the stapes footplate of the middle ear, usually performed to improve hearing in patients with otosclerosis.

stapes. Bone in the ossicular chain that articulates with the incus and inserts, via its footplate, into the oval window to transmit vibrations into the inner ear.

staphyloma. Weakening or thinning of the outer tissue in the globe.

stapler, stapling. Use of fasteners in surgical closure; the staples may be steel (skin surface), titanium (internal organs), or absorbable synthetic (all uses).

stem cell. Undifferentiated cell that can develop into various types of cells.

stenosis, stenotic. Abnormal narrowing or stricture of a canal or orifice.

stent. Implantable device to provide support to a lumen.

stereotactic, stereotaxis. Three-dimensional medical imagery used to inform surgical or radiological procedures.

stereotactic radiosurgery. Use of external radiation to deliver a beam of radiation directly to an internal structure, such as a brain tumor, after precisely locating the structure using three-dimensional computer images.

sternal split. Surgical incision of the midline sternum for access, usually describes an incision into the superior sternum to provide access to the thymus, thyroid, or portions of the esophagus.

sternotomy. Surgical incision into the sternum, usually describes the bisection of the sternum medially for access to the heart.

sternum. Bony plate overlying the center of the chest that articulates with the first seven ribs and the clavicle; also called breastbone.

stimuli. Any activity or substance that produces a sensation that is received and transmitted.

stoma. Surgically constructed connection from a urinary or gastrointestinal organ to the skin surface for the elimination of waste; the lining of the connection is composed of natural tissue, eg, a loop of intestine or a ureter.

stone. Abnormal deposits of mineral salts or other naturally occurring elements that form an unattached concretion; also called calculus or lithiasis.

strabismus. Condition in which the eyes are not aligned, causing both cosmetic and visual symptoms.

strangulated. Separated from a blood supply, usually by constriction.

strapping. Placement of adhesive strips to hold a musculoskeletal structure in place following injury or surgery.

stricture. Narrowing of a lumen.

stricturoplasty. Surgical reconstruction to widen an abnormally narrow lumen, eg, surgical reconstruction of a segment of small intestine to alleviate stenosis caused by scar tissue.

stroboscopy. Use of a lighted device to directly visualize the vocal cords during speech.

styloidectomy. Surgical resection of the styloid bone to eliminate impingement on the scaphoid in the wrist.

subarachnoid. Referring to the space between the arachnoid and the pia mater of the lining of the spinal cord and brain.

subcapsular. Within or inferior to a capsule.

subcostal. Inferior to the ribs.

subcutaneous. Beneath or within the skin.

subdiaphragmatic. Near the inferior surface of the diaphragm; also called subphrenic.

subdural. Occurring or situated between the dura mater and the arachnoid in the lining of the brain and spinal cord.

subepithelial. In a layer beneath the epithelium.

subfascial. In a layer beneath the fascia.

sublaminar. Beneath the plate of bone on the pedicle of the vertebral arch.

sublingual. Beneath the tongue; also called hypoglossal.

subluxation. Abnormal positioning of a bone at a joint, eg, a partial dislocation.

submandibular. Beneath or below the mandible; also called inframandibular.

submental. Beneath or underneath the chin.

submucosa. Beneath or underneath the mucosa.

suboccipital. Inferior to the occipital lobe of the brain, at the base of the posterior skull and superior to the level of the second cervical vertebra.

subphrenic. Near the inferior surface of the diaphragm; also called subdiaphragmatic.

subpulmonic. Inferior to the lungs; in transposition of great vessels, referencing left ventricular outflow, eg, a subpulmonic obstruction.

subserosal. Beneath the serous membrane.

substernal. Behind the sternum.

subtemporal. Behind the temporal bone superior to the ear.

subtotal. Less than all.

subureteric. At the distal end of the ureter where it empties into the bladder, usually referencing an endoscopic implant injection site for treatment of vesicoureteral reflux.

subxiphoid. Behind the cartilage that extends inferior to the sternum.

superficial. At or near the surface.

superior. Situated above or toward the top.

supinator. Muscle that has the function of turning back or turning up an extremity, eg, a muscle at the radius that moves the hand to a palm-up position.

suppository. Dissolvable medication lozenge that is inserted into the rectum, vagina, or urethra.

supracardiac. Above the heart.

supracervical. Above the neck or above the cervix uteri.

supraciliary. Relating to the eyebrow.

suprahyoid. Superior to the hyoid bone in the neck; below the chin.

suprapubic. Superior to the symphysis pubis.

suprasternal notch. Anatomical indentation in the superior margin of the sternum.

supratentorial. Situated above the tentorium cerebelli in the brain.

supravalvular. Above the valve, usually referencing a heart valve.

supraventricular. Above the ventricular level in the heart.

surgical excision. Removal of all or part of an organ or body part.

surgical margin. Edge of healthy tissue excised with a lesion to ensure the entire lesion has been removed.

suture. Stich that secures the position of tissue or a series of stitches to repair a wound.

symblepharon. Adhesion of the palpebral conjunctiva to the bulbar conjunctiva.

sympathectomy. Surgical excision of a sympathetic nerve or surgical interruption of sympathetic nerve pathways that results in dilation of blood vessels or a decrease in perspiration, depending on the nerve affected.

sympathetic. Describing a nerve that is part of the autonomic nervous system that constricts blood vessels, raises blood pressure, accelerates heart rate, or causes perspiration.

symphysiotomy. Surgical division of the symphysis pubis.

symphysis. Slightly mobile cartilaginous joint that does not have a synovial membrane, eg, the pubic symphysis or cartilage between vertebrae.

syndactylization. Correction of foot or hand deformity so that toes or fingers are evenly spaced.

syndactyly. Soft tissue fusion of fingers or toes.

syndesmosis. Natural joint secured by connective tissue and without articulation, eg, the tibia and fibula at the ankle.

synechia. Adhesion of iris to the cornea (anterior) or lens capsule (posterior).

synosteotomy. Surgical entry into a joint; also called arthrotomy.

synostosis. Fusion of bone.

synovectomy. Surgical excision of all or part of the synovium.

synovial joint. Articulating joint contained in a capsule of lubricating fluid.

synthetic. Not biological in origin.

syrinx. Abnormal, oblong cavity filled with cerebrospinal fluid in the brain or spinal cord.

T cell. White blood cell that protects the body against foreign or malignant cells; also called T lymphocyte.

tag. Small outgrowth of skin.

take-down. Surgical revision of a previous surgery, usually a reversal of the surgery.

talectomy. Surgical excision of all or part of the talus bone of the ankle joint; also called astragalectomy.

tamponade. Closure or blockage.

tandem. Long, narrow tube designed to fit inside a lumen, eg, the urethra or cervical os.

tarsoconjunctival flap. Tissue of the eyelid, including conjunctival tissue, that is incised but still retains its own blood supply and is repositioned for grafting.

tarsorrhaphy. Surgery in which upper and lower eyelids are sewn together.

tattoo. Multiple punctures of skin or cornea to infuse color, or in the case of the cornea, stimulate growth.

telangiectasia. Chronic condition in which dilated capillaries cause raised, red spots on the skin.

temporal bone. Bilateral skull bone that forms the side and base of the skull; temporal bone has four segments: mastoid, petrous, squamous, and tympanic segments.

tendon. Tough, fibrous connector of muscle to bone.

tenodesis. Suture of tendon to bone.

tenolysis. Surgical incision of scar tissue or adhesions that are impairing a tendon.

tenoplasty. Surgical reconstruction of a tendon.

tenorrhaphy. Surgical repair of a tendon.

tenosynovectomy. Excision of all or part of a tendon sheath.

tenotomy. Severing of a tendon.

testosterone. Hormone largely responsible for male characteristics.

thenar. Referring to the fleshy bulb of skin at the edge of the palm proximal to the thumb.

therapeutic. With the goal of improving the patient's condition.

thermoablation. Surgical destruction of tissue using heat.

thermocauterization. Use of heat to cut, burn, or seal.

thermoplasty. Endoscopic ablation of bronchial tissue as a treatment for severe asthma.

thermoregulatory. Relating to the regulation of body temperature.

third-order branch. Third branch off of the second branch of the aorta or the initial access vessel, as described in vascular catheter placement; branch vessel emanating from a second-order vessel.

thoracentesis. Aspiration of fluid from the thoracic cavity; may be a diagnostic or a therapeutic procedure.

thoracic. Relating to the thorax.

thoracic cavity. Chest area bounded by the rib cage, diaphragm, and neck; also called thorax.

thoracic duct. Main duct of the lymphatic system, located in the lower left neck; it arises posterior to the internal jugular vein and anterior to the phrenic and transverse cervical artery; the anatomy is variable, and the duct has multiple interdigitated channels.

thoracolumbar. Relating to the thoracic and lumbar spine.

thoracoplasty. Remodeling or reshaping of the thoracic cavity, including removal of ribs; used as a treatment for chronic infections of the pleural space.

thoracoscopy. Examination of the pleural cavity by means of an endoscope.

thoracostomy. Creation of a communication between the chest cavity and the skin that requires an incision and usually with insertion of a drainage tube.

thoracotomy. Incision into the chest wall.

thorax. Chest cavity bounded by the rib cage, diaphragm, and neck; also called thoracic cavity.

thrombectomy. Surgical removal of a blood clot from within a blood vessel.

thromboendarterectomy. Excision of a blood clot (thrombus) along with the lining of the artery in which it is lodged.

thrombolysis. Procedure to dissolve a blood clot in situ.

thrombolytic. Describing an agent that acts to dissolve blood clots.

thrombose, thrombosis. To clot; the act of clotting.

thrombus. Intravascular clot of blood that remains in the location where it was formed; plural of thrombus is thrombi.

thymectomy. Surgical removal of all or part of the thymus gland.

thymoma. Tumor that originates in the thymus gland.

thymus gland. Bilateral lymphatic organ located behind the sternum; site of T-cell origin.

thyroglossal duct cyst. Abnormal remnant of fetal development arising in the throat; congenital condition may be asymptomatic or cause dyspnea and neck nodule.

thyroidectomy. Removal of all or part of the thyroid gland.

thyrotomy. Incision into the thyroid gland.

tissue expander. Temporary subcutaneous implant equipped with a port that can be infused to increase the implant size; over time, the skin overlying the implant stretches in preparation for final reconstructive surgery.

tissue volume reduction. Endoscopic application of heat to destroy tissue.

tocodynamometer. Electronic device that measures the length and frequency of uterine contractions.

tocolysis. Medical inhibition of uterine contractions, usually in preterm labor.

tonsil tag. Tonsil tissue that remains after a tonsillectomy.

TORP. Total ossicular reconstruction prosthesis; artificial replacement for the malleus, incus, and stapes in the middle ear.

torsion. Twisting action or a static twist; the risk is ischemia.

torticollis. Painful muscle contraction disorder that causes twisting and/or jerking of the neck.

trabeculoplasty. Alteration of tissue of the trabecular meshwork.

trabeculotomy ab externo. Cutting of the trabecular meshwork with an approach from the exterior of the eye.

trachelectomy. Surgical excision of all or part of the cervix uteri.

trachelorrhaphy. Suture repair of the cervix uteri.

tracheobronchial. Relating to the trachea and bronchi, eg, all major airways.

tracheobronchoscopy. Endoscopic examination of the trachea and bronchial tubes.

tracheoesophageal fistula. Abnormal communication between the trachea and the esophagus.

tracheomalacia. Congenital condition of abnormally flexible cartilage in the trachea, which can lead to tracheal collapse.

tracheoplasty. Surgical reconstruction of the trachea.

tracheoscopy. Endoscopic examination of the trachea, including the larynx.

tracheostoma. Surgically created communication between the trachea and the skin of the neck through which a patient breathes.

tracheostomy. Surgical creation of a communication between the trachea and the skin of the neck through which a patient breathes.

tracheotomy. Surgical incision into the trachea.

tracheotomy tube. Synthetic tube placed during a tracheotomy to keep the incision open; the tube is used because a stoma has not yet been permanently formed.

trachoma. Eyelid infection caused by *Chlamydia trachomatis* bacterium.

traction. Pulling force, as in tension that pulls the retina away from the blood-rich choroid layer of the eye or therapeutically directed tension placed on the musculoskeletal system as a therapy.

tractotomy. Surgical transection of a sensory nerve tract in the spine or brain stem as a treatment for intractable pain.

transabdominal. Through or across the abdomen, usually referencing an approach.

transanal. Using an anal approach.

transantral. Using an approach through the maxillary sinus wall (antrum).

transaortic. Through the aorta or aortic valve.

transarticular. Spanning across a joint.

transbronchial. Using a bronchial approach.

transcanal. Through the external auditory meatus.

transcatheter. Through a catheter advanced to the operative site.

transcoccygeal. Through or across the bone at the base of the spinal column.

transcochlear. Through the inner auditory canal with entry through the cochlea.

transcondylar. Across a rounded projection of bone; in the skull, describing an extension of a suboccipital surgical approach, and in the femur and humerus, describing a fracture of the condyle at the proximal knee or elbow joint.

transcranial. Through the cranium.

transcutaneous. Through or across the skin (usually referencing an approach).

transduodenal. Performed by surgically incising the duodenum.

transection. Cut made across the long axis of a structure; a cross-section.

transendoscopic. Through an endoscope, usually referencing an approach.

transfacet. Through or across a vertebral facet, usually referencing an approach.

transfer. To convey or shift something from one place to another.

transfixion. Surgical method in which a cut is made from within outward.

transforaminal. Across the opening at the side of the spine where a nerve root enters.

transfusion. Transference of blood components from a donor to a patient in order to replenish lost blood or improve the quality of the patient's blood.

transhepatic. Across or through the liver.

transhepatic cholangiography. Radiographic imagery of the biliary ducts with injection of contrast media into a bile duct of the liver.

transient. Temporary.

translabyrinthine. Across the labyrinth of the ear.

translocation. In transposition of the great vessels, a technique in which the native aortic root is excised from the ventricle infundibulum and transplanted into the left ventricular outflow as part of the repair.

translumbar. Through or across the back.

transluminal. Through a lumen, or tube, eg, a vessel or intestine, usually referencing an approach.

transmastoid. Across the mastoid bone, usually referencing approach.

transmural. Across the wall of an organ or structure, including the entire thickness of the wall.

transnasal. Across or through the nose, usually referencing approach.

transnephric. Across or through the kidney.

transoral. Through the mouth, usually referencing an approach.

transorbital. Through the eye socket, usually referencing an approach.

transpalatine. Through the roof of the mouth, usually referencing an approach.

transpedicular. Across or through the segment of vertebra between the vertebral body and the transverse process (pedicle).

transperineal. Through the perineum, usually referencing an approach.

transperitoneal. Through the peritoneum, usually referencing an approach.

transpetrosal. Access to the brainstem through an extended middle foss approach.

transplant. Transfer or graft of tissue from one location to another or from one entity to another.

transplantation. Surgical transfer and grafting of tissue from one location to another or from one entity to another.

transposition. Surgical movement of tissue from one place to another.

transpubic. Through or across the pubic bone, usually requiring excision of a piece of bone.

transrectal. Through the anus and into the rectum.

transsacral. Through or across the portion of spine that is proximal to the coccyx.

transseptal. Through a septum, eg, from the right side of the heart to the left through the ventricular or atrial septum.

transsphenoidal. Through or across the sphenoid bone, located posterior to the ethmoid sinus bilaterally.

transtemporal. Through the temporal bone and mastoid, posterior to the ear.

transthoracic. Across or through the thorax.

transtracheal. Through or across the trachea.

transtympanic. Entering the middle ear by incising the eardrum (tympanic membrane).

transureteroureterostomy. Transplant of the transected end of one ureter to the other ureter for urinary diversion.

transurethral. Through the urethra.

transvaginal. Across or through the vagina, usually referencing an approach.

transvenous. Through the vein.

transventricular. Through or across the right or left ventricle of the heart.

transverse. Horizontal, or on a plane perpendicular to the sagittal frontal plane.

transverse rectus abdominis myocutaneous flap (TRAM). Surgical reconstruction of the chest wall and breast following mastectomy; this is done transferring a flap of skin, fat, and muscle from the abdomen to the chest.

transvesical. Across or through the bladder.

transzygomatic. Through the zygoma bone to the anterior cranial fossa, lateral to the eye.

trephination, trephine. Surgical removal of a disc of skull to enable access to the dura or brain; trephine is a circular saw for that purpose.

trichiasis. Condition in which eyelashes grow toward, rather than away form, the eye.

tricuspid valve. Three-leaf valve that regulates the flow of blood from the right atrium to the right ventricle.

trigger point. Anatomic site that is causing symptoms.

trigone. Triangular section of internal posterior wall of bladder delineated by the points of the two ureteral openings and the urethral orifice; trigone tissue carries the sensors that alert the brain when the bladder is reaching capacity and needs emptying.

trocar. Sharply pointed tube that fits inside a cannula and is used to withdraw fluid from a cavity or for use in paracentesis.

truncus arteriosus. Congenital heart defect in which a single vessel exits the right and left ventricles instead of the normal pulmonary artery and aorta, usually accompanied by a septal defect that mixes oxygenated and deoxygenated blood.

tubercleplasty. Surgical reconstruction or repair of a tubercle on the tibia at the knee joint.

tubercle. Small, knobby process on a bone for attachment of a ligament.

tuberosity. Rounded projection on a bone for muscle or ligament attachment.

tubouterine. Relating to the uterus and fallopian tube(s).

tumor. New growth of tissue.

tunneled, tunneling. Extending beneath the skin, eg, a catheter that is inserted into a vessel but tunneled through subcutaneous tissue so that its portal is in a safer or more convenient location than the catheter insertion site.

turbinate. Thin, spongy sets of bone covered in epithelium that segment the nasal airway and warm and moisturize air before it enters the pharynx; also called concha.

tympanic membrane. Membrane between the exterior and middle ear that vibrates as sound passes through it; also called the eardrum.

tympanolysis. Surgical excision of adhesions or scars from the eardrum.

tympanoplasty. Operation to repair the eardrum and/or middle ear structures with removal of disease from the middle ear, eg, cholesteatoma; it may be combined with mastoidectomy surgery.

tympanostomy. Surgical incision into the eardrum with placement of a small ventilating tube or grommet through the opening so that the middle ear communicates with the external ear; performed to treat chronic middle ear effusion, otitis media, and dysfunction of the Eustachian tube.

tympanotomy. Incision into the eardrum.

ulcer. Open circumscribed lesion on the surface of the skin, or on serous or mucous membrane, due to destruction of tissue; characterized by necrosis, sometimes suppuration, and slow healing.

ultrasonography. Diagnostic technique that uses ultrasound; when ultrasound waves are passed over a body area, the reflection, or echo, of the sound waves as they pass over the junction of tissues of differing intensities is converted into a visual pattern.

ultrasound. High-frequency sound waves reflected in differing degrees by various tissues to create an image, as seen in ultrasonography.

umbilectomy. Surgical excision of the navel; also called omphalectomy.

umbilical hernia. Bulging or protrusion of abdominal contents at the navel due to weakened muscles.

umbilicus. Navel, which is a scar remaining from the site of the fetal umbilical cord attachment.

undermining. Surgical division of a cutaneous or subcutaneous layer so that it is freed from its moorings and can be repositioned to cover a defect, eg, for a flap.

unilateral. Including or affecting one side of a bilateral body part.

uniplane. Referring to a fixation device that is applied in one direction, or along one plane, as seen in long-bone fractures.

unipolar cautery. Hemostasis achieved using an electrocautery tool that releases electrical current into the patient to complete the current cycle; also called monopolar cautery.

unroofing. Surgical excision of a portion of an enclosed cyst or other structure to permanently open it.

urachal cyst. Fluid-filled, anomalous cavity in the urachal sinus or ligament dorsal to the umbilicus.

ureterectomy. Surgical excision of all or part of the ureter.

ureterocalycostomy. Surgical excision of the lower pole of the kidney to expose the lower calyceal system, with anastomosis of healthy ureter to a calyx after excision of a segment of diseased or obstructed proximal ureter.

ureterocele. Ballooning of the ureter; a congenital anomaly.

ureterocutaneous. Relating to the skin and the ureter.

ureteroenterostomy. Surgical diversion of urine with the anastomosis of the ureter(s) to the wall of the intestine.

ureterography. Radiographic imagery of the ureter with injection of contrast media.

ureteroileal. Relating to the ureter and the ileum.

ureterolithotomy. Surgical incision into the ureter to retrieve a urinary calculus.

ureterolysis. Surgical severing of scars or adhesions of the ureter.

ureteroneocystostomy. Anastomosis of a severed distal ureter end to a new site in the bladder for urinary drainage.

ureteropelvic junction. Location where the ureter connects to the renal pelvis of the kidney.

ureteroplasty. Surgical reconstruction of the ureter.

ureteropyelography. Radiographic imagery of the ureter and renal pelvis with injection of contrast media.

ureteropyelostomy. Anastomosis of healthy ureter directly to the renal pelvis, usually after excision of a segment of diseased or obstructed proximal ureter.

ureterorrhaphy. Suture repair of the ureter.

ureterosigmoidostomy. Surgical diversion of urine with the anastomosis of the ureters to the wall of the sigmoid colon, usually performed in patients who have undergone cystectomy.

ureterostomy. Surgical creation of a communication between the urinary system and the skin by suturing the ureter to an incision in the abdominal wall for urinary diversion to an ostomy bag; also called the stoma.

ureterotomy. Surgical incision into the ureter.

ureteroureterostomy. Surgical anastomosis of two segments of ureter.

urethral vesicular junction. Site at which the urethra opens to the bladder.

urethrocele. Sagging of the urethra; commonly associated with cystocele but not a cause of urinary incontinence; inability to control the flow of urine.

urethrocystography. Radiographic imagery of the urethra and bladder with injection of contrast media.

urethromeatoplasty. Surgical reconstruction of the urethral canal.

urethropexy. Surgical fixation of the urethra, usually to the public symphysis.

urethroplasty. Surgical reconstruction of the urethra.

urinary diversion. Surgical redirection of the flow of urine, usually due to disease in distal urinary structures.

urinary tract. Group of organs that perform the functions of urinary production and elimination; organs include the urethra, urinary sphincter, bladder, ureter, and kidneys.

urodynamics. Diagnostics and measurement of urinary flow, pressure, continence, and capacity.

uroflowmetry. Recorded measurement of urinary flow; measured as cubic centimeters per second.

urostomy. Surgical creation of a communication between the urinary system and the urinary diversion to an ostomy bag; also called the stoma.

utricle. Fluid-filled sac within the labyrinth connected to the semicircular canals of the ear.

uvula. Pendulous, fleshy protuberance that hangs from the soft palate above the base of the tongue.

uvulectomy. Surgical excision of all or part of the uvula at the back of the soft palate.

uvulopalatopharyngoplasty. Surgical reconstruction of the soft palate and pharynx to remove excess tissue that may contribute to obstructive sleep apnea and to reposition other tissues in the oropharynx; the goal of uvulopalatopharyngoplasty is to enlarge the size of the airway; also called palatopharyngoplasty or uvulopharyngoplasty.

uvulopharyngoplasty. Surgical reconstruction of the soft palate and pharynx to remove excess tissue that may contribute to obstructive sleep apnea and to reposition other tissues in the oropharynx; the goal of uvulopharyngoplasty is to enlarge the size of the airway; also called palatopharyngoplasty or uvulopalatopharyngoplasty.

vaginectomy. Surgical excision of all or part of the vagina.

vagotomy. Surgical incision into the vagus nerve with the purpose of reducing stomach acid secretions.

vagus nerve, cranial nerve X (CNX). Providing sensory nerves to the ear, tongue, pharynx, and larynx; motor nerves to the pharynx, larynx, and esophagus and parasympathetic nerves to the thoracic and abdominal viscera.

valvectomy. Surgical excision of all or part of a valve.

valve. Anatomical leaflet or skin flap that prevents backward flow of fluids along a lumen or within an organ system.

valvotomy. Surgical incision into a valve.

valvuloplasty. Surgical reconstruction of a valve.

van Hoorne's canal. Duct that collects lymph in the chest.

varicocele. Anomalous enlargement of the venous plexus along the spermatic cord in the scrotum.

varicocelectomy. Surgical excision of an anomalous enlargement of the venous plexus along the spermatic cord in the scrotum.

varicose vein, varicosity. Chronic dilation and tortuous vein, commonly seen in the saphenous veins of the lower extremity but also in the genitalia or esophagus; plural of varicose vein is varices.

vascular family. All vessels that branch off a main vessel coming off the aorta.

vascular resistance. Impediment to blood flow caused by blood vessels; a component in high blood pressure.

vascularized. Describing a site where new vessels have formed.

vasectomy. Surgical interruption of the lumen that carries spermatozoa (vas deferens) as a means of contraception.

vasoactive. Affecting blood vessels by causing the lumen to decrease or increase in diameter.

vasoconstriction. Reduction in the size of a vascular lumen.

vasogram. Radiographic imagery of the vas deferens with injection of contrast media.

vasospasm. Sudden constriction of a blood vessel, reducing blood flow; also called angiospasm.

vasotomy. Incision into the vas deferens.

vasovasorrhaphy. Suture repair of the vas deferens.

vasovasostomy. Surgical reversal of a vasectomy by reanastamosis of the vas deferens.

vein stripping. Surgical excision of segments of vein, usually saphenous vein, through small incisions in the leg as a treatment of varicose veins.

velopharyngeal inadequacy. Functional disorder of the soft palate in which the soft palate fails to close off the nose during speech or swallowing; commonly seen in patients with cleft palate.

velum. Flexible, fleshy portion of the posterior roof of the mouth; also called soft palate.

vena cava filter. Surgical implantation of a basket designed to capture emboli from the lower extremities in the inferior vena cava.

venipuncture. Insertion of a needle into a vein, usually for the withdrawal of blood into a syringe.

venography. Radiographic imagery of veins with injection of contrast media.

venotomy. Incision into a vein.

venous congestion. Pooling of blood in veins due to backflow caused by faulty valves; may be accompanied by edema.

venous stasis. Slowing or stoppage of return blood flow from the veins of the lower extremities.

venous valves. Small directional folds in the inner lining of veins that restrict backflow of blood, especially in the legs.

ventilating tube. Small synthetic tube or grommet inserted into the tympanic membrane so that the middle ear communicates with the external ear; performed to treat chronic middle ear effusion, otitis media, and dysfunction of the eustachian tube.

ventral. Relating to the front; may be called anterior.

ventricle, ventricular. Hollow chamber, eg, in the brain or in the heart; ventricles of the brain contain cerebrospinal fluid, and the right and left ventricles of the heart pump blood to the lungs (right) and throughout the body (left).

ventricular fibrillation. Irregular, rapid, and ineffectual contractions in the ventricles; life-threatening arrhythmia.

ventricular tachycardia. Paroxysmal tachycardia that originates from an ectopic or reentrant focus in the ventricle.

ventriculomyotomy. Surgical incision into the muscle wall of the ventricle of the heart.

venule. Small vessel that carries oxygen-depleted blood from the capillaries to the veins.

verge. Distal boundary of the anal canal.

vermilion. Darker colored skin around the mouth; the lipstick area.

vertebral body. Weight that supports oval bone that forms the anterior vertebra.

vertebroplasty. Surgical reconstruction of the vertebra.

vertex. Head, eg, a vertex presentation for childbirth is one in which the head is facing down and will be delivered first.

vertical. Along the sagittal plane.

vesical neck. Distal bladder near the ureteral orifice.

vesicocentesis. Insertion of a tube or catheter through the skin and into the bladder for urinary drainage.

vesicostomy. Surgical creation of a communication between the anterior wall of the bladder and the skin of the abdomen; the communication that is created; may be temporary or permanent.

vesicoureteral reflux. Backflow of urine from the bladder into the ureter toward the kidney.

vesicourethropexy. Surgical fixation of the urethra, usually to the posterior surface of the pubic bone.

vesiculectomy. Surgical excision of all or part of the seminal vesicle.

vestibular nerve. One of two nerves forming the eighth cranial nerve (CNVIII) that transmits information relating to sound and balance to the brain.

vestibule. Body cavity that serves as the entry into another space.

vestige. Remnant, usually referencing a congenital anomaly that existed during fetal development that should have resolved.

virus. Infectious agent that is too small to be seen through a microscope and that multiples inside of living cells.

viscera, visceral. Internal organs of the chest, abdomen, or peritoneum; singular of viscera is viscus.

visual acuity. Sharpness and clearness of vision.

vitrectomy. Surgical removal of vitreous from the eye.

voiding. Urination.

volvulus. Twisting of a loop of intestine around its mesenteric attachments.

vomer. Thin bone that forms the posterior portion of the nasal septum.

von Recklinghausen disease. Genetic disorder manifested by the development of tumors along the nerve pathways; also called neurofibromatosis type 1.

vulvectomy. Excision of all or part of the vulva.

walking tube. Skin used for grafting that is formed into a cylinder that remains attached to the donor site on one end while being anastamosed to the recipient site or a site closer to the recipient site on the other end; walking tubes have largely been replaced by microvascular methods.

wedge biopsy. Diagnostic excision of a pie-shaped tissue block.

wedge resection. Therapeutic excision of a pie-shaped tissue block.

Z-plasty. Local skin graft technique in which a Z-shaped incision facilitates coverage of a defect.

zygote. Fertilized egg during its first days of rapid cell division.

◈ APPENDIX B ◈

Surgical Acronyms

AAA	abdominal aortic aneurysm
AC	acromioclavicular
ACA	anterior cerebral artery
ACL	anterior cruciate ligament
ANS	autonomic nervous system
ARM	anorectal malformation
ART	assisted reproductive technology
ASD	atrial septal defect
ATFL	anterior talofibular ligament
AV	atrioventricular
AVF	arteriovenous fistula
AVM	arteriovenous malformation
BAHA	bone-anchored hearing aid
BBB	bundle branch block
BPH	benign prostatic hyperplasia
BPI	brachial plexus injury
BPP	biophysical profile
BSO	bilateral salpingectomy/oophorectomy
CAA	coronary artery anomaly
CABG	coronary artery bypass graft
CAD	coronary artery disease
CAT	computer axial tomography
CBD	common bile duct
CFA	common femoral artery
CFL	calcaneofibular ligament
CHA	congenital heart anomaly
CIN	cervical intraepithelial neoplasia
CMC	carpometacarpal
CMG	cystometrography
CNS	central nervous system
CNV	cranial nerve V, trigeminal nerve
CNX	cranial nerve X, vagus nerve
COPD	chronic obstructive pulmonary disease
CS	compartment syndrome
CSF	cerebrospinal fluid
CST	contraction stress test
CT	computed tomography
CTS	carpal tunnel syndrome
CVI	chronic venous insufficiency
CVS	chorionic villus sampling
CWL	Caldwell-Luc. *See also* Eponyms.
DBS	deep brain stimulator
DDD	degenerative disc disease
DIP	distal interphalangeal
DJD	degenerative joint disease
DLI	donor lymphocyte infusion
DNS	deviated nasal septum

DRIL distal revascularization and interval ligation

DSF depressed skull fracture

E/M evaluation and management

EBUS endobronchial ultrasound

ECCE extracapsular intraocular extraction

ECLS extracorporeal life support

ECMO extracorporeal membrane oxygenation

ED erectile dysfunction

EEJ electroejaculation

EGD esophagogastroduodenoscopy

EMG electromyography

ERCP endoscopic retrograde cholangiopancreatography

ESRD end-stage renal disease

EUS external urinary sphincter

EVAR endovascular aortic aneurysm repair

FB foreign body

FCU flexor carpi ulnaris

FDP flexor digitorum profundus

FDS flexor digitorum superficialis

FESS functional endoscopic sinus surgery

FLM fetal lung maturity

FNA fine needle aspiration

FTSG full-thickness skin graft

GERD gastroesophageal reflux disease

GFR glomerular filtration rate

GHJ glenohumeral joint

GIFT gamete intrafallopian transfer

GPI globus pallidus interni

GSV great saphenous vein

GTD gestational trophoblastic disease

HPS hematopoietic progenitor cell

HPV human papilloma virus

HRA high-resolution magnification

HSV highly selective vagotomy

I&D incision and drainage

ICA internal carotid artery

ICCE intracapsular cataract extraction

ICD implantable cardioverter-defibrillator

ICP intracranial pressure

IDEA intradiscal electrothermal annuloplasty

IDET intradiscal electrothermal therapy

IJV internal jugular vein

IOL intraocular lens

IOP intraocular pressure

IP interphalangeal

IPG implantable pulse generator

IUD intrauterine device

IUS internal urinary sphincter

IV intravenous

IVC inferior vena cava; intravenous cholangiography

IVF in vitro fertilization

LAD left anterior descending

LAGB/lap-band laparoscopic adjustable gastric band

LBBB left bundle branch block

LBP lower back pain

LCA left coronary artery

LCX left circumflex

LEEP loop electrical excision procedure

LLETZ large-loop excision of the transformation zone

LMP last menstrual period

LP lumbar peritoneal

LPA left pulmonary artery

LVRS lung volume reduction surgery

MCA middle cerebral artery

MCL medial collateral ligament

MCP metacarpophalangeal

MMK Marshall-Marchetti-Krantz. *See also* Eponyms.

MMS Mohs micrographic surgery

MPA main pulmonary artery

MPR multifetal pregnancy reduction

MRND modified radical neck dissection

MTP metatarsophalangeal

NFB nasal foreign body

NG	nasogastric
NPT	nocturnal penile tumescence
NSS	nephron-sparing surgery
NST	nonstress test
NSV	no-scalpel vasectomy
NTD	neural tube defect
OCR	oocyte retrieval
OCR	ossicular chain reconstruction
OG	orogastric
OMC	ostiomeatal complex
ORIF	open reduction internal fixation
OSA	obstructive sleep apnea
PAD	peripheral artery disease
PCL	posterior cruciate ligament
PCV	parietal cell vagotomy
PDA	patent ductus arteriosus
PE	pressure equalization
PEG	percutaneous endoscopic gastrostomy
PFA	partial foot amputation
PGV	proximal gastric vagotomy
PICC	peripherally inserted central catheter
PIP	proximal interphalangeal joint
PL	pharyngolaryngectomy
PLND	pelvic lymph node dissection
PNS	peripheral nervous system
POP	pelvic organ prolapse
PORP	partial ossicular replacement prosthesis
PROM	premature rupture of membranes
PTA	peritonsillar abscess
PTB	patellar tendon bearing
PTCA	percutaneous transluminal coronary angioplasty
PUBS	percutaneous umbilical blood sampling
PUD	peptic ulcer disease
PV	portal vein
pVAD	percutaneous ventricular assist device
PVR	post-voiding residual
RBBB	right bundle branch block
RBL	rubber band ligation
RCA	right coronary artery
RCC	renal cell carcinoma
RF	radiofrequency
RFA	radiofrequency ablation
RND	radical neck dissection
RP	radical prostatectomy
RPA	right pulmonary artery
RRP	radical retropubic prostatectomy
SA	sinoatrial
SAN	spinal accessory nerve
SC	sternoclavicular
SCA	sudden cardiac arrest
SCC	squamous cell carcinoma
SCM	sternocleidomastoid
SDH	subdural hematoma
SEPS	subfascial endoscopic perforator surgery
S-ICD	subcutaneous implantable cardioverter-defibrillator
SIS	saline infusion sonohysterography; small intestine submucosa
SLAC	scapholunate advanced collapse
SLAP	superior labral tear anterior to posterior
SMAS	superficial musculoaponeurotic system
SNS	somatic nervous system; sympathetic nervous system
SPK	simultaneous pancreas–kidney
SRS/SBRT	stereotactic body radiation therapy
SSV	small saphenous vein
ST	scapulothoracic
STN	subthalamic nucleus
STSG	split-thickness skin graft
SUI	stress urinary incontinence
SV	selective vagotomy
SVR	surgical ventricular restoration
TAA	thoracic aortic aneurysm
TAH	total abdominal hysterectomy
TAP	transversus abdominis plane
TAVR/TAVI	transcatheter aortic valve replacement/ transcatheter aortic valve implantation
TGA	transposition of great arteries

TGV	transposition of great vessels
TIPS	transvenous intrahepatic portosystemic shunt
TMC	trapeziometacarpal
TMJ	temporomandibular joint
TMR	transmyocardial laser revascularization
TOCO	tocodynamometer
TOF	tetralogy of Fallot
TOLAC	trial of labor after a cesarean birth
TORP	total ossicular replacement prosthesis
TRAM	transverse rectus abdominis myocutaneous flap
TV	truncal vagotomy
TVOR	transvaginal oocyte retrieval
UCO	ureterocalycostomy
UCL	ulnar collateral ligament
UES	upper esophageal sphincter
UFR	uroflowmetry
UP	uterine prolapse
UPJ	urtereropelvic junction
UPP	urethral pressure profile
UPPP/UP3	uvulopalatopharyngoplasty
USSR	ulnar superficialis slip resection
UTI	urinary tract infection
UVJ	urethral vesicular junction
VAD	ventricular assist device
VAIN	vaginal intraepithelial neoplasia
VATS	video-assisted thoracic surgery
VBAC	vaginal birth after cesarean
VCF	vertebral compression fracture
VIN	vulvar intraepithelial neoplasia
VP	ventriculoperitoneal; voiding pressure
VPI	velopharyngeal inadequacy
VSD	ventricular septal defect
VUR	vesicoureteral reflux
ZIFT	zygote intrafallopian transfer

◆ APPENDIX C ◆

Procedural Eponyms

A

Abbe–Estlander procedure. Creation of a local full-thickness flap that includes skin, labial artery, and mucosa for reconstruction of medial defects of the opposite lip, as seen in cleft lip repairs.

Addam operation. Resection of palmar fascia at multiple sites to treat Dupuytren's contracture.

Akin operation. Removal of a bony wedge from the proximal end of the proximal phalanx of the big toe to treat hallux valgus (bunion).

Albee–Delbert operation. Insertion of a bone peg into a hole through the trochanter and neck of the femur to treat a fracture of the neck of the femur.

Albee's operation. Stripping of the surface of the femur and corresponding acetabulum and immobilization of the hip in order to allow the bones to fuse, creating ankyloses of the hip joint.

Alexander's operation. Shortening of the round ligament to secure a displaced uterus.

Altemeier procedure. Excision of a segment of prolapsed rectum with the anastomosis of the remaining distal and proximal ends of the rectum.

Anderson–Hynes pyeloplasty. Excision of the ureteropelvic junction and part of the pelvis with reattachment of the ureter to the remaining pelvis; a surgical correction for redundancy of the renal pelvis.

Anderson tibial lengthening. Use of an external fixation system on one leg to achieve tibial lengthening in a patient with legs of unequal length.

B

Babcock operation. Ligation of the saphenous vein using a long probe inserted through a small incision; the probe retrieves the vein, which is removed and its proximal end ligated.

Baker tube. Intestinal tube inserted through the jejunostomy and fed distally to decompress the bowel.

Baldy–Webster operation. Surgical shortening of the round ligaments by fixing them behind the uterus to treat retroversion of the uterus.

Bankart procedure. Surgical placement of drill holes and sutures to repair the integrity of a glenohumeral joint with recurrent dislocation.

Bardenheuerer operation. Ligation of the innominate artery with partial sternoclavicular and rib resections using both transverse and vertical incisions.

Barkan's operation. Incision into Schlemm's canal under direct visualization; glaucoma treatment.

Bassini repair. Suture of transversus fascia and conjoined tendons to the inguinal ligament to relocate muscles to cover a defect in the inguinal canal as part of the repair of an inguinal hernia.

Belsey fundoplication. Surgical treatment of gastric reflux disease by wrapping the fundus of the stomach around the lower esophagus; the esophagus is treated with a two-thirds wraparound.

Bennett procedure. Surgical lengthening of the quadriceps (femoris, vastus intermedius, vastus medialis, and vastus lateralis muscles) by releasing fibrous or scarred tissue.

Bilhaut–Cloquet procedure. Combining or winnowing of soft tissue and/or bone to form a single fused thumb in congenital bifurcation of the thumb.

Billroth I or II. Surgical excision of part of the stomach. In Billroth I, the pylorus is excised and the proximal stomach is sutured to the duodenum. In Billroth II, the antrum of the stomach is excised and the greater curvature is sutured to the jejunum.

Bischof procedure. Surgical treatment of leg spasticity with a laminectomy followed by longitudinal incision of nerve roots to disrupt nerve impulses.

Blalock–Hanlon procedure. Surgical treatment for hypoxemia associated with transposition of the great vessels through the creation of a septal defect to improve oxygen levels in arterial blood.

Blalock–Taussig procedure. Surgical treatment for hypoxemia associated with tetralogy of Fallot; performed by severing a branch of the subclavian or carotid artery and anastomosing it to the pulmonary artery in order to improve oxygen levels in arterial blood.

Blom–Singer prosthesis. Indwelling device for restoration of speech abilities post laryngectomy; it is inserted through a fistula created in the trachea.

Bonney test. Manual elevation or deviation of the bladder neck during cough or strain to detect stress urinary incontinence; also called Marshall test or Marshall–Marchetti test.

Borthen operation. Surgical stretching of the tissue of the iris as a treatment for glaucoma.

Bost fusion. Surgical fusion of the wrist joint using grafts of cancellous bone.

Bosworth operation. Surgical treatment of acromioclavicular joint dislocation using a screw to facilitate ligament repair.

Boyce operation. Incision into the renal parenchyma to access the calyces between the anterior and posterior branches of the renal artery for the removal of calculi.

Boyd hip disarticulation. Trans-iliac or trans-pelvic amputation with an anterior racquet-shaped incision and suture of a gluteal flap to the pectineus and adductor muscles.

Brent ear reconstruction. Four-stage reconstruction of the external ear to treat microtia, includes creation of cartilage framework, lobe transposition, elevation, and tragus construction.

Bricker procedure. Creation of a urinary diversion in which the ureters are anastomosed to a short segment of intestine, which is brought to the skin surface to establish a stoma; the diversion is not continent.

Bristow procedure. Treatment of recurrent anterior instability of the shoulder by transferring the coracoid process through a horizontal slit in the subcapsularis tendon and fixed with sutures onto the neck of the scapula, where it serves as a block in front of the humeral head.

Brock operation. Surgical reconstruction of a stenotic pulmonary valve with excision of part of the valve, approach through the right ventricle.

Brostrom procedure. Stabilization of the ankle with repair of the anterior talofibular ligament.

Browne operation. Hypospadias repair with urethroplasty using the intact strip of epithelium to form the roof of the urethra; the stripped floor of the urethra heals secondarily.

Brunelli procedure. Correction of wrist instability by securing a tendon through a hole drilled in the scaphoid bone.

Brunschwig operation. Pelvic exenteration with resection of the bladder, urethra, rectum, reproductive organs, anus, and support structures, with creation of urinary and digestive stomas; usually reserved for stage IV pelvic cancers.

Burgess amputation. Trans-tibial amputation with a long posterior flap technique.

Burhenne procedure. Insertion of a catheter and wire basket into the bile duct to retrieve a gallstone.

Burow operation. Excision of a small triangle of tissue at the corner of a skin flap to facilitate movement and enable better cosmetic results; also called Von Burow operation.

C

Caldwell–Luc approach. Incision high in the gum line in the anterior maxilla and through the underlying bone to approach the maxillary antrum; access used for sinus surgery or orbital blowout fracture.

Callander knee disarticulation. Amputation at the knee level with removal of the patella; soft tissue forms long posterior and anterior flaps for closure.

Camey enterocystoplasty. Creation of a neobladder from intestine.

Campbell procedure. Splitting of the patellar tendon and pulling of the lateral half to the medial side where it is attached to the inner portion of the patella; performed to treat recurrent dislocation or subluxation of the patella.

Cecil repair. Hypospadias repair in which a new urethral segment is constructed and secured in the scrotum and then separated from the scrotum.

Chambers procedure. Calcaneal osteotomy shift of the heel bone medially or laterally for patients with offset hindfoot alignment.

Chiari osteotomy of the pelvis. Acetabular osteotomy for patients with inadequate femoral head coverage; hip capsule is interposed between acetabular roof and femoral head, with soft tissue adjacent to the joint for coverage.

Collis gastroplasty. Esophageal lengthening by splitting the stomach; stomach tissue is used to create a segment of neo-esophagus.

Colonna procedure. Surgical reconstruction of an intracapsular femoral neck fracture with acetabular reconstruction.

Cunningham shoulder reduction. Nonsurgical reduction of a dislocated shoulder.

D

Dana operation. Incision of a sensory nerve root to relieve intractable pain or spasms; posterior rhizotomy.

Darrach's procedure. Excision of the ulnar head to treat pain in the distal radioulnar joint; usually reserved for elderly patients because it limits functionality.

Denis Browne operation. Hypospadias repair with urethroplasty using the intact strip of epithelium to form the roof of the urethra; the stripped floor of the urethra heals secondarily.

Denver–Krupin procedure. Placement of an aqueous shunt into a subconjunctival extraocular reservoir for glaucoma.

Dor fundoplication. Surgical treatment of gastric reflux disease by wrapping the fundus of the stomach around the lower esophagus; the esophagus is treated with a one-half wraparound.

Dwyer procedure. Making two cuts into the calcaneus, started on the outside calcaneus and converging to a point on the inside of the heel; bone is removed and remaining bone is secured with two screws; performed to correct an orthopedic defect of the foot.

E

Elliot's operation. Use of a corneoscleral trephine to create a subconjunctival fistula for drainage of aqueous humor.

Estes' operation. Autotransplant of an ovary to the uterine cornu; fertility procedure for patients with absent or defective fallopian tube.

Estlander procedure. Creation of a switch flap with mucosal advancement for repair of a lip defect.

Evans technique. Suturing of the peroneus brevis muscle to the peroneus longus muscle and relocation of a tendon to reduce foot inversion; performed to improve instability of the lateral ankle ligaments.

Eversbusch operation. Correction of upper eyelid ptosis by shortening the levator muscle.

F

Fasanella–Servat procedure. Tarsal and conjunctival resection using an internal transconjunctival approach to repair mild to moderate ptosis.

Finney pyloroplasty. Side-to-side gastroduodenostomy with pylorus incision; the goal is to increase the diameter of a narrowed or thickened pylorus.

Foley catheter. Self-retaining urinary catheter with an inflatable balloon tip in the portion of the catheter that resides in the bladder.

Foley operation. Surgical reconstruction of the pelvis (pyeloplasty) of the kidney; performed to treat stenosis of the ureteropelvic junction.

Fontan procedure. Palliative treatment of complex congenital cardiac defect by directing systemic venous blood to the lungs without first passing through a ventricle.

Fothergill operation. Fixation of the cardinal ligaments to treat uterine prolapse.

Frazier–Spiller operation. Destruction of the trigeminal nerve; approach is through the middle cranial fossa.

Fredet–Ramstedt operation. Longitudinal incision into the anterior wall of the pylorus to the level of submucosa; for treatment of stenosis; also called Ramstedt operation.

Furlow palatoplasty. Double Z-plasty to close a cleft soft palate or to lengthen the palate for velopharyngeal dysfunction; one type of Z-plasty involves oral mucosa, another involves nasal mucosa.

G

Gaskin maneuver. Placement of a patient in labor on her hands and knees to reduce shoulder dystocia.

Gavriliu operation. Surgical reconstruction of the esophagus using part of the stomach.

Gifford's operation. Nonpenetrating corneal incision along the boundary of an ulcer to limit its growth.

Gillies operation. (1) Reduction of zygomatic fracture including an incision in the temporal region; (2) surgery for ectropion with augmentation of the skin surface of the eyelid with skin graft.

Girdlestone's procedure. Salvage procedure for chronic infection following a failed total hip arthroplasty (THA); the infected bone is excised and a new THA may be attempted, once eradication of infection is verified.

Gonin's operation. Retinal detachment sealed with cautery using a device inserted through a puncture in the sclera.

Grondahl–Finney cardioplasty. Esophagoplasty to enlarge the opening into the stomach as a treatment for dysphagia.

Gundersen flap. Transfer of conjunctival tissue to replace damaged corneal tissue.

Guyon's amputation. Trans-tibial amputation just above the malleoli.

H

Halsted's operation. (1) Repair of inguinal hernia; (2) radical mastectomy.

Hartmann's operation. Resection of the rectosigmoid colon with creation of a colostomy.

Hartmann's pouch. Closing of the distal anus and rectum at the proximal end to create a pouch that can be accessed only through the anus.

Heineke–Mikulicz pyloroplasty. Longitudinal incision along the pylorus that is closed transversely; the goal is to increase the diameter of a narrowed or thickened pylorus.

Heller operation. Esophagomyotomy in which the muscle of the lower esophageal sphincter is cut, usually to treat alachalsia.

Henderson procedure. Transconjunctival myotomy and incremental release of the levator aponeurosis from the anterior tarsal surface as a surgical treatment of eyelid retraction in Grave's disease.

Heyman capsule. Radioactive cylinder inserted into the uterus or vagina (intracavitary) for the delivery of targeted, therapeutic radiation in a patient with a malignancy; placement is temporary.

Heyman procedure. Transfer of all five extensor tendons to respective metatarsal heads with anastomosis of distal stumps of long extensor tendons to short; fourth and fifth to short extensors of fourth.

Hoffmann apparatus. Four-pin device for percutaneous external skeletal fixation following closed reduction.

Homans–Miller procedure. Excision of subcutaneous lymphedematous tissue in the treatment of upper extremity lymphedema.

Huggins operation. Excision of testes in patients with metastatic prostate cancer to reduce serum testosterone levels in the patient.

Hummelsheim operation. Split-tendon transposition technique for strabismus repair.

I

Ilizarov procedure. Attachment of external circular fixation system to underlying bone via multiple wires; for the correction of limb length discrepancies through distraction or treatment of fracture.

Irving sterilization. Ligation, division, and burial of the proximal stump of the fallopian tube into the myometrium in female sterilization, usually at the time of a cesarean delivery.

J

Jaboulay operation. Creation of an expanded opening between the distal stomach and the duodenum by surgical gastroduodenostomy between the antrum and the stomach and the duodenum; the pylorus is not incised.

Jaboulay pyloroplasty. Side-to-side gastroduodenostomy; the goal is to increase the diameter of a narrowed or thickened pylorus without incising the pylorus.

Jaboulay–Winkelmann operation. Excision of tunica vaginalis to reduce a hydrocele.

Jantene operation. Arterial switch operation of the aorta and the pulmonary artery; surgical treatment of transposition of the great vessels.

Johansen/Johanson procedure. Two-stage urethroplasty to repair a stenotic or injured male urethra; an indwelling catheter remains while the tissue around it scars to create the lumen.

Jones procedure. Transection of the extensor halluces longus at interphalangeal joint of hallux; it is then rerouted through a hole in the first metatarsal head and sutured back to itself proximally; distal stump is sutured to extensor halluces brevis and interphalangeal joint fusion is performed to prevent hammertoe; performed to release retrograde plantar buckling.

Joplin procedure. Fusion of the proximal phalanx and metatarsal bone with transplant of the extensor tendon to the head of the metatarsal bone; treatment for hallux valgus (bunion).

K

Kausch–Whipple procedure. Radical pancreaticoduodenectomy.

Kelikian procedure. Syndactyly procedure with skin incision and repair that eliminates the webbing and resection of the proximal half of each adjacent digit proximal phalanx.

Keller procedure. Excision of the proximal end of the proximal phalanx to line it up with the metatarsal shaft, with placement of a temporary wire or pin; treatment for hallux valgus (bunion).

Keller–Mayo procedure. Treatment for hallux valgus (bunion) with resection of joint and joint prosthesis in proximal phalanx.

Kocher maneuver. (1) Mobilization of the duodenum during abdominal surgery to expose structures of the retroperitoneum; (2) closed reduction of a shoulder dislocation using traction and external rotation of the humerus.

Kocherization. Mobilization of the duodenum during abdominal surgery to expose structures of the retroperitoneum.

Kraske procedure. Excision of the coccyx and part of the sacrum in a sacral approach to rectal cancer surgery, with partial proctectomy and anastomosis.

Krause operation. Exposure of the trigeminal ganglion and nerve root of the cerebellopontine angle for decompression.

Kroenlein procedure. Lateral orbitotomy, usually to access a lesion or for decompression.

Krukenberg procedure. Amputation of the hand with creation of a pincer from the forearm stump.

Kuhnt–Szymanowski procedure. Lower blepharoplasty for ectropion with wedge excision.

L

Lapidus procedure. Fusion of the first metatarsal and first cuneiform joint and the first and second metatarsal bases with a tenotomy releasing the metatarsal bone; treatment for hallux valgus (bunion).

Laroyenne operation. Puncture of the posterior wall of the vagina to access the Douglas cul-de-sac for evaluation and treatment of infection.

Larrey's amputation. Amputation at the shoulder joint.

Latarjet procedure. Surgical treatment of recurrent shoulder location by excising and securing the corocoid and its muscle attachments a few centimeters to the anterior shoulder socket.

LeFort I procedure. Treatment of upper jaw malocclusion and cleft palate by separating the maxilla and palate from the skull above the roots of the maxillary teeth and fixing the maxilla in a new position.

LeFort II procedure. Treatment of facial malformation by severing the maxilla, nose, and medial aspects of the orbit from the skull and fixing the maxilla and nose in a new position.

LeFort III procedure. Treatment of facial malformation by severing the maxilla, nose, and zygoma from the skull and fixing the maxilla, nose, and zygoma in a new position.

Lembert's fenestration. Drilling a small window into the semicircular canal and placing a skin flap over the hole to treat otosclerosis.

LeVeen shunt. Shunt surgically implanted into the peritoneal cavity to drain peritoneal fluid into a vein, usually the internal jugular or superior vena cava.

Limberg flap. Four skin flaps that surround a rhomboid-shaped defect; flap angles are 60° and 120°.

Linton procedure. Excision of varicose vessels using an open approach and with subfascial interruption of perforating veins.

Lisfranc operation. Disarticulation of the midfoot between the tarsal and metatarsal bones, with a closure of dorsal and plantar flaps.

Lord's procedure. (1) Eversion of the tunica vaginalis to reduce hydrocele; (2) dilation of anal muscles to treat hemorrhoids.

Lynch procedure. Sinusotomy performed by entering the frontal sinus through the medial orbit, with the removal of diseased tissue.

M

Marshall–Marchetti–Krantz procedure. Surgical reinforcement of the bladder by suturing the neck of the bladder to the pubic bone or local fascia to correct female urinary stress incontinence.

Marshall test. Manual elevation or deviation of bladder neck during cough or strain to detect stress urinary incontinence; also called Bonney test or Marshall–Marchetti test.

Marshall–Marchetti test. Manual elevation or deviation of bladder neck during cough or strain to detect stress urinary incontinence; also called Bonney test or Marshall test.

Mayo operation. Stripping of varicose veins using an extraluminal ring that cuts the venous tributaries along the way.

Mayo procedure. Resection of the head of the first metatarsal to treat hallux valgus.

Maze procedure. Multiple surgical incisions into right and left atrial tissue; the goal is to alter the neural pathway of abnormal electrical impulses that are causing atrial fibrillation.

Miles operation. Resection of the distal colon through an abdominoperineal approach.

Monticelli procedure. External uniplane fixation by attachment to underlying bone via multiple wires; for the correction of limb length discrepancies through distraction or treatment of fracture.

Moschcowitz operation. Correction of a femoral hernia using an inguinal approach.

Mule's operation. Evisceration of the eyeball with use of artificial vitreous to fill the void.

Mumford procedure. Excision of the distal clavicle to reduce pain in the acromioclavicular joint, usually following trauma.

Mustard procedure. Correction of transposition of great vessels by construction of an atrial baffle to shunt blood from the pulmonary veins to the right ventricle and systemic drainage to the left ventricle.

N

Naffziger operation. Orbital decompression with removal of lateral and superior orbital walls for relief of severe exophthalmos.

Nagata ear reconstruction. Two-stage reconstruction of the external ear for microtia; includes construction of cartilage framework, lobe transposition, elevation, and tragus construction.

Nicoladoni's operation. Thumb replacement by transplantation of the second toe to the first metacarpal.

Nissen fundoplication. Surgical treatment of gastric reflux disease by wrapping the fundus of the stomach around the lower esophagus; the esophagus is treated with a complete wraparound.

Nuss procedure. Surgical reconstruction of the thoracic wall to repair congenital chest wall malformation of pectus excavatum or carinatum; a curved pectus bar is implanted into the intercostal space across the chest posterior to the sternum.

O

Ober–Yount procedure. Release of the iliotibial band of fascia that runs from the hip to the knee in patients with contracted fascia who are wheelchair bound; incisions are made in the fascia at the hip and at the knee to release the tension.

O'Connor operation. Strabisus surgery in which a stitch is placed in the lateral rectus muscle to allow for postsurgical lengthening of muscle, if necessary.

Ollier–Thiersch graft. A thin, split-thickness skin graft; also called Thiersch graft.

Olshausen suspension. Shortening of the round ligaments to elevate the uterus.

Orringer procedure. Esophagectomy with proximal stomach brought through the diaphragm to be anastomosed to remaining esophagus; requires both neck and abdominal incisions.

P

Partsch's operation. Marsupialization of a dental cyst.

Patey's operation. Radical mastectomy in which the pectoralis minor is excised while the pectoralis major is preserved.

Peans' operation. Disarticulation of the hip joint with intraoperative ligation of vessels.

Pereyra procedure. Surgical reinforcement of the bladder by suturing the paraurethral tissue near the bladder neck to the abdominal fascia to correct female urinary stress incontinence.

Pirogoff procedure. Amputation of the foot through the ankle, with retention of part of the calcaneus.

Polya gastrectomy. Modification of the Billroth II operation with partial gastrectomy and posterior gastrojujunostomy.

Pomeroy's operation. Sterilization of the female by excision of a segment of each fallopian tube.

Ponseti method. Sequential casting of an infant with clubfoot to stretch ligaments and correct the deformity; bones of the foot and ankle are brought into proper alignment; manipulation and cutting of the Achilles' tendon is part of the therapy.

Potts–Smith procedure. Insertion of a shunt from the descending aorta to the pulmonary artery for palliation of tricuspid atresia.

Pregl's test. Cystourethroscopic examination of the urethra and into the bladder.

Prentiss operation. Surgical correction of undescended testes using an inguinal approach and division of fascia transversalis to shorten the distance to the scrotum.

Puestow procedure. Side-to-side anastomosis of the pancreatic duct and jejunum (pancreaticojejunostomy) to provide drainage in chronic pancreatitis.

Putti–Platt procedure. Surgical treatment of an unstable shoulder joint by layering muscle anterior to the joint and shortening the subcapsularis.

R

Ramstedt operation. Longitudinal incision in the anterior wall of the pylorus to the level of submucosa; for treatment of stenosis; also called Fredet–Ramstedt operation.

Rastelli procedure. Repair of transposition of great vessels, pulmonary stenosis, and ventricular septal defect.

Ray amputation. Amputation of a toe and part of the corresponding metatarsal bone.

Raz procedure. Surgical correction of urethral and bladder neck hypermobility by anterior suspension; approach is through the vagina; for treatment of female stress incontinence.

Reed technique. Shortening of the circumference of posterior leaflets in a mitral annuloplasty to treat mitral incompetence.

Ridell operation. Sinusotomy with removal of anterior and inferior walls of the frontal sinus.

Ripstein operation. Proctopexy for rectal prolapse using a transabdominal approach and a mesh sling to secure the bowel.

Risser jacket. Hinged plaster or fiberglass and turnbuckle removable cast that extends from chin or upper chest to hips and, in some cases, one leg to the knee; the cast immobilizes the patient's spine and is a treatment for scoliosis.

Ritgen maneuver. Delivery of a fetal head by pressing on the perineum behind the anus so that the fetal head extends upward and forward through the vulva between contractions.

Ross procedure. Total aortic root replacement with pulmonary valve autograft for aortic valve stenosis; pulmonary valve receives homograft valve.

Roux-en-Y anastomosis. Y-shaped anastomosis of the small intestine; the small intestine is severed, and the distal end of the intestine is attached to the upper stomach while the proximal end of the small intestine is sutured end-to-side to the distal end of the intestine.

Rubens flap. Deep circumflex iliac artery perforator flap for breast reconstruction; a fat-pad free-flap alternative to transverse rectus abdominus myocutaneous flap.

S

Schanz operation. Palliative femoral valgus osteotomy as a treatment for irreducible hip dislocation, usually in cases of cerebral palsy; results in pain relief and improved range of motion.

Schauta operation. Hysterectomy with resection of adnexa, lymphatics, and other tissues, with approach and removal of tissue via the vaginal orifice.

Schede procedure. Thoracoplasty in which necrotic bone and tissue is removed to unroof an empyema and promote the growth of healthy granulation tissue.

Scheie procedure. Peripheral iridectomy with scleral cauterization to treat glaucoma.

Seldinger technique. Insertion of a needle into the target in order to place a catheter; a guidewire is passed through the needle, the needle is removed, and a catheter is passed along the guidewire.

Senning procedure. Surgical construction of two interatrial channels for crossing the systemic and pulmonary venous circulations in transposition of the great vessels.

Shirodkar operation. Placement of purse-string sutures in the cervix uteri to prevent dilation of the cervix; a treatment for incompetent cervix that may be performed during early pregnancy or before pregnancy.

Sistrunk operation. Surgical excision of thyroglossal cysts and sinuses.

Smith operation. Intracapsular cataract removal for immature cataract.

Smithwick operation. Surgical resection of a sympathetic nerve.

Soave procedure. Transanal single-stage surgical excision and endorectal pull-through procedure to treat Hirschsprung's disease; diseased distal bowel is excised and the end is sutured to form a new rectum.

Ssabanejew–Frank operation. Gastrostomy with suture of a cone of stomach wall to the skin as the stoma site.

Stamey procedure. Surgical suspension of the urethra of each side, with sutures placed into anchoring tissues of the bladder neck or pubic bone using a vaginal approach; for female stress incontinence.

State operation. Excision of a segment of diseased colon with end-to-end anastomosis of the rectum and colon, usually as a treatment for congenital megacolon.

Sugiura procedure. Devascularization of the abdominal esophagus and proximal stomach performed with esophageal transection and stapling to treat esophageal varices.

Swanson's arthroplasty. Silicone interpositional arthroplasty for the proximal interphalangeal joint.

Swenson procedure. Ileoanal pull-through procedure with preservation of the anal sphincters after excision of the rectum and segment of diseased colon; performed to repair congenital megacolon.

Syme's amputation. Removal of the malleoli in amputation of the foot at the ankle.

T

Tanzer ear reconstruction. Six-stage reconstruction of the external ear for microtia; includes construction of cartilage framework, lobe transposition, elevation, and tragus construction.

Thiersch graft. A thin, split-thickness skin graft; also called Ollier–Thiersch graft.

Thiersch operation. Removal of a small and thin split-thickness skin graft by razor, knife, or dermatome to cover a small recipient site.

Tommy John surgery. Reconstruction of the ulnar collateral ligament using a tendon autograft.

Toupet fundoplication. Surgical treatment of gastric reflux disease by wrapping the fundus of the stomach around the lower esophagus; the esophagus is treated with a half to two-thirds wraparound.

Traverso–Longmire procedure. Pylorus-preserving pancreaticoduodenectomy.

Trendelenburg operation. Ligation of the great saphenous vein as a treatment for varicose veins of the lower extremity.

U

Uchida procedure. Sterilization of the female by excision of a segment of each fallopian tube, with subserosal injection of saline and suture of the amputated ends.

Urban procedure. Resection en bloc for malignancy, including regional lymph nodes.

V

Vineberg operation. Anastomosis of the internal mammary artery to coronary artery to revascularize an ischemic heart muscle.

Von Burow operation. Excision of a small triangle of tissue at the corner of a skin flap to facilitate movement and enable better cosmetic results; also called Burow operation.

W

Waldius procedure. Total knee replacement using a single-axis hinged prosthesis that allows no rotation in the longitudinal axis and no abduction.

Wassmund procedure. Maxillary osteotomy via tunneling of palatal and labial mucosa.

Waterston procedure. Creation of a shunt from the ascending aorta to the pulmonary artery for palliation of congenital tricuspid or pulmonary valve atresia or stenosis.

Weaver–Dunn procedure. Reduction of dislocated acromioclavicular joint with nonabsorbable sutures that secure the clavicle in place.

Weil's osteotomy. Metatarsal osteotomy with screw fixation and release of the extensor tendons as treatment for toe clawing or pain in the ball of the foot.

Wertheim's operation. Radical abdominal hysterectomy, usually including the upper vagina.

Whipple procedure. Pancreatoduodenectomy, gastro-jejunostomy, and choledochojejunostomy with excision of the head of the pancreas, distal third of the stomach, and the duodenum; for pancreatic cancer.

Whitehead operation. Circumferential excision of internal hemorrhoid vessels and mucosa with repair.

Whitman astragalectomy. Excision of the astragalus as a treatment for paralytic deformity of the foot.

Winter procedure. Insertion of a large biopsy needle into the glans penis to create fistulas between the corpora cavernosa and the glans penis for detumescence of priapism.

Witzel operation. Incision through the abdominal wall and into the stomach or pylorus; may include placement of a feeding tube.

Y

Young's operation. (1) Creation of mucocutaneous flaps to treat atrophic rhinitis; (2) formation of a neo-urethra to treat epispadias; (3) excision of the prostate using a perineal approach.

Z

Zadek's procedure. Surgical excision of the root of a nail to treat ingrowing toenail.

Zavanelli's maneuver. Gentle push of an infant's head back into the vagina when bilateral shoulder dystocia prevents vaginal birth; the infant is delivered by cesarean section.

Ziegler procedure. Creation of a window in a secondary cataract using an open approach; largely replaced by laser discission.

Subject Index

A

C

D

E

M

N

O

R

S

T

U

V

W

Z